THE SCIENCE AND ART OR THE PRINCIPLES AND PRACTICE OF MEDICINE.

BY J. C. PETERS, M.D.

VOLUME I.
No. 2.

New-York:
WILLIAM RADDE, 300 BROADWAY.
Philadelphia: RADEMACHER & SHEEK.—*Boston:* OTIS CLAPP.—*St. Louis, Mo.:* R. & H. LUYTIES, M. D.—*Chicago, Ill.:* HALSEY & KING.—*Cincinnati, O.:* J. M. PARKS, M.D.—*Cleveland, O.:* JOHN B. HALL.—*London:* BALLIERE, 219 Regent-st.—*Manchester*, Eng.: TURNER, 97 Picadilly.

HENRY LUDWIG, STEREOTYPER AND PRINTER, NO. 39 CENTRE-STREET.

NOTICE.

—o—

The diseases first to be treated of will be *Fevers*, and every experienced and studious physician is most earnestly requested to furnish communications on the practical treatment of simple, irritative, catarrhal, rheumatic, intermittent, remittent, congestive, bilious, typhus, typhoid, and all other fevers. Our aim is to draw out, not merely the theoretical treatment of these diseases, but their actual practical treatment at the bedside, and such as has been found to be most effectual and satisfactory by experience. All such communications may be addressed to J. C. PETERS, M. D., No. 19 East Fifteenth-street, New-York.

Due credit will be given to every contributor. It is most cordially desired that all minor differences of opinion will be waived, and that many unselfish and earnest and practical men will unite in making this work a national, liberal, and truthful exposition of the best practice of honest, learned, and experienced men. It is not intended to prostitute this work to the selfish ends of any one man, or small clique of men; but, if possible, to make it the faithful exponent of the views and practice of as many able and modest medical men as practicable.

WM. RADDE,

No. 300 BROADWAY, NEW-YORK.

A

TREATISE ON THE SCIENCE AND ART,

OR,

PRINCIPLES AND PRACTICE OF MEDICINE.

INTRODUCTORY REMARKS.

SKETCHES FROM THE HISTORY OF MEDICINE.

AUTHORITIES.—Renouard's History of Medicine, (1). Scott's Lectures on the History of Medicine, (2). Good's Study of Medicine, (3). Watson's Medical Profession in Ancient Times, (4). Bartlett's Discourse on the Times, Character, and Writings of Hippocrates, (5). The British and Foreign Medical Review, (6). Malgaigne's Essay on the History and Philosophy of Surgery, (7). Carpenter's Physiology, (8). Paris' Pharmacologia, (9). Bigelow, (10).

Renouard's Synoptical Table best exhibits the great chronological divisions of the History of Medicine:

1st.—*The Primitive, or Instinctive Period,* terminating with the Fall of Troy, B. C., 1184.

2d.—*The Sacred, or Mystic Period,* including the Egyptian, Jewish and Greek clerico-medical systems, and terminating with the dispersion of the Pythagorean Society, B. C., 500.

3d.—*The Philosophical Period,* including the times of Socrates, Plato, Aristotle, and Hippocrates.

4th.—*The Anatomical Period,* commencing at the foundation of the Alexandrian Library, B. C., 320; and terminating at the death of Galen, A. D., 200. Herophilus and Erasistratus were the founders of this school. It is also sometimes called the Egypto-Greek Period.

5th. *The Greek-Roman Period,* from A. D., 200, to A. D., 650.

6th.—*The Arabic-Greek Period,* commencing at the destruction of the Alexandrian Library, A. D., 640, and terminating at the revival of literature in Europe, A. D., 1400. Rhazes and Avicenna were the leaders in this school.

7th.—*The Erudite Period,* comprising the 15th and 16th centuries.

8th.—*The Reformatory Period,* including the 17th, 18th, and present centuries.

§1. That an acquaintance with the chief particulars in the history of medicine should be regarded as indispensible to the well-informed physician, all must be willing to admit; yet it is much neglected. Apart from the interest which necessarily pertains to the subject, a knowledge of medical history is calculated to secure the establishment of what alone is true, or, at all events, well founded; and that physician who has undergone the additional mental culture it implies, is undoubtedly in a better position for the avoidance of error, and for the rejection of unsound views. The consideration of the doctrines, theories and practice of former races of physicians will also be eminently serviceable. The student of history will be apt to agree with Hufeland that medical art is eternal; systems transient; there is only one art of healing, and that rests on the eternal laws of nature; but there are many systems which merely mark the spirit of inquiry, prevailing at the time, and the degree of knowledge in some one direction, which we have attained. We have had systems enough to know that medicine does not reside exclusively in scholastic systems. Every one has always claimed to be the only true one, the only saving one, until it was superceded by a new one which makes the same pretensions as its predecessor. This will and must always continue to the end of time.

The student of medical history can conjure up the dead, mighty in medical art and science; he may pass them before him as in a panorama. The shadowy forms of Egyptian priests will head the array; then will follow the scarcely less shadowy Greek priesthood, and the silent and contemplative disciples of Pythagoras. The Cnidians, and then the Asclepiades, marshalled by Hippocrates, will follow these; Socrates, Plato and Aristotle mingling in their ranks. Then, once more, a long array of Græco-Egyptian sages will appear, headed by Herophilus and Erasistratus, the masters of the Alexandrian school, flanked by those of Pergamos, with a multitude of disciples—Pagan and Christian, Asiatic and Latin. Close upon these, tread the Arabians, led by Rhazes, Haly Abbas, Avicenna, intermingled with Greeks of the declining empire; and misty forms bring up the rear, a motley, commingled multitude. On they pass, until, again, Greek and Roman figures are visible, marshalling on the men of the dawning middle ages. Strange is their array; bearded and gowned necromancers, cowled priests, short-frocked bathmen, and barbers, and hooded women. Motley, too, their banners! The symbols of astrology and Christianity are written on them, with the names of Hippocrates, Aristotle, and Galen, of Plato, Avicenna, and Paul of Egina, of Celsus, Boetius, and Cælius Aurelianus. But the light dawns much more brightly as the panorama moves on, and Galileo, Bacon, Vesalius, Harvey and Sydenham, and sages, whose names should be as familiar to the medical student as his own, appear in the scene. They are intermingled, however, with Rosicrucians, and alchemists, pretenders and fantastic dreamers, among whom we recognize Paracelsus, Brown, and Mesmer. (6). Or, as Dr. Scott truly says, the study of the history of medicine is not one of mere antiquarian curiosity, but of great practical importance; for, if we would attain an enlarged and liberal view of any subject, and emancipate our minds from the temptations of our own age, we must patiently incur the labor of investigating its origin, and of carefully tracing it down, from the infancy of its being to the state in which it reaches us. We must give an impartial ear to apparent error, as well as to truth; systems and theories, which seem to bear the impress of inconsistency, must be weighed as candidly as those whose completeness and apparent truth gains our immediate admiration. So long as we merely compare ourselves with ourselves, we shall do no more than flatter our own vanity and the vanity of our age, while our controversies, instead of being noble rivalries in search of truth, will be trivial personal debates of no present importance, and of no future interest. No medical education can be deemed complete, however accurate the views imparted, which does not embrace the department of medical history; for thus we may become acquainted with remedial measures which time and fashion have thrown into oblivion; we are more likely to discover the principles in virtue of which all such measures are effectual, that common relation between medicines and diseases which constitutes the appropriateness of the one to the other; and we shall be fortified against the fascinations of ingenious but baseless theories, by observing the fleeting character of those which have passed successively through the ordeal of time and experience. At the same time, we will doubtless discover that almost every theory and system contains something which is eminently true and useful; the only, or the greatest mistake of the founder being, that he has mistaken a partial, but brilliant truth, for the sum of knowledge. The proper study of the history of medicine will fortify the student's mind against a *too* ready reception of any exclusive theory, or a slavish or bigotted adherence to any. He would estimate them at their proper value as subsidiary, and even essential to the progressive advancement of medicine; as the means, and not the end. He would almost be prevented from fixing his faith upon any one theory or system exclusively, whether physiological, or therapeutical. He would not be a medical sceptic, and indifferent to all opinions and systems alike; for he would learn that some truth is in all. Thus, the student would be trained to be a true and cultivated, liberal eclectic, to seek and find truth in every system and every theory; he would find truth in the allopathic, hydropathic and homœopathic systems; and in bio-chemical, dynamical and histriological theories.—*Brit. and For. Med. Rev.*, Jan., 1847. P. 106.

§2. The first man must have been the first physician, for the evils to which he was exposed must have led to efforts for their relief, and all means employed for this purpose may be regarded as medicinal; hence the first common-sense medicine must have been domestic, household, or popular.

Bacchus, king of Assyria, Lybia and India, has been considered the author of medicine; or rather medicine first commenced to flourish in his time. To Ham, or Hammon, son of Noah, has been attributed the same honor; it is now probable that they first taught the use of wine, rather than that of any purely medicinal substances. The Tubal Cain of the Scriptures is supposed to have been the originator of the art or writing, arithmetic, geometry, astronomy, music, laws, religious ceremonies, surgical instruments and books on medicine. In the course of time he was transformed by the Egyptians and Greeks, into Thot, or Hermes, or Mercury Trismegistris. (2). However this may be, in the beginning of medicine, instinct, intuition, accident and random experiments must have been the principal resorts of the people. But neither of these will teach us the best management of a broken or dislocated limb, nor of a severe rheumatism, pneumonia or small-pox.

In a multitude of cases it could easily be shown that the suggestions of *instinct* were faulty and pernicious—although it is possible that the senses of our forefathers, before they were contaminated with the smells of perfumery, distilleries, chemical works, and vile cooking, may have been as acute as those of the camel, who smells water at a great distance; or of the dog, who tracks his master, or his prey by the scent alone. Among some savage tribes, at the present day, whose senses are more cultivated, in a few directions, than those of civilized nations, the scent is almost as acute as in the lower mammalia; according to Carpenter, it is asserted by Humboldt, that the Peruvian Indians in the middle of the night, without the aid of sight, can distinguish the different races, whether European, American Indian, or Negro, by the sense of smell alone. Carpenter also cites the well-known case of James Mitchell, who was deaf, blind and dumb from his birth, yet the sense of smell alone enabled him at once to perceive the entrance of a stranger; he also says it is recorded that a blind gentleman, who had an antipathy to cats, was possessed of a sense of smell, so acute that he perceived the proximity of one that had been accidentally shut up in a closet adjoining his room. The black Bushmen of Australia, it is well-known, will follow a person, not merely by his tracks, like the North American Indians, but by smell, like a hound. Carpenter finally says that he has been assured, by a competent witness, that a lad in a state of somnambulism, had his sense of smell so remarkably heightened as to be able to assign, without the least hesitation, a glove placed in his hand to its right owner—in the midst of about thirty persons, the boy himself being blindfolded.

But even if the instincts and senses of our forefathers were more acute and accurate than ours, that alone would not have made them good physicians. Instinct is only adapted to a few essential and recur ring necessities; while the acute senses of dogs, Indians, &c., &c., have not enabled them to become able physicians.

§3. Instinct, in animals, has its counterpart in *intuition* in man; in instinct all is blind, necessary and invariable, somewhat like the operations of the vital power in building and maintaining the human body; thus the beaver which builds his cabin, the bird which constructs his nest, the bee or wasp his comb, or the spider his web, act only from instinct, which may be regarded as an extraneous and visible operation of the vital power. In intelligence all is elective, conditional and modifiable, while intuition holds a medium place between intelligence and instinct; it is often more far-reaching and exact than intelligence, generally less blind and necessary than instinct. Intuition is defined as the faculty by which the mind perceives the truth of things immediately, or the moment they are presented, without the intervention of other ideas, or without reasoning, or deduction, argument or testimony. Intuition is the power of seeing with the mind immediately, directly and clearly, or of discovering truth without reasoning. All instinct is innate; intuition is nearly so; thus the beaver builds without having learned it; all in him is fated or from necessity; he builds in a masterly manner, from a constantly irresistible impulse. Intuition is almost as perfect in its sphere; while in intelligence all results from observation, experience and reasoning. Intuition, like instinct, however perfectly it may work in its sphere, is limited; intelligence knows no limits, and what is generally called intuition is often simply an exceedingly quick intelligence, powerful memory, and rapid and accurate reasoning.

Animals have intuition, as well as instinct, and a limited amount of intelligence; at least, in some cases, they seem to learn that, by intuitive perception, which man could not arrive at by the most refined processes of reasoning, or by the careful application of the most varied experience; thus, a fly-catcher, for instance, just come out of its shell, has been seen to peck at an insect, with an aim as perfect as if it had been all its life engaged in learning the art. It is possible, however, that this bird has a neck and muscles of such arrangement as to make pecking motions the most natural and ordinary uses of them; just as young partridges and quails will run fleetly and judiciously as soon as they are out of the shell.

A large portion, however, of what are considered intuitions in man are merely impressions more or less reliable, or acts of involuntary recollection; thus a woman, during the delirium of fever, continually repeated sentences in languages unknown to those around her, but which proved to be Hebrew and Chaldaic; of these she was perfectly ignorant, but on tracing her former history, it was found that, in early life, she had lived as a servant with a clergyman, who had been accustomed to walk uo and down the passage, repeating or reading aloud sentences in these languages, which she must have retained in her memory *unconsciously* to herself. (8).

A physician who is without intuition will never feel those sudden unlooked-for inspirations which reveal to the man of genius the character of a disease, complicated in its progress and diagnosis, and enable him to discover in untrodden paths, the means of overcoming its violence and obstinate resistance. Thus he loses in deliberation the favorable opportunity which may never return, and the right moment of acting with advantage. Such a physician may not kill his patients, but he lets some of them die; in vain nature often commences a favorable result, still trembling, he dares not second her. (6).

But it is very evident that neither simple instinct or intuition will enable us to sail a ship from here to China, nor to discover a new disease or a new remedy; neither Bright's disease or any other was discovered by pure intuition; nor was vaccination, Peruvian-bark, Sulphur, Mercury, or any other specific discovered in this way. Observations frequently and carefully repeated, i. e., true experience, and rational deductions rigidly and thoroughly tested, are the only safe guides for the majority of physicians; and a practice founded on them is the only safe and reliable mode; but it is a slow, cautious, and difficult method, for "Art is long, life is short, system transient, experience often deceptive, and judgment difficult." If this is all that can be said of the best experience and judgment, what can be said of the ordinary loose experience of many practitioners, and their imperfect reasoning as applied to practical medicine? But from times immemorial, many physicians have carried out a species of antagonism between theory and practice, and between reason and experience. The theorist *may* proceed according to logic, but the practitioner *must* be guided by experience; thus false theories and an imperfect or deceptive science may prevail for generations without misleading practitioners too much, and a physician may often reason badly without injury to his patient, and without depriving himself of the best light of experience. (1).

§4. Doubtless, after having experienced, thousands of times, the danger of trusting to such unsafe guides as instinct and intuition, in cases to which their use was not adapted, a surer method was sought in the lessons of simple *experience*. The best physicians of primitive times doubtless reasoned very little on morbid phenomena, or the effects of remedies; they contented themselves with observing which were the remedies that had healed certain diseases, and in employing thereafter the same means in like cases.

Renouard says that Hippocrates, Celsus, Galen, and all the historiographers of medicine agree in saying that, before the introduction of philosophy into this science, i. e., before the age of Pythagoras, there was no other rule than *simple empiricism*, sometimes called *instinctive*, or *natural empiricism*.

The first therapeutic axiom was: *Remedies which have cured a disease, must be equally efficacious in curing identical cases, and may be very useful in similar or analogous cases.*

Renouard says, nothing is clearer, nothing is truer than this aphorism—it has all the infallibility of a mathematical axiom. (1).

But this good rule was quickly departed from, and is yet very carelessly carried out; physicians sought simply for somewhat analogous cases, and constantly failed to treat them rightly, and cure them. Those cases which are identical for all practical purposes are comparatively rare; for instance, two true Hunterian chancres, contracted from the same woman, by two equally healthy, temperate and non-scrofulous men, may be regarded as identical, as far as practical medical purposes are concerned, and will be cured by the same remedy, provided the diet, exercise, physical and mental condition, &c., &c., of the two patients be similar.

But two chancres, contracted by two men of widely different modes of thinking, acting and living, from two women, the one as decent as a fallen woman can be, and the other as debased and debauched as only a prostitute can be, will be widely different things, and require different treatment. The same holds true with fever and ague, occurring in healthy and unhealthy subjects, and all other diseases. In fact, it is exceedingly difficult to apply rigorously, a past fact in treatment to a case in hand, for whatever may be the degree of similarity that exists between two pathological states, as there is never an absolute identity, and rarely a degree of similarity sufficient for practical purposes, it follows, that a course of medication which has succeeded perfectly in one case, *may*, strictly speaking, fail in another apparently very similar case; and certainly *will* often fail in many only somewhat or apparently similar cases.

It is evident that the best means of avoiding, or rather of diminishing this permanent cause of failures and mistakes, consists in perfecting the diagnosis of diseases and remedies, or pathological diagnosis, and therapeutical diagnosis, as much as possible. The importance of a correct diagnosis has been recognized by the great and good physicians of all ages; for how can *similar diseases* be treated by *similar* remedies, unless the diagnosis of both be established.

The first plan of establishing a diagnosis, according to Renouard, was to take account of all the symptoms that presented themselves in the course of a disease, and to record them, in regular succession, as they appeared. According to this plan, a great number of ancient nosological tables were formed, so that for any disease, a comparison of the phenomena that appeared, was made with the symptomatic tables that had been framed, and from this comparison an appropriate treatment was deduced.

Renouard continues to say: This method, which appears at first sight so natural and exact, is at bottom extremely defective. In the *first* place, it has the serious inconvenience of attributing an almost equal value to all the symptoms, while daily observation proves that notable differences exist:

2d.—In the *second* place, a long enumeration of morbid phenomena, recorded one after another, without choice or discernment, is no more a portrait of a disease, than proper colors thrown at hazard upon a canvass, will be that of a person sitting for his likeness:

3d, and lastly.—All classification of diseases becomes impracticable on this plan, for, before attempting a work of this kind, it is necessary to inquire how many analogous symptoms, of the first magnitude, would be required to place two affections in the same class, and assign them a like treatment. Renouard says it would be absurd to attempt to answer this question.

It is highly interesting to observe that Hahnemann instinctively followed the same primary and necessary plan, in studying the effects of remedies, which the primitive physicians were obliged to follow in their first studies of disease. Hahnemann rejected the major part of the materials of all the physicians who preceded him, and as the human mind will always act in the same manner under like circumstances, he naturally took the identical primary and elementary steps, in the study and diagnosis of remedies, which the ancient physicians took in their first studies of disease and its diagnosis. (1).

This method prevailed before the time of Hippocrates, especially among the Asclepiadæ of Cnidus. Hippocrates strongly felt the deficiencies of this manner of observing and describing morbid processes, as it led the Cnidian physicians to multiply innumerably the division of diseases. He says, those who have collected the sentences that are termed Cnidian, have well traced the morbid symptoms as they are exhibited, but any one may do as much as this without being a physician, by asking sick persons the pains and sensations they experience. Much has been neglected in the Cnidian sentences which it is important for the physician to know, without questioning his patient, and which is essential to the exact appreciation of the disease. Errors are easily committed, if distinctions are made in diseases from mere shades of difference, and if other names are given to all those which are not identical! One would almost suppose that Hippocrates was talking directly to some modern physicians. (1).

§5. The Egyptian nation was the instructress of the human race; Egyptian medicine is the source from whence the Jews and Greeks drew the first elements of this science.

As was common among other people of high antiquity, such as the Babylonians and others; the Egyptians commenced in the first place, according to Strabo, (as quoted by Houdart and Renouard), by exposing the sick in public, so that any of those who passed by, who had been similarly attacked and cured, might give their advice for the benefit of the sufferers. At a later period, all who were cured of any important disease were required to go and make an inscription in the temples, of the symptoms of their disease and the medicines which had been beneficial to them. The temples of Canopus and Vulcan, at Memphis, became the principal depots of these registers, and they were kept with the same care as the archives of the nation. For a long time the truly liberal and republican plan was adopted, of allowing every one the privilege of going to consult these registers, and of choosing, for his sickness or that of his neighbors, the medicines of which experience had confirmed the value. The whole practice of medicine then rested entirely on simple observation, and every person had an equal, or at least a good opportunity of acquainting himself with the entire records of Egpytian practical medicine. In this way, it is asserted, a prodigious quantity of facts were collected, from which some correct principles at least might be and were adduced.*

After the lapse of a little time, the Egyptian priests, who were charged with the preservation of these observations, did not hesitate to seize upon the exclusive practice of the art. For it is almost an instinctive idea, with many persons and priests, that the anger of the gods is the principal cause of disease, and it seems to belong to the functions of the priests to attempt to appease this. When they had collected a great mass of facts, they formed a medical code, the fruit of the experience of ages, called the Sacred Book, from the directions of which they subsequently pledged themselves not to vary. If, in following the rules there laid down, they could not save their patients, they were not held responsible; but they were punished with death, if, after departing from them, a favorable result did not justify their course. We would regard such a law as an atrocious one, if made by modern rulers; it must have arrested all subsequent progress of medicine; it virtually assumed that the experience which had gone on before was good and sufficient, and that which might follow was either bad, or unnecessary. Still, we must recollect that the law was not made before the correctness of those principles had apparently been well proven and established. Diodorus of Sicily says, that the design of a law so severe, was, that a practice confirmed by long and careful experience, and supported by the autho-

* But little of their experience has come down to us; but we know that they used Squills in dropsy, for which it is still used, and for scarcely anything else than some coughs and urinary troubles

rity of the greatest masters of the art, was preferable to the limited experience of each particular physician. At a later period, they were allowed to depart from the code on the fifth day, if the result was not satisfactory. (1).

Renouard asks, what judgment would we pass upon that sovereign or senate, who would attempt to re-establish and execute a law as foolish and iniquitous as this Egyptian one, under the pretext that the present medical code is the fruit of the experience of ages, and that the solidity of the principles which serve as its base, is sufficiently established. Renouard says, that we doubtless could not sufficiently curse such a senseless tyranny, so contrary to the progress of science, and the best interests of the sick. It would then seem just to bless, in some exceedingly moderate and homœopathic degree, those powers, and societies, and colleges who pass a virtual sentence of scientific death or perpetual banishment upon all those who do not believe and practice as they do. The Egyptian age seems not to have entirely passed by in some quarters, as I fear some of my readers may or will experience.

The Egyptian Sacred Book fortunately was lost, although I, for one, would take great pleasure in reading it; still I would rather forego that treat, than to have it thrust forever upon the medical world as the sacred and all-sufficient book of medicine. But it is not only Egyptian priests, medical authorities and societies who are guilty of intolerance, and would be of oppression if they could; almost every reformer in medicine and founder of a system, and his enthusiastic followers, have been guilty of the greatest intolerance towards their fellows who disagreed with them, and have heaped scorn, abuse and satire upon them, have almost regarded them as fools and murderers.

§6. Among the Greeks, MELAMPUS is the first physician who immortalized himself by his extraordinary cures, and to whom altars were erected from gratitude. He lived nearly 200 years before the Trojan war. He is said to have cured Iphiclus of impotency, by giving him the rust of iron in wine for ten days. But he is more particularly celebrated as the originator of the Helleborism of the ancients, a method of cure which has been rescued from oblivion by the industry and erudition of Hahnemann. The most famous of the cures of Melampus, were those of the daughters of Prœtus, King of Argos. These princesses, having taken vows of celibacy, became subject to fits of hysteria or monomania, and would leave their father's palace to run wild in the woods, lowing, and acting as much like cows or great calves as they could. Many other women became affected sympathetically in the same way. Melampus, who had noticed that goats were purged, and their venereal appetites lessened by eating white Hellebore, or *Veratrum Album*, gave these young princesses milk in which this plant had been infused; then caused some robust young boys to chase them over the fields until they were thoroughly fatigued; then enchanted, we hope not ravished, them, (for enchanting and ravishing are sometimes almost synonymous terms), and made them bathe in a fountain of Arcadia, called the Clitorian, (which certainly has a very suspicious sound,) and thus completed their cure. Such is the origin of the use of Hellebore in mental derangement and many nervous, bilious and hypochondriacal affections. We would advise every physician to glance over Hahnemann's celebrated treatise on the Helleborism of the ancients;* for it is truly a stupendous monument of industry and erudition, and, withal, exceedingly interesting to those fond of the history of medicine. It is right to add, that since Hahnemann's time, the Hellebore of the ancients has been traced to the *Helleborus orientalis;* which is neither the ordinary white, green or black Hellebore, but a different species, which is found growing in the localities where the plant used by the ancients is known to have been most abundant. In honor of its first discoverer, Melampus, it has, from time immemorial, been called *Melampodium.*

Chiron, the Centaur, is said to have had Hercules, Jason, Theseus, Castor, Pollux, Ulysses, Nestor, Æneas and Achilles, or the majority of the heroes of the Trojan war, and captors of the golden fleece, among his pupils. It would be curious to discover what surgical instruments were invented by Hercules, Achilles, &c. But he was more distinguished as a surgeon than a physician, although he cured blindness, and his renown in the treatment of ulcers was so great, that the name of "chironians" was given to all obstinate and malignant ulcers which resisted the treatment of other, and less distinguished doctors. Chiron is also said to have been the instructor of Esculapius, who is more generally regarded as the father, or even the god of Greek medicine.

Esculapius obtained an almost universal veneration in his times; his worship, which passed from the Greeks to the Romans, extended into all countries penetrated by the arms of these two nations.

Podalirius, one of the sons or followers of Esculapius, furnishes the first example of blood-letting in the annals of medicine. The daughter of Dametus, the king of Caria, having fallen in a fit, or, as others say, from the top of a house, lay senseless and motionless, and was already supposed dead, when this surgeon bled her from both arms, and had the happiness of seeing her restored to life. (1).

§7. The practice of medicine in the temples of Esculapius was modelled after that of Egypt; for colonists from Egypt arrived in Greece, when the earliest Greeks yet lived on the acorns of their forests, and were clad in the skins of wild beasts. The first Egyptian colony laid the foundation of the city of Argos, 1856 years before Christ; several ages later, Cecrops fled from the banks of the Nile, landed on the

---

* Republished by William Radde, No. 300 Broadway, New-York.

shores of Attica, and became the founder of Athens; Cadmus came from Tyre, and built the walls of Thebes. Fifty years after the Trojan war, the first temple of Esculapius was erected in Greece; but very soon others were raised in Italy, Asia and Africa. The priests attached to the temples of Esculapius were called asclepiadæ, which signifies descendants or followers, but not necessarily children of Esculapius. They formed a particular caste, governed by so-called "sacred" laws, like the priests of Egypt, one of which says: "It is not permitted to reveal sacred things except to the elect." (1).

The temples of Esculapius, as is well known, were generally very salubriously situated; sometimes on the summit of a hill, as at Schooley's, Catskill, or the White Mountains; on the declivity of a mountain like West-Point; sometimes on the shore, like Newport, Nahant, Rockaway, Cape May, or Long Branch; sometimes distant from the sea, and near to a warm or medicinal spring, like Saratoga, Virginia Springs, St. Catharine's Well, or Sharon; and sometimes simply near a fountain of living water, as at Brattleboro'.

Groves of trees refreshed the sight of the sick, and afforded them cool and solitary retreats in their beautiful and spacious avenues; people came from all quarters on pilgrimages to these places, as now to Baden-Baden, Hombourg, Nassau, Aix la Chapelle, Ems, Wiesbaden, Carlsbad, Bath, Cheltenham, &c. The sick and the convalescent found there both agreeable and healthful diversions; the wholesome regimen to which they were subjected, the pure and temperate air they breathed, the salutary waters they drank and bathed in, the faith and hope by which some of them were animated, it is supposed, wrought more cures than are now effected at the majority of our fashionable watering-places, where the diet is often anything but plentiful and wholesome, the air of the ball- and dining-rooms anything but pure and temperate, the groves of trees anything but beautiful and spacious, the diversions anything but healthful.

Sceptics were not wanting, even in ancient times, who saw through some of the mummeries of the priests. Among other quackeries, snakes of a yellowish-brown color, and large size, whose bite was not venomous, and which were easily tamed, were much employed by the priests in those performances which filled the people with astonishment and superstition. Aristophanes, in one of his comedies, put the following words in the part of one of his characters. (1):

"The priests of the temple of Esculapius, having extinguished all the lights, told us to go to sleep, adding, that if any one should hear a hissing, which indicated the arrival of the god, he should not move in the slightest manner. So we all laid down, without making any noise; but I could not sleep, because of the smell of an excellent broth, belonging to an old woman near me. Desiring most earnestly to get at the broth, I raised my head very quietly, and saw the priest taking away the votive offerings from the sacred tables, and going the round of the altars, putting into his bag everything he could find. I believed I had a right to follow his example, so I quickly attacked the old woman's pot of broth, fearful that the priest might get at it before me. The old woman hearing me, stretched forth her hand to save her food; but I hissed and seized her fingers with my teeth, as if I were an esculapian snake, when, snatching back her hand, she lay down quickly, and covered up her head; while I swallowed her broth and retired to rest." (1).

According to Schulze and Plutarch, there were more than eighty of these temples of Esculapius, and, at the founding of new temples, specimens of the esculapian serpent, which were only originally found at Epidaurus, were always transferred from the old to the new abodes. So great was the veneration for these snakes, that, in the year of Rome, 461, to arrest the progress of pestilence in that city, commissioners were sent to transfer a sacred serpent from Epidaurus, to the island in the Tiber, where the first temple to Esculapius was erected among the Romans. Snake-worship is supposed to have had its origin from a heathen perversion of the ancient records of the doings of the snake in the Garden of Eden, or of the brazen serpent, which Moses raised on a pole, in the wilderness, to cure the Israelites who were bitten with fiery serpents. However this may be, it was the earliest emblem of the god of medicine, and was supposed to image that vigilance, wisdom and subtlety, or circumspection which should characterize the true physician. Afterwards, the cock was added, as an emblem of vigilance at early morn, and of courage; and the dog, as an emblem of fidelity by night, and of honesty and courage combined. (1).

The statues of Esculapius usually represented a bearded and aged man, indicative of experience and wisdom; sometimes bare-headed, sometimes crowned, as representative of the storms and trials through which he must pass, or the victories which he had gained; sometimes erect, as the good physician requires no support but an approving conscience, and the blessing of God; sometimes leaning on his staff, around which the serpent is seen winding in spiral folds, as emblematic of the dreadful and poisonous influences, whether of plant or animal, which he could turn aside and control for the benefit of man; sometimes the staff was knotted, to indicate the difficulties of practice, or the hard blows which heroic physicians thought it necessary to inflict upon disease; sometimes he is alone, as if the healing art were all-sufficient, more frequently attended by his daughter Hygea, robed in white, as indicative of the purity and simplicity of hygienic rules, with a serpent in one of her hands, as emblematic of her power over evil influences, and a shallow cup in the other, of some pure water, or healing drink, to which the serpent is directing his attention, in reverence. Not unfrequently, between the figures of Esculapius and Hygea, a noble child is seen standing, representative of that fruitfulness, beauty and health which medicine and hygea so often bestow. (1).

Sometimes the genius of medicine was indicative of thought and silence; it sat pensive and alone, with its finger pressed upon its lips, as if admonishing its votaries to solitary study, deep thought, and to bury within its own bosom the confidential disclosures of the sick; or as if assuring that the wise and experienced physician thinks much and speaks little. (4).

Stripped of its heathenish devices, how grandly does the ancient idea of the true physician seem—sage, modest, faithful at night, vigilant in the morn, courageous and discreet at all times, fatherly, the friend of the young, the comforter of the old, cleanly, abstemious, and the preventer of disease and pestilence.

In Hippocrates' words, a physician should be clean in his dress, grave in his manners, moderate in all his actions, chaste and reserved; he should neither be envious or unjust, nor fond of dishonorable gain; affable, but not a great talker; modest, sober, patient, pious without superstition; prudent, diligent; not ashamed to solicit the assistance of other physicians; and thoroughly impressed with reverence for the Deity. He ought not to be ashamed of receiving information from the meanest persons, about remedies that may have been given with success; for the most skilful physicians are sometimes disappointed, and all medicine was originally derived from the populace; he ought never positively to assert that such or such a remedy will cure; he ought to visit his patients with sufficient frequency, and pay strict attention to all their complaints.

How different is all this from the actions of the impulsive, impatient, loquacious, conceited, arrogant and intolerant masses who have crowded into the profession.

§8. The ancient practices, in the Greek temples of Esculapius, as before said, were derived from those of Egypt; the Egyptian Esculapius is said to have flourished eleven centuries before the Greek, and to have been synonymous with Thot, or Hermes, who became transformed by the Greeks into Mercury, and both are said to have had the Tubal Cain, of the Scriptures, or the first worker in brass, for their prototype. Mineralogy and metallurgy, and, in some measure, chemistry must have made considerable progress before Moses was able to fashion a brazen serpent, and the Jewish idolaters golden calves.

The Esculapian temples at Cos and Epidaurus, according to Strabo, the historian, were always filled with patients, and along their walls the tablets were suspended, upon which were recorded the history and treatment of the individual cases of disease. (1).

One of these tablets has been found on the island in the Tiber, near Rome, at the site of the ancient temple before alluded to. It has the following inscription in Greek :

"*Lucius* was attacked with pleurisy, and every one despaired of his life; the god ordered that the warm ashes of the altar be mingled with wine, and applied to his side. He was saved, and gave thanks to the god before the people." Warm alkaline cataplasms are probably more useful than the flax-seed poultices of the French.

"*Julian* vomited blood, and appeared lost; the oracle ordered him to take the pine seeds of the altar, and eat them for three days, mingled with honey." Turpentine is still used in hæmorrhages.

"A blind soldier, Valerius Aper, was directed to take the blood of a white cock, mingle it with honey and make a collyrium, to be applied for three days; he was restored to sight." In the Scriptures, the gall of a fish was ordered for the same purpose, and although blood contains iron, Phosphorus, Natrum-muriaticum, and many other medicinal substances, we cannot withhold the suspicion that the blindness of Valerius was not an amaurosis, but some film, or slighter trouble.

"Caius, who was blind, was obliged to perform adoration at the sacred altar; he passed once from the right to the left, rested his fingers on the altar, raised his hands and applied them to his eyes, and recovered his sight immediately, and in the presence of the people." Although this cure is not more astounding than those said to be effected by sacred pictures, bones, relics, and winking virgins in some modern churches; and the votive tablets, in the shape of silver hearts, heads, legs, arms, breasts, and little babies, of the same churches, are almost as good descriptions of the diseases cured, as those recorded on the ancient votive tablets; still, we think, the Esculapian priests used other means in their miraculous cures than those publicly recorded. Narratives of this kind were well calculated to fortify the piety of the faithful; but they certainly do not serve any great end in the advancement of science. It is pretty well established, that the asclepiadæ wrote down, in secret, the history of each disease, and the means employed to combat it. The immense number of practical facts obtained by the Egyptians, and recorded in their sacred book of Hermes, were known to the Greek priests; and the exquisite taste and precision which characterize some of the books of Hippocrates, who was a priest of Esculapius, show that they had, for a long time, been in the habit of closely observing, and clearly describing diseases. (1).

§9. We also believe that some very important cures, of serious diseases, may have been effected in the temples of Esculapius, *by faith* alone. It is a well-attested fact that, as soon as the powers of *nitrous oxide*, or laughing gas, were discovered, Dr. Beddoes at once concluded that it must necessarily be a specific for paralysis. A patient was selected by him for the trial, and the management of it was entrusted to Sir Humphrey Davy. Previous to the administration of the gas, Davy inserted a small pocket-thermometer under the tongue of the patient, as he was accustomed to do upon such occasions, to ascertain the degree of heat, with a view to future comparison. The paralytic man, wholly ignorant of the nature of the mysterious process to which he was to submit, but deeply impressed, from the representations of Dr. Beddoes of the certainty of its success, no sooner felt the thermometer under his tongue than he concluded the talisman was in full operation, and, in a burst of enthusiasm, declared that he already experienced the effect of its benign influence throughout his whole body. The opportunity was too tempting to be lost; Sir Humphrey Davy cast an intelligent glance at Coleridge, who was present, and Dr. Beddoes, and desired the patient to renew his visit on the following day, when the same ceremony was performed, and repeated every succeeding day for a fortnight—the patient gradually improving during that period—when he was dismissed as cured, no other application having been used. It is next to impossible to suppose that the Esculapian priests did not witness many such recoveries, from their more complicated and more impressive ceremonies. The invalid, on his arrival at a temple, was first submitted to purification, by fasting, ablution, sacred inunction and prayer; and we must recollect that the belief of the Greek of the fifth century, B. C., in the constant, immediate, all-controlling agency and interference of the gods in human affairs, was as implicit and as unqualified as that of the Hebrew in the one true God. Not only all their temples, but almost every house and street, and market-place had its tutelary divinity, its fonts of lustral water, and its altars for sacrifice. All the great games and festivals were either for formal and solemn religious purposes, or they had something of a religious significance and end. No great enterprise was undertaken without solemn consultation of oracles, sacrifices and libations. Private and public conduct, the actions of individuals and the movements of fleets and armies were constantly governed and directed by what were believed to be the immediate and visible interposition of the gods. Even Plato held the sun and stars to be gods, animated each with its special soul, and every Greek, instead of an ordinary sun, thought he saw the great god Helios mounting his chariot in the morning in the east, reaching at noonday the solid heaven, and arriving in the evening, in the western horizon, with horses fatigued and desirous of repose.—The patients in the temples reposed upon the skins of sacred, sacrificed rams, in order to procure celestial visions; they heard music at night, and hissings, which they thought celestial or infernal; and a priest, cloaked in the dress of Esculapius, imitating his manners and often accompanied by females, who represented Hygea and Panacea—that is, young actresses, thoroughly tutored in their parts, entered and solemnly delivered an oracular medical opinion; while the hissing serpents prevented the majority of the patients from entertaining any other feeling but that of awe. It is probable that the cures by faith were, at one time, so numerous, that many of the priests were led to neglect more material means. (1, 6).

In our own most sacred record, we read that a woman, who was diseased with an issue of blood or uterine hæmorrhage, for twelve years, came behind Jesus and touched the hem of his garment; for, she said, within herself: "If I but touch his garment, I shall be whole;" and, when Christ saw her, he said: "Daughter, be of good comfort; thy faith hath made thee whole;" and she was well from that hour. We do not think it necessary to go further than the simple enunciation of our Saviour, that it was *faith* which made her whole. Again, when he saw that the man, sick with the palsy, had *faith*, he commanded him to take up his bed and walk; and he arose and departed. There are other cures and restorations effected by the divinely miraculous power of our Saviour alone; in this place, I wish merely to allude to those which were accomplished by faith. If faith in the glass bulb of a thermometer will cure palsy in two weeks, that infinitely glorious, all-absorbing, and intense *faith*, which our Saviour excited, could accomplish the same in a moment of time.

To return to the less sacred cures, we must recollect that the priests of Esculapius, although great cheats in many respects, had some belief in common with their patients. Such miraculous recoveries must, at first, have impressed them powerfully; there must have been moments when some of them, at least, had more faith in their blind gods than even they were aware of. Everybody has experienced the excitement produced by a new discovery, or a new and striking idea, whether his own or another's; and the judgment and approbation of the bulk of mankind are more prone to be influenced by what acts on their feelings and imagination, than by that which merely and coldly appeals to their understanding. Our feelings, thus wrought upon, we are no longer what we were, or what we ought to be for a calm investigation; the stimulus is all the more powerful, if excited by apparently supernatural events, or religious belief; it influences our observation, conception, and judgment, and we cease to preserve that calmness of examination which we may possess in reference to other matters, and which is so essential in our practical observations and researches. But the frequent repetition of these apparently miraculous cures must finally have convinced the priests of their true nature; in place of honestly and frankly attributing them to faith, they used them to play still more powerfully upon the imaginations of their patients—the blind Caius, who was only obliged to make adoration at the altar, probably was an impressible subject, with simple intolerance of light, which is often called blindness, even by very sensible persons—they cannot endure the light and think they are blind; a powerful mental impression will enable them to bear the light for a short time, at least, just as an aching tooth becomes stilled when the dentist is near. The blind soldier was a more hardy subject, and with a more material disease of his eye; hence simple adoration was dispensed with, and the blood of a pure and rare esculapian bird, a white cock, was an ingenious addition to a collyrium which was applied to his eyes for three days.

Thus the priests went on, deceiving themselves and others; and some of them, doubtless, becoming more rascally each day, and others, like Hippocrates, becoming more and more enlightened, and more and more honest, not only by contrast, but from a clearer perception of what knavery was, and a more hearty detestation of it. Aristides the just, was the dupe and victim of knavish asclepiades for ten successive years; he was alternately purged, vomited and blistered; made to walk barefoot under a burning sun, in summer; and, in winter, he was doomed to bathe his feeble and emaciated body in the icy river. All this severity, he was made to believe, was exercised towards him by the express directions of Esculapius himself, with whom he was cheated to fancy he conversed in his dreams, or his midnight vigils, and frequently beheld in nocturnal visions. Upon one occasion, the god, fatigued with the earnest and frequent importunities of his obstinate votary, ordered him to lose one hundred and twenty pounds of blood; the unhappy man not having so much blood to spare at one time, with infinitesimal wisdom, took the liberty of interpreting the oracle in his own way, and parted with no more than he could conveniently spare. This reminds us of some of the pranks of the "modern spirits." (1).

§10. The earliest writers in the Alexandrian school of medicine, on the pharmaceutic branch, were Zeno, Andreas, Appollonius, surnamed Mus, and several others, who, however, only treated of medicines incidentally. *Pamphilius*, in the reign of Ptolemy Philometor, was the author of a treatise on herbs, of which he speaks in *alphabetical* order, treating of their agricultural, as well as their medicinal uses. He compiled largely from the Egyptian Hermes, or Thot, the well-known great medical authority of the ancient Egyptians. (1).

Nicander, who was a contemporary, wrote, in verse, a treatise on poisons, and the bites and stings of venomous creatures. The musical training of the ancient physicians is evident here; but what would we think, in our times, of having an Orfila, or "Christison on Poisons," in rhyme?

It is said that the improvements in pharmacy, and additions to the materia medica, were as much due to the commercial intercourse of Alexandria with India and southern Asia, as the scientific enterprise of its physicians.

The older *Heras*, who flourished in the reign of Attalus II., and belonged to the school of Pergamus, was among the earliest, if not the very first, to introduce those compound confections, which, under the name of theraica, or antidotes, were afterwards in almost universal use among the ancients. Anodyne liniments or embrocations, were also among his inventions. We doubt not, that he had some as effectual as our opiate, and other anodyne liniments; for his king, Attalus, was not only a patron of the medical profession, but was himself actively employed in the cultivation and employment of medicinal plants. Plutarch says, that in his gardens were planted *Hyosciamus*, *Hellebore*, *Cicuta*, *Aconite*, and other poisonous herbs, all of which he collected with his own hands, at proper seasons, for the purpose of experimenting with the expressed juice, their fruit and their seed, and determining their respective properties. This first medical botanic-garden was evidently not cultivated as a mere rarée-show, nor merely to exhibit to students specimens of the plants, either living or dried, but for experiments upon the well and the sick. A more philosophical use of a medical botanic-garden than, perhaps, was ever afterwards made, up to the time of Hahnemann. (1).

Mithridates, king of Pontus, it is well-known, experimented upon himself with poisonous plants, in order to habituate himself to their use, and thus become insusceptible to their deleterious effects. A much less noble object of experimentation than that of Storck and Hahnemann, who experimented upon themselves to aid sick people. His composition, afterwards known as the *Mithridaticum*, and employed as an antidote, was among the most celebrated nostrums of antiquity. *Pompey*, after overcoming this prince, ordered diligent search to be made among the archives of his palace for the recipe of this famous formula; and very erroneously supposed that he had discovered it in a confection, consisting of twenty leaves of *Rue*, a few grains of salt, two walnuts, and a couple of dried figs, which was to be taken, fasting, every morning, and followed by a draught of wine. This more simple compound somewhat resembles the more modern confection of Senna. Rue is used, in modern times, as an emmenagogue, to produce abortion; as a nervous stimulant, in hysteria, in the colics and convulsions in children. Hence it is probable that Mithridates used it as a preventive of belly-ache, in himself and children, or to regulate the monthly turns of his wives and concubines. (1).

§11. The Romans, we have seen, were later in their advances in medical knowledge than Egyptians and Greeks; the first Roman physicians, if we can call them so, were slaves, taken in foreign wars, who had, or pretended to have, more knowledge of medicine than their masters. The first regular physicians in Rome were Greeks, who had emigrated there; and the people of Rome, on the authority of Pliny, were slow in relinquishing their prejudices against Greek scholars and doctors, and indisposed to forget the humble position of those slaves, among themselves, who were devoted to the healing art. They, hence, were foolish or prejudiced enough to suppose that polished Greek scholars and physicians were escaped slaves, who aped the manners of their superiors.

Cato, the censor, was celebrated for his opposition to all sciences not of native growth, and especially to Greek physicians. It is true that some of these were only intriguants, without instruction or manners, having no other aim than to make a fortune, and capable of any baseness to attain it. But a man of Cato's acumen should have been able to separate the true from the false; to distinguish between an instructed Greek, and those medicasters of a low grade, those herbalists, or holders of some panacea, or family-recipes, which resemble our modern patent-medicine venders.

Still, we have seen that all practical medicine originally sprang from the populace; even the knowledge of the Egyptian priests was originally obtained from the common people, who were forced to record all the cures effected at their own homes, and with medicines of their own discovery, in the temples. Specimens of all newly-invented surgical instruments were also obliged to be deposited there.

In Rome, the second stage of medicine was not the *priestcraft* stage, but the *patriarchal;* the oldest and best-instructed of the family treated the diseases of his family, as he understood them; and it does not appear that the Romish priests at first assumed this function more than others. Cato, the censor, was much engrossed in this domestic medicine; he even wrote a book on the subject, in which he recommends *cabbage* as a sovereign remedy in many cases. This, perhaps, is scarcely more ridiculous than the tar-water mania of Bishop Berkeley, of much later times, or the blue-pill of Abernethy, or the leeches of Broussais. But Cato did not even disdain to transmit to posterity the magical words which he believed useful to repeat for the reduction of luxations and fractures. For curing a luxation, or fracture at the hip, says he, take a green diving-rod, four or five feet long, split it in the middle, and let two men hold it at the hip and sing: "*In alio, s. f. motas, vœta daries dardaries, astataries dissunapitur,*" until the injured parts are again replaced. The luxation being reduced, or the fracture set, and properly adjusted in splints, repeat the incantation every day, as at first, or change to the following:

"*Huat, hanat, huat ista, pista, sista dominabo damnaustra;*" or, if this fails: "*Huat, haut, haut, ista, sis, tar, sis, ardannabon dunnaustra.*"

Cato thought, or determined to think, that the Greeks had sworn to kill all the Roman barbarians, by means of medicine, and yet, were cunning enough to require pay from those whom they treated, in order to gain their confidence, and thus ruin them more easily. In short, he says to his son: "Remember that I have forbidden you to employ physicians." Every country, even our own, at the present day, contains many such patriotic souls, who condemn everything foreign; who reject every French, German, or even English medical innovation. (1).

§12. *Antonius Musa*, according to Pliny, is said to have owed his first success, in Rome, from having recommended *Lettuce* to the emperor Augustus, which his former attendant, Camilius, had prohibited. The sedative powers of *Lactuca Sativa*, or Lettuce, were known, as we have just seen, in the earliest times; and allusions to this plant, frequently occur in the medical writings of antiquity. Galen, in the decline of life, suffered much from morbid vigilance, until he had recourse to eating a lettuce every evening, which cured him. Among the fables of antiquity, we read that Venus, after the death of Adonis, threw herself upon a bed of lettuces, to lull her grief and repress her desires. Lactucarium, the active principle, or concrete milky juice of lettuce, is sometimes called *lettuce-opium*, from its inducing composure and drowsiness, and its narcotic odor strongly recalling that of opium. Unfortunately, it is very uncertain in its action, and is often collected and prepared carelessly; besides, it is quite as unpleasant as opium to the taste; yet, it is still used to calm nervous disquietude, relieve pain, cough, and cause sleep, even in febrile diseases; as it is said to diminish the force and frequency of the pulse, and the temperature of the body, somewhat like Digitalis. It has often been used in chronic rheumatism, colic, gastralgia, and morbid sensibility of the eyes. A small treatise, attributed to Musa, is said to be still extant, in which, in the short space of eight octavo pages, he treats of the plant *Vetonica*, and its application to forty-seven different ailments. I am not ashamed to admit, that I do not know what Vetonica is; I can find *Veronica*, or Speedwell—which is said to have a warm, bitter, and astringent taste—and was once a very favorite remedy against incipient consumption, mucous states of the lungs, humid asthma, blood-spitting, &c. It was also used against chronic skin-diseases, in nephritic complaints, in the treatment of wounds, to purify the blood, and in scurvy. It originally grew in the south of Europe, and was imported into this country. The *Veronica-virginica* or *Leptandra*, or *Culver's Physic*, is almost as extravagantly praised by the botanic physicians of this country, as Vetonica ever was by Antonius Musa. The brother of this physician was highly esteemed by Juba II., king of Numidia, a man of great learning, and author of the first Greek history of Rome. The Numidian king, on discovering a new medical plant, near Mount Atlas, named it after this physician; and it is still known by the name first assigned to it—the Euphorbia. The gum or resin of Euphorbia, is still much used in continental Europe, as a perpetual vesicatory; it takes the place of the Sabina, or Savine ointment, of the English and American physicians; it is variously used, in the proportion of half a drachm to an ounce of lard or Basilicon ointment; or mixed with Lard, Turpentine, Cantharides, Mastich, Rosin, or even Sandaracha, or Arsenic. It was formerly used as a purgative in dropsy. It is a most powerful remedy, and readily causes the most violent colics, with peculiar and intense hiccough, cold sweats, and prostration. Æneas gave it in honey, with some unknown herb, (Margoldsaft), as an expectorant in chronic coughs. Cælius Aurelianus gave it in dropsy, not so much to carry off the water, *as to prevent its return*, (if it possesses this property, it is one of the most valuable remedies of antiquity); in tetanus, he rubbed it on the spine. *Archigenes* gave the formula of a plaster, which, with some alterations, is the basis of the modern Italian and Swiss perpetual blisters.

Cassius, who lived near the time of Celsus, was the first to use *cold water*, plentifully, in fevers.

Themison, the founder of the Methodic sect, was familiar with the use of Opium, or Lettuce, Hyosciamus, and other narcotics; and his name is associated with a confection of poppies, which he employed in diseases of the respiratory organs.

Apuleus Celsus wrote a treatise on herbs, still extant, "*De Medicaminibus Herbarum*," partly popular, and much taken up with the bites and stings of venomous creatures.

Scribonius Largus, who flourished in the reign of the emperor Claudius, whom he accompanied in his campaign into Britain, wrote a treatise, "*De Compositione Medicamentorum*," which is devoted rather to the composition and uses of medicines, than to the consideration of the diseases to which these are applied—hence, approaches to a materia medica. Many of his compound confections are quoted by later writers. He abounds in remedies for particular ailments, and, as usual, his antidotes, plasters, and embrocations are highly illustrative of the polipharmacy of the times. He gives the formula for the celebrated Mithridaticum, an antidote against all kinds of poisons, before alluded to, as invented or employed by Mithridates, king of Pontus.

Scribonius Largus copied largely from Apuleius, his preceptor, without acknowledgment. But he tells us, that many of his compositions he had prepared himself and used, and that the rest were obtained mostly from his friends, among which he must have regarded his preceptor as one, although he does not mention him by name. Plagiarism seems to have been as common in the quite olden times, as later ones. (1).

Andromachus, the elder, was physician to the emperor Nero, and the first Roman doctor to enjoy the official distinction of *Archiater*. He was celebrated for his Theraica, into which he introduced the flesh of vipers—to which, at that time, were ascribed wonderful powers—as an antidote to disease and poison.

The art of healing, which some affirm to be still a conjectural art among ourselves, has, by all accounts, made but little progress among the Chinese, and the art of surgery still less. Among the number of pharmaceutical preparations recommended by the Chinese practitioners, and which are derived from the animal kingdom, must be numbered a variety of ingredients furnished by various species of the snake and serpent tribes, which the Chinese use as remedial agents, as well as for food. The viper, more particularly, is exposed for sale, either alive, in small baskets of twisted bamboo, or dead and reduced to soup, or pickled and preserved, with seasonings of various sorts, in jars or barrels. It is on record, that the physicians of ancient Europe, fed their patients, for a long time, upon vipers grilled on the fire; that they made them drink wine of vipers, and thus cured the most obstinate diseases of the skin, such as elephantiasis, leprosy, &c. Might it not be worth while to ascertain whether the Chinese doctors do not also employ the flesh and juices of the viper to cure these frightful maladies, which are the only ones for which hospitals have been established in China? These travelling quacks generally exhibit a board, inscribed with the curative virtues of the reptiles they sell. In this respect, they do not imitate the more pretentious shop-keepers of the same profession, who are apt to exhibit a long list of the different sorts of snakes they have on hand. It is the practice of these traders to write up, after or under their names, on the sign-board, the words, "pu-hu," which may be translated, "no cheating here;" but, alas! corroborative evidence is much wanting to substantiate the truth of the declaration. In latter years, Hering, of Philadelphia, has revived the use of snake-poisons, in his celebrated Lachesis.

Philomenus, who also lived in the time of Nero, was the first to recommend *Assafœtida*, and frictions with tepid oil, for the treatment of tetanus.

Archigenes, a Syrian physician and surgeon, who flourished in Rome, in the reign of the emperor Trajan, was the first to use *Castor*, and to recommend Hellebore, in mentagra and other cutaneous affections. The mentagra of the ancients was a much more severe affection, than the modern variety, except some of the worst examples of barber's itch. It first appeared in Rome, during the reign of the emperor Claudius, and spread, especially among the male nobility, sparing women and persons in humble life; it was communicated, among other ways, from one individual to another, by the act of kissing, which, as is well-known, is much more common among continental males than with us; it appeared first on the chin, lips, and face, and afterwards spread over the body, in the form of eruptions, which degenerated into foul and offensive ulcers. It was called lichen, by Pliny, who says it had previously existed in the East, and that its contagion was first imported into Rome by a Roman knight, who communicated the infection to other individuals in his class of life. Homœopathists regard it as significant of its benefits in mentagra, that Hellebore, in its recent state, is so violently acrid as to produce inflammation, and even blistering, when applied to the skin; and infer, as the dried root loses much of its power, even large quantities may have been almost infinitesimal in power. (1).

Antyllus, another surgeon, in the reign of Valerian, treated humid asthma with *inhalations* or suffumigations, placing the patient in such a position, as readily *to inhale the fumes of Aristolochia* or *Clematis*, sprinkled over burning coals, in a chafing-dish or brazier. In this connection, we may mention that *Cœlius Aurelianus*, a Numidian physician, while writing on diseases of the throat, takes occasion to criticise Hippocrates, in reference to his recommendation of the inhalation of vapors, medicated with Hyssop, Sulphur, or Bitumen, *by means of a tube introduced into the fauces*, for the relief of threatened suffocation; a practice, against which he speaks in the strongest terms, judging it impossible to introduce a tube into the fauces, already so much obstructed as not to admit even air; or to inject thick smoke, where thin air is unable to penetrate. (1). It would seem, that Hunters and Greens were not wanting, even in ancient times.

It may be well to mention that Soranus, Cœlius Aurelianus, Asclepiades, Themison, and Thessalus, the originators and champions of the Methodic sect, which prevailed at this period, confined themselves as much as possible to general remedies, to the exclusion of specifics, or particular remedies for particular ailments. The primary education of ancient physicians was general and abstract, rather than specific or particular; but we do not know how their patients would have relished the information, that their physicians, instead of confining themselves to the treatment of their own individual and peculiar ailments, were endeavoring to effect a cure of that huge conglomerate of diseases, of which it requires, perhaps, many dozens of examples to furnish one general description.

Among the remedies used by these medical Methodists, were the juice of *Plaintain*, *Portulacca*, and *Sempervirens*; a diet of barley-meal, of lentils, or of quinces, or toasted bread moistened with vinegar. They rarely resorted to purgatives, except in dropsy, which, some homœopathists say, is merely producing a serous discharge from free surfaces, to relieve serous effusions into shut sacs. The Methodists were equally opposed to diuretics, sudorifics, irritating injections, opiates, and bleeding to the extent of fainting.

In diseases attended with distinct remissions and intermissions, they employed *recuperatives*, which we possibly term fortifying or strengthening means, or *tonics*; and *analeptic* agents, which resembled our antiperiodics; for analepsia was a species of epilepsy, which proceeded from the stomach, and with which the patient was apt to be seized, often and suddenly; hence, analeptic remedies were those which were thought to prevent the paroxysms. The most modern analeptic pills are those of Dr. James, celebrated as the inventor of James' powders; the pills consist of James' powder, Gum-ammoniac, Myrrh, Aloes, and Castor.

To check profuse sweating, the ancient Methodists sprinkled the surface of the body with powdered chalk, Alum, and other astringents.

As Alcohol was not yet discovered, to preserve plants and make tinctures, the culinary art was more intimately related to that of the apothecary, in olden times, than now. The principal Roman writer on cookery, was *Apicius Cœlius*, and many of his preparations were useful to the sick. He lived chiefly in Minturnæ, in Campania, during the reign of Trajan. His book is said to be larger and more complete than most modern cookery-books. Alcohol was probably discovered in the time of Pliny the elder, as he speaks of a strong Falernian wine, which was inflammable. (1).

The most noted Greek writer of this period, was *Dioscorides*, who lived in the reign of Claudius, although some suppose he was physician to Cleopatra. His great work on the materia medica was the only complete treatise which had yet appeared, and was the result of much personal inquiry and experience. What he did not know himself, he drew from the most reliable sources. Galen speaks highly of his accuracy, and, as an authority, his name is hardly yet obsolete among the writers on the materia medica. His work was in five books, and he published another on poisons. He was the first to group his remedies according to their therapeutic actions, and their application to particular ailments. It is more esteemed than those of Pliny or Galen, for its order, clearness, and exactness. He was the first who made mention of aromatic substances, and *mineral* remedies. All primitive medicine is originally botanic, as plants are much more readily procured than mineral preparations. As a specimen of the practice of his times, he advises *Nettles*, bruised with Myrrh, to be applied as a pessary, to provoke the menstrual flux. He says: "If introduced to the womb, fresh, it enables it to assume its natural position, when prolapsed or retroverted; also, that it opens the mouth of the womb. The seeds, boiled in wine, excite wanton desires; drank with Myrrh, it brings on the menses."

"Used sparingly with honey, it was said to be useful in complaints of the chest, pains in the side, and inflammation of the lungs. It was thought to purge the chest; applied to the side, with wax to remove diseases of the spleen; the leaves were used to increase the urine, and relieve flatulency; rubbed up with syrup, and applied to the nostrils, it was used to relieve bleeding of the nose; rubbed up with salt, it was supposed to form a good salve for bites of dogs, gangrenous sores, chancres, open ulcers, which are difficult to heal, tumors, and opened abscesses, especially parotidean."

Among the botanic physicians of this country, Nettles are regarded as valuable in diarrhœa, dysentery, hæmorrhoids, various hæmorrhages, and scorbutic affections, in gravel and other nephritic complaints; summer-complaints of children, and bowel-complaints of adults; and as an excellent styptic to bleeding surfaces. Large doses cause lethargic sleep; fourteen or sixteen seeds, three times a day, have removed goïtre and excessive corpulence, and are anthelmintic; in uterine hæmorrhage, as a rubefacient, and in paralysis.

It will be seen that the descriptions and recommendations of the modern botanic physicians, are but little or no better than those of the quite ancient physicians. It will also be evident, that all primitive medication was vegetable or botanic, as it still is, among all rude nations, like the Indians, Tartars, &c. Civilization must have made considerable advances, before minerals can be used as remedies. It is easy for the common man to pick up a plant, and make some random trials with it; but, to obtain mineral remedies, metallurgy must be well understood, and chemical science have made some progress. The rejection of mineral remedies, in the treatment of disease, can proceed from three causes only: first, ignorance, or a rude state of medicine; second, a reaction against the excessive use or abuse of such remedies; and third, a desire to make a new sect or party, in medicine, and thus make capital and fame out of the opposition and abuse of other physicians. All these reasons are unworthy ones. It is, undoubtedly, true that the indiginous vegetable remedies of many countries are much neglected by regular physicians; and we can easily imagine an honest and enthusiastic preference, on the part of simple herbalists and botanists, for vegetable remedies; but this preference becomes either a narrow-minded or dishonest one, when it leads to the rejection of other useful remedies, and this exclusion is used as a means of reproach and of injury to the business of other practitioners.

Dioscorides was preceded by Theophrastus.

Aristotle, the instructor of Alexander the Great, made the first collection of the products of nature undertaken with a scientific aim. His attention was directed particularly towards zoology, and he made, in that branch of the science of natural history, discoveries which would have been sufficient to immortalize his name. After him, *Theophrastus*, the inheritor of his manuscripts and his museum, continued to direct his school, in natural historical studies. He did for botany what his master had done for zoology. He studied the internal and external conformation of vegetables, their modes of nutrition, flowering, and fructification; in a word, he created vegetable physiology. He described the physical qualities, and medicinal virtues of more than five hundred plants. (1).

The name of Theophrastus is interesting to homœopathists, simply because Hahnemann quoted largely from him, in his article on the Helleborism of the Ancients. A celebrated Leipzig physician, wishing to criticise Hahnemann's essay, applied at the University Library for a copy of the work of Theophrastus, supposing that it was written by Theophrastus Paracelsus; and was much annoyed at finding that Theophrastus was an ancient Greek writer, instead of a German author of the middle ages.

§13. In the New World, we find the same kind of rude progress, among people who had had no species of communication with the inhabitants of the Old World. Renouard states that Antonio de Salis says that Montezuma, emperor of Mexico, possessed gardens, where great numbers of plants were cultivated, whose properties were well-known to the physicians of the country, who employed them with success. Cortez, having been attacked with a severe disease, Montezuma assembled a council of the most skilful native physicians, who employed various remedies, and, in a short time, restored the eminent patient to health. (1).

The Chinese appear early to have cultivated the materia medica, and pharmacology in particular. At an early period, they possessed more than forty works on these subjects, of which one alone, the most complete of all, is composed of fifty-two quarto volumes. There have never been any regular apothecaries in China, but they daily retail, in the markets, considerable quantities of drugs, and various compositions, which are boasted to have an efficacy against a host of diseases. The physicians, too, are accustomed to prepare and administer their own remedies. Some of the most distinguished doctors, however, simply give a formula, and leave to other physicians, of less rank, the task of executing it.

§14. Tartar physicians are purely *botanic* doctors—the Tartar pharmacopœa rejecting all *mineral* remedies, like our modern botanic doctors. The llamas are the physicians, and their medicines consist entirely of vegetables pulverized, and either infused in water or made up into pills. The patients, also, have a most exalted faith, in which the physicians may share sometimes. For, if the llama-doctor does not happen to have any medicine with him, he is by no means disconcerted; he writes the names of remedies upon little scraps of paper, moistens the paper with his saliva, and rolls them up into pills, which the patient tosses down, with the same perfect confidence as though they were genuine medicaments. To swallow the name of a remedy, or the remedy itself, say the Tartar physicians and patients, comes to precisely the same thing. It would require an ingenious calculation to define the difference between a Tartar thought of a remedy, and the suspicion of the two-thousandth dilution of one!

The Tartar method of collecting their vegetable remedies, or simples, is not an unmethodical one. According to Huc, towards the commencement of September, the llamas of the faculty of medicine all repair to Tchogortan, for the purpose of botanizing. Every morning, after they have recited their prayers, drunk their buttered tea, and eaten their barley-meal, all the students of medicine tuck up their garments, and go forth to the mountains, under the guidance of their professors. They are each provided with a long, iron-pointed stick, a small pick-axe, and a leathern bag. They spend the entire day on the mountains, but before sun-set, the llama-physicians return, laden with perfect faggots of branches, and piles of plants and grasses. As you see them weariedly descending the mountains, supported by their long staves, and bearing these burdens, they look more like poaching wood-cutters, than like future doctors in medicine. Those who have special charge of the aromatic plants, are often obliged to have an escort or guard; for their camels, attracted by the odor, always put themselves in pursuit of these aromatic personages, tumble them over, and, without the smallest scruple, devour those precious simples, destined for the relief of suffering humanity. The remainder of the day is occupied in cleaning, and spreading out on mats, these various products of the vegetable kingdom. The different articles are then selected and classified; a small portion only is given to each student, for his labor in collecting the whole of them, the great bulk remaining the property of the faculty of medicine. The drugs, thus collected at Tchogortan, are deposited in the general drug-room at Kounboum. When they have been thoroughly dried, in the heat of a moderate fire, they are reduced to powder, and then divided into small doses, which are neatly enveloped in red paper, and labeled with Thibetian characters. The pilgrims who visit Kounboum, buy these remedies at exorbitant prices. The Tartar Moguls never return home without an ample supply of them, having an unlimited confidence in whatever emanates from Kounboum. On their own mountains and prairies, the same plants, the same shrubs, the same roots, and the same grasses are found; but, then, how different must the plants, shrubs, roots and grasses, that grow and ripen in the birth-place of Tsang Kaba.

§15. Almost every nation has unlimited confidence in the virtues of some particular, perhaps inert, medicine, or system of medicine. The Chinese believe in the Ginseng-root. Incomparable virtues are attributed to it; among others, that of putting off the infirmities of age and prolonging life beyond the ordinary term. The people, who believe in its fabulous properties, buy it, literally, with its weight in gold.

As the right of gathering this root is monopolized by the emperor of China, the most extensive precautions are taken, by him, to prevent an encroachment on this privilege. The places where the Ginseng is known to grow are guarded with great vigilance, and a whole province, that of Twantong, bordering on the desert, is surrounded by a barrier of wooden stakes, about which guards continually patrol, to keep the inhabitants within bounds, and prevent them from making excursions into the woods in search of the prohibited drug. Notwithstanding this vigilance, their eagerness after gain incites the Chinese to wander by stealth in the desert, often to the number of two or three thousand, in search of the root, at the hazard of losing their liberty and all the fruits of their labor, if they are taken. The emperor employs his own servants for the purpose of collection, and, in the year 1709, had ten thousand Tartars engaged in scouring the woods in pursuit of the plant. Each man, so employed, was obliged to present his majesty two ounces of the best he should collect, and to sell him the rest for its weight in pure silver. At this rate, it was computed that the emperor would get, in a year, about twenty thousand Chinese pounds, which would not cost him above one-fourth of its value, at the common rate of selling it. The army of herbalists, in order to scour the country effectually, divide themselves into companies of one hundred each, which proceed forward, in a direct line, every ten of them keeping at a little distance from the rest. In this way they overrun an extensive wilderness in a short space of time. (10).

The Chinese physicians have written many volumes upon the qualities of Ginseng. It is made an ingredient in almost all the remedies which they give to their nobility, its price being too great for common people. The sick take it to recover their health, and the healthy to make themselves stronger and more vigorous. They affirm that it removes all fatigue of body or mind; dissolves humors, cures pulmonary diseases, strengthens the stomach, increases the vital spirits, and prolongs life to an old age. Its price, at Pekin, is eight or nine times its weight in silver. Father Jartoux found it to quicken and strengthen his pulse, improve his appetite, and enable him to bear fatigue better. Once, when so fatigued and wearied, as to be scarce able to sit on horseback, half of a root rendered him insensible of any weariness in an hour. The green leaves, chewed, produce nearly the same effects.

It is needless to add that Gingseng is one of those huge medical delusions which occasionally possess nations and ages. In 1718, Lafiteau, a Jesuit missionary among the Iroquois, found a plant answering to the description of it, in Canada; soon after this, the French commenced the collection of the root in Canada, for exportation. For this purpose they employed the Indians, who brought it to the merchants, and, at one time the Indians about Quebec and Montreal were so wholly taken up in the search for Ginseng, that their services could not be engaged for any other purpose. In 1748, the common price of the root at Quebec was from five to six livres a pound, or $1 to $1.20. The first shipments to China proved very profitable; but, in a short time the market was overstocked, and the Chinese began to think the American Ginseng inferior to the Tartarian, and its value depreciated, so that it has never since been a very profitable article of commerce. (10).

The root of Ginseng is derived from the Panax Quinquefolium. It has an agreeably sweet, bitter, and aromatic taste. So far as it has been tried, medicinally, in this country and Europe, its virtues do not appear by any means to justify the high estimation of it by the Chinese; for it approaches more nearly to liquorice than any other medicine, and a whole root may be eaten without inconvenience. Its place in the materia medica is among the demulcents. In tedious chronic coughs, it has occasionally proved useful as a lubricating mucilage, combined with some degree of aromatic warmth. In this country it is principally sold by the druggists as a masticatory, many people having acquired a fondness for it, and it is regarded as one of the most innocent articles for this purpose. The confidence of the Chinese in Ginseng is a pregnant example of the blind faith of many lay-persons and physicians, in comparatively inert means. Many of the great theorists and systematists, in medicine, with a little more show of science, are scarcely a step removed above the insufficient platform of Chinese belief.

§16. Among the Jews, the first medicine mentioned is Mandrakes. Rachel was less fruitful than Leah, both wives of Jacob. We are told, that Reuben went in the days of the wheat-harvest, and found Mandrakes in the field, and brought them unto his mother Leah. Then Rachel, having heard of it, said to Leah: "Give me, I pray thee, of thy son's mandrakes." And Leah said unto her: "Is it a small matter, that thou hast taken my husband from me and wouldest thou also take away my son's mandrakes?" And Rachel said, "Therefore, Jacob shall lie with thee to-night, for thy son's mandrakes." When Jacob came out of the field in the evening, Leah went out to meet him, and said, "Thou must come in unto me; for, surely, I have hired thee with thy son's mandrakes. And he lay with her that night." The record goes on to say, that in consequence of taking the mandrakes, the mouth of Rachel's womb was opened, and she conceived and bare a son, and her reproach of barrenness was taken away. That son's name was Joseph.

The Mandrake is supposed to be the *Podophyllum Peltatum*, or May-apple, or wild lemon, which has been found, it is said, by our botanic physicians, very beneficial in dysmenorrhœa, amenorrhœa, and some affections of the bladder. But the Jewish Mandrake was, doubtless, the *Mandragora Officinalis*, or Atropa Mandragora, a narcotic remedy, somewhat similar to Belladonna and Stramonium in its properties, and to which it is botanically allied. It is a perennial European plant, with a spindle-shaped root, which is often forked beneath, and has, therefore, been compared in shape to the human figure. In former times, the root was supposed by some to possess magical virtues; others infer that the doctrine of signatures led to its medical use; it was also used as an amulet, and to promote fecundity, which superstition is said to be still cherished by the vulgar, in some parts of Europe. It is conjectured to have been used as an anæsthetic agent, by the ancients, in surgical operations, from its narcotic effects; and it had also been given in scrofulous, scirrhous and syphilitic tumors.

The writings of Moses are said, by Renouard, to constitute a precious monument for the history of medicine; for they embrace hygienic rules of the highest sagacity, but which may be regarded as a detached fragment of Egyptian science, as Moses studied in Egypt. It is proven that Moses always gave his instructions, concerning leprosy and other infirmities, to the priests only, for the Levites joined the practice of medicine to their sacerdotal functions. Renouard says that they maintained, for a long time, this double relation to society, as there is no mention made of lay-physicians among the Jews, except in the book of Ecclesiastes, the author of which lived in the third century before Christ.

§18. The next step forwards in therapeutics, after the resources of instinct, the senses, simple observation, intuition, mysticism, knavery, and priestcraft had been exhausted, was to *rational empiricism.* Both the intellect and the senses were used; but in ancient Greece, the gymnasiums, which, at first, were places devoted entirely to bodily exercise, gradually became surrounded by halls and porticos, where philosophers, rhetoricians, artists, and physicians assembled, to hold their schools and dispute on questions of art, hence philosophy soon became too much mixed up with medicine."

It would also have been strange, if the gymnasiums had not been used, at an early period, not only to exercise the strong and healthy, but to strengthen and cure the feeble and sick.

Herodicus was the first medical gymnast. Renouard writes, that in the Third Dialogue on the Republic, Socrates, speaking to Glaucus, says: "It was not before Herodicus that the art of treating and curing diseases, as now attempted, was put in practice. Herodicus was the master of a gymnasium, and becoming a valetudinarian, he combined gymnastics and medicine, by which combination he tormented himself, and many others after him."—In what way?

"By producing a slow death, for, as his disease was mortal, he followed it, step by step, without being able to cure it, and neglected every thing else to take care of himself. Distressed by anxieties, if he varied ever so little from his regimen, by force of art he reached an old age, through a life of real agony.

His art rendered him excellent service, if it prolonged his life.

"Not so. In every well-ordered government each citizen has a task to fulfil, and no one has the right to linger a life of sickness, and in taking care merely of himself. These considerations led Esculapius to prescribe heroic treatment, suitable only for the diseases of persons of strong constitutions and good habits; but, in regard to those radically unsound, he was not willing to assume the responsibility of prolonging their lives and sufferings, and put them in condition to beget other beings, destined, most likely, to inherit their diseases. He thought it was not required of a physician to treat and patch up those who could not fulfil the career nature had marked out for them, because it was neither advantageous to themselves, nor to their country."

Thus it seems that the Lings, Roths, Taylors, and other practitioners of gymnastics and the movement-cure, had their counterparts in olden times.

The death of Socrates is highly interesting in a medical point of view. He, like many others who were condemned to death by the tribunal of Areopagus, was poisoned with the juice of Conium; his death has conferred a notoriety upon Conium, which time will never efface. The account of his death, as narrated in the *Phœdon* of Plato, affects the mind, by its tender touches and by a consideration of the blind and delusive impulses which can stimulate a popular faction to destroy the best of men. (10).

"The man who was to administer the poison, brought it ready bruised, in a cup. Socrates, beholding the man, said: 'Good friend, come hither—you are experienced in these matters—what is to be done?' 'Nothing,' replied the man, 'only, when you have drank the poison, you are to walk about until a heaviness takes place in your legs; then lie down—that is all you have to do;' at the same time, he presented him the cup. Socrates received it from him with great calmness, and regarding the man with his usual aspect, asked: 'What say you of this potion? Is it lawful to sprinkle any portion of it on the earth, as a libation, or not?' 'We only bruise,' said the man, 'as much as is barely sufficient for the purpose.' 'I understand you, said Socrates, but it is certainly lawful and proper to pray the gods that my departure hence may be happy, which I therefore beseech them to grant!' So saying, he carried the cup to his lips, and drank it without a gesture." (10).

"Thus far, most of us had been able to refrain from weeping. But, when we saw that he was drinking, we could no longer restrain our tears; and from me they issued with such violence, that Crito and Apollodorus, who had been incessantly weeping, now broke forth into loud lamentations, which infected all who were present, except Socrates. He said: 'What is it you do, my excellent friends? I have sent away the women, that they might not betray such weakness. It is our duty to die cheerfully, and with expressions of joy and praise. Be silent, therefore, and let your resignation be seen.' We suppressed our tears, and Socrates, after walking about for some time, told us his legs were beginning to grow heavy, and laid down, for so he had been ordered. The jailor examined his feet and legs, touching them at intervals; at length he pressed violently upon his foot, and asked if he felt it; to which Socrates replied, that he did not. The man then pressed on his legs, showing us that he was becoming cold and stiff; and Socrates, feeling it himself, assured us that when it reached his heart he would be gone. And now, the middle of his body growing cold, he spoke for the last time: 'Crito, we owe a sacrifice to Esculapius. Discharge this, and neglect it not!' His eyes became fixed, and he was dead. Crito closed his eyelids and mouth." (10).

§19. Pure experience was retarded somewhat by Pythagoras, the philosopher. He was the last of the sages who have transmitted their doctrines in an unusual language, and who made use of hieroglyphical writing. He travelled in Egypt, Phœnicia and Chaldea, and also pushed his journeys into India, where he communed with the Brahmins and Magi, and was initiated into the secrets of their worship, laws, and doctrines. He instituted a strange complex of jesuitism, and radicalism. His disciples were noted for the simplicity of their costume, their symbolical language, their habitual silence, their avoidance of pleasure, and the purity of their lives; they ate in common, used a very frugal diet, and executed the orders they received without any observations. His doctrines held the key to the pretended occult sciences, the reign of which, among the illuminati, extended down as far as the eighteenth century. The Pythagoreans, strange enough, first introduced the custom of visiting their patients in their own houses, going from house to house, fulfilling their duties as physicians, as is done at present; whence they were called periodic or ambulant physicians, in contradistinction to the Asclepiadæ, who consulted and treated the sick only in temples.

The doctrine of numbers was first made public by Pythagoras. He, and his masters and disciples designated God by the figure 1, and matter by 2; and they expressed the universe by 12, as 1 before 2 made 12; then, as 12 was the multiple of 3 by 4, they conceived that the universe was composed of a trinity, each of which was developed in four concentric spheres; the ineffable being was placed in the common centre of these twelve spheres, which corresponded to the twelve signs of the zodiac. The trinity, in man, was represented by soul, spirit and body—manifested by thought, intelligence and sensibility; the trinity, in God, was represented by love, power and wisdom. This complex system of numbers was finally so degraded as to be supposed to have analogues in diseases, especially in diurnal, tertian and quartan fevers; and all diseases were supposed to have a tendency to terminate on numerical or critical days; viz: on the 3d, 4th 7th, 11th and other days. Then twice 7, or 14 days; 3 times 7, or 21 days; or 4 times 7, or 28 days, &c., were also regarded as critical days, in prolonged diseases; while 7+9 was regarded as the grand climacteric of sixty-three years, &c. This system of Pythagoras exerted some influence of Hippocrates, quite necessarily, as it almost immediately preceded his advent; and nearly every founder or reformer is influenced by the absolute knowledge, or attractive theories which immediately precede his times. He adopts part, and dissents from the rest; assimilates some and opposes the remainder; gains the platform of his predecessors, and advances beyond or opposes some of their views; i. e. he thinks and acts somewhat similar to them on some points, alters and opposes others.

§ 20.

"Diseases are sometimes cured by contraries, sometimes by similars, and sometimes by remedies which have neither similitude or antagonism."—HIPPOCRATES.

"A combination and a form, indeed,
Where every god did seem to set his seal,
To give the world assurance of a man."

"B. C. 460, a great medical leader appeared, in the person of a physician from the island of Cos, and in the form of a priest, from one of the temples of Esculapius. He was endowed by nature with the most wonderful and accurate powers of observing both the phenomena and effects of disease. He was gifted with a sound judgment, ripely matured by extensive converse with the sick, which were, in his day, brought in crowds to the temples of Esculapius; while his prejudices, in treatment, had been blunted by extensive travels over many countries, in which he had observed and helped to stay many far-spreading plagues and pestilences. He commenced by teaching moderation, and urged the physicians to slacken in their hot and active pursuit of disease. He told them how frequently he had seen the malign powers draw off reluctantly from before some equally invisible and unknown powers that worked for the good of men. He taught them that all the commotions and disturbances which they noticed in the sick were not solely the effects of disease, but were rather the result of a conflict between benign and malign powers; and insisted that although the former were frequently not so powerful as the latter, yet they persevered with such earnest good-will that physicians might safely draw the conclusion that most acute fevers, inflammations, &c., were not necessarily fatal, but, on the contrary, had a great tendency to get well of themselves. Hence he condemned all officious intermeddling, and advised, when physicians knew of no certain means of aiding the benign, or of counteracting the malign powers, that they should watch and wait, and not think that they were idle; for the benign powers, working silently and efficiently, would frequently reduce the malign to such terms, that medical art might easily complete the conquest. He urged them to disregard the fragments of philosophy, poetry and theory that had misguided them, and to cast their reliance upon rational empiricism; for it was evident that their notions of the nature and treatment of disease ought not to flow out of poetical dreams and scholastic definitions, but from careful observation, ripe experience, and from such principles as arise immediately out of facts, and which are not contradicted by other and better substantiated facts and principles. And, finally, he taught them that it was far better to learn how to cure one disease, well and quickly, than to waste their time in endeavoring to arrange their imperfect experience and principles into necessarily imperfect systems and theories."

Need we wonder that his name has been handed down to us through long and dim ages, both time-worshipped and time-honored, when in the writings of *Hippocrates* we find all the principles of the inductive philosophy—it is evident that a physician showed Lord Bacon the road to immortality—STOKES. It is wonderful to note how far-seeing and true-seeing this great and good physician was. His descriptions of disease are yet perfectly unrivalled; his predictions of the course of disease are still unequalled; his treatment of acute diseases is so complete that it is said that the allopathic experience of two thousand years has scarcely improved upon it; and, above all, he was far superior to the superstitions of his benighted age.

Need we wonder that he has been styled the "prince and father of physicians," and that his thrice-honored name has been held in reverential piety through various stagnations of science; through the gloomy periods of the Dark Ages; through noisy and tumultous reformations; and through all the pomp and ascendancy of numerous brilliant theories and schools, when, in addition to all these great and glorious things, we find him abounding in precepts, inculcating propriety of conduct and purity of morals, and even binding his disciples with an oath, "never to indulge in libertine practices, nor to degrade their art by applying it to criminal purposes;" while he makes them swear, by Apollo the physician, by his servant Esculapius, and by his daughters Hygea and Pomona, that they will treat the sick to the best of their judgment and power, and in the most salutary manner, and without injury or violence; that they will neither be prevailed upon to administer pernicious remedies, nor be the authors of such advice; that they will make the good of the sick their principal aim; and that they will avoid all voluntary injury and corruption. And again he bade them call the gods to witness, that they might prosper in life and business, and be forever honored and esteemed, or despised and condemned by all men, as they observed or violated this their solemn oath.

To Hippocrates is generally attributed the merit of having separated medicine from false philosophy; others have attributed to him the glory of having united true philosophy with medicine. It is certain that medicine had been too much philosophized upon before Hippocrates; it is also equally true that Hippocrates theorized, somewhat after the manner of Socrates and Pythagoras, and that he necessarily shared the prejudices of his age in some particulars; but, in many respects, his philosophy is distinguished from that of his cotemporaries by greater and much more profound wisdom. He reminded philosophers and physicians continually of the maxim, too often neglected by them, and sometimes even by himself, "*that the nature of man and his diseases cannot be well known without the aid of accurate medical observation, and that nothing can be affirmed concerning that nature, until after having acquired a certainty of it, by the aid of the senses;*" a maxim diametrically opposed to the dogmas of Pythagoras, the great leader of the philosophy of his times, and which includes the germ of an entirely new philosophy, which Plato misconceived, and of which Aristotle only had a glimpse, but which Bacon, centuries after, developed in the inductive method.

The great pathological theory of Hippocrates was that of *coction* and *crisis*. He regarded many acute diseases as an association of phenomena, resulting from the efforts made by the conservative principle of life, to effect a coction of the morbific matter in the economy. He thought this could not be advantageously expelled until it was properly prepared; that is, until after its elements were separated from the natural humors of the body, and united with the excretive matters, so as to form an excrementitious material. He taught that when the morbid process approached its maturity, nature often seemed to redouble her efforts; the fever was augmented, the patient might seem overwhelmed, and all the symptoms aggravated, yet a salutary crisis was approaching; that the physician should respect the critical labor of nature, provided it proceeded properly, and never disturb it with too violent or heroic remedies, but to help the vital principle only when there was a clear and urgent necessity. When the coction was effected, which might be known by the amendment of the symptoms, it only remained to evacuate the heterogeneous and excrementitious materials. Nature often accomplished this last effort herself, and then the disease terminated with a critical sweat, urination, or stools; but it also frequently happened that the vital principle became fatigued and broken down by the efforts of the crisis, and required aid, when the physician must come to its relief, by means of proper strengthening food and medicines, and should also help to urge the excrementitious matter towards those emunctories to which it naturally tends; that is, he must give sudorifics, diuretics, or purgatives, according to the indications of nature, whose faithful attendant and minister he must show himself to be, in all things. This practice is very different from the ordinary dosing and drenching of sick people, in season and out of season, with powerful evacuating remedies, thus degrading the physician almost to the level of scavengers and chambermaids, rather than elevating them to the position of handmaids of nature.

The therapeutic principles of Hippocrates were liberal and broad. He says: "*Diseases are sometimes cured by contraries, sometimes by similars, and sometimes by remedies which have neither similitude nor antagonism.*" In other words, diseases are sometimes cured by antipathic medicines, and sometimes by those which are homœopathic, and sometimes by those which are allopathic. Hippocrates endeavored to give remedies which either opposed the hurtful operations of the disease, or aided and acted similar to the curative endeavors of the vital powers; or, in default of these, such as would change or alter the whole action of the disease for the better,—forming a wise and broad variety of alterative treatment, very different from the petty and contracted alterative mode of later and even present times.

The pathological and therapeutical views of Hippocrates were in strict accordance with his physiological opinions. He always maintained the existence of a ruling principle, a so-called vital principle, vital dynamism, or vis-naturæ, by which all the normal functions of the body were performed. Its manner of action was by attracting that which is good and suitable, retaining, preparing, changing, or, according to need, rejecting the superfluous or injurious; to which power was added a kind of affinity, by which the various congenial substances acquired a tendency to unite, and the uncongenial to separate, whilst, also, a general sympathy was maintained throughout the body. In disease, the animal economy still endeavored to carry out its original design and functions. It was accustomed to separate and eject effete matters, and to reject injurious ones, and sometimes completed these operations still more powerfully in disease, than in health; hence the province of the physician was to aid in removing or opposing noxious agents by contrary remedies, to sustain the vital powers and restorative processes by similar remedies.

As many of these processes were very subtle and concealed, he was distinguished by the faculty of minute observation of the apparently most trivial circumstances; he examined all discharges from the body, not forgetting the tears, wax from the ears, mucus from the nose, expectoration, perspiration, urine, fæces, &c. It would be difficult to point out any field of examination which he omitted. His prescriptions were efficient, but eminently simple. He felt that the healing art was the most noble of all arts, but that the ignorance of many who practice it often made it the least worthy. He said there were many physicians in name, but few in reality; for, to acquire a high degree of medical knowledge, it is necessary to possess a natural inclination for it, the means of instruction, study and application from youth up, a docile spirit, diligence, and a long time.

Thirty years after Hippocrates, was born another great philosopher, Plato, who preferred pure reasoning to pure experience. Thus, Hippocrates was preceded and followed by great theorists or philosophers, viz.: Socrates, Pythagoras, Plato, and Aristotle; and his views, and those of his followers, were necessarily modified by the prevalent philosophical notions of their day. But Hippocrates probably derived some part of his high moral principles from Socrates and the Pythagoreans; and his love of truth and of virtue, his patriotism, his unwearied benevolence and unflinching disinterestedness have contributed to render his name immortal, quite as much as his scientific and practical knowledge.

Hippocrates lived in an age of progress. The earliest historians, the profoundest philosophers, the wisest legislators, the ablest generals, the greatest architects, painters, and sculptors of Greece, were all men of the same epoch. And, while other sciences and arts were thus springing into life, and rising at once to maturity, it is not surprising that some man of genius should appear in the ranks of medicine, to give to its principles form and utterance. This man was Hippocrates. According to Bartlett, the birth of Hippocrates corresponds almost exactly to the secure establishment of national independence in Greece. The battle of Marathon was fought thirty years before he was born. He had listened to the stories of Thermopylæ, and Salamis, and Platæa, from the living lips of the survivors of those fields. He had been told of that day of humiliation, when the Persian monarch, with the kings of Tyre and Sidon, held their synod in the Acropolis of Athens, to deliberate upon the fate of Greece, and to portion its territories. But, during the period between the defeat of the great army of Xerxes and the birth of Hippocrates, the Persian power had been utterly swept from the Grecian territory. It is sufficient to say of the period in which Hippocrates lived, that it was "the age of Pericles." Greece was covered with those architectural structures, which are still in their ruin, as much the wonder and admiration of the world as they were the pride and glory of Athens on the day they were finished. Phidias' great gold and ivory statue of Minerva was dedicated when Hippocrates was twenty-three years old; Eschylus, the founder of Greek tragedy, died when he was a child; Sophocles and Euripides were only twenty-five and thirty-seven years his senior; Socrates was but ten years older; Herodotus and Thucydides, the great historians, were only twenty-four and eleven years his seniors, while Xenophon was fifteen years younger. The first comedy of Aristophanes was exhibited when Hippocrates was thirty-three years old; the death of Socrates took place during his life-time; the latter period of his career was illustrated and made immortal by the teachings of Plato, and its close was lighted up by the dawning sun of Aristotle The father of Demosthenes died when Hippocrates was eighty-two years old, and he, doubtless, had heard the voice of the greatest orator of any age. When he was eighty-seven, he witnessed the brief but splendid career of the great Theban, Epaminondas. Pericles and Alcibiades were among his friends and patients. (5).

The Greek philosophers, previous and up to the times of Hippocrates, had speculated upon almost every subject of human thought and inquiry—on morals, ethics, metaphysics, and politics; also on the material creation, man and nature. The philosophies about the latter embraced what their authors intended for comprehensive and complete schemes of creation, and systems of nature, including, in their vast scope, the entire universe in all its relations, and, of course, all the sciences, such as astronomy, physics, mathematics and medicine. These pure theorists had speculated upon the origin of things, the nature and composition of matter, the causes of physical phenomena, &c. Each of these philosophers had indulged in speculations peculiar to himself; each had framed his own system of nature, the general character of which is obvious enough; for mingled with the slenderest and scantiest material of positive knowledge, they consisted of vague, hypothetical, *a priori* speculations and conjectures, in relation to external nature and all physical subjects. But there was one most important result of this speculative inquisition into the economy of nature: the tendency to scepticism, which it engendered, tended to the overthrow of heathen mythology, and led, in its stead, to the conception of a single supreme intelligence, acting through all nature by a fixed and invariable system of laws. Before it the Homeric hosts, heroes, demi-gods, and gods, the gods of Ida and Olympus, were soon destined to fall. It was in the midst of this transition-movement in theology that Hippocrates lived—subject to all its influences, and taking an active part in all its interests. The two most illustrious of these philosophers were Socrates and Plato, and their philosophy was only partially emancipated from the old religious faith. The teachings of Moses and the prophets had not yet influenced these men, although it was now only about four hundred years before the advent of Christ.

The doctrines and practice of Hippocrates were derived from three principal sources: First, and the most important, was the experience, traditional and recorded, of the Asclepiades, the priest-physicians of the temples of Esculapius; the second source of his medical knowledge was found in the studies and teachings of the philosophers, who included, in their comprehensive system of nature, the organization and functions of animals, human physiology and diseases. Among the most celebrated of these were the Pythagoreans. The third source of this ante- and cotemporary Hippocratic medicine was found in the gymnasia, which developed and perfected the forms that were embodied in marble by Phidias and Praxitiles, those manly and heroic shapes that were represented by Apollo, Antinöus and Mercury, and that superb and consummate physical womanhood embodied in the Junos, Hebes, Minervas and Dianas of Greek art and religion. The effect of this methodical physical training—the bodily exercise, exposure, ablutions, the dietetic discipline and control of the appetites and passions, upon the preservation of health and prevention of disease was very great, carried on, as they were, under the direction of experienced guides and teachers. In this way was established a code of sound hygienic doctrine. Under Herodicus, the gymnasia became establishments for the formal and methodical treatment of disease. The nervous votary of fashionable life in Greece, the victim of ennui, indolence, and an aimless, frivolous existence often went to the gymnastic cure.

Bartlett supposes that the appearance and manners of Hippocrates were in keeping with the elegance of the times in which he lived. In describing the sickness of Silenus, he says: "At the head of the bed, watching steadfastly and earnestly the appearance of his patient, is seated his physician, the already celebrated Hippocrates, of Cos. He is thirty years old, and in the very prime and beauty of early manhood; his face is dignified, thoughtful and serene; and his whole aspect, manner, and expression are those of high antique breeding, of refined culture, and of rather studied and elaborate elegance. His hair is long, and both this and his beard are kept and arranged with scrupulous neatness and care. He wears, over his tunic, a large flowing mantle, of light, fine woollen, suitable to the season, and not unlike the later toga of the Romans; it was fastened at the neck with a cameo of Esculapius, and fell, in graceful folds, nearly to his feet. His sandals have been taken off, and his feet washed by a slave, in the vestibule." (5).

It is a sad consolation to find that the "father of medicine" was almost powerless to relieve some cases. Young Silenus was sick with a fever,—the fiery *causus* of the climate. Hippocrates' examination of his patient was long, anxious and careful. He saw, at once, that the gravity and danger of the disease had increased since his last visit. He inquired very minutely into the manner in which the night had been passed, and was told by the watchers that the patient had had no sleep; that he had talked constantly, had sung and laughed, and had been agitated and restless. He found the hypochondria tumefied, but without much hardness. The stools had been blackish and watery, and the urine turbid and dark-colored. He noticed the temperature and feel of the skin, and he studied, for a long time and with great solicitude, the general manner and appearance, the decubitus, breathing, motions, and especially the physiognomy of the patient. No examination of the rational symptoms of the disease could have been more thorough and methodical. Having satisfied himself, as to the state of his patient, he retired to an adjoining room, followed by some of the attendants, to give directions in regard to the remedies he intended to use. The patient had already been bled, and had had a purgative of black Hellebore. His physician could do but little more, and with a sad, but decided expression of his fears as to the issue of the case, and a few kind and pious words to the young, weeping wife, about the dignity, the solace, and the duty, in all our trials, of submission to the will of God, he gathered his mantle about him, and proceeded on his daily round of visits."

Again, Bartlett transports us to the house of Pericles—to the death-bed of that great and venerable Archon. It is only a year or two later, and Hippocrates is but thirty-two years old. Everything in the spacious apartment indicated the pervading presence of stately elegance, of high, various, many-sided luxury, culture and refinement. Philosophy and letters are represented; a statue, from the chisel of Phidias, stands in the room, and the walls are covered with pictures fresh from the pencils of the great Greek masters. Raised, and resting in solemn and august serenity upon its last pillow, lies that head of Olympian grandeur, which, after the lapse of nearly twenty-three centuries, has found no fitting representative and likeness, except in that of our Webster. Pericles was sinking under a protracted and wearing fever, the result of an attack of the plague; his long and glorious life was about to close—many of his near personal friends and relatives had already fallen victims to the pestilence; both of his sons had perished; Phidias, the sculptor, and his old teacher, Anaxagoras, had died a little while before. Those who were left, had now gathered round the bed of the dying Archon, to pay to him the last solemn and kindly offices of life. Socrates was there, and Sophocles, his old companion in arms, also a grandson of Aristides the just; generals, admirals, statesmen, orators, artists, poets, and philosophers are clustered around, and the youthful Alcibiades stands aside, subdued, for the first time in his life, and probably the last, at the spectacle before him, of his dying relative and guardian. Conspicuous among them all—their equal and associate in rank, fortune, in social position, in reputation, in learning, culture and refinement—was the young physician of Cos. Unlike Galen, who fled when pestilence reached Rome, Hippocrates had been summoned from his island home, in the Ægean Sea, to stay the march of the pestilence which was now desolating Athens.

Many physicians, both of the olden and of more modern times, have endeavored to develop themselves after the model of Hippocrates; of these, Sydenham (1650—1690) has, by universal acclaim, been pronounced the most successful in the attempt. He paid very little attention to the prevailing medical doctrines of his time, being early persuaded that the only correct method of acquiring an exact knowledge of his art was to observe diligently the progress and course of diseases, whence the natural curative indications—i. e., such as were *similar* to or in accordance with the intentions of nature—might be derived. He first applied this inductive method to acute febrile diseases, and it cost him many years of anxious attention to satisfy himself as to the proper method of treating them; finally, by closely imitating the operations of nature, he was enabled to introduce many essential improvements in the medical art of his day, which he described as having been invented by specious reasoners, and to be rather the art of *talking* than *healing*, although he bitterly lamented his want of knowledge of *specific* remedies, and adds that: "Certain it is, that a true specific is of that real value that a person would be amply rewarded for his pains, who, by making a diligent inquiry after this kind of medicines, should discover but one in his whole life; for, though that should seem a good method of curing acute diseases, which, after nature has pitched upon a certain method, or kind of evacuation, assists her in promoting it, and so, necessarily, contributes to cure the distemper, yet it is nevertheless to be wished that the cure might be shortened by means of specifics, and, what is of more importance, that the patient might be secured from the evils which are the consequence of those errors that nature cannot help committing, in expelling the cause, even though she is assisted, in the most effectual and skilful manner, by the physician."

He ever, like his great prototype, Hippocrates, maintained the character of a generous and public-spirited man, and conducted himself without that arrogance and vanity which too often accompanies original talent, so that he has, with one accord, been proclaimed the first physician of his age, and received the title of the "English Hippocrates."

§21. It has been supposed that it would, perhaps, have been well for the world if the physicians, at this precise juncture, had hit upon the ancient Egyptian idea of establishing a sort of absolutism in medicine, with the right of hereditary descent and primogeniture. This idea was not so far removed from the minds of men, at the period of which we write, as it is at present, for Hippocrates derived his descent from Esculapius, the supposed god of medicine, and his family, the Asclepiades, had devoted themselves, from time immemorial, exclusively to the service and cultivation of the medical art. We know full well how extremely difficult it has proven, as yet, for emperors, kings, princes, or even presidents, to learn the secret by which they might retain the greatest amount of wisdom and virtue in their own families; but it seems possible to us that, by the aid of some internal centralization of power, the art of medicine might have been kept from retrograding behind the state of development it had attained by the exertions of Hippocrates.

As it was, they preferred remaining a democracy—even the lowest of their number, if he possessed enterprise and talent enough, might, perchance, force his way to the very summit of his profession; but, occasionally, the majority considered it fair to annul the rights of the minority, and even to degrade some of their members, if they attempted to teach the majority wholesome but unpalatable truths. In fact, they tested the adage, "in the multitude of counsellors there is wisdom," to the utmost, for they soon began to depart from the precepts and example of Hippocrates, and most of them were soon as over-zealously and hotly engaged in the pursuit of death and disease as ever. A small, crudely-conservative party, however, remained, but they, too, retrograded widely from the teachings of Hippocrates; for he had taught that, in many diseases, certain internal curative processes, called *coction* and *crisis*, assimilated, changed, or concocted the disease, and then completed its work by expelling its products, in the so-called "critical evacuations," and that, at the proper times, it was the highest aim of the physician to imitate these processes, and aid the critical discharges—in a word, to become the ministers, not the masters of nature. But the routinists only saw the terminations in bleeding from the nose, vomiting, purging, sweating, &c., and hence bled, vomited, purged, sweated and urinated their patients, until a portion of the lay-world began to suppose that they had mistaken their vocation, and become the "chambermaids of nature," rather than ministering angels to her.

§22. After the time of Hippocrates, ancient medicine, like the modern, was divided among experimentalists, theorists, and eclectics. The experimentalists, or empirics, maintained that *experience* might be gained in three ways: First, from accident or chance; second, from experiments, instituted by design; and third, from an imitation of the results of chance or experiment. When this last method had been repeated, with sufficient frequency to prove or disprove certain opinions, or lines of treatment, it was regarded as constituting the established art of medicine.

The theorists, or dogmatics, maintained that it was necessary to know the *hidden* causes of disease, as well as the manifest. It is impossible, said they, to cure a disease rationally unless we know whence it arises; they did not deny the necessity of experience, but maintained that it could not be obtained accurately without reasoning. On the other hand, the empirics professed to know only the manifest causes of diseases, and all questions concerning the hidden causes and natural functions were regarded as superfluous, since nature and life itself are incomprehensible. They stated, with truth, that even when the causes of disease are manifest, as in wounds, it does not necessarily follow that the means of cure are equally manifest; that simply to know the disease, such as cancer or tubercle, does not imply that we know how to cure it. If, then, the knowledge of evident causes does not always suggest the right remedy, why should such as are hidden?

When these two parties had pushed forward their experience and reasoning as far as the advances of the times would admit, *eclectics* chose from each what seemed best established, and thought and practiced according to that light; for they saw that the controversy between the experimentalists and theorists owed much of its acrimony to the determination of each party to consider itself wholly right, and its opponents wholly wrong, instead of willingly recognizing the existence of some truth, some deficiency, and some error in both. To theorize and speculate on the *hidden causes* of diseases is very different from true investigation; but speculation may, or may not lead to true examination. The office of theory or reasoning, is simply to explain the facts which experience establishes, not to supersede or interfere with them; and its still higher office is to discover the laws which unite those facts. New facts may require a new law, or a modification of an old rule, to unite the new facts with the old; hence the ultimate achievement of extensive experience and true and broad reasoning is essentially a uniting process, and is, necessarily, *anti-sectarian*—for a sect is something limiting and limited. True progress requires the breaking of the bounds and bonds of a stationary system or sect; hence it is evident that theory, experience, and eclecticism must alternately prevail and be superseded by a newer and better theory, newer and riper experience, and newer and broader eclecticism.

It was shortly after the establishment of the Alexandrian school, that is about three hundred and twenty years before Christ, that the first schools of the dogmatists or theorists, and the experimentalists or empirics arose. These rival sects disputed with each other, with tenacity and keenness, for centuries.

The true ancient empiric was not a quack, but an experimental and experienced physician. Philenus, of Cos, and Serapion, of Alexandria, were probably the founders of this sect. They asserted boldly that the doctrines of elementary qualities, cardinal humors, and essences of diseases were all false and hypothetical; they even rejected the fundamental, antipathic, therapeutical law—*contraria contrariis curantur*—for they confined themselves entirely to the results of experiment and observation, and were the determined opponents of all spiritualism, all *a priori* general ideas, and all hypotheses, both about disease and its treatment. Medical skill and science were to be acquired, the empirics said, by three modes. The first was personal observation of the sick and dead, (autopsy); the second, the study of observations recorded by others, (history of disease); the third consisted of deductions, drawn from observation and history, which enabled them to make discoveries, or led to further and more minute observation. The examination and autopsy of the empiric was made with the greatest care; that errors in observation might be avoided, it was necessary that a disease should have been carefully watched, under every variety of complication and circumstance, and a method of treatment carefully followed, in the same manner, before the autopsy of that disease was considered complete. In short, they almost appear to have used a numerical or inductive method. The practitioner who had thus carefully observed a disease, and preserved a perfect record of its course, termination, and treatment, had arrived at a theorem; and he who had accumulated a sufficient number of theorems was then, only, first regarded as an *experienced* or *empirical* physician. The next step of the ancient cultivated empiric was the application of the experience of known diseases to unknown, by means of resemblances or analogies, (epilogism and analogism); that is to say, a new disease was treated according to the method established for one to which it had the closest resemblance—proper allowance being made, in some of the accessory medication, for the differences between the two diseases; and the same plan was adopted in substituting one remedy for another. The cultivated empirics observed, generalized, and doubted; thus following the three great systems of Plato, Aristotle, and Pyrrho. With Aristotle, they observed and inferred, (autopsy and theorem); with Plato, they generalized and inferred, (theorems, epilogisms, and analogisms); with Pyrrho, they doubted both the accuracy of their observations and of their generalizations, for they believed that the men who wish to learn, must first know how to *doubt*—for science is nothing else than the *solution* of antecedent doubts. Their doubts kept the empirics within the bounds of common sense, and they appear to have been the truly rationally-practical men of the day. They adopted the methods best calculated to attain to a true natural history of disease, and to improve therapeutics. They may be taken as the best models for imitation, by the moderns, to be found among the ancient sects.

§23. The first great theory in medicine, after the time of Hippocrates, was that of Asclepiades and Themison. They paid particular attention to two great causes of disease, which they designated as *strictum* and *laxum* Themison, especially, showed himself to be a very master in strategy, for he went to work, rather jesuitically, to oppose these two diseases, or rather their agents against each other. When laxum, or debility, was at his sneaking and malicious sport, it was not difficult to direct strictum, with his burly allies, tonics, and stimulants, upon laxum, as he was sapping the strength, and undermining the constitution of his victims, under the name of debility. And, in return, when strictum was over-crowding mankind, laxum was easily made to insinuate his troop of relaxants, reducents, evacuants, &c., so as not only quickly to cool down the turbulent strength of his sturdy enemy, but to spirit away the life of the patient. Themison, of course, gained great credit by his so-called methodic, or methodistic procedure, and he soon became so inflated with his success, that he insisted that he could overcome disease and death themselves. The world was soon convinced to the contrary, for they found that almost as many of the sick died now as before; but, when he became more and more one-sided, and, in order to sustain his position, falsified many truths, then they became disgusted with, and distrustful of him, and of strictum and laxum, and soon neglected them all too much. As in empiricism, each suite or combination of symptoms, not hitherto described, was deemed a new disease; and as, in the course of time, their species were constantly multiplying, without any attempt at generalization being made, eventually the greatest confusion was produced; hence the simple mode of viewing science, presented by Asclepiades of Bythinia, a distinguished professor of rhetoric at Rome, founded upon the philosophy of Epicurus, met with general favor. According to his views, the human body is formed of highly permeable tissues, perforated by invisible pores, through which pass and repass, continually, certain atoms, of different shapes and volumes, incommutable, indivisible, and impalpable in their nature—being perceptible alone to the mind's eye. Health depended upon the exact, symmetrical correspondence between the pores and the atomic molecules. However unsatisfactory his physiology, his therapeutics, from their simplicity, possessed a great attraction for his patients. His object was simply to enlarge the pores when too contracted, and vice versa; and his means of effecting it were chiefly of a hygienic character, such as various exercises, frictions, and the use of wine—to the exclusion of all remedies having a violent action. It is obvious that measures of this description could only prove useful in a limited class of affections, and, accordingly, Asclepiades' reputation was but ephemeral. His disciple, Themison, may be looked upon as the true founder of the methodic sect. He divided acute and chronic diseases each into three genera—the constricted, fluxionary or relaxed, and the mixed—basing his distinctions, not on the hypothesis of porosity, but on the sensible characters derived from observation. Thus, swelling, tension, induration, suppression of natural evacuations, were esteemed characters of the constricted genus. The classification of the species of disease under these genera, was, however, of a very arbitrary character—diseases, possessed of few or no characters in common, being grouped together, while different professors were at issue as to what genus certain maladies should be referred to. Nevertheless, his essay at a pathological classification, founded upon the obvious characters of diseases, and not on their imaginary qualities, was a great step. The methodists had but two *therapeutical indications* to fulfil; to relax when there was constriction, to constringe when there was flux or relaxation—and all their agencies were arranged in one or other of these classes. Bleeding, emollient cataplasms, tepid and laxative drinks, sudorifics, temperate air, sleep, and moderate exercise acted as relaxants. Darkness, cool air or drinks, red wine, vinegar, alum, &c., operated as astringents. They rejected all specific operations of medicines, such as the purgative, diuretic, excepting the emetic, which, however, they did not use to evacuate bile, or phlegm, but for the shock they imparted to the economy, opening and modifying the condition of the pores. The methodists never troubled themselves with any researches for *causes,* whether occasional or approximate; since, from the moment these have taken effect, it is the disease induced by them which is to be cured; and it is from it, its nature, character, and progress, and not from anterior circumstances, which no longer exert any influence, that indications must be drawn. They attached, also, little importance to a knowledge of the precise seat of the disease, or part affected, or to concomitant circumstances, as age, habits, general strength, season, &c., believing all such details superfluities, which should not modify the treatment pursued.

Thus, they would treat, in the same manner, mania, jaundice, amenorrhœa, because they belonged to the constrictive genus, &c. They paid no attention to the natural tendency of the vital forces, coction or critical days, and they studied anatomy and physiology even less than the empirics. So great was their desire for simplicity, that all their patients were put upon a uniform regimen, in which the extent and duration of fasting were rigidly regulated.

So simple a method much facilitated the acquisition of a superficial knowledge of the medical art, and Thessalus boasted he could teach the whole science in six months. This, doubtless, contributed also to the rapid progress the sect at first made. It likewise satisfied the very prevalent love of generalization, so characteristic of this epoch, and, in some sort, offered itself as a medium between the extremes of dogmatism and empiricism. With the former, it adopted rationalistic truths, but deduced from sensible phenomena; and with the latter, it took observation for its guide, but unencumbered by a multitude of precepts. Galen was no dupe of the pretensions of the methodists, but vigorously employed himself in unmasking the sophisms, and demonstrating the insufficiency of their theories, and the dangers of their practice—bestowing on the professors themselves, any epithets his satirical disposition suggested. The arrogance of some ancient physicians reached an extraordinary degree. Necomachus, the father of Aristotle, was physician to the father of Philip of Macedon; cotemporary with whom, was Menecrates, who, before undertaking a case of disease, required that the patient, on recovery, should attend him wherever he went, decorated with insignia, while Menecrates, in a purple robe and crown of gold, should personate Jupiter. He once wrote to Philip of Macedon: "Menecrates Jupiter to Philip, greeting: Thou reignest in Macedon, and I in medicine; thou givest death to those in health, I restore life to the sick; thy guard is composed of Macedonians, mine is constituted of grateful souls." In order to treat him with all the honor due to divinity, Philip invited him to a feast, where he was placed at an altar, and regaled with perfumes and libations, while the merely mortal guests enjoyed the more substantial pleasures of an earthly banquet. Paracelsus, in later times, was scarcely less arrogant or insulting than Menecrates.

The doctrine, that all diseases consist either in excess of strength or tone, or in debility, is very simple and plausible. Accordingly, we find it revived and predominating at several various times. Thus Hoffmann, in 1718, after spending twenty years in the formation of his "*Medicina Rationalis Systematica*," ended by declaring strictum, or spasm of the capillary vessels, to be the cause of fever. Again, Brown, in order to keep true the old adage, "that one one-sided theory generally calls out just its opposite," gave forth, in 1770, in his "*Elementa Medecinæ*," that ninety-seven out of one hundred diseases arose out of a modification of laxum, which he called indirect debility. In fact, the same doctrine, variously modified and simplified, is frequently applied in practice in the present age; some always stimulate, others always deplete; some stimulate with one hand, while they deplete with the other; while a third party always reduce a patient to the brink of the grave, and then suddenly stimulate him into a drunkard for life. The doctrines and practice of methodism were so general and simple, that one of the ancient sect, Thessalius Trallianus, declared he could teach the whole of medical science in six months. Another physician once threatened to write the whole art on a sheet of paper.

§24. Next, Erasistratus assumed that phlogosis, or inflammation was at the bottom of the majority of diseases; all fevers were decreed to proceed from previous inflammation, and antiphlogistic treatment became the prevalent method of managing disease; although, singularly enough, Erasistratus rarely employed bleeding—he preferred abstinence or fasting, dieting, mild injections and baths. He was not very partial to purgatives, and did not believe, with Hippocrates, that certain of these remedies had the specific power of eradicating some particular humor exclusively. Erasistratus and Herophilus were the great leaders of this new Alexandrian school of medicine; and it is well known that anatomy was first sedulously cultivated by these men; hence it is probable that the frequency with which signs of inflammation were found in the bodies of dead men, led, as in the times of Broussais, to this over-rating of inflammation as the only cause of disease.

As all the more important medical doctrines seemed to have been destined to be revived one or more times, we find that the notion of Erasistratus, that almost all diseases grow out of inflammation, had been previously advanced by *Diocles;* and, as is well known, has been quite lately thrust forward again, and carried to a still more revolting extent by Broussais, and Bouillaud. It is a singular fact, that the more simple the doctrine, and the more bold and dangerous the treatment the more followers will they have. Thus, when Brown cut the Gordian knot, by asserting that numerous diseases, even many of the most acute fevers and inflammations were the result of debility, and required decidedly stimulating treatment, he carried, for a time, almost the whole medical world with him. Again, when Broussais strenuously insisted that all disease was but inflammation, and that of the stomach and bowels, and taught that the anatomist's scalpel was all that was necessary to discover, while the lancet and gum-water was all that was required to cure disease, almost every physician believed him, for a time, and followed his precepts. Future ages will hold up the horrid vampirism of the "*Ecole Physiologique*" to the horror and detestation of the whole world. We have no hesitation in asserting that no country but France, and no city but Paris, and that only when rendered bloodthirsty by the excesses of the French Revolution, would have originated such a theory, or tolerated such practice. It was, no doubt, reaction against this excessive bloodshedding, which led Hahnemann, shortly afterwards, to teach exactly the opposite doctrine, viz.: That the human system never contained a drop of blood too much; that the lancet was never necessary; and that blood-letting was always injurious. "All extremes are error. The reverse of error is not truth, but error. Truth lies between these extremes." In modern times, Professor Gross is remarkable for his obstinate adherence to the childish notion that the majority of diseases arise from inflammation.

§25. Next, the physical and natural historical sciences began to be cultivated, and the world had come to the conclusion that organic bodies were exclusively composed of atoms and pores. It now became very easy for Asclepiades (B. C. 100) to imagine that he saw some of the emissaries of disease prowling around, and stealthily stopping up the pores of men, just as fox-hunters stop up the holes of poor Reynard. He also imagined that another affection, which he called disorder, disarranged the atoms, and left the benign powers, which had now received the names of *vis medicatrix naturæ*, or vital powers, to open the pores and re-arrange the atoms as best they could. Laxum, the memory of which had been revived again, was quickly called in play, with a host of baths, sweats, purgatives, relaxants, phlemagogues, melanagogues, cholagogues, and what not, in order to loosen the pores. At the same time, emollients and ointments were used, to make the atoms slide more easily, and frictions, which rubbed the atoms almost every way except the right one.

It will strike every one that Asclepiades' doctrine of the atoms and pores was revived nearly seventeen hundred years afterwards, viz.: in 1679, by the mathematical school of Borelli; and was again brought forward by Bœrhaave, in 1709, in his celebrated doctrine of *error loci*, in which the blood-globules were supposed to enter blood-vessels which were too small to allow them to pass through, whence obstruction of the circulation of blood, and the cold stage of fever ensued.

§ 26.

"Prove all things and retain the best."

Menzel says that the history of medicine, in a nut-shell, is that one one-sided system generally calls forth just its opposite, and, when these two have exhausted themselves in combat, sound physicians institute an eclectic mode of procedure, and select from each what suits them best. Accordingly, about the commencement of the Christian Era, Thessalus, and a numerous sect, who called themselves *eclectics*, without professing attachment to any particular theory, or claiming to have discovered any new principles, founded their doctrines and treatment upon such selections from the opinions and practices of all cotemporary and previous authors, as their reason or fancy dictated. Hence, they bled and purged, in order to subdue phlogosis; revived the doctrine of strictum and laxum; unstopped the pores, and attempted to rub the atoms into place again; and, as they found all these means insufficient, they began to cull, and that not very discriminatingly, from the secrets and mummeries of the quacks and sorcerers, who still abounded. As, notwithstanding all these improvements, they still frequently found themselves at a loss, they began to use all the different methods and means at the same time, in the same disease. They were guided, no doubt, by the fact that an indifferent marksman, with a wide-mouthed cannon, heavily loaded with grape and canister, may, perchance, hit a mark, which it would require a very experienced rifleman to reach with a single bullet. This method has something for itself, for it is not every one who has natural powers or application sufficient to become a good shot; but, at the same time, it called down much abuse upon the medical profession, and led the world to compare a physician to a man with a large club, who strikes about at random, in a dark room where there is a sick man. The consequence is, he sometimes hits the disease, at others, brains the patient. Cullen also says that this sect also first gave origin to those senseless and incongruous mixtures and compounds, which, he says, still disgrace the prescriptions of many physicians. Thessalus could not help becoming elated at his success, hence he assumed the title of the "conqueror of physicians." Hippocrates thought that the highest honor the physician should aspire to was to be a "minister of nature."

§ 27.

"Health is maintained by supplying similars with similars. Disease is overcome by opposing contraries to contraries."—GALEN.

Just previous to the Dark Ages, another great medical leader arose. Claudius Galen, born in the one hundred and thirty-first year of the Christian Era, was a native of Pergamos, a city of Asia Minor, celebrated for its temple of Esculapius, its school of medicine, and its library. which, in richness, was only second to that of Alexandria. His father placed him under professors distinguished in all the sciences, and he profited by the instructions of the stoics, academicians, epicureans and peripatetics, with extraordinary success; he was soon able to dispute with the most erudite, on grammar, history, mathematics and philosophy. He also undertook several voyages, for instruction, and remained some time in Egypt; afterwards he went to Rome, where his easy and brilliant elocution, his profound and varied erudition, secured him the esteem of the highest personages. But soon his boasting, his disdain for his colleagues, which he took no pains to disguise, and his natural jealousy against every other prominent physician, justly raised up against him a crowd of enemies; he accused the Roman physicians of base jealousy, and stupid ignorance, and applied to them such epithets as thieves and poisoners. He was, undoubtedly, a most accomplished and very learned man, still, more of a theoretical than practical physician; but he, no doubt, had too high an opinion of his own merits, and, like all such as over-estimate their own good qualities, he expressed himself with a bitterness and contempt which frequently became untrue, besides unjust, of his personal opponents and cotemporaries. For this failing, on the part of Galen, but little apology can be found, living at the time he did, and unsoftened, as he undoubtedly was, during the greater part of his active life, by the amenity and genial influence of Christianity, which had become exceeding prevalent in his age. He also seemed to have had some other mean traits of character, as the charge has frequently been made that he fled from Rome to avoid the plague. The fact that he left Rome, just as the pestilence reached it, is undoubted. Such was the man who ultimately attained a rank in the medical world, and swayed the opinions of physicians and of the public, on all points connected with medicine, in a manner before and since unknown. For thirteen centuries after his decease, the doctrines and tenets of Galen were regarded very much in the light of oracles, which few persons had the courage to oppose. Galen asserts that he was not attached to any of the sects that divided the physicians of his times. He treats as *slaves* those who followed any one system or master, and, with immense modesty, asserts: "No one, before me, has given the true method of treating disease." This so-called true method consisted in the exclusive adoption of the axiom, which says that "*diseases are cured by their contraries.*" He endeavored to discover the essence of diseases, in order to apply to it a treatment whose action would be *diametrically opposite*. He is the originator and "father of the antipathic school."

When Galen entered on the field, the medical world was divided into many sects, such as the dogmatics or theorists, the methodics, pneumatics, episynthetics, eclectics and empirics. At his time, the empirics were most esteemed. Galen was educated in the tenets of all these sects; he commenced his medical career as a student in the temple or Asclepion of Pergamos, under Satyrius, the pupil and successor of Quintus, who was a consummate anatomist, and the ablest physician of his time. He also studied under Thatonicus, a Hippocratic rationalist, and under Eschiron, a renowned experimentalist or empiric; he had already mastered the Platonic philosophy, under Albinus, and spent much time at Alexandria, which was still the most celebrated school of medicine.

The rival sects of the rationalists, or dogmatists, or theorists, and the experimentalists or empirics, had existed and disputed for centuries. The methodic sect had arisen about thirty years before Galen's time, while, very shortly before his birth, there had been established the eclectics, pneumatics, and episynthetics. The bright feature of Galen's career is that, unlike all the physicians who had preceded him, and unlike all the physicians of Rome who were his cotemporaries, he attached himself to none of these sects. He chose from the tenets of each what he believed to be true, and most generally useful; but, in no way, did he connect himself with the pneumatic or the eclectic school, with the dogmatists, empirics, or episynthetics. As already seen, he despised those who attached themselves exclusively to any particular master.

Health was maintained, he said, by supplying similars with similars, whilst disease is overcome by opposing contraries to contraries. These two propositions furnish the key to his whole system of medicine. His method professed no great originality in its individual parts, being made up of the doctrines of his predecessors, of every sect. In all his works, amounting to not fewer than two hundred, Galen delights to display his erudition, and, notwithstanding their vast number, they are mostly written in a polished style. Hippocrates wrote with the terseness, modesty, and truthfulness of a philosopher; Galen with the flowing redundancy of a rhetorician—allowing nothing to remain unsaid, and adorning his discourse with criticism, biography, anecdote, personal narrative, and incidental allusions of every sort, and disfiguring them with sarcasm, and vainglorious boasting. His brilliant errors, no less than his sterner truths, gave popularity and influence to his writings. But authority, however transcendent, to be enduring, must be founded on truth alone. The authority of Galen was not thus founded, and, after a reign of more than twelve centuries, he has fallen from his high estate. He who looked upon himself as superior to Hippocrates; who held that the latter had merely commenced what he himself had been able to carry to completion, lies buried in the accumulation of his own labors; whilst Hippocrates, drawing his inspiration from the simple study of nature, and from his own truthful and liberal soul, may still be studied with edification. It is a just punishment, although a very late one, of a man who vehemently and systematically condemned the opinions and practice of others. Still, Galen had his uses. In respect to the history of medicine, he has rendered immense service; for he has preserved for us the opinions of a great number of physicians, whose works have perished, and especially of the chiefs of the sects. Thanks to him, we are enabled to raise a corner of the veil which conceals the great struggles and disputes of the dogmatists or theorists, the empirics or experimentalists, and the methodists. He lived on the borders of a period—"the Dark Ages"—when physicians prided themselves more by shining in the subtleties of dialectics and the display of a vain erudition, than on their practical wisdom, so that the very faults of this author secured the sceptre of medicine in his hand; for, as regards erudition, subtlety, and reasoning, and universality of acquisitions, he only yields the palm to Aristotle, whom he again surpassed by the elegance, purity and strength of his style. His primary studies enabled him to do this, for we have seen that, even in his younger days, he was competent to dispute with the most erudite on grammar, history, philosophy and mathematics. At an early period, he had also been instructed in all the subtleties of dialectics, and, like Plato, he assigned to dialectics the first rank in the sciences. One of the earliest positions he took, was, that "no precept can be legitimate, in medicine, but on the triple condition of being true, useful, and in accordance with principles already laid down"—as if it were not sufficient that they should be true and useful. Galen was gifted with a facility of conception and an extraordinary love of labor, sharpened by hard studies in medicine and philosophy, and, being practiced in all the subtleties of dialectics, he overwhelmed his adversaries by the extent of his acquirements, the number of his productions, the force of his logic, the bitterness of his sarcasms, and the immensity of his pride. At his time, the minds of physicians were fatigued by that long anarchy, which, during six ages, had buffetted them about; and they only sought a doctrine brilliant enough to rally them, and a master strong enough to rule over them.

When Hippocrates appeared, Socrates had just proclaimed a rational method; philosophy had found a leader, and medicine had to follow the impulse. The characteristic of the Socratic philosophy is the rejection of mere speculation, and the admission of only ascertained facts and positive premises as the basis of all science and reasoning; he set no store on those things which tend to no useful or practical end; in fact, above all, Socrates attached himself to three things: *reality*, *morality*, and *utility*, and Hippocrates followed his example. The system of Hippocrates rested upon necessarily incomplete, and as yet uncertain observations, and his principles did not allow him to conceal any deficiencies of observation or practice, but, on the contrary, forced him to make them more apparent, so that others might complete them, and true progress be made. His system was menaced also with an approaching and formidable struggle with the philosophy of pure reasoning, aided by all the eloquence of Plato. To Galen, no peril of this sort presented itself, for he gave the preference to Plato, whose philosophy, so long combated by rival sects before the advent of Christ, gradually regained its ascendency just before Galen's time, and borrowed from Christianity a new power, while lending it a useful support. Hence, Plato's system, which he contributed to strengthen, and which was about to reign supreme in all the schools, secured to him, during a long succession of ages, a superiority without a contest, and a domination without a rival. It was no part of Galen's system to point out his own errors and deficiencies, but to make the medical and lay-public believe that he knew and understood everything. Hippocrates recorded all of his failures and his losses; Galen only now and then relates the history of a patient, with the evident object of exhibiting the superiority of his diagnosis, and the excellence of his theory. We do not observe in his recitals, as in those of Hippocrates, the plain and impartial historian, relating his facts without bias or intentional deceit, but we meet with a subtle and prolix dialectician, who lets no phenomenon escape without distorting it, or interpreting it according to a preconceived system; or, at least, lengthily and not impartially discussing it. He no sooner commences his mental journey, than he seems to take pleasure in losing himself; from anatomy itself—that somewhat gross anatomy of the ancients, which only requires eyes to see it—he often turns away his sight. Preoccupied with final causes, he is so long searching for what he thinks ought to be, that he mistakes what is. Thus Galen, who was a good anatomist and experimenter, and should have been a truthful observer and practitioner, was led to strengthen and cause the prevalence of a system foreign to all positive observation. Still, Galen admired Hippocrates, and did some justice to the experimental or empiric sect. He enumerates the names of many authors who professed it, and, at the time he wrote, the term had not become an injurious epithet; and he, who was never very measured in the terms he employed against his adversaries, and loaded the methodists with those of contempt, speaks of the empirics with much respect, and more than once admits being staggered by their reasoning, even while opposing it. The methodist, Aurelianus, also speaks of them in honorable terms, and the eclectic, Celsus, does so still more favorably. After the downfall of ancient empiricism, it remained downcast for ages, and its very name became synonymous with ignorance. Nevertheless, we shall see it rise again from this humiliation, and aspire, even boldly, under the title of the experimental method, to a universal dominion over the sciences, when the works of Bacon, Locke and Condillac shall have somewhat simplified its characteristics.

The personal character of Galen is seen in the numerous incidental allusions and amusing anecdotes scattered through his writings, some of which are of sufficient importance to be given in his own manner:

"Soon after my arrival in Rome," says he, "Glauco, the philosopher, took a great fancy to me, in consequence of my reputed skill in diagnosis. Meeting me, accidentally, in the street, and shaking hands with me, he remarked:

"'I have fallen upon you opportunely. I wish you to visit with me a patient, in this neighborhood, whom I have this moment left—the Sicilian physician whom you saw walking with me some days since, and who is now ill.'

"I inquired of him what ailed his friend, when, with his habitual candor, he replied, that Georgias and Apulas had spoken to him of my skill in diagnosis and prognosis, which appeared to them more like the result of divine inspiration than of medical science, and that he wished to know for himself whether I was really thus skilful. He had hardly done speaking before we reached the door, so that I had no opportunity of replying to his request, (what I have often said to you), that, on some occasions, the signs of disease are certain; at others, they are ambiguous, and require to be considered again and again. But, as we entered, I observed a servant, carrying from the chamber a vessel, containing a thin, bloody sanies, like the recent washings of flesh—a sure evidence of diseased liver. Without appearing to notice this circumstance, I proceeded with Glauco to the patient's apartment; when, placing my fingers on the wrist of the sick man, I examined his pulse, in order to determine whether the attack was inflammatory, or simply a weakness of the affected viscus. As the patient was himself a physician, he remarked that he had recently been up, and that the effort at rising might have accelerated the pulse; but I had already discovered the evidences of inflammation, and seeing, on a recess in the window, a jar, containing something like a preparation of hyssop in honey and water, I knew that he had mistaken his disease for pleurisy, in which, as in inflammation of the liver, there is usually pain under the false ribs. He had been led to this opinion, as I at once perceived, by experiencing this pain, by his short and hurried breathing, and by a slight cough. Understanding the case, therefore, and turning to good account what fortune had thrown in my way, in order to give Glauco a high opinion of my ability, I placed my hand over the false ribs, on the right side of the patient, and, at the same time, declared this to be the seat of pain, which the sick man admitted to be correct. Glauco, supposing I had made this discovery merely by examining his pulse, began to express surprise. But, to increase his astonishment, I added:

"'Inasmuch as you admit the existence of pain at this spot, I wish you further to say whether you are troubled with a slight cough, and whether your cough is not dry, without sputa, and occurring at long intervals.'

"While I was yet speaking, the sick man was seized with a cough, such as I had described, whereat Glauco was exceedingly excited, and, no longer able to contain himself, began to vociferate in praise of my abilities.

"'Do not think,' said I, 'that these are all the discoveries my art enables me to make; there are others, yet to be mentioned, which will elicit the testimony even of the patient.' Then, turning to the latter, I resumed: 'Is not the pain in this part increased, and accompanied with a sense of weight in the right hypochondrium whenever you take a full breath?'

"At hearing this, the patient also was surprised, and was as loud in my praise as Glauco. Seeing fortune still smiling upon me, I was desirous of making some remark in reference to the shoulder, which appeared to me to be drawn downward, as often occurs in severe inflammations, as well as in indurations of the liver; but I did not venture to speak on this point, fearing to diminish the admiration which I had already excited. Nevertheless, I touched upon it cautiously, saying to the patient:

"'You will not long feel the shoulder drawn downward, if, perchance, you do not find it so already.' When he admitted this symptom also, seeing him greatly astonished, I said: 'I will add but one other word, to show what you conceive to be the nature of your complaint.'

"Glauco declared that he would not be surprised if I should do even this. But the patient, overcome with wonder at such a promise, observed me closely, waiting for what I should say. I told him he had taken the disease to be pleurisy. This, with a further expression of surprise, he admitted to be the fact, as it was also the opinion of his attendant, who had been fomenting his side with oil, for the relief of that disease.

"From this time forward, Glauco entertained the highest opinion of me, and of our art; for, having never before come in contact with a physician of consummate ability, he had hitherto formed but an humble estimate of the profession. I have related to you these particulars," he adds, as if addressing a class of students, "in order that you may understand that there are symptoms peculiar to particular diseases, and others common to several diseases, and, further, that there are some symptoms inseparable from the disease, some usually accompanying it, others again of an uncertain character, or of rare occurrence; so that, if fortune at any time offers to you a good opportunity, as in the instance just related, you may know how to take advantage of it, remembering that fortune often presents to us the means of acquiring fame, which, through ignorance, many are unable to turn to good account." (1).

§28. During the Dark Ages, the Arabian physicians transmitted the medical discoveries of the Greeks, enriched by a few discoveries of their own, to the nations of Europe, during a period of about five centuries—from the seventh to the twelfth—and thus contributed to sustain the light, which, however obscured, was never wholly extinguished. They are said to have acquired their knowledge originally from Egypt, though they generally copied the Greeks. They introduced several simple remedies, such as Manna, Senna, Rhubarb, Tamarinds, Cassia, Musk, and also various syrups, juleps, and confections, also preparations of gold and silver. But their most remarkable discoveries were due to the science of chemistry, of which they were among the earliest students, though some processes now called chemical, appear to have been conducted as early as the first century, for, even in the time of Dioscorides, Mercury was obtained from Cinnabar by sublimation. Arabian medicine dates from the capture of Alexandria, in A. D. 638. Some works of merit were preserved, and among these the writings of the earlier Greek physicians; these were translated into Syriac, which introduced them to the notice of the Arabians.

The oldest and most complete account of Arabian medicine and medical authors is given by Haly Abbas, who wrote, about A. D. 980, a complete system of medicine, in which he gives the pith of the writings of Hippocrates, Galen, Oribasius, Paulus Egineta, &c. Rhazes, Avicenna, Avenzoar of Seville, Averhoes of Cordova, and Albucasis, also a Spanish Moor, were the principal Arabian medical authors. If these writers contributed much imperfect chemical lore to the stock of knowledge, they certainly, also, did much good, by handing down to posterity the wisdom of their predecessors. For several centuries, they held almost undivided and undisputed authority in the medical schools; even as late as the sixteenth century professors read and explained Avicenna and Rhazes in the European schools more than they did the works of Hippocrates, Galen, and Dioscorides.

Paracelsus derived some of his knowledge of alchemy, chemistry, of Opium, Mercury, Sulphur, and Antimony, from the Arabians, who had prosecuted chemistry during all the foregoing period, and occasionally rendered its results available in the treatment of disease.

As late as 1610, the Rosicrucians revived the system of Pythagoras, associated with the mystery, magic, and alchemy of the Arabs.

§ 29.

"'*Contraria contrariis curantur*' is false, and never did hold true in medicine. It is well done when we oppose like to like. Know all men, that like attacks its like, and never its contrary."—PARACELSUS.

"Great wit to madness nearly is allied,
And thin partitions do the bounds divide."

"Nay, what are all errors and perversities of his, even those aimless, confused miseries and vagabondisms? If we will interpret them kindly, they are but the dazzlements, and staggerings to and fro, of a man sent on an errand he is too weak for, by a path he cannot yet find."—CARLYLE's "Heroes in History."

Beyond the Dark Ages, we have seen Galen standing, like one of the Pillars of Hercules; upon this side, and, upon their very verge, we find Paracelsus standing like the companion pillar. When the gloom and mystery of the Dark Ages began to roll away, and just after the discovery of America by Columbus, (1492), and at the commencement of the Reformation by Luther, (born 1483), a man of giant intellect (born 1493—died 1541) shook himself from the sleep of ages, and gazed abroad upon a world convulsed with reformations and new discoveries. Straightway he began to strut and stagger, stride and stumble, and bawl and fume about like one in whom sleep and liquor are still struggling for the mastery, or like one who is still perplexed with dreams and fantastic imaginings, and thickly beset with night-mares, moon-calves, and all unclean things. However, drunkards and sleep-walkers often get into situations where no amount of ingenuity or daring would conduct them in their wakeful and sober moments. But, such are just as apt to stride toward the infernal regions, as toward truth and fame. In point of fact, they may advance, to a certain extent, in each direction, and this is exactly what Paracelsus did. His legs, too, like his thoughts, were great wanderers, and led not only over Europe, but even into Asia and Africa; while his inclinations led him alike to house with professors or quacks, alchemists or physicians, astrologers and sorcerers, or experienced old women, mountebanks or nurses. From all these he gleaned their stores of medical knowledge, and began to think and preach that ancient medical lore, quack remedies, astrological mummeries, chemical retorts, gallipots and crucibles, and very active chemical drugs and poisons might be used with just as much, if not more advantage in the cure of disease, than the lancets, knives, scissors, hot irons, bleedings, Senna, bran-soup, and Liquorice, of the predominant Galenical school, which was composed almost entirely of Catholic priests, who had taken upon themselves to give medical advice, merely because they were the only persons who were able, at that time, to read the Greek and Roman authors on medicine. Cullen says: "It is well-known to have happened in all ages, that of the persons who apply themselves to science, the greater part implicitly believe and receive the doctrines delivered them by their masters; which, having once imbibed, they adhere to them, with a degree of bigotry that opposes every attempt towards innovation and improvement." If this be the case with laymen, how much more easy was it for priests, nurtured in the infallibility of the Romish Church, to proceed still further, and elevate the writings of Galen and Avicenna into infallible and almost holy scriptures in medicine. If some rude handling and contemptuous sneering is ever necessary and useful under such circumstances, it was doubly required here, and Paracelsus was admirably fitted to apply the scourge. Besides, Luther had now commenced his Reformation, and it had become, in some measure, fashionable to attack the clergy. As, like many doctors, he was not over-burthened with piety, Paracelsus did not mince matters, but commenced at once by asserting that, if the representatives of God on earth, the clergy, could not impart more useful knowledge of the secrets of physic than those contained in the musty works of Galen and Avicenna, it was even justifiable to consult the devil; and, in order more completely to signify his contempt for them, he publicly burnt the works of Galen and Avicenna at the stake.

To add to the difficulties of the Galenical priest-doctors, they were now forbidden, by a papal bull, to leave their cells in order to visit the sick, under pain of excommunication; so that the friends or servants of the sick had to carry their urine and fæces to the cloisters, together with as good a verbal account as they could give. If we call to mind the fact that they had always been forbidden to dissect, and hence, could acquire but a very imperfect knowledge of the human frame, it will be evident that the clerico-Galenists made but sorry doctors, and that it was high time for them to confine themselves to their own proper avocations. As if the fates had willed that Paracelsus should succeed, syphilis, which, it was supposed, was introduced into Europe by the soldiers of Columbus, on their return from America, began to cause frightful devastations, which could not be controlled by bleeding, senna, bran-soup, or liquorice. On the other hand, Paracelsus, to whom the credit is due of being the first physician who boldly employed Mercury internally, and who had learned its use in syphilis from an Italian quack, began to use it with immense success, and teach his followers to do the same. It is not to be wondered at that he became still more arrogant and abusive, but we own that it does surprise us to find him asserting that the very down upon his bald pate had more knowledge than all the priest-doctors; that the buckles on his shoes had more learning than Galen and Avicenna, and his beard more experience than all their university-taught priests.

By the bold and free use of such powerful drugs as Opium, Antimony, and Mercury, which he had the merit of introducing into practice, and which the Galenical school were too prejudiced to use, Paracelsus was enabled to effect so many remarkable cures, that his reputation soon became so great, that he was consulted even by the most learned, and finally the magistrates of Basle engaged him, at a great expense, to fill the chair of medicine at their university. The Galenists, of course, insisted that his mode of practice was dangerous and absurd in the extreme. They instanced the use of Mercury in syphilis, saying that it produced ulcers and rottenness of the bones, and other effects very similar to those caused by the venereal disease. Paracelsus, however, immediately began to teach that the Galenic dogma, "*contraria contrariis curantur*," was false, and never did hold true in medicine; that a hot disease had never been cured by cold remedies, nor cold diseases by hot remedies. "*But it is well done*," says he, "*when we oppose like to like. Know all men, that like attacks its like, but never its contrary.*" Yet he was too shrewd an empiric to blind himself by his own prejudices and dislikes; hence we find that "*Plumbum purgat febres*" was one of his most favorite maxims. Still, although the quarrel seemed to turn about abstract principles—to be whether *contraria contrariis*, or *similia similibus curantur* were the true law—in point of fact, the case was very different. We have already seen that the Galenists did not apply their law correctly and accurately, and neither did Paracelsus; the real question at issue was, whether bleeding, Senna, bran-soup and Liquorice, or Mercury, Lead, Opium, Antimony and Sulphur were the more powerful and better remedies. The result would not have been doubtful, for an instant, if Paracelsus had not become so quackish and intolerant as to render himself hateful, so that he was finally shunned by the better classes of society, and, in consequence, began to lead a life of extreme dissipation in the very lowest company. Ultimately, he rushed from one extreme of folly to another, until he succeeded, to his own satisfaction, in discovering an elixir of life which would render men immortal. Disease and death were, of course, close upon his heels, and overtook him, one day, while in a drunken fit, so that he died at the early age of forty-six years, before he was able to drink of his elixir.

Long and loud was the exultation of the Galenists at his fall; long and loud did it resound and reverberate for upwards of three hundred years, at the end of which period, however, the fool's cap was torn from the skull of Paracelsus, in order to crown it with laurels. So successful, however, were the slanders of the Galenists, after his death, that, even in the present age, he is regarded, by the majority, as the "prince of quacks." Even the more enlightened, like Paris, content themselves with saying that, "in contemplating the career of this extraordinary man, it is difficult to say whether disgust or astonishment is the most predominant feeling. His intolerance and unparalleled conceit, his insincerity and brutal singularities, and his habits of immorality and debauchery are beyond all censure; whilst the important services he has rendered mankind, by opposing the bigotry of the schools, and by introducing powerful remedies into practice, cannot be recorded without feelings of gratitude and respect; and, in whatever estimation he may be held, there can be no doubt that he exerted the most powerful influence upon the age in which he lived, by exciting the envy of some, the emulation of others, and the industry of all." Such was the man who gave the most important remedies to the allopathic school, viz.: Mercury, Antimony, Opium and Sulphur; and gave a law to the homœopathic school, viz.: *similia similibus curantur.**

§30.

"Honor the physician, for necessity sake."

After the death of Paracelsus, the clerico-medical body grew more and more intolerant. They were in sole possession of the universities, which, in fact, for the most part, were originally ecclesiastical corporations, instituted chiefly, if not solely, for the education of churchmen. They were founded by the Pope, and were so immediately under his protection, that their members, whether masters or students, were exempted from the civil jurisdiction of the countries in which they were situated, and were amenable only to ecclesiastical tribunals.

But the Pope, Honorius III., about 1235, ordained that no ecclesiastic should prescribe blood-letting, practice that operation, or be present where it was performed; and that no sub-deacon, deacon, or priest should exercise any branch of surgery, or give the right of benediction to any who did. In consequence of these restrictions, a few laymen were encouraged to study surgery, and these the clerico-Galenical doctors forthwith commenced to persecute. In order to oppose the lay-physicians the more effectually, they began to teach their own servants, who also acted as their barbers, to dress wounds, and perform the various minor operations in surgery. It happened, about this time, that Pope Alexander III. revived the canon respecting clerical tonsure, or shaving the head. The priests, in consequence, had their attention strongly directed to the efficacy of cold applications to the head, previously shaved, in many acute diseases, especially of the brain. The *barber-surgeons*, as they now styled themselves, of course acquired fresh importance, although the more capital operations were commonly entrusted to the lay or surgical scholars of the universities. The medical scholars were all obliged to take the vow of celibacy, and hence generally became priests after they had finished their studies; but the opposition of the clerico-medicasters to the surgeons frequently led them to intermeddle with surgical operations. In consequence, Pope Clement V., soon after the commencement of the fourteenth century, positively forbid the priests to practice surgery, under pain of excommunication. It is an old proverb—"like master, like man." The more the popes restricted the priests, the more the latter oppressed the surgeons; and the universities henceforth *refused to receive any student into the faculty who did not solemnly abjure surgery.* Thus ex-

---

* I have been to his grave, at Salzburg, in Austria, in company with Rokitansky and Skoda.

cluded from the universities, the surgeons were obliged to look to themselves, and, with the aid of Louis IX. of France, formed themselves into a college in honor of St. Cosme, and began to establish schools of surgery in the different countries.

The clerical physicians at once began to treat them as if they were rebels from established authority, and forthwith set in operation all the arts and manœuvres that power and craft could devise, to oppress and degrade the surgeons. They encouraged the barbers in private, promised them their protection, and began to give them secret lessons in surgery, (an art which they themselves were strictly forbidden to learn or practice), and succeeded, by these means, in elevating the barbers, in common opinion, to the rank of surgeons, whilst they almost degraded the surgeons, in public opinion, to the rank of barbers. But their malignity did not rest here—they procured a decree passed, which denied the surgeons the right of instructing their own pupils; and while anatomy was almost exclusively taught by the surgeons, the clerico-medical profession uniformly and strenuously maintained that they were the only good, fit, and competent teachers of surgery, although their vows precluded them from studying this art. The absurdity of having surgery taught by a set of men who were strictly forbidden to dissect, even bleed, or perform the least surgical operation, or be present where one was performed, seems too gross to need pointing out. But this arrogance and folly, absurd as it now appears to us, and pernicious as t always has been, had its origin in that spirit of domination, exclusion, and monopoly, which has always characterized the ruling parties of the world. In consequence, the colleges of surgeons were repeatedly, interdicted by the clerico-medical body, and by their protector, the Pope, from teaching publicly the art which they professed and practiced. Thomson says he has been unable to find any better reason for this than the maxim, "the clergy abhors blood," which is so often expressed in the decrees of the Church of Rome, but never, he believes, acted upon but in this instance, as they generally made but little scruple of murdering obnoxious rivals, or of burning reputed heretics alive.

They went still further—had old decrees reversed and new ones passed, which conferred upon them not only the right of instructing the surgeons, but of determining the cases in which surgical operations were necessary; of being present at these operations, and of directing in every particular the conduct of the operator. Nor did they stop here. The clerico-medical faculty contended that surgeons should not be permitted to publish any work on the subject of their profession, till it had been examined and had received their approbation and licence. Even Ambrose Paré, the father of French surgery, perhaps the most distinguished surgeon that France has ever produced, and the man who had the merit of introducing the most valuable improvement into surgery that has ever been made, viz., that of tying arteries after amputation, was forbidden to publish his little work, which contained an account of it. After years of solicitation, he was only enabled to do this by means of a licence, extorted directly from the king, in the face of the hot opposition of the priest-doctors.

Another point, which was keenly contested, was the right of preventing the surgeons from using internal remedies, even in surgical cases. For writing a prescription for some slight complaint, or even a certificate of bad health, the offending surgeon was usually punished by being obliged to pay a heavy fine, or by making the most humiliating submissions. Finally, the surgeons were forced to take an oath of fealty to the priest-doctors, and pay a small piece of money annually, as marks of their inferiority and dependence.

Not a friend exerted himself in the favor of the surgeons, except Henry II. of France, who ordained that all physicians who took fees should be bound to taste the excrements of their patients, and perform to them all other kind offices, otherwise they should be adjudged to have been the cause of their death.

The apothecaries also came in for their share of persecution, because they prepared and sold Mercury and Antimony, then becoming introduced into practice. Guy Patin writes, in 1640: "Antimony is detested by all honest persons, having only on its side charlatans, empirics, and apothecaries, and such like rabble. The Antimonians play with the lives of men, and impudently send their poor patients into the other world; they, and the chemists, apothecaries, and charlatans are, in their kind, the demons of the human race. The pretended demon of the infernal regions kills not so many as does this chemical demon, and chemical poison. Those who give Antimony are imposters, charlatans, stibial-torturers and executioners."

Patin was a good example of the Galenical doctor of the times. He made little or no use of drugs, save purgatives, and sternly prohibited the use of Opium, Cinchona, or Antimony, then beginning to be introduced, under any circumstances whatever; but he was, perhaps, the most daring phlebotomist on record, for he treated his own son, for a continued fever, by means of twenty free bleedings from the arms and feet, and at least a dozen good purgations, with Cassia, Senna, and syrup of Pale Roses. About the year 1633, the king of France was bled sixty-four times in eight months, and then his physicians began to purge him. Patin says: "Sennertus knows nothing about bleeding old persons and young children; the miserable fellow excites my pity. A day does not pass in Paris, in which we do not bleed several infants at the breast, and we cure patients more than eighty years old by bleeding them. To prevent the pitting of small-pox, the best remedy is a bold venesection from the commencement of the disease. There is not a sensible woman in Paris, who would refuse to allow her infant to be bled for the fever of measles, convulsions, or teething. A young gentleman, seven years of age, who fell ill of a pleurisy, was bled thirteen times."

In opposition to this practice, the chemists tried to procure the admission of some of the various mineral preparations, especially of Mercury and Antimony, into the materia medica; but, to this the Galenical physicians opposed the stoutest resistance, and were long successful in their opposition, especially in France. Guy Patin repeatedly refers, with pride, to the two solemn decrees by the faculty of medicine, in 1566 and 1615, against Antimony, as a virulent poison; decrees which were afterwards sanctioned by Parliament, and it was not until 1666, that the opponents of the Galenists were strong enough to obtain a formal reversal of the obnoxious edict. In speaking of Dr. Guneant, Patin says: "When his daughter was sick, her hangman of a father ordered her to take Antimonial Wine," and exclaims, "I think the man is mad, or possessed of a devil!" Patin also attempted to countermine the chemists and apothecaries, by publishing a small work, entitled the "Charitable Physician," to instruct the public in preparing the few purgative potions and enemata he employed; in fact, his pharmacopœia, and that of the Galenists, seem to have been limited to Manna, Senna, Rhubarb, Cassia, and the syrup of Pale Roses, by the help of which, bleeding, and an appropriate regimen, he maintains all curable diseases were to be treated. He endeavored to make the people understand that the grocers could sell them Rhubarb, Senna, and syrup of Pale Roses, with which remedies they could do without the apothecaries, and save themselves from the tyranny of the "Arabic cooks or chemists." Of apothecaries, he again says: "We ought to hate them as a pest, inasmuch as they have corrupted and endeavored to destroy true medicine."

Patin contemptuously called the surgeons and barber-surgeons, the booted lackeys of the physicians, and exulted that they could not order either a purgative, or an anodyne, or any other medicine, except on the prescription of a physician. The surgeons were obliged to pay one hundred *sous tournois*, as an annual tribute to the physicians, and swear to pay the same honor and respect to the doctors that scholars owe to their masters; not to divulge the secrets of the faculty, and that they would prescribe no purgative, alterative, or cordial medicine, and, in fact, merely carry out the manual operations of surgery.

The only excuse for this harsh treatment of the chemists was that Antimony, Mercury, Opium, &c., were frequently given in such massive doses, that they often caused the evil effects, which Patin represents as always following their use.

§ 31.

"Gentlemen, some physiologists will have it, the stomach is a mill; others, that it is a fermenting vat: others, again, that it is a stew-pan. But, in my view of the matter, gentlemen, it is neither a mill, a fermenting vat, nor a stew-pan, but a *stomach,* gentlemen—a *stomach!*"—JOHN HUNTER.

In 1640, about one hundred years after the death of Paracelsus, Van Helmont, who had graduated with great honor to himself, happening to be troubled with a slight itch, could not get rid of it by means of the Galenical priest-school method; afterwards, he was easily cured by means of one of Paracelsus' so-called quack remedies, Sulphur, which so disgusted him with the study of medicine, that he repented that he had wasted so much time in the study of it, and threw it up in despair, in order to apply himself with ardor to chemistry. He spent fifty whole years in distillations, and examined, with great pains and incredible industry, all kinds of bodies, fossil, vegetable and animal, in a chemical way, and thus furnished a new body, or course of chemical knowledge. In fact, chemistry grew under his hands, and he rapidly and steadily metamorphosed alchemy into it. Astrology had already been expanded into astronomy, and, of course, as soon as its mystery was stripped away from it, it was no longer applicable in medicine. But chemistry was something tangible and efficient, and Van Helmont soon began to apply it to the cure of disease. We have already seen that Paracelsus had loudly proclaimed the insufficiency of priestcraft and Galenism, and we know that Van Helmont was deeply convinced of the same; hence, it does not surprise us to find him attempt to bring about a reformation in medicine. The Galenists were as used to conflict, as they were to success, and, hence, were not slow in making themselves felt. They commenced moderately, by merely refusing licences to practice, or sheep-skin letters of marque, to those who were affected with a zeal for improvement. In order to carry this out with some show of law and right, they instituted the most close and rigid examinations into the qualifications of candidates, and those who were tinged with the chemical doctrines were rejected, and their characters were attempted to be destroyed, under the color of having been found "mere lewd and unlearned empirics"—as the phrase then was—although, by their own shewing, these very persons had received a university education, had travelled abroad to the best medical schools, and were celebrated for their scientific acquirements. The chemists soon saw, however, that mere scientific disputation would not answer, and came to the conclusion that, as the errors of the Galenic school were bolstered up by the experience of sixteen hundred years, they must, like Luther, appeal to an enlightened public. In a short time, a predilection in favor of the chemical doctrines was brought about, and the merited success which attended the use of active chemical remedies, aided by the heroic trio of Paracelsus—Mercury, Opium, and Antimony—soon kindled a more general influence in their favor.

The Galenists now resorted to more severe measures, and, this revolt from orthodox authority was, in a great measure, attributed to the mischievous introduction and unmerited success of antimonial remedies, which they had always regarded with great abhorrence, since the time that one of their own number, Basil Valentine, having noticed that Antimony fattened pigs, gave it to a whole brotherhood of priests, who had become thin from vigils and fasting, in order to restore their fair proportions again, but with the effect of killing them all off, whence they gave the drug the name of *Anti-moine*, or *Anti-monk*, or *Antimony*. They denounced antimonial remedies with all the virulence of party spirit and private hate combined, and extorted a decree from the Supreme Council of Paris, proscribing, under severe penalties, the use of Antimony, under any circumstances, and actually expelled Besnier from the faculty of medicine, for having once administered it to a patient.

Among the common epithets applied to the chemical physicians, were those of "Arabic cooks," and "stibial torturers." The priests were finally driven from the schools of medicine, and, in 1644, chemistry was gradually engrafted into the theory of medicine, and too soon, alas, became the exclusive guide in the treatment of disease.

The stomach then came to be regarded as a sort of Papin's digester, or else as an alembic, retort, or stew-pan. Almost all diseases were located in alterations of the fluids, and finally were looked upon as only growing out of an excess, either of acid or alkali. The nervous system, and the solids of the body were entirely forgotten. Of course, the chemical school carried within it the seeds of its own destruction; and the fatal errors, into which such a one-sided hypothesis is liable to betray the practitioner, is said, by Paris, to have received an awful illustration in the history of the memorable fever which raged in Leyden, in 1669, and which consigned two-thirds of the inhabitants of that city to an untimely end: an event which, in a great measure, is to be ascribed to Sylvius de la Boe, who, having just embraced the chemical doctrines of Van Helmont, assigned the origin of this distemper to a prevailing acid, and declared that its cure could alone be effected by the copious administration of alkaline remedies—an extravagance, which Paris truly adds, Van Helmont himself would hardly have fallen into; and continues: "Thus it is in every science, as in politics, the partisans of a popular leader are frequently more sanguine, and less reasonable than their master; they are not only ready to delude the world, but most anxious to deceive themselves, and, while they warmly defend their favorite doctrine from the attacks of those who assail it, they willingly close their own eyes, and conceal from themselves the different points that are untenable." Or, to borrow the figurative language of a French writer, "They are like the pious children of Noah, who went backward, that they might not see the nakedness which they approached for the purpose of covering."

§ 32.

"Man's body's like a house: His greater bones
Are the main timber, and the lesser ones
Are smaller splints; his ribs are laths, daubed o'er,
Plastered with flesh and blood; his mouth's the door;
His throat's the narrow entry; and his heart
Is the great chamber, full of curious art;
His midriff is the large partition-wall,
'Twixt the great chamber and the spacious hall;
His stomach is the kitchen, where the meat
Is often but half sod, for want of heat;
His spleen's the vessel, nature does allot,
To take the scum that rises from the pot;
His lungs are like the bellows, that respire
In every office, quickening every fire;
His nose the chimney is, whereby is vented
Such fumes as with the bellows are augmented;
His bowels are the sink, whose parts to drain
All noisome filth, and keep the kitchen clean;
His eyes are crystal windows, clear and bright,
To let in the object, and let out the sight.
And as the timber is—or great, or small,
Or strong, or weak—the house is apt to stand or fall!"

DEATH'S DOINGS.

The above poetical effusion gives even a favorable opinion of the notions of physiologists and physicians in those times. In the meantime, as the chemical theory was a humoral theory, and busied itself with the fluids only, as a matter of course, the next theory busied itself solely with the solids of the human body. The wonderful discoveries and advances made by the application of the principles of mechanics to astronomy and other branches of natural philosophy, but, in particular, the increasing popularity of the corpuscular theory of Descartes, and the discovery of the circulation of the blood, in 1628, which was thought to be most easily explained on mathematical and mechanical principles, all led the profession of physic to the study of mechanics. Hence we find Borelli, in 1679, attempting, in his "*Motu Animalium*," to explain all muscular actions by a series of mathematical propositions. But Bellini soon outstripped Borelli, in adopting, as a general principle, that the living system, in all its operations and functions, was strictly obedient to the laws of gravity, and that the same reasoning applied to it as to hydraulics, hydrostatics, &c. And now, instead of acidity and alkalinity, the fermentation and putrescency of the chemical school, we find nothing but calculations respecting the size of atoms, the diameters of the pores and vessels, of the friction of bodies against each other, the impulse of the fluids, &c. The stomach, instead of being regarded as a stew-pan, a retort, or a still, was now compared to a mortar, or a mill, and it was thought that its muscular coat played the part of a pestle or grindstone. Thus Pitcairn estimated the power of the muscular coat as equal to a force capable of moving 12,591 pounds; the power of the diaphragm at 248,335 pounds —it should be recollected that neither of these muscles is over one-eighth of an inch in thickness. Again Borelli estimated the power of the heart at 180,000 pounds, although Reil, shortly after, placed it as low as several ounces. Bellini also attempted to explain the operation of medicine on mechanical principles, and, having imprudently regulated his practice accordingly, he was generally unsuccessful, and soon lost the confidence of the public.

§ 33.

"Observe how system into system runs!"—POPE.

Menzel has so admirably depicted the origin of the next system that we draw largely from him. Of course, as the last or mechanical theory busied itself entirely with the solid parts of the body, and made out the living body to be a mere hydraulic machine—provided with mechanical instruments, including pullies, levers, pumps, suckers, bellows, strainers, &c.—and evinced an extreme of materialism, directly the opposite extreme that of spiritualism was run into by the celebrated Stahl, who became the leader of a sect of physicians in opposition to the mechanical theorists. He taught that the soul was extended through the whole body by means of the nerves; that it not only originally formed the body, but that it was the sole cause of its motions and functions, and like a faithful guardian, calls such powers of the system into action, as are qualified to remove, or obviate the noxious impressions, and to preserve its salutary operations; hence, he generally regarded diseases as salutary efforts of the rational and presiding soul to avert the destruction of the body. As the practice of the chemical and mechanical schools had been extremely bold and active, he made his quite inert, and zealously opposed the use of the most efficacious remedies, such as Opium, Mercury, Bark, &c., and even became exceedingly reserved in the employment of bleeding, vomiting, purging, &c. Menzel ingeniously supposes that Stahl was led to the adoption of his system, by matters entirely foreign from medicine. The Reformation in religion had passed through its most turbulent period, and pietism, or a wholly passionless, but, at the same time, expectant repose in God had been instituted; hence, Stahl originated the *expectant* mode of treating disease, according to which the physician should expect everything from nature and the soul, and should not dare to interfere in any rude or violent manner. If the above conjecture be true, Stahl had his attention strongly drawn, at another time, in a different direction; for, at a later period, we find him teaching that the soul endeavored to cure most diseases by producing piles, and find him and his disciples giving frequent doses of Aloes, in order to bring about this fundamental change in the operation of the soul. Man was defined of old as a chicken without feathers. Stahl doubtless thought this too gross, and, in order to represent the union of spirit and matter in a striking manner, defined man as something with a soul and piles.

§34.

"An old friend with a new face."—Old Song.

Of course the medical profession relapsed quickly into materialism, and Hoffmann, who was a professor in the same university as Stahl, again revived our old friends strictum and laxum, and began to teach that every form of fever consisted in a *strictum* or spasm, of the capillary or minute arteries; that all diseases consist in an excessive, irregular, or diminished action; that when the action was irregular or violent, *strictum*, spasm or convulsion ensued; when weaker than natural, that *laxum* or atony of the muscular fibres was the effect. At the birth of our old friends, strictum and laxum, the nervous system had not yet been discovered, and as Hoffmann located them in the nerves, he has the merit of first turning the attention of physicians to the diseases of the nervous system, instead of wasting their time in framing mere mechanical and chemical theories.

§35.

"Another old friend with a new face."—Old Song.

The solids, by this time, were a hackneyed theme, and, notwithstanding that Fernelius had already taught that the fluids must be regarded as something foreign to the body, and not at all necessary to its existence, this did not deter the celebrated Boerhaave from reviving the old humoral doctrines, and, along with them, our quondam friends, the atoms and pores. Menzel says the age of Boerhaave (1668 to 1737) was one of poli-history and micrology, in which everything was carried on with microscopic minuteness. That the Dutchmen, Ruysch and Lowenhœck showed, by the most minute dissections, the wonderful texture of the vascular system of the human body—that tree with a hundred thousand living branches—while Swammerdam discovered over one hundred thousand muscles and nerves in a caterpillar. The theologians dissected the Scriptures with the same minuteness as did the philologians the profane writings; hence a new word was introduced into the lexicons, with as much ceremony as the Dutch, in those days, added a new tulip to an already voluminous catalogue. And the historians traced out gigantic genealogical trees—trees of the imperial families, and even of the lowest patrician families—with the same care as in the present age they trace out the pedigree of horses and even jackasses of noble blood, and did not even forget the stillborn children. Hence it is perfectly natural that Hoffmann (1660 to 1742) should find out our old friends, strictum and laxum, and be able to point out their residence with microscopic minuteness and accuracy; and that Boerhaave should do the same for the atoms and pores, and should derive all diseases from disturbances of the most delicate globules or atoms, in their passage through the most delicate arteries which nourished the larger arteries, viz., the *vasa vasorum;* and thus arose the celebrated theories of spasm of the extreme vessels, and *error loci* of the blood-globules.

§36.

"Theory is as necessary to amuse physicians, as a tub to amuse a whale."—CULLEN.

As Cullen had such an exalted opinion of the uses of theory, he, of course, endeavored to supply one with the least possible trouble, and accordingly, brought forward that of Hoffmann, viz: "That spasm of the extreme vessels was the cause of fever." According to him, debility of the brain proved an indirect stimulus to the vascular system, and caused spasm of the extreme vessels; next, the debility and spasm of the extreme vessels induced increased action of the heart and arteries, which served to restore the energy of the brain, which, in its turn, overcame the spasm of the extreme vessels. Brandy and water ought certainly to be the best cure for fever, according to this theory. But, although the greater part of the fame of Cullen is based upon his stolen theory of spasm of the extreme vessels, his great merit really consists in profound powers of observation and practical tact. His histories of diseases are inimitably explicit and correct. He excels even the acute and celebrated Sydenham in his descriptions of those symptoms by which one disease may be distinguished from another. The accuracy and comprehensiveness of his definitions are peculiar to himself, and the generality of his practical rules are carefully selected from his own extensive experience, and that of the most judicious and successful of his cotemporaries. (CURRIE.) Cullen experienced some of the intolerance of his cotemporaries. He preferred the then more modern system of Hoffmann, to that of Boerhaave, which then prevailed in Scotland. His disregard of the aphorisms of Boerhaave, caused him to be called a new Paracelsus, a Van Helmont, and a whimsical innovator. Great efforts were made to disparage him and his opinions, both publicly and privately; he was even requested, by the Lord Provost of the University of Edinburgh, to avoid differing from Boerhaave in his lectures. Dr. Simpson seems to have taken pattern after the Lord Provost.

§37.

"The curse of growing factions and divisions still vex your counsels."—Venice Preserved.

Boerhaave and Cullen were still tainted with humoralism, but a personal pique of Brown (1735—1786) against Cullen, led him to form a new system of medicine, in which the fluids were entirely forgotten, and which put the finishing stroke to the downfall of all humoral doctrines; and, since his time, until quite lately, solidism has reigned triumphant. Although Brown's chief object was to reduce the medical art to the utmost simplicity, no one succeeded in perplexing it more. Strictum and laxum were again ushered on the field in a new guise; all diseases were arranged in two great divisions, viz.: sthenic and asthenic. Diseases which were usually considered as proceeding from an excess of strength, were declared to have their origin in indirect debility, and debility was declared to be strength. Opium was elevated into a stimulant, and Alcohol pronounced a sedative.

John Brown, the author of the celebrated Brunonian doctrine, was born in 1735. Before he had completed his fifth year, he had read almost the whole of the Old Testament, and, at grammar-school, he soon reached the head, not only of his class, but of the school. His father died soon after, and he was left so poor that he was apprenticed to a weaver, but had such an insuperable aversion to the loom and shuttle, that his previous teacher offered further tuition to him gratuitously, and he resumed his studies, with the view of becoming a preacher. Hahnemann was put in a grocery store, from which he was also rescued by his former tutor. Brown first became an usher to a school, and had abundant opportunities of making an acquaintance with the best Latin classics. His memory was very retentive. He was also enthusiastically fond of Greek, and eagerly perused every Greek author he could procure. He then went to Edinburgh, entered the philosophy classes, and supported himself by giving instruction to his fellow-students in Greek and Latin. Hahnemann also supported himself by teaching languages —not only Greek and Latin, but English, French and Italian. Brown's mode was so successful, that numbers flocked to him for improvement. He also advanced so far in his divinity studies, as to deliver a divinity lecture in the hall of the University, preparatory to taking orders.

Accident turned his attention to medicine. He was employed by a medical student to put an inaugural medical thesis into Latin, and took such a fancy to medical studies that he henceforth devoted himself to medicine. He was able to support himself by private tuition, but was unable to pay the fees for medical lectures, and was presented with free tickets. Hahnemann also had free tickets presented to him by the University of Leipzig. Brown's progress was remarkable. His accurate preliminary knowledge of classics, mathematics, logic, and philosophy, highly qualified him to avail himself of medical knowledge, and he became a great favorite with the professors. His vivacity, wit, great conversational powers, and facility for maintaining an argument, rendered him an especial favorite with the pupils, and his society was much courted, especially at convivial meetings. In this latter, he differed from Hahnemann. He now became a tutor or grinder of medical students, and prepared students for holding disputations in the Latin tongue, on the subject of their theses. In 1761, he became a member of the Royal Medical Society of Edinburgh; president of it in 1776, and again in 1780, where he shone as his oratorical powers were very great. His reputation increased, his finances improved, and he obtained the friendship of Cullen, but was led into too great love for the pleasures of the table, and into habits opposed to frugality, and thus got much in debt.

He next became private secretary to Cullen, conducted his correspondence—most of which was in Latin—as Cullen was deficient in classical acquirements. Cullen named several of his children after him, and Brown adopted the system of Cullen with all that ardor which characterizes a generous mind towards a benefactor. Brown also paid particular attention to anatomy and botany, to qualify himself for a professor's chair in some of the new colleges in America, and went to Holland to perfect himself still more in these branches. But Brown was so useful to Cullen, that he persuaded him to abandon his intention of going abroad, and promised to exert himself in obtaining the first vacant Edinburgh professor's chair. This he did not try properly to do, and Brown became angry and left Cullen, and soon commenced his independent career as a lecturer in Latin, upon a text book he had prepared, and in promulgation of his own doctrines, contained in the "Elementa Medicinæ." The opposition of Cullen gave him notoriety, and his lectures were attended by many pupils of distinguished ability. Cullen and Brown also carried on a tremendous war in the Royal Medical Society, in the debates, which were remarkable for their vehemence and intemperance of speech.

His doctrines now began to spread abroad, and the excitement on the Continent was great. His name became celebrated in France, Spain, Italy, even in Poland and Russia; but in Germany especially, his opinions had great and very numerous supporters, and he was looked upon as a medical Luther. At the University of Göttengen, the discussions of his doctrines became so violent that the students broke out in rebellion, and had to be put down by the military. All this happened before Brown had graduated, and his quarrel with Cullen rendered it impossible for him to graduate in Edinburgh, so he went to St. Andrew's, and took his degree on September 21st, 1779, when he was forty-four years, and Hahnemann, twenty-four years old; Hahnemann graduated in the same year and about the same time as Brown.

The war between the Cullenists and Brownists still continued. The attacks and retaliations on both sides were absolutely malignant. Brown's intemperance began to injure him in the opinion of many, and to right himself somewhat in public opinion, he published his "Elementa Medicinæ," in 1780, when he was forty-five years old; but the publication of this work only increased the bitterness against its author.

All students who were tainted with Brown's doctrines were unceremoniously rejected by the University of Edinburgh. The effect of this on his classes was soon visible; his income was diminished, and he was even obliged to deliver some of his lectures while in jail, or some place of confinement for debtors. Assailed on all sides by the friends and adherents of Cullen; imprudent, if not intemperate in his habits; oppressed by debt, and disappointed in his hopes of obtaining a professor's chair in Edinburgh, he removed to London in 1785, when aged fifty-one years, and Hahnemann was thirty-one years old. His progress to London was a triumphant one. In almost every village and town he had former pupils. Convocations of the neighboring gentlemen were called together to give him dinners, where the profundity of his conversation and the brilliancy of his wit fixed the attention and raised the admiration of the company. His progress to London, hence, was so slow that, finally, he had to give his friends the slip. He had a wife and eight children, most of them daughters, to support. His love of society and pleasures of the table were his greatest enemies.

In London, patients did not flock to him at first in crowds, but his house was thronged with admirers. It became the resort of many ingenious and able men who wasted his time and substance. He next gave lectures at his own house to a few pupils, and also three courses in Fleet-street, at the Devil Tavern. He translated his "Elementa" into English, for £50, in twenty-one days—rising at four o'clock in the morning, and he never lay beyond five. He also drank less and looked better in health than he had for years; but he was soon arrested for debt, while planning various medical works. His patients now increased in number; almost every day brought him a new accession, for he was beginning to be esteemed by London physicians, and his opinion, in consultation, sought after. He had made a contract to write a book on Gout, for £500, and was projecting a Medical Review, when he was struck with apoplexy, and died October 7th, 1788, in his fifty-third year, when Hahnemann was thirty-three years old. The students of Vienna and Pavia went into mourning for him. Dr. Parr had a high opinion of the learning of Brown, often spoke of him in eulogistic terms, and thought him the first Latinist in Europe.

Brown was an honorable man, and had great rectitude of feeling; he was also a man of genius, learning and wit. His domestic conduct was unexceptionable; he was devotedly attached to his wife and children; gave deep attention to their education himself, even instructing his daughters in Latin and Greek. He had great goodness of heart, he despised riches, and hated everything base; in short, he had such openness of heart, that he could be taken in by every knave.

His "Elementa Medicinæ" was published after he had studied medicine twenty years. The first idea of his system broke on him in a fit of gout, while in his thirty-sixth year, after he had lived low for six months, his usual, previous habit being to live too freely. At the end of six years he had another fit of gout, and again, after living low for five or six months; he was then put on low diet and strict regimen for an entire year, and had no less than four attacks of gout, and passed the whole year, with the exception of fourteen days, between limping and excruciating pain. This experience gave rise to the "*Brunonian doctrine.*"

He traced his acute attacks, not to excess of vigor, but to *indirect debility*, and treated himself accordingly, with favorable results. He soon extended this practice to other diseases, and established two classes of diseases only—sthenic and asthenic; and two classes of remedies, viz., stimulating and debilitating. He thought he had simplified medicine, and reduced the doctrine and practice of it to scientific certainty and success.

He considered all speculations about vitality as incomprehensible, and as even having proved the bane of medical philosophy; hence, he directed his attention simply to the phenomena of life. He endowed all animate nature with a certain amount of excitability, variable in different persons, and at different times. He regarded all extraneous agents as exciting powers, and considered life as a forced state, dependent upon the presence of internal and external exciting powers, and capability of excitability. If the excitement were too great, secondary weakness was occasioned; this constituted what he called *indirect debility*. If the excitement be withheld, then weakness is induced of a different nature, viz., *direct debility*.

The powers acting on the body were regarded as exciting or stimulant, and he thought they produced excitement by expending excitability; that the seat of excitability was in the medulla of the nerves and in the muscles. All diseases he regarded as occasioned by either *direct* or *indirect debility*, in consequence of too much or too little stimulus. The general diseases, arising from excessive excitement, he called *sthenic*. Those that arose from a deficient excitement, he regarded as *asthenic*. The indication for the cure of the sthenic diathesis was to diminish; that for the cure of the asthenic was to increase the excitement, till that degree which constitutes the mean betwixt its extremes and which is suited to good health is restored. Such is the doctrine contained in the "Elementa Medicinæ."

The system of Brown went far to abolish the humoral pathology. Hypotheses have often led the way to great improvements in medicine; they frequently precede the confirmation of truth, and the supposition is, of itself, of great utility.

In 1781, he published, anonymously, under name of Robert Jones, M. D., "An Inquiry into the State of Medicine, on the Principles of Inductive Philosophy." Beddoes says it is ill-arranged, tedious, uncouth, arrogant and illiberal, yet, admits that it contains passages presenting juster views of medicine, than he had seen elsewhere, and conceived in the genuine spirit of Bacon.

In 1787, he published "Observations on the Principles of the Old System of Physic," exhibiting a compend of the new doctrine—also anonymously.

Brown's notions about indirect debility led to the treatment of many diseases, fevers, &c., by stimulants, which had previously been managed by antiphlogistic and debilitating remedies. This was, in some respects, a crude kind of homœopathy, practised with large doses; it familiarized the medical world with the treatment of some kinds of fevers, with stimulants; even Bark, which is a tonic and healing remedy, is not the kind of remedy one would select, *a priori*, to combat so feverish a disease as intermittents. Physicians were becoming familiarized with the treatment of some diseases, in an opposite manner to what ordinary reasoning would lead them to adopt. This, doubtless, paved the way to the more easy reception of the law, *similia similibus*, in Hahnemann's mind; for Hahnemann was profoundly versed in Brown's doctrines—his studies in the history of medicine also aided him.

§ 37.

"It is an error to suppose that blood is necessary to the preservation of life; a patient cannot be bled too much."—SANGRADO.

"After so many vacillations in its march, medicine at length follows the only path which can conduct it to truth."—BROUSSAIS.

Medicine would not have been true to itself if the next theory had not been as different as possible from its predecessor. It was perfectly natural for Brown, who was as poor as poverty itself, a charity scholar in the University of Edinburgh, and often in want of a meal of victuals to attribute ninety-seven diseases out of a hundred to debility, which required large quantities of the most active stimulants—wine, brandy, and Opium—in order to cure them. It was equally natural for an army-surgeon, Broussais, (1808–38), who had passed through the horrors of the French Revolution, and had followed the victorious armies of Napoleon, to believe and teach exactly the reverse of this doctrine, viz., that ninety-seven diseases out of a hundred arose out of inflammation, and required the most active blood-letting. We have already seen that Diocles, Erasistratus, and Screta had taught this identical doctrine. They advised free bleeding, followed by large draughts of *cold* water; Sangrado, in more modern times, pushed bleeding, followed by large draughts of *warm* water, to the extreme; Broussais improved still further, and used free bleeding, followed by large draughts of *gum* water.

Brown's doctrine was so exceedingly simple that a physician of the commonest capacity could practice it; hence he, for a time, carried the whole medical world with him. Broussaisism is infinitely more simple and easy than Brunonianism; a student of any common talents might learn it in a fortnight, and thus become a physician superior to all others, ancient or modern, those of the Broussaian school alone excepted. Inflammation of the stomach and bowels was dictatorially pronounced the cause of all diseases; the scalpel served to prove this, and the lancet was sufficient to cure all diseases. All drugs were forbidden, for they must necessarily irritate the stomach and bowels, and increase the inflammation of them; even the gum-water, which was used for a drink, must be made of gum-tragacanth, as the coloring matter of gum-arabic was too irritating to the stomach and bowels. It is said that the French conscripts let light and civilization into benighted Europe through the gaps made by the lance and bayonet; as Broussais undoubtedly did much to forward the study of morbid anatomy, it has been said that he did so at the point of the lancet. Napoleon attempted to overcome Russia with one million men, while Broussais volunteered to master the Walcheren fever, backed by five hundred thousand leeches. Thus it is: in 1731, Sauvages calculated that there were ten classes, forty orders, more than three hundred genera, and an almost innumerable number of species of diseases. "What a prodigious number of enemies!" exclaims M. de Ratte. A few years after, Vogel insisted there were five hundred and sixty genera; but soon Pinel reduced the number to three hundred and fifty-one. And, again, Cullen reduced the forty orders of Sauvages to twenty; his three hundred and fifteen genera to one hundred and fifty-one, and also carried his pruning-hook into the field of species. Brown and Broussais reduced this prodigious number of enemies, the first to two, the latter to one; thus bringing the wish of Nero true, that his enemies might have one neck that he might exterminate them at a blow. The promises to teach writing in six hours are nothing in comparison to this endeavor to make medicine easy. And then what changes were made in the materia medica—the long line of emetics, cathartics, diuretics, sudorifics, expectorants, stimulants, sedatives, narcotics, &c., &c., all swept away, and their place supplied with a ptisan and a leech. The learned and accomplished physician was degraded into a bleeder, cupper, and leecher, and giver of gum-water.

And how are we to account for all the success which this doctrine met with among medical men? Merely by casting an eye on the personal qualifications of Broussais. They were much like those of other great medical systematists—he was vigorous, energetic, and severe; hardy, resolute, and threatening. His look, bold, imperious, and confident to his fellow-physicians, while he was mild and encouraging to his patients; to the former he was a truly terrible assailant and dialectician, to the latter he had his moments of winning and almost infantine sweetness.

§39. As a reactionary movement against this almost total neglect of symptoms, we soon find Louis asserting that the most trivial symptom is of importance when it throws light upon the diagnosis and prognosis. He and his followers instituted long, most minute and accurate examinations of their patients; a half-dozen rose-pimples on the abdomen, but two or three times the size of a pin's head, were found sufficient to mark typhus fever, when far graver symptoms did not suffice to distinguish it from other diseases. The somnolence of typhus was found never to occur before the fourth day, while that of small-pox sets in by the third day; hence a fever, with somnolence on the third day, we may predict, with much probability, will prove to be small-pox. The rose-spots were found never to be present before the sixth, nor be later in appearing than the ninth day, nor to last longer than the seventeenth day; while sudamina never appear before the twelfth day, &c. With the aid of hundreds and thousands of such signs, the physician, who is versed in the numerical method, may often, without putting a question, diagnose a disease, tell with much certainty how long the patient has been sick, and predict a favorable or fatal termination. Thus, in thirty-three cases of membranous croup, small or large patches of false membrane were found on the tonsils or throat, thirty-three times; in one hundred and sixty-two cases of inflammatory, catarrhal, or spasmodic croup, these patches were not present in a single instance. Of the one hundred and sixty-two cases none died; of the thirty-three cases thirty died. This diagnostic and prognostic sign, hence, only failed once in one hundred and ninety-five times, and we may predict, with great accuracy, that nine out of ten cases of croup, with these patches, will prove fatal; and that every case in two hundred of the other forms will recover.

Thus we have seen that the study of symptoms and physical signs, as applied to diagnosis and prognosis, have been carried to a very high state of perfection. Nor were chemical signs long neglected. Every well-read physician is acquainted with the labors of Lecanu, Andral, Gaverret, Berzelius, Liebig, Simon, Lehmann, Dumas, &c. But it seems that whenever anything novel and true is started in medicine, that a number of physicians cheat themselves into the belief that it is the whole truth, and neglect everything else. While laboring under this hallucination, however, they apply themselves, with untiring zeal and singleness of purpose, to the development of their favorite speciality, and, in an incredibly short space of time, force it onward to a very advanced state of perfection. Thus it is with chemical diagnosis at the present day; a late, pert, French writer says: "Nothing can now be done, in the way of diagnosis, without the aid of chemistry, the test-tube, and the microscope. The scalpel, physical explorations, the pulse, &c., &c., are now almost forgotten, while chemical re-agents, little furnaces, and glass tubes and retorts have usurped their once honored place. Enter a French or German hospital, and the first thing which strikes the eye is a little table, upon which is arranged all the means and instruments of chemico-analytical medicine. The pulse is touched, perhaps the lungs are examined, all, however, for mere form's sake, and then the serious business of the day commences. An experimental bleeding is made, not because the patient's state requires it, but the blood has to be weighed, measured, calculated, formularized, and atomized, and then from the excess or deficiency of one one-hundred-thousandth part of a milligramme, the physician supposes that he is enabled positively to distinguish the blood of rheumatism from that of consumption, or that of jaundice from that of small-pox. Blood is now necessary to the sick man, not to sustain his life, or to solve the problem how much of it may be taken from him without destroying him, but merely that his physician may discover what disease he is laboring under.

§40. For a time, all systems of medicine were neglected, but no science has so intimate a connexion with the alterations in nature, seasons, times, and the domestic world; hence, it constantly presents a new physiognomy, and, from one decennium to another, exhibits new phases and development. The public, who only see the practical application and results at the bedside of the sick, often attribute these changes to caprice or fashion. This charge is most galling to the scientific physician, viz., that of treating his patients according to transitory, superficial, and daily-changing influences. The public no longer hear of the profuse blood-letting and leeching, that characterized the medical practice of the last ten years, hence it assumes that bleeding is out of fashion. The Pyrmont springs are still overflowing with the same waters, once so highly prized as all-healing, but are now comparatively deserted for Kissingen, or some other waters; hence, the layman thinks that the former is out of fashion among physicians. But how would the case stand if neither physicians nor fashion made these changes, but nature itself loudly called for them? If atmospheric, telluric, and cosmic influences should, at one time, stamp an inflammatory character upon diseases, which would then require antiphlogistic treatment? And if, at another time, atmospheric or social conditions should impress a typhoid or nervous character upon the majority of diseases, which, hence, during that epidemic, would not bear lowering or antiphlogistic treatment, and would oblige the physician to give stimulating or nervine remedies? Again, for a length of time, almost all diseases may bear an erysipelatous, or gastric, or bilious character, and the treatment of disease must have a mixed character, between the moderate antiphlogistic and stimulant, aided by anti-gastric and anti-bilious means—such as emetics, purgatives, &c. Does medicine, then, always deserve to be reproached as a fickle art? Does not, rather, this ever-changing physiognomy of practical medicine prove, that faithful followers of the indices of nature are pursuing her, step by step, now tracking her trail into some by-path, and, ever and anon, returning with her upon the old, well-beaten road? Does there not seem to be an absolute necessity for these apparently arbitrary changes in the curative methods? Does it not seem as if only the very fewest of medical systems were the product of mere speculative reasoning, and the major portion of them were a convolution of scientific aphorisms upon the then predominant character of disease, which soon grew and lengthened into a new method or system? These systems could only prevail while they were the actual product of an accurately comprehended, but still only transitory character of disease. Thus we may infer that Brown lived in a time when the typhoid or nervous type of disease was the prevailing one, and he, mistaking the transient for the permanent, created anew the doctrines of sthenia and asthenia, and, supposing the asthenic variety to be of the most frequent occurrence, revived the almost universal use of stimulating, irritating, or exciting remedies, around which practical medicine revolved, for a time, as a common and almost the only centre. The stimulating method was first tested at the bedside when almost all diseases bore an asthenic type, and many surprising cures and recoveries were effected, and the Brunonian system rapidly gained the temporary confidence of all practical men, while a crowd of blind worshippers placed Brown and his doctrines as the head, and centre, and substance of all systems. But gradually the type of disease changed, the inflammatory character grew apace, and Brown's maxims were found to be no longer of such generally useful application; still, the royal road had been opened up, a new generation of physicians had commenced their life-career upon it, confident that it alone led to health and truth, and bitterly opposed, for a time, the newer antiphlogistic doctrines of Broussais; but shortly, a large portion of the medical world followed in his train.

May we not, hence, assume that all, or, at least, many other systems had a similar origin, rise and fall. At present, no system is perhaps predominant, except it may be the rational eclectic. The views of the English Brown, the French Broussais, the Italian Rasori, and the German and Dutch mystical and natural-philosophical schools of Haller and Boerhaave are fast being lost in the gloom of the past. But we are far from thinking that the age of systems and theories in medicine, has forever passed by; rather, we are most thoroughly convinced that soon some genial mind will again master, with an adept's skill, the prevailing character of disease, and build up a system which will have all the usual advantages, faults, and good and bad consequences of systems in general, but which will, almost necessarily, find much favor with the medical public for a time.

§41.

" Similia similibus curantur."

HAHNEMANN, Christian Frederick Samuel, the well-known founder of homœopathy, was born on the tenth of April, 1755, at Meissen, near Dresden, in Saxony, and died on the third of July, 1843, at Paris, aged eighty-eight years.

His father was a fortuneless painter on porcelain, in the celebrated manufactory at Meissen, where all the so-called Dresden china is made. The only sign of literary taste which his father exhibited, was the production of a little treatise on painting in water-colors, although he assiduously required his son to learn geometry and designing. The father and mother of Hahnemann gave him his first instruction in reading and writing; subsequently, he went to the town-school at Meissen, and, when only twelve years of age, was selected by his teacher to give some of the other scholars their primary instruction in Greek. In his sixteenth year he went to the high-school, and soon obtained the love of his teacher, the rector Müller, who was celebrated in his own neighborhood, at least. His father did not wish him to devote himself to study, and hence removed him from school, for several months at a time, but it is a well-authenticated fact that Hahnemann made himself a small lamp out of clay, and pursued his studies at night, fearful that his occupation would be discovered if he used one of the house candlesticks. Finally, his father placed him in a grocery-store, in Leipzig; but the life of a merchant's clerk was so insupportable to him, that, in a few weeks, he ran quietly away, and returned to his father's house, where he was concealed several days by his mother, until his parent's anger could be appeased. His old teacher, Müller, now came to his rescue, and insisted that he should study under his own supervision, without pay, which he did for eight years more, or until he was twenty years of age.

A peculiar bond of love arose between young Hahnemann and his generous instructor; they both frequently suffered in health, it is said, from the severity of their studies, which were continued by day and by night; and both began to take an interest in the study of medicine. Müller allowed Hahnemann to dispense with those studies, of which he was not particularly fond; did not oblige him to attend some of the lectures, nor insist upon the completion of certain dry-written tasks; on the contrary, he even allowed him to read books on natural science and medicine during lecture hours; received visits from him at all times of the day, and insisted upon his being present at the sessions devoted to his private scholars and boarders, during which he often discussed the ancient Greek, Latin, and Hebrew authorities with him.

On leaving the school, it was the custom to write a Latin essay on some subject, and Hahnemann selected the somewhat unusual one of "The wonderful structure of the human hand," although, while yet a boy, he had employed some of his leisure hours in reading the aphorisms of Hippocrates.

The moral instruction of Hahnemann was not uncared for. His father is universally described as virtuous, steady, and energetic; he is said to have early taught his son to think and act for himself, to exercise his independent judgment in all cases; not to take anything on trust, but, in every instance, to act as reflection told him was for the best; "*to act and to be, not simply to seem*," was the most constant of his exhortations.

In the year 1775, when he was twenty, and Napoleon six years old, Hahnemann went to the University of Leipzig, with just fourteen dollars in his pocket, to study medicine. This money was the last he received from his father, whose income was not only very small, but who had several other children to support.

By the intercession of the counsellor of the mines, Börner, of Meissen, he was presented with a free admission to the lectures of all the professors in Leipzig. He supported himself by giving lessons, in German and French, to a rich young Greek, from Jassy, in Moldavia, and by translating medical works from the English into German. Although he labored much by night, still it was not possible, nor did he desire to attend all the medical lectures, but merely the best and most important ones. After remaining in Leipzig two years, *as there was no public hospital yet*, he determined to go to Vienna, in order to become practically familiar with disease. It speaks much for the industry and economy of Hahnemann, that he was able to do this at his own expense. In Vienna, he obtained the friendship of the celebrated Quarin, physician to the emperor and the hospital of the Brothers of Charity, in the faubourg Leopoldstadt. Hahnemann was the only young physician whom Quarin took around with him in his private practice. He loved and instructed him as if he were the first and best of his scholars. Here Hahnemann was robbed of the larger portion of his little funds, so that he was obliged to live for nine months on the miserable pittance of thirty-eight dollars. Then Quarin strongly recommended him to the Baron von Brückenthal, Governor of Siebenburgen, or Transylvania, who selected him as his physician and librarian. He arranged the baron's incomparable collection of antique coins, and his valuable library and manuscripts, practiced in the baron's family, and in the populous town of Hermannstadt, for one and three-fourths of a year. Then he went to Erlangen, to obtain his degree of Doctor of Medicine, which he did on the tenth of August, 1779, when in his twenty-fourth year, and at his own expense. Bonaparte was then just ten years old, having been born on the fifteenth of August, 1769.

He commenced practice in the small mountain town of Hettstadt, but moved to Dessau in 1781. His leisure time he devoted to chemistry and made several trips into the mountains for improvement in mineralogy and metallurgy. From thence he was called to Gommern, near Magdeburg, as district physician, where he married Miss Henrietta Kuchlerin, daughter of an apothecary; wrote his first book on medicine, which gives the result of his experience of medical practice in Transylvania, and is remarkable for a desponding view of medicine in general and of his own practice in particular, as he candidly admits that most of his cases would have done better had he let them alone. After remaining nearly three years in Gommern, "where," he naïvely observes, "no physician had ever been before, and whose inhabitants had no desire for one," he removed to Dresden.

In Dresden he obtained the confidence of the health officer, Dr. Wagner, who gave him much instruction in legal medicine and medical jurisprudence, of which he was an acknowledged master. Finally, Wagner became ill, and, with the consent of the city authorities, appointed Hahnemann physician to those infirmaries or hospitals over which he had supervision, and employed him as his assistant or substitute, in his private practice, for one year. Still, Hahnemann says, he did not play a very important part in Dresden, and adds, "probably, because I did not want to." Through the friendship of the celebrated librarians, Adelung and Dassdorf, he enjoyed free access to the Dresden libraries, of which he made most extensive use, in enlarging his fund of medical knowledge. During the following three years, he published many medical works, the most celebrated of which is "A Treatise on Poisoning with Arsenic," which is quoted to this day, as an authority, by the best writers on toxicology; his valuable chemical tests, for ascertaining the purity of wine, are also well known.

As we happen to possess a copy of Hahnemann's original treatise on Arsenic, published in 1786, we will give a specimen of his style at that time. It may be well to add that the treatise of Harless, of which Trousseau and Pidoux think so highly, that they follow and copy it quite servilely, is based on that of Hahnemann. This little duodecimo, of two hundred and seventy-six pages, is characterized by that immensity and accuracy of learning which distinguished Hahnemann's earlier writings. Among the authorities consulted by Hahnemann, were Bergmann, of Vienna, (1783); Navier, of Paris, (1776); Scheele, of Sweden; Logan, of St. Petersburg, (1783); Aucante, (1775); Gagliani, of Italy; Plenk's Toxicology; Hoffmann's Med. Rat. System; Wepfer's Toxicology, (1733); Haller, Gmelin, La Force, (1716); Letters of Madame de Sevigne, on the poisonings of the Marchioness de Brinvilliers, Merveau, Maret, and Durande, of France; Paracelsus, edition of 1679; Bonet, Van Helmont, Stahl, Storck, Peter Von Abano,

Sala, Sennert, Musgrave, Brocklesby, of England; Rounow's Swedish Transactions, (1778); Alphonius and Massaria, of Italy; Amatus Lusitanus, Baccius, Borelli, and at least twice as many more authorities, of all ages and languages.

Hahnemann's third chapter is devoted to the consideration of three degrees of poisoning with Arsenic:

"The first degree is, where a large quantity is taken, under circumstances favoring its full effect, viz.: on an empty stomach, or with heating liquors; in persons with irritable nerves and choleric temperament, subject to spasmodic and inflammatory affections, or shattered by anger, grief, jealousy, or fear, overloaded with acrid bile, or affected with chronic disease. If several or many of these favoring influences are present, the most violent and rapidly fatal form of arsenical poisoning, in the first or highest degree, will occur, and death may ensue in from three to thirty hours.

"*Symptoms.*—1. The poisoned person first experiences a cold shuddering, which seems to pervade the whole body, while an inexpressible anxiety or nausea, which seems to oppress the chest as well as the stomach, a cold, deathlike sweat, and a general trembling of the limbs, alternate with one another, in frequent paroxysms.

"2. The hands, feet, and tip of the nose become cold, blue circles form around the eyes, while the oppressed pulse gains in hardness and quickness.

"3. Now follow violent attempts at vomiting, which, although very forcible, are not fruitful at first, and finally become almost ineffectual, from spasmodic closure of the cardiac orifice, and emptiness of the stomach of everything but Arsenic, which is tenaciously plastered on its walls. The patient complains of burning and tearing pains in his throat, œsophagus, and stomach, and knows not what to do with himself.

"4. The Arsenic continues to ravage and destroy the stomach, without compelling it to full and beneficial vomiting; it clings fast to the villi of the mucous membrane, and contracts it as boiling water would, and irritates the blood-vessels to progressing inflammation, without having previously induced beneficial and judicious evacuations. The whole nervous system trembles and struggles, and we see greater evidences of involuntary or intentional destruction than of prosperous reaction. Nature seems to feel her dreadful enemy too oppressively to gather strength and courage to oppose and overcome it, yet she attempts it, from time to time, in repeated ineffectual struggles.

"5. The fruitless retchings, the fever, the frightful chills, the anxiety, the internal heat and unquenchable thirst increase; the breathing becomes quicker and hotter, more spasmodic and violent; and the glistening eyes project from their sockets. The inexpressible anxiety, and the burning, rending, and overpowering pain in the epigastrium tortures the patient with a progressive increase.

"6. At first, the abdomen is contracted; afterwards, when inflammation and irritation of the stomach, liver, and spleen occur, it becomes hot and distended; the attempts at vomiting become irresistible and incessant; the panting and gasping lungs, the dry, parched tongue, and gaping mouth seek refreshment from cool air and water. The stools and urine are suppressed; the vomits have a disgusting smell and color, and may be mixed with blood. Cutting and griping pains in the bowels ensue, especially around the navel; the patient is beside himself, so that he does not hear and see correctly, while his expression is frightfully anxious and fearful.

"7. We now see evidences of the omnipotence of the corrosive destroyer—which persists in its internal ravages without check or mercy, —in the livid, frothy lips, the swollen and trembling tongue, the agonized expression of the bloated face, the viscid sweat on the cold forehead, and the lead-colored circles around the staring eyes.

"8. The miserable sufferer no longer looks like himself, but seems a wretched and tortured stranger from another sphere. He screams frightfully, or wimpers despairingly, in broken or angry words, for help from agony, fire, and death; then tosses and struggles violently.

"9. Soon after this, we see signs of loss of feeling and sensation; he becomes more quiet; his breast heaves less frequently; the vomiting ceases; his black, parched lips tremble, and his pulse becomes extinguished, and involuntary putrid stools of a most offensive smell and appearance occur.

"10. The pupils dilate; the death-rattle is heard in the throat of the dying and unconscious sufferer; jerks and spasms convulse his stiffening limbs and icy-cold features; his stertorous breathing becomes fearfully slower and slower; and, finally, with a last spasmodic gasp, a ghastly corpse alone is left, the staring eyes and gaping mouth of which fill us with horror.

"The first stage of the affection, as described in paragraphs 1 to 5, occupies about one-half of the whole duration of the attack; the second stage, described in paragraphs 6 to 8, about three-eighths of the last half; and the last stage (see paragraphs 9 and 10) occupies only the last eighth of time. All the sufferings are increased if acids, stimulating drinks, or Opium are used."

It should be borne in mind that Hahnemann was but thirty-one years of age when the above minute and graphic description of the effects of Arsenic was given. He has described the gastro-enteric and paralytic varieties of arsenical poisoning with great truthfulness. He has not dwelt so fully upon the more obscure and larvate forms as some later writers have done.

He now took so much more delight in chemistry and literature than in the practice of medicine that he almost retired from the medical profession in disgust. But, in 1789, he removed to Leipzig, and in that year published his "Treatise on Syphilis," which shows an intimate acquaintance with the best works of that period on the subject. But this book is chiefly remarkable for its description of a new mercurial preparation, known to this day, in Germany, by the name of "Hahnemann's Soluble Mercury," and for some novel views relative to the treatment of syphilis; the dose of Mercury being remarkably small, the signs when enough Mercury has been ingested, for the cure of the disease, being peculiarly astute, and his denunciations of the local treatment of the primary sore being peculiarly severe and positive. During the next year, 1790, when Hahnemann was thirty-five years of age, he obtained the first glimpses of the well-known law of homœopathy, *similia similibus curantur*, and commenced his career as a reformer in medicine. Brown had died two years before, in 1788; Cullen died in 1790, and Napoleon was made a captain of artillery in 1792.

In order to form a fair opinion of Hahnemann and his labors, he should be judged by a comparison with the labors and advances of the men of his, not our times. While Hahnemann was in his cradle, according to Hering, Voltaire and Madame Pompadour were just in their prime; Frederick and Maria Theresa were not yet known as the Great; Lessing was just studying Shakespeare, and Lavoisier was yet engaged in his boyish sports. Cullen, Brown and Darwin were the medical luminaries of his time. Thus, Cullen died in 1790, aged seventy-seven; Brown in 1788, aged fifty-three, and Darwin in 1802, aged seventy-one. Hahnemann's theory and practice, we repeat, should be judged in comparison with those of his cotemporaries. His industry and devotion to literature and science, and to the medical profession, both theoretically and practically, we have seen, were unusually great; but his changes of place were as frequent as his changes of studies, and must have retarded his progress as a practical physician very much. Still, he accomplished more than many a less restless and dissatisfied man has done. He was master of Greek, Latin, Hebrew, and, we believe, of Arabic; he was equally well acquainted with English, French and Italian. He had translated "Ball's Modern Practice of Physic;" also, "Cullen's Materia Medica;" "Monro's Materia Medica," and "Brown's Elements of Medicine." Also, "Stedtman's Physiological Essays;" "Nugent on Hydrophobia;" "Falconer on Mineral Baths and Waters;" "Ryan on Consumption," and "Grigg's Advice to Females"—all from the English. From the Latin, he had translated "Haller's Materia Medica." From the French, "Demachy's Procedés Chymiques Rangés Methodiquement et Definis;" Sandés' "La Falsification des Medicaments Devoilée," and Metherie's "Essay sur l'Air pur, et les Different Especes d'Air." But his translations were not all confined to medical subjects. "Young's Annals of Agriculture;" "Demachy's Art of Distilling Liquors," and "The Art of Making Vinegar," from the French; and Fabroni's "Dell arte di fabe il Vino," from the Italian, were among his labors. Many affirm that his studies tended to render him a learned, rather than a purely practical physician.

His original writings had been about spasmodic affections; directions for curing, radically, old sores and indolent ulcers, with more appropriate treatment of fistulas, caries, cancer, white-swelling, and spinal disease; on bile and gall-stones; on the means of checking putrefaction; unsuccessful experiments with some new discoveries; observations on the astringent principle of plants; exact mode of preparing Soluble Mercury; means of preventing salivation, and the disastrous effects of Mercury; on the preparation of Glauber Salts; "Handbook for Mothers, on the preservation, and physical and moral education of young children," &c., &c.

Mixed up with all these, we have translations of "The Lives of Abelard and Heloise;" "Chemical Observations on Sugar;" "A New Collection of Medical Prescriptions;" "A Treatise on Poisoning with Arsenic;" "On the Preparation of Soda from Potash and Kitchen Salt;" "A Treatise on Coal Fires, and the use of Coal in Heating Baker's Oven's;" "Tests for Iron and Lead in Wine;" "On Baryta and Plumbago;" "On the Insolubility of some Metals and their oxydes in Caustic Ammonia," and "On the Preparation of Cassel Yellow," &c., &c.

He had gained the respect of classical scholars, of librarians, of men of literature, of some of the first physicians of his times, of hospital physicians and surgeons; he was acquainted with almost every ancient and modern language, with the literature of the medical profession, both of his own and ancient times; he was an able chemist, a careful, if not a very experienced physician; he was a good mineralogist and botanist; he had studied the effects of impure air, of improper food, of faulty exercise; he could aid the baker, wine-merchant, the mechanic, or artizan in their peculiar pursuits, almost as readily as he could converse with the man of science and literature.

In all this period, we find but two charges against Hahnemann. First, in his "Treatise on Ulcers," he mentions that he has invented a certain "Strengthening Balsam," for the treatment of old ulcers, whose composition he does not reveal, but which he offers to supply, genuine, to any one. Perhaps, as Dudgeon suggests, like Shakespeare's starved apothecary, it was his poverty, and not his will that consented to this unprofessional bit of retail trade. Second, he thought that he had discovered a new salt, which afterwards turned out to be simple Borax; in the meantime, he had sold specimens of it at the rate of a ducat a drachm. His followers claim that he honestly returned the money thus obtained by his mistake. We may lose some of our confidence in his infallibility as a chemist, but this is not enough to make us impeach his honesty; and Berzelius is manifestly unjust when he says, that Hahnemann would have been a great chemist if he had not turned a great quack.

In 1790, Hahnemann translated "Cullen's Materia Medica," and, dissatisfied with the explanation given of the manner in which Peruvian Bark cured intermittent fever, he determined to experiment upon himself, while in good health, with Peruvian Bark, in order to compare its effects in health with its effects in disease. He claims to have discovered "that Bark, given in large doses to sensitive, yet healthy individuals, produces a true attack of fever, very similar to the intermittent fever." This discovery, Dudgeon says, was to him what the falling apple was to Newton, and the pendulum, in the baptistery at Pisa, to Galileo. From this single experiment, his mind seems to have been strongly impressed with the conviction that the pathogenetic, or disease-producing effects of drugs, would give the key to their therapeutic or curative powers. He quickly came to the conclusion that every powerful medicinal substance produces in the human body a peculiar kind of disease; that physicians should be acquainted with the peculiar effects of each drug upon the healthy before they experimented upon the sick. Up to his time, with the exception of a few experiments with drugs on the healthy, by Storck and a few others, most of the effects and virtues of medicinal substances had been discovered by *accidental and experimental*, or *empirical* experience, and by *chance*. The effects of remedies, in health and disease, were often first observed by non-medical persons; then bold, often over-bold physicians, gradually made trial of them. Hahnemann mournfully observes: "Sad is the thought, that the noblest, the most indispensable of arts is built upon *accident* and *experiment*, which always presupposes the endangering of many human lives. Will the chance of such discoveries suffice to perfect the healing art, to supply its numerous desiderata? Sadly must we look forward unto future ages, when a peculiar or specific remedy for this or that particular form of disease may, *perhaps*, be discovered by chance, as was Bark for intermittent fever, or Mercury for syphilitic diseases! Such a precarious construction of the most important science, could never be the will of the wise and most bountiful Preserver of Mankind. How humiliating is it for proud humanity, if its very preservation must depend on chance alone. No! it is exhilirating to believe that for each particular disease, for each peculiar morbid state, there are specific and directly-acting remedies, and, that there is also a way in which these may be *methodically* discovered. We must observe: first, what is the pure action of each drug, by itself, on the healthy human body; second, we must note what is its action in this or that simple or complex disease."

At first, Hahnemann contented himself with hunting up, in the works of ancient and modern authors, hints respecting the physiological action of different drugs; and, in his researches, to have looked more for the peculiar and striking effects of the drugs, than for those excessively and ridiculously minute shades of symptoms, which we find he so carefully recorded in his later years. In fact, he seems rather to have searched for parallels to those abstract forms of disease described in the works on nosology, than for analogies to the individual concrete cases of actual practice. He, at first, paid much attention to the histories of designedly or accidentally swallowed drugs and poisons, and such as have been taken by persons in order to test them. He truly remarks, that a complete collection of such observations would, if he mistake not, be the foundation-stone of a new and true materia medica."

But to return to our history. Hahnemann seems to have had little or no opportunity to test his ideas, by practice, in Leipzig, and the little village of Stotteritz, close by; he occupied himself too much with his chemical lucubrations, and was obliged to continue his translations, in order to support his increasing family. Dudgeon exclaims: "How his great, but impatient soul must have been chafed and fretted at the oppressive clog of poverty, and the necessity of providing bread for the daily wants of his children, which prevented him from pursuing the investigations of which he had discovered the clue. The poverty of Hahnemann often amounted to an actual want of the common necessaries of life; for, about this time, after toiling all day long, at his task of translating works, he frequently assisted his brave-hearted wife to wash the family clothes at night, and, as they were often unable to purchase soap, they used raw potatoes for that purpose. The quantity of bread he was enabled to earn, by his literary labors, for his numerous family, was so small that, in order to prevent grumbling, he used to weigh out to each an equal proportion. At this period, one of his daughters fell ill, and being unable to eat the portion of daily bread that fell to her share, she carefully put it away in a box, hoarding it up, child-like, till her appetite should return. Her sickness however, increasing, she, one day, told her favorite little sister, that she knew she was going to die; that she never would be able to eat any more, and solemnly made over to her, as a gift, the accumulated fragments of hard, dried-up bread, from which she anticipated such a feast had she recovered."

With eagerness, Hahnemann accepted, in 1792, the offer of the Duke of Saxe-Gotha, to take charge of an asylum for the insane, in Georgenthal, which would give him a present competency, and, above all, leisure to pursue his now painfully interesting investigations, and an opportunity of putting his discovery to the test. A cure that he made of the insane Hanoverian minister, Klockenbring, created some sensation, for he was a man who, in his days of health, attracted the admiration of a large portion of

Germany, not only by his practical talents for business and his profound sagacity, but also by his knowledge of ancient and modern lore, and his acquirements in various branches of science. Klockenbring's almost superhuman labors in the department of state police, for which he had great talent, his constant sedentary life, the continued strain upon his mind, and a too hearty diet, finally made him deranged. Hahnemann here proved himself one of the earliest, if not the very first advocate for that system of treatment of the insane, by mildness, which has now become almost universal. Dudgeon says: "He never allowed any insane person to be punished, 'since,' says he, 'there can be no punishment where there is no sense of responsibility; such patients,' he says, 'deserve our pity, and cannot be improved, but must be rendered worse by rough treatment; their physicians should never feel offended at what they do, for an irrational person can give no offence; the exhibition of their unreasonable anger should only excite our sympathy, and stimulate our philanthropy to relieve their sad condition.'"

Singularly enough, Hahnemann did not remain long in his situation at Georgenthal, for, in the same year, he removed to the village of Walschleben, where he wrote the first part of the "Friend of Health," a popular miscellany on hygienic principles, and the first part of his "Pharmaceutical Lexicon." We are utterly at a loss to account for these frequent changes of place on the part of Hahnemann; it sometimes makes us fear that he must have naturally been a very discontented man, or else of a quarrelsome disposition. They must have interfered very much in his studies, and, more especially, with his opportunities of studying disease practically.

In 1794, he went first to Pyrmont, a little watering-place in Westphalia, and during the same year to Brunswick. In 1795, he emigrated to Wolfenbuttel, and in the same year to Königslutter, where he remained until 1799. During this period of comparative settlement, he gave out the second part of his "Friend of Health," and "Pharmaceutical Lexicon." He also wrote, in 1796, for *Hufeland's Journal*, that remarkable "Essay on a New Principle for Ascertaining the Remedial Powers of Medicinal Substances," wherein he firmly expresses his belief that, for *chronic diseases* at least, medicines should be employed that have the power of producing similar affections in the healthy body. During the following year, while Napoleon was carrying on his first campaign in Italy, and just about the time that he married Josephine, Hahnemann published, in *Hufeland's Journal*, an interesting case illustrative of his views, and wrote another essay on the irrationality of complicated systems of diet and regimen, and complex prescriptions. About this time he also published an "Essay on Antidotes," and others on the treatment of fevers and periodical diseases. Hahnemann had now abandoned the complicated medication of the dominant practice, forbore to write prescriptions, and himself gave the medicines, which he now invariably admininistered singly and alone. It will be very interesting for us to get some idea of the doses which Hahnemann administered at this period. In his essay on "Some Kinds of Continued and Remittent Fevers," we find him giving Ignatia, (see "Lesser Writings," American edition, p. 330*), in large doses, every twelve hours, viz.: to children from nine months to three years of age, from one-half to two-thirds of a grain; to those between four and six years, from one to one and one-half grains; to those between seven and twelve years, from two to three grains. He describes the good effects produced as truly surprising, and says the fever terminated in two or three days, without leaving any traces or any weakness; it also removed completely, or nearly so, the dyspnœa and suffocating cough in those that had these symptoms.

In another variety of fever, attended with immobility of the pupil, sopor, occasional perspiration, clay-colored stools, he gave Opium, in doses of one-fifth of a grain, to children of five years; three-tenths to those of seven or eight years; seven-twentieths to those of ten years, and he himself took half a grain. He says the symptoms disappeared completely in the course of the day; but twelve hours after, in the evening, he gave a still weaker dose, and then the fever certainly did not return. The constipation likewise ceased—they were cured.

In a typhoid influenza, which occurred in 1782, Camphor, he says, surpassed all the expectations which could have been formed of it. It was efficacious and almost specific in all stages of the disease, accompanied or not by fever, especially when given as early as possible, and in *large doses*. At first, Hahnemann was what he calls cautious in its use, and did not give to adults more than from fifteen to sixteen grains per day; but he soon thought he perceived that, in order to produce a speedy recovery, it was necessary to give, even to weak subjects, thirty grains, and to more robust individuals forty grains in the twenty-four hours. The favorable result, he says, was never long delayed; the constipation ceased, the bad taste in the mouth went off rapidly, together with the nausea and discomfort; the weight and pain in the head diminished from hour to hour, the febrile rigor was smothered in its birth, the heat diminished, a general, mild diaphoresis occurred, with a diminution of all the drawing, tensive pains in the external parts; the strength of the patient soon returned, along with appetite and sleep; the despondency changed into strength and hope, and the patient recovered his health without a drawback. The disease, he says, would yield under this treatment in four or six days at most, and there did not remain a single morbid symptom behind—not even lassitude. He knew of only one case, out of more than a hundred, where the Camphor failed. Among

* Republished by William Radde, No. 300 Broadway, New-York.

others, he relates the following case: while this epidemic was raging, a child of twelve years of age was seized with the characteristic tearing pains in all the limbs, with headache and intolerable pains in the eyes; after a chill, all signs of the disease ceased, but the child lost its sight. Fifteen grains of Camphor were given daily, for a fortnight, by Hahnemann, and the vision was rapidly restored.

In a different form of influenza, in which the pains occurred either without fever, or accompanied by a kind of intermittent fever, without the lassitude, prostration, faintness, and sweating characteristic of nominal influenza, the heat being moderate, and the chill all the more obstinate, Camphor failed completely, while Cinchona, but better still, Ignatia, removed the febrile symptoms only, while the pains became constant; then Ledum-palustre, in doses of from six to seven grains, three times a day, for adults, produced permanent relief.

In a case of intermittent asthma, which recurred regularly every Monday afternoon, he gave Cinchona-bark, in doses of half a drachm in the morning, and a drachm after an early dinner, every Monday. The fit was suppressed completely, and, after two more doses, all traces of the affection disappeared.

In 1797, in a case of colicodynia, he gave four powders, each containing four grains of Veratrum-album, and told the patient to take one powder per day. The patient, however, took two powders, instead of one, daily, thus taking sixteen grains in rather less than forty-eight hours. The artificial colic, produced by this heroic treatment, increased to such a dreadful extent that the sick man wrestled with death, was covered with a cold sweat, and almost suffocated. He had no attack for six months after, although he partook, from time to time, but in moderation, of food which had always brought on similar attacks before.

As late as 1815, in a case of gastric disease, he gave one dose only, of a full drop of the pure juice of Bryonia-root, to a patient with dyspeptic troubles, with directions to come again in forty-eight hours; at the end of which time, he felt confident the patient would be cured, although she had already been sick for three weeks. The cure took place on the next day.

Other instances could easily be adduced, especially from his article on antidotes, in which Hahnemann effected cures with comparatively large and even massive doses; but these will suffice for the present. Although he thought fit to change to excessively infinitesimal doses at a later period, that cannot vitiate his former good experience with larger quantities of medicine. Neither he nor his followers have a right to deny these cures, nor to object to those who prefer to cure in like manner. There are many able physicians who cannot believe in infinitesimal doses, who have studied homœopathy as faithfully as any of those who profess to be the only true disciples of Hahnemann. They have the authority and example of Hahnemann for their practice. The great peculiarities of Hahnemann's medical practice, at this period, were the careful and discriminating use of numerous comparatively new remedies, such as Bryonia, Veratrum, Ledum-palustre, and many others, and the administration of these remedies in a simple or uncompounded form, and in moderate doses.

It was between 1796 and 1799 that he first came in collision with the laws by dispensing his own medicines. The apothecaries of Königslutter brought an action against him for interfering with their rights, and it was in vain that Hahnemann appealed to what he asserted was the letter and spirit of the law, arguing that their privileges only extended to the compounding of medicines, and that every man, and, still more, every medical man had the natural right to give or sell uncompounded drugs, which were the only substances he employed, and which he, moreover, administered gratuitously. It was all in vain; contrary to justice and common sense, but not to the laws of Germany, Hahnemann, who had shown himself a master of the apothecaries' art, by his learned and laborious "Pharmaceutical Lexicon," and was also a thorough chemist, was prohibited from administering his own simple medicines.

The law was and is: "No one shall prepare and dispense medicines, except a regularly-legalized apothecary, and then only from the prescription of a regularly-legalized physician. Therefore, the physician shall not dispense medicines, nor the apothecary prepare and dispense medicine of his own accord for patients, without the prescription of a legally-qualified physician."

The apothecaries were allowed to sell innocent medicinal substances to any one that asked for them, such as Rhubarb, Peruvian-bark, Jalap, Aloes, Asafœtida, Valerian, and all other simples that are not dangerous in small quantities; also the simple preparations of these drugs in alcohol, sugar, or water, such as tincture of Rhubarb, Peppermint-lozenges, &c. Ignorant herbalists were also allowed, by law, to sell, in the public weekly market, medicinal roots and herbs to all who asked for them. But neither apothecaries nor herbalists were allowed to sell dangerous herbs or minerals, such as Arsenic, Stramonium, &c., without a physician's prescription. Hahnemann claimed the privilege of dispensing infinitesimal doses of Arsenic, Mercury, Prussic-acid, Nux-vomica, &c., &c., insisting that they were single or simple remedies, and the quantities were so small that they were also innocent medicines. But the government refused to permit Hahnemann and his disciples to dispense Arsenic and other powerful drugs, fearing, perhaps, that they might at times, at least, give other than infinitesimal and innocent doses.

Apart from that spirit of monopoly and pride of caste and guild, which is so prevalent in Europe, the right to prepare, compound, and dispense medicines from the formulas of physicians was conceded, by law, to the privileged apothecary, in order that none unconversant with this work, or having a bad stock of medicines, might bungle with the prescriptions; and because the physician, who is at all engaged in practice, would often possess neither the skill to make the often elaborate mixtures himself, nor the great amount of time requisite to devote to their preparation. As an offset to the advantage of the physician, apothecaries were not allowed to sell any but the most simple and innocent remedies, except on the prescription of a medical man. The public were protected, inasmuch as none but well-educated and legalized apothecaries were allowed to sell medicines; their stock of medicines were obliged to be submitted to examination yearly, by government inspectors, and all poor drugs were condemned and destroyed. The public were thus prevented from poisoning themselves or others, except with the connivance of a physician; neither were they allowed to dose themselves or their families, except with the most innocent remedies, without consulting and paying a medical man. With many disadvantages, these arbitrary laws have a few good points about them, and it could hardly be expected that the ancient laws of the land should be abrogated without good reasons. For my own part, I think that sufficiently small homœopathic doses can be prescribed from many good apothecary establishments, and almost regret that the laws did not prevent excessively infinitesimal doses from becoming, for a time at least, an integral portion of homœopathy. The apothecary laws, in Germany, date as far back as 1551. In his war against the laws and the apothecaries, Hahnemann used a great deal of ingenuity. Thus he says: ("Lesser Writings," p. 710,) "The words *medicine* and *medicament* are never employed in any laws relative to medicine, except as signifying *a medicinal mixture composed of several medicinal ingredients*, and the preparation of this alone is exclusively entrusted to the privileged apothecary, who is to prepare and dispense it according to the prescription of a legitimate physician." Hahnemann also adds, "In like manner, the physician of the old-school is *enjoined* to prescribe several medicinal ingredients in his recipe, which are to be mixed together by the apothecary." He continues: "Thus, it is certain that, *according to law*, the prescription *must* direct *several* medicinal ingredients to be united together, so as that they shall constitute one medicament, in the dispensing of which compounds or mixtures the apothecary's privilege solely and alone consists."

Hahnemann seemed inclined to force allopathic physicians to give none but compound medicines, and to allow allopathic apothecaries to dispense no others. I admit that it was a great hardship and injustice that so well qualified a physician, chemist, and pharmaceutist as Hahnemann should not be allowed to dispense his own medicines, if he pleased; but he used doses at this time, in 1797, which might easily have been prescribed from the apothecaries, for, even as late as 1820, he sometimes used the first and second attenuations. Hahnemann also attempted to change the significance of the word "simples" in his own favor. It was allowed, by law, to any one to deal in innocent herbs and simples. In the materia medica, the word "simple" is the general denomination of an herb or plant, as each vegetable is supposed to possess its particular virtue, and therefore to constitute a simple remedy. To simple, in the materia medica, means to gather simples or plants. He endeavored to apply this word, or its Latin synonym, "*simplicia*," to his remedies, which were single, or uncompounded medicines, and, in one sense, simple, although Arsensic, Corrosive Mercury, &c., are not generally regarded as innocent or simple medicines, in another sense. In later years, he claimed that by dilution they were rendered innocent or simple. And he asks triumphantly, (p. 699), "Where is a syllable to be found, in all the royal ordinances relating to medicine, that distinctly forbids physicians to administer "*simplicia*" with their own hands to their patients?" From one sentence it would seem that Hahnemann was somewhat unwilling to divulge his prescriptions to the apothecaries, for he speaks of his medicines (p. 699) as "preparations that are known to me (Hahnemann) alone, but not to any chemist, and, consequently, not to any apothecary."

Still more singularly, he confuses the word "dispense" with "compound." On page 698 of his "Lesser Writings," he says: "Homœopathy does not *compound*, and, consequently, does not dispense." On page 697, he says, "Where the laws relative to medical affairs speak of preparing medicines and of dispensing, they always and invariably imply thereby the compounding of several medicinal substances into one formula or prescription." On page 702, "Homœopathy, far from dispensing, that is, making up prescriptions composed of several powerful medicines, (the preparation of which belongs of right to the apothecary), only uses small doses of single or simple medicines." Hahnemann frequently used the words dispense and compound as synonymous terms, and drew the conclusion that, as homœopathic physicians do not compound their medicines, they also do not dispense them, in the legal sense, when they give or sell them to their patients.

Hahnemann's articles on the preparation and dispensing of medicines are powerful and ingenious, like everything which proceeds from his pen; but they had little or no effect on the government officials, whom he in vain requested "To keep the Leipzig apothecaries within the limits ot their privileges, and to notify them that their rights did not extend to a new method of treatment which has never before been practiced—which only requires small doses of simple medicines, consequently, only *simplicia*, which no ruler ever yet forbade scientific physicians to administer to their patients, and which consequently are, as we may naturally suppose, not prohibited in any regulations of medical police."

During the last year of Hahnemann's residence in Königslutter, viz., in 1799, when he was forty-four years old, and when Napoleon had lately finished his campaign in Egypt, and had just been proclaimed first-consul, he witnessed a severe epidemic of scarlet-fever, and made his discovery of the prophylactic power of Belladonna in this disease. In a family of four children, three sickened with scarlet-fever, but the fourth, who was taking Belladonna at the time, for an affection of the finger-joints, escaped, though she had heretofore always been the first to take any epidemic that was going about. Hahnemann was already acquainted with the power of Belladonna to produce a state similar to that of the first stage of scarlet-fever, and he had already used it with success at that period of the disease; he was now led to suppose that it was not only a curative, but also a preventive remedy for scarlet-fever. An opportunity soon presented itself of putting its prophylactic powers to the test, for, in a family of eight children, three were seized with the epidemic, and he immediately gave Belladonna to the remaining five children, in small doses, and, as he had hoped, all these five escaped the disease, notwithstanding their constant exposure.

As a preventive against scarlet fever, two drops of a very weak solution of Belladonna were given to a child one year old; three drops to two-year-old children; four drops to those three years old; five or six drops to four year old; six or seven drops to those five years old; seven to eight to those six years old; nine to ten to those seven years old; eleven to thirteen drops to those eight years old; fourteen to sixteen drops to those nine years old; and so on, up to forty drops for a person between twenty and thirty years of age. The doses were generally to be repeated only every seventy-two hours, but, in severe epidemics, every twenty-four hours; if violent mental emotions had occurred, or the child had become chilled, one or two extra doses had to be given.

In fully-developed scarlet-fever, Hahnemann still relied upon Opium and Ipecac. He says, the burning heat, drowsy stupefaction, agonizing tossing about, vomiting, diarrhœa, and even convulsions were subdued in a very short time, at most in an hour, by a very small quantity of Opium, either internally or externally. Internally, he gave one drop to a child four years old, and two drops to one of ten years old, every four or eight hours in severe cases, in milder ones, only every twenty-four hours. If Opium was used externally, a piece of paper, from one-half to one inch in length and breadth, moistened with the strong tincture of Opium was laid on the pit of the stomach, and left there until it dried.

When there was increase of fever towards evening, with sleeplessness, total loss of appetite nausea, intolerable lachrymose peevishness and groaning, he gave Ipecac., from one-tenth to half a grain, in fine powder, or from one to ten drops of the tincture. The above symptoms were removed in a few quarters of an hour, by Ipecac., and he states that he found these two remedies, Opium and Ipecac., indispensable, as they were generally completely sufficient, not only to ward off the fatal termination, but also to shorten, diminish and alleviate the scarlet fever and adds, *that he cannot imagine a more suitable mode of treatment, so rapid and certain in its results, as he had found it.*

The mode which Hahnemann adopted, of drawing the attention of physicians to his newly-discovered prophylactic, was somewhat singular. He announced for publication a book on the subject, and advertised for subscribers, promising to publish the work which should reveal the prophylactic, as soon as he got three hundred subscribers at one Friederich d'or each. In the meantime, he contracted to supply to each subscriber a quantity of the unknown prophylactic for trial, with the proviso that the results should be communicated to him. This unusual proceeding, which, Dudgeon says, may only be justified on the plea that Hahnemann wished to have the prophylactic tested more impartially than it would have been had he at once revealed the name of it, gave rise to much opposition from physicians, who made little or no response to his offer, and too frequently loaded him with accusations of avarice and selfishness. The hostility of the physicians and apothecaries of Königslutter finally drove him from that town in 1799, where fortune for the first time had begun to smile upon him, and he turned his steps towards Hamburg, but finding little or nothing to do there, he removed to the adjoining town of Altona. In 1800, Napoleon took possession of the Tuilleries, and shortly after carried on his second Italian campaign, and fought the battle of Marengo. In order to leave Königslutter for Hamburg, Hahnemann purchased a large wagon, in which he packed all his property and family, and with a heavy heart bade adieu to Königslutter. A dreadful accident befell the melancholy cortege. Descending a precipitous part of the road, the wagon was overturned, the driver was thrown off his seat, his infant son so injured that he died shortly afterwards, and the leg of one of his daughters was fractured. He himself was considerably bruised, and his property much damaged by falling into a stream that ran at the bottom of the road. With the assistance of some peasants, they were conveyed to the nearest village, where he was forced to remain upwards of six weeks, on his daughter's account, at an expense that greatly lightened his not very well-filled purse

Hahnemann alludes thus to this point in his letter "On Professional Liberality in the Nineteenth Century," (p. 365) he says: "At the end of the century that has just expired, (1700), *my zeal for the welfare of mankind* misled me to announce a prophylactic remedy for one of the most destructive of children's diseases, scarlet-fever. Scarcely a fourth part of the number I might have expected subscribed for it. This lukewarm interest, shown for such an important affair, discouraged me, and I arranged that the subscribers should receive a portion of the medicine itself, in order to satisfy them, in case my book on the subject should not be published. The subscribers consisted chiefly of physicians, who had epidemics of scarlet-fever in their neighborhood. At least thirty of these, whom I begged, by letter, to testify to the truth, and to publish the result, be it what it might, in the *Reich's Anzeiger*, made no reply. A good many private individuals got the medicine sent them, but the advice of their ordinary medical attendants prevented them from saving their children by its means. Only two physicians wrote upon the subject; one, Dr. Muller, of Plauen, in the epidemic of 1800, found that no child took scarlet-fever who had used this medicine (name not given) for two or three weeks. Some time after, one child took the scarlet-fever, and Dr. Muller thought that this one case proved more against the efficacy of the remedy than five hundred which seemed to be protected by it. The other physician, Dr. Jani, of Gera, gave it to ten families, with thirty-six children in all. Three children, in one family, were attacked by scarlet-fever while using it. Of the thirty-three children in the remaining nine families, who used it for a month, none were attacked with scarlet-fever; but, as far as was known, none of them were immediately exposed to the infection."

Hahnemann expressly desired physicians to publish their experience with his preservative, whether adverse or not; but was particularly severe on poor Dr. Jani, for asserting that the thirty children who escaped were not exposed to the infection, as far as was known, when he admits that the scarlet-fever was universally prevalent. Hahnemann supposed that when an epidemic of scarlet-fever was universally prevalent in a place, it did not generally spare two children out of a hundred, and that the mere circumstance of not having been directly exposed to infection, as far as known, does not suffice to preserve them.

It is evident, from the above, that Hahnemann, wished his preservative given to all children, indiscriminately, in the town and village in which scarlet-fever prevailed, and not merely to those who were living in the same house in which scarlet-fever was epidemic, and to those who had really been exposed to the disease. It is true, that scarlet-fever is propagated in two ways; viz., by *epidemic influence* and *contagion*. Meigs even asserts that he has not the least doubt that epidemic influence is by far the most active cause, and, to prevent its influence, a preservative must be applied to all those who breathe the air of the place in which it prevails. Meigs is also convinced that it is much less contagious than either small-pox, measles, whooping-cough, or chicken-pox; for he has quite frequently known children exposed directly, and for a considerable time, to the infection, and yet escape.

It is evident that these children must have been proof both against the epidemic influence and the contagion. Hence, it is no proof of the efficacy of Belladonna, as a preservative, if some children escape while using it; but it certainly would be if not only large numbers escaped, but almost every one did. Meigs—an allopathist, who may be regarded as a model of fairness and candor—says, that he has used it for four years, and his impression of it is decidedly favorable. In one family, he gave it to nine children, exposed directly to the disease, either from their being in the house in which it was prevailing, or in the very room of the patient; yet eight escaped the disease entirely, and the one who took it, had it very mildly and safely. Dr. Porcher—another allopathist of this country, quoted by Meigs—from an examination of about four hundred volumes, pronounces decidedly in its favor. He says the evidence is overwhelming, from its cumulation, from the careful way in which some observers conducted their inquiries, and that he cannot but regard the neglect to avail ourselves of its use as a violation of those sacred obligations which force us to leave nothing untried which may contribute so largely to the mitigation or eradication of one of the severest inflictions of the hand of God.

This important question should be decided, calmly and dispassionately; the abuse, stupidity, and bigotry of many dominant-school physicians, on this point, is only a little less offensive than the enthusiastic and over-zealous manner in which some homœopathists insist upon its universal value, and distort or magnify every fact which speaks in its favor.

But, to return to Hahnemann's career. He did not better himself by his removal to Hamburg and Altona, and, not long after, removed to Mollen, in Lauenberg. From thence, he soon went to Eulenburg, in Saxony; but the opposition of the superintendent physician of that place drove him out, after a short sojourn. He wandered first to Machern and thence to Dessau, where he published his "Monograph on Coffee," which he considered the source of many chronic diseases, such as chronic inflammation of the eyes, disease and caries of the bones, fluor albus and menstrual disorders, destruction of the teeth, impotence, piles, &c. Subsequently, Hahnemann attributed most of these diseases to psora. We only allude to this matter here to call attention to the fact that Hahnemann occasionally changed opinions which had been most positively expressed and insisted upon.

During this period, before 1803, he had also, during his wanderings, translated several books from the English, and written various articles on medical reform in *Hufeland's Journal*. In 1806, he translated the "Materia Medica" of the great Albert Haller, from the Latin. The years 1805 and 1806 were also eventful ones for the development of the doctrine, as he published his masterly little work, entitled "Esculapius in the Balance;" the "*Fragmenta de Viribus Medicamentorum*," in Latin; his "Essay on the Medicine of Experience," also the latter in *Hufeland's Journal*, in 1806. They were also eventful years for the whole of Europe; we need also say that the battle of Jena was fought October 14th, 1806.

From Dessau he went to Torgau, and, from thenceforward, ceased to write for medical journals, and published his strictures on regular medicine, and his projects for its reformation, in a magazine of general literature and science, called the *Allgemeiner Anzeiger der Deutschen.* During the years 1808 and 1809 he published a succession of papers, among which are his "Essay on the Value of the Speculative Systems of Medicine," his earnest letter to Hufeland, and, finally, in 1810, he published the first edition of his "Organon," and removed to Leipzig, where he lectured in the University, and remained stationary for ten or twelve years. While Hahnemann was thus separating himself from the ordinary ties which bound him to the dominant profession, Napoleon was divorced from Josephine, in 1809, and married Maria Louisa, in 1810.

The "Organon" must be regarded as Hahnemann's decree of final separation from the regular medical profession. His second entrance into Leipzig was comparatively triumphant; he appeared in the University before an array of professors, learned men, and enthusiastic students. He read and defended his "Essay on the Helleborism of the Ancients" with marked success, and was handsomely and warmly congratulated by the Dean of the University. Almost at the same time, Napoleon entered the Russian territory. The first French army-corps was met by a single Cossack, who asked for what purpose they entered the Russian territory; on receiving his reply, the solitary sentinel struck spurs to his horse and disappeared in the forest. At the first step which Napoleon made on Russian ground, his horse stumbled, and he fell to the ground—which, of course, was regarded as a bad omen.

Hahnemann's second residence in Leipzig formed a most important period in his career. We have seen that he arrived there in 1810—he, consequently, must have been fifty-five years of age. He had scarcely passed his prime, either in bodily or mental strength; his virtues must have been confirmed, his faults have been now almost unchangeable. Hahnemann, we have seen, was born in eventful times: those of Frederick the Great, Maria Theresa, and Catharine of Russia. The middle of his career, we have also seen, was still more marked by great persons and events, namely, those of Napoleon and his times. At this period, the campaign in Spain had just been finished, and that of Russia, we have seen, was about commencing. The revolutionary element was now uppermost; the simple dependence upon old times, institutions, and authorities was fearfully shaken. Besides, a new power in popular medicine had come upon the field: Anthony Mesmer commenced his career in animal magnetism in 1774, consequently when Hahnemann was nineteen years old, and we shall see that the latter paid much attention to this subtle and mysterious subject. It has been thought very probable that some of Hahnemann's views about infinitesimal doses and potencies were derived from his studies of mesmerism, while some have been spiteful enough to hint that Cervantes was the first discoverer of infinitesimal doses, for he says, in chapter third of "Don Quixote," that "In the plains and deserts, where knight-errants fought and were wounded, no aid was near, unless they had some sage enchanter for their friend—who could give them immediate assistance, by conveying, in a cloud through the air, some damsel or dwarf, with a phial of water, possessed of such virtue that, upon tasting a single drop of it, they should instantly become as sound as if they had received no injury."

The religious world had also been struck to its core by a new system of theology. Emmanuel Swedenborg was born on the 29th of January, 1688—i. e., sixty-seven years before Hahnemann's birth, in 1755—and died on the 29th of March, 1773, aged eighty-five, when Hahnemann was eighteen years old. We can readily imagine that Swedenborg might have been a very attractive character to Hahnemann. He was as learned in many languages as was Hahnemann; he was a naturalist, a mineralogist, a good mathematician, an inventor and builder of machines and fortifications, and, withal, a poet. He was an ardent, studious, and fearless man; a reformer, in every sense of the word, and one as well skilled in the physical sciences as in the intellectual, moral, and religious. Still we have no absolute proof that Hahnemann paid more attention to Swedenborg's theological opinions than those of other reformers. It has been stated by some one, however—we know not on what authority—that Hahnemann received his first hint about infinitesimal doses from a clairvoyant, and Swedenborg must be regarded as a clairvoyant, *par excellence.*

It may be as interesting to others as it was to me to hear in what way Swedenborg's mission commenced. Swedenborg was asked (see Sandal's "Eulogium," and other tracts) in what manner he first began to have his revelations:

"I was at London," said Mr. Swedenborg, "and dined late at my usual inn, where I had a room kept for me, that I might have the liberty to meditate in peace on spiritual things. I had felt myself pressed by hunger, and was eating very heartily. Towards the end of the meal, I perceived that a kind of mist came over my eyes, and I saw the floor of the room covered with frightful reptiles, such as serpents, toads, caterpillars, and others; their number appeared to increase as the darkness did, but both soon passed away. After that, I saw clearly a man, in the midst of a bright and shining light, sitting in a corner of the room. I was alone, and you may judge of the consternation I was in when I heard him pronounce distinctly, and in a sound of voice very capable of striking terror:

"'*Eat not so much!*'

"After these words my sight began to grow obscure; but came to, little by little, and then I saw myself alone in the room. Still a little frightened at what I had seen, I made haste to my own apartment, without speaking to any one of what had happened to me. I there reflected seriously on it, and could find no reason to suppose it to be an effect from chance or any physical cause.

"The following night, the same person appeared to me, in a strong, shining light, and said:

"'*I am God the Lord, the Creator and Redeemer; I have chosen thee to explain to men the interior and spiritual sense of the Sacred Writings. I will dictate unto thee what you ought to write.*'

"I was not at all frightened now, and the light with which he was encompassed, although very bright and resplendent, occasioned no painful impression on my eyes. He was clothed in purple, and the vision lasted a full quarter of an hour. That same night, even the eyes of my spirit opened, and disposed so that I might have a spiritual sight of heaven, the world of spirits, and the hells; and I found everywhere many persons of my own acquaintance—some of them deceased a long, and others but a short time.

"From that day, I gave up all my worldly occupations, that I might have leisure to employ myself in spiritual ones, in conformity to the command I had received. It happened often unto me, after that period, that my spiritual sight was opened so far that I could see, in the most clear and distinct manner, what passed in the spiritual world, and converse with angels and spirits, in the same manner as I speak with men."

I do not wish to express any harsh opinion about the revelations of Swedenborg; but De Boismont says, if we regard him as an *ecstatic*, none can refuse him credit for an enthusiasm full of faith, and a great elevation of thought. M. Denis (quoted by De Boismont) thinks it is, perhaps, the most poetical and religious transport that has been manifested by a soul initiated into the mysteries of the Kabbala; and cites, as a proof of the intimate relations which exist between Swedenborg's system and the ancient Kabbala, is, that the object, to which he purposes to lead us, is the science of correspondences known to the ancients. More material physicians and psychologists regard his visions as mere hallucinations, similar to those of Nicolai, the Berlin bookseller; while some spiritualists suggest, that the apparition which appeared to Swedenborg, was an angel of darkness, transformed into an angel of light, to seduce and deceive him. Others suppose that he had hallucinations, similar to those produced by Haschisch, Opium, Stramonium, and Alcohol.

Whatever may be the truth of this matter, I merely wish to call attention to the fact that Swedenborg's writings and teachings tended to foster a belief in immaterial or spiritual things, in preference to material ones; in potencies, rather than materialities; in mysticism and supernaturalism, more than in tangible and natural ideas. Still, I repeat, we have no proof that Hahnemann was a Swedenborgian; his family and friends throw no light upon his religious views, while his writings would lead us to suppose him a simple and earnest Deist.

Again, in 1784, when Hahnemann was twenty-nine years old, animal magnetism had made such strides that the Marquis of Puysegur—an honest man, and owner of a considerable estate—finding it too hard work to magnetize all who came to him, hit upon a clever expedient. He had heard Mesmer say that he could magnetize bits of wood, why should not he magnetize a whole tree! There was a large elm, on the village-green at Busancy, under which the peasant girls used to dance on festive occasions, and the old men to sit, drinking their wine, on the fine summer evenings. M. de Puysegur proceeded to this tree and magnetized it, by first touching it with his hands and then retiring a few steps from it; all the while directing streams of the magnetic fluid from the branches toward the trunk, and from the trunk toward the root. This done, he caused circular seats to be erected around it, and cords suspended from it in all directions. When the patients had seated themselves, they twisted the cords round the diseased parts of their bodies, and held one another firmly by their thumbs, to form a direct channel of communication for the passage of the fluid. He thought he was very useful, and imagined he produced many salutary effects on all the sick poor in his neighborhood, who flocked around his tree. Sometimes there were more than one hundred and thirty patients there in a morning, and he thought that all of them felt, more or less, the good effects of his magnetic tree—every leaf of which seemed to him to communicate health—and he was delighted to see the charming picture of humanity which the elm-tree scene daily presented. Loutherberg, the well-known painter, and his wife, practiced animal magnetism, in London, about the same time—but for money, charging from one to three guineas for tickets of admission; and it is said that, at times, upwards of three thousand persons crowded around their house, unable to gain admission. While such mysteries were in vogue, it was comparatively easy for Hahnemann to believe in the efficacy of infinitesimal doses.

We will return to the subject of potentization and infinitesimal doses at some other time—it is sufficient, at the present period, to indicate some of those influences which rendered their discovery more easy

We will merely mention that the Marquis de Puysegur was a man of great wealth, also an honorable and philanthropic man; he used his elm-tree as a plaything, if you will, but, as he supposed, solely for the benefit of the sick poor. Hahnemann was equally honest and enthusiastic with his spiritual or magnetic doses of sugar of milk and alcohol —we have a right to say, much more honest and enthusiastic; for he did not magnetize or potentize his medicines only once, as did the Marquis Puysegur his elm-tree, but thirty times. Neither did he endeavor to make one potentized or magnetized substance a sort of universal remedy, like the Marquis' elm-tree, but he, with great pains and labor, endeavored to find out a special potentized remedy for each individual case of disease. Like Swedenborg, Hahnemann was one of the most learned men of his time. We may differ from Hahnemann, Swedenborg, and Puysegur, but we have no right to impeach their honor or honesty; churchmen and physicians may regard them as dangerous innovators, and as enthusiastic and poetical, rather than practical men, but the purity of their lives, and the earnestness of their exertions, for what they supposed the welfare of mankind, should forever remain undoubted.

It may be right to add here that some of Hahnemann's discoveries and opinions were modifications of previous discoveries. Thus, he says, "A precipitated Mercury, very similar to my Soluble Mercury, was first used internally in 1693, by Gervaise Ucay;" and Black's Pulvis Cinereus is also very similar.

We have seen, Paracelsus had previously taught that the Galenic dogma, "*contraria contrariis curantur*," was false, and never did hold true in medicine; that a hot disease had never been cured by cold remedies, nor cold diseases by hot remedies. "But it is well done," said he, "when we oppose like to like. Know all men, that like attacks its like, but never its contrary." So well known is this that Menzel, in his "Review of Medical Science," says, "The celebrated physician, Hahnemann, returned to the system of Paracelsus, somewhat modified."

Again, Autenreith published a work on internal eruptions, especially on internal itch, or psora, before the time of Hahnemann, and the older authors laid much stress upon them. The celebrated baron and physician, Anthony Storck, principal consulting physician to the Empress Maria Theresa, had distinguished himself, from 1760 to 1771—when Hahnemann was sixteen years old—by a long and assiduous course of experiments, with Conium, Hyosciamus, Stramonium, Aconite, Colchicum, &c., &c., both upon the sick and healthy, and in their simple and uncombined state. It is probable that Hahnemann got his notions of experiments with drugs on the healthy, and the use of only one remedy at a time, from Storck, and a more noble example he could not have selected. It is equally probable that Swedenborg, Mesmer, Puysegur,

Paracelsus, Cullen, Brown, and others, exerted some influence upon other of Hahnemann's opinions and practices.

To return to our subject. If we divide Hahnemann's life into five periods, his second residence in Leipzig falls into the *third*, which, like the third act of a drama, is the most important of the five, as it always controls the final development of the whole. He, himself, always regarded it as the most important portion of his eventful life. He had determined to appear as an academic teacher; to explain his views and system, by means of lectures in the University, and obtain disciples and apostles for its expansion. He regarded it as the turning-point for himself and his system; he felt convinced that he would either increase vastly in fame and consequence, or his star would set forever.

He also intended to take a stand as a prominent practicing physician, and to induct others into his mode of practice. He determined to expose his views of disease and its treatment to the critical examination of the medical public, and decide the question whether it could stand a collision with the laws governing physicians and apothecaries. The points for which he was determined to contend were, for the untrammelled practice of homœopathy at the bedside of the sick; for its recognition and application in judicial or medico-legal cases; for the free dispensing of medicines; for an independent professor's chair in all the universities; for the establishment of dispensaries and hospitals, or, at least, wards in hospitals; for the compulsory or legal examination of students in homœopathy; for the appointment of homœopathic physicians to posts of honor, usefulness, and emolument; in short, for the recognition and legal reception of homœopathy by the authorities, and endowment of it with all the rights and advantages which the dominant-school physicians possessed.

In order to obtain the right to lecture in the University of Leipzig, he was required to pay the sum of thirty-five dollars to the institution, and to read and defend a dissertation on some medical subject, in the Latin language, before the assembled faculty and invited guests. This done, he would not only have the right to lecture on any subject he pleased, but the privilege of announcing his lectures in the university catalogue or prospectus, and of advertising and posting placards in the University and elsewhere.

On the twenty-fourth of June, 1812, the Grand Imperial French Army began the passage of the Nieman, into Russia, and Napoleon's great campaign in Russia was fairly commenced, and, on the twenty-sixth of June, 1812, Hahnemann delivered and defended his celebrated "Lecture on Hellebore; or, a historico-medical dissertation on the Helleborism of the Ancients." His son, Frederick Hahnemann, was his respondent, or so-called opponent. A translation of this literally stupendous literary effort will be found in "Dudgeon's Collection of

Hahnemann's Lesser Writings," republished by Mr. Radde, of this city. We would earnestly request every medical man at least to look over this production. It will enable us to form a very just estimate of the learning and genius of Hahnemann. It proves him a profound linguist, intimately conversant with Hebrew, Greek, Latin, Arabic, Italian, French, and English; a most astute philologist and critic, and a skilled medical historian. In order to compose it, he must have read, in their original languages, the works of Avicenna, Galen, Pliny, Oribasius, Herodotus, Hippocrates; Ctesias the Coan, a cotemporary of Hippocrates; Theophrastus the Eresian, who lived three hundred years before the Christian Era; Haller, Pallas, Vicat, Lucretius, Celsus, Scaliger, Dioscorides, Murray, Jacquinus, Salmatius, Antyllus, Grassius, Muralto, Gesner, Bergius, Greding, Unter, Lorry, Reimann, Scholzius, Benivenius, Rödder, Lentilius, Strabo, Stephanus the Bysantine, Rufus, Ætius the Amideman, Rasarius, Archigenes, Aretæus of Cappadocia, Plistonicus, Diocles, Themison, Cælius Aurelianus, Alexander of Tralles, Paulus of Ægina, Johannes, surnamed Actuarius, Massarius, Petri Belloni, Pausanius, and many others.

Most of these names are honorably known to every one familiar with the history of medicine; still, very few modern physicians have ever even seen any of the works above alluded to. Hahnemann did not quote them in a second-hand, or underhand manner; he had read and pored over many of them understandingly. We can prove this in a very few words: thus, on page 603,* he says: "This word, 'sesamoides,' does not occur in the genuine writings of Hippocrates; the first writer that mentions it is Diocles, who flourished twenty years after Hippocrates' death." On the same page, he tells us, in referring to the dose of Hellebore, that Dioscorides teaches a more definite quantity; also, Pliny is wrong in stating the Phocian Anticyra to be an island, for it was situated on the continent, half a mile from the port. On page 600, we read, "In a passage in Antyllus we find so and so, and Oribasius quotes the same passage." In quoting a line from Persius, Hahnemann tells us that it is an imitation of Horace; on another page, 596, we read, "Hippocrates seems to me to allude to this, when he says, so and so." In speaking of Mesue, he tells us that he flourished in the reign of the Caliph Al Raschid, about the year 800; that he was a man of such celebrity that he was termed the "evangelist of physicians," and goes on to say that, in his book, "De Simplicis," chapter 30, he tells us there are two kinds of Hellebore, &c. In speaking of Cælius Aurelianus, he tells us that his dialect is African, not pure Roman, but rude and rough. He also tells us that Galen explains the operation of Hellebore in a much

* See "Hahnemann's Lesser Writings," republished by Wm. Radde, 300 Broadway, New-York.

too mechanical manner; that Cælius Aurelianus, in his barbarous language, improperly applies the term Helleborism to the decoction of Veratrum. In another place we find, "The following are the words of Menesitheus, quoted by Oribasius: he tells us of a peculiar mode of giving Hellebore, recommended by Pliny; that Celsus, who wrote in the time of Augustus, always called Hellebore, Veratrum-album; that the description of Hellebore by Pliny is evidently taken from Theophrastus and Dioscorides, and he accuses Pliny of translating and copying whole passages from Dioscorides, without ever mentioning his name." In making clear a passage from the Greek Theophrastus he says: "I have only added these two words; the remainder of the text of Theophrastus I have preserved in its integrity, only somewhat changing the order of the words. Again, Herodotus does not say a word about the remedy used by the physician Melampus, in the cure of the daughters of Proetus. Again, the Prænotiones, attributed to Hippocrates, are written in such a hard, rough, and abrupt style, that they were probably the writings which, long before the time of Hippocrates, were preserved in the temple of Esculapius, at Cos."

Dozens more of instances might easily be given, but these will suffice to prove that Hahnemann actually studied the authorities he alluded to and quoted from in the most painstaking and critical manner; yet this is the man who has been termed an "illiterate quack." Well may we exclaim, if Hahnemann was illiterate, who is or can be learned!

It is needless to add that the delivery of this dissertation covered Hahnemann with glory; he quickly gathered around him a circle of very estimable men, some of them were not insignificant lecturers and professors, more were enthusiastic students of medicine, and impressible physicians. From this time onward, he gave regular semi-annual lectures in the University, for which his "Organon" served as a basis, and which he kept up on Wednesdays and Saturdays, from two to three o'clock, in the afternoon. We understand that Professor Mutter, of Philadelphia, was one of his hearers. Hartmann attended these lectures for about two years, and says that Hahnemann might, perhaps, have introduced his doctrines more easily to the physicians and students, if he had more dispassionately discussed the principal points of his "Organon" than was his custom in his lectures. His manner, unfortunately, was not calculated to gain for himself and his doctrines many friends and adherents; for, whenever it was in his power, he poured forth a flood of invectives and abuse against the established system of medicine and its advocates, so that the number of his hearers hourly diminished, till, at length, only a few of his pupils attended. Still, he continued these lectures several years undisturbed. Hahnemann's conduct in this matter is the more inexcusable if we recollect that he had been a charity-scholar, in this very University of Leipzig, in 1775 and 1776.

We have, also, a little information about Hahnemann's habits of life and study while in Leipzig, which, although it may be trivial, is more or less interesting. He rose in the morning at six o'clock, in summer, and at seven, in winter; drank several cups of warm milk, lighted his pipe, and walked for a short time in his garden, then prescribed for his patients or answered letters. About ten o'clock, he almost always ate some fruit, without much interruption to his hours of audience, which were from nine to twelve. At twelve o'clock, punctually, he dined—usually upon strong beef-soup, very tender beef or mutton, game, larks, fowls, pigeons; he rather disliked veal and pork; he liked his stewed fruit very sweet. With the exception of green beans, cauliflower and spinage, he rarely ate vegetables or greens; in place of bread, he often took cake. His daily drink was sweetened "gose," a light kind of white Saxon beer. After dinner, he took a nap of an hour on the sofa, then attended to his patients until seven o'clock, when he took tea, or rather drank warm milk, in winter, and, in summer, a peculiar Saxon drink, called "gosenkaltschale," i.e., a cold beverage, made with light beer or wine, with grated bread, sugar, lemon, &c., or with fruit, such as strawberries, currants, &c. At this period of his life, when he was fifty-five or fifty-seven years of age, he took a short walk, either in his garden, or in the town, accompanied by a little dog, which, also, had a place beside him at table. Then he retired to his study, and wrote and read until eleven, twelve, or one o'clock at night. Occasionally, he joined his family-circle in the parlor, at ten or eleven o'clock, and very rarely took a drive during the day to a near relative's or friend's house.

As Hahnemann approached towards sixty years of age, he received patients from nine to twelve, A. M., and from two to four, P. M., only. After the clock struck twelve in the morning, and four in the afternoon, no visit, from any quarter, was received; at twelve, to the minute, he was called to dinner. After four o'clock in the afternoon, it was then the daily custom of himself and family, in all weathers and at all seasons, to take an hour's ramble on the beautiful ramparts which surround Leipzig, or in the city; he walked on before, arm and arm with his wife, while his crowd of daughters walked behind, also arm in arm. Occasionally, only, a more extended walk was taken to some neighboring place or village.

In the house, he always wore a black velvet skull-cap, a black silk cravat and vest, a dressing-gown, short knee-breeches, with cotton stockings and Turkish slippers; in winter, he used a fur coat, woollen stockings, and fur boots. In the street, he wore an ordinary round black hat, and overcoat. It was only on festive occasions that he wore a dress or frock coat, long pantaloons, silk stockings, and shoes. In winter, he wore a fur cap, fur coat, and fur boots. He rarely used silk pocket-handkerchiefs and silk gloves.

He always burned tallow candles—no oil lamps; the candles often served to light his pipe, for he smoked much. It is said that, in the earlier part of his career, he sat up every other night at his studies, and then acquired the inveterate habit of smoking, which he persisted in until he went to Paris. He was very careful of his pipes and tobacco; if his pipe went out, he never relighted it, but always took a fresh pipe and tobacco. He took no interest in any game but chess; but that he rarely spared time to play. He never slept in an artificially-warmed room.

He had a very good knowledge of astronomy—had globes and illustrated planetary systems, was fond of the telescope, and often discussed astronomical matters with Counsellor and Astronomer Schwabe. He was a good meteorologist, and, with the aid of hygrometers, barometers, and thermometers, many of which he had in his house and garden, became a very good judge of the weather. He was well versed in geography, both ancient and modern, and had a large collection of maps and charts. His library was large, and he had books upon almost every science, language and subject. His translations prove that he had a good acquaintance with all the ordinary modern and ancient languages, but he was also a skilled philologist. One of his favorite recreations was to receive an evening visit from his friend, Adam Beyer, Professor of Philology in the University of Leipzig. They often entered upon the higher and more intricate philological criticism in the Latin and Greek languages, and the Professor is said to have listened, with pleasure and profit, to Hahnemann's opinions on the current philological controversies. Professor Beyer was celebrated for his profound study of Cicero, and his "*Officia Ciceronis*" had a place of honor in Hahnemann's library. Perhaps, the *London Lancet* would like again to stigmatize Hahnemann as an "illiterate quack."

In addition to these, Hahnemann, according to the testimony of his daughters and friends, paid much attention to mesmerism and animal magnetism, and employed them both in his practice. It is very probable that these latter studies exerted a baleful influence upon his views of disease and treatment, although, in his writings, he only occasionally advises a few mesmeric passes, and the application of the north or south pole of the magnet. The theories of potentization, by rubbing or trituration, and of immaterial or infinitesimal doses, probably grew out of Hahnemann's attention to animal magnetism and mesmerism. Mesmer was in Vienna as late as 1778. Hahnemann was in the same city in 1777, aged twenty-two years. Mesmer did not die until 1815, aged eighty-one. Hence, Hahnemann witnessed the commencement and progress of mesmerism, also, that of clairvoyance and the dawn of spiritualism.

Hartmann, while a student of medicine, became intimate with Hahnemann. He says that Hahnemann conversed readily with him upon the studies which he was pursuing and the lectures he was attending, especially about the materia medica and therapeutics; at times he became so excited that it seemed as if his pipe would burst. Hartmann fed the flame carefully, as he not only enjoyed the excitement which he had caused, but gained many practical hints from these explosions. He says it was very interesting to see this short, thick-set man, who was usually so dignified and even rigid in his attitude and walk, get into a state of excitement in which the blood rushed to his head and face, his eyes sparkled, and he was obliged to take off his skull-cap, in order to cool his heated head. It was only scientific subjects, and, especially, his own peculiar system of medicine, which thus aroused and interested him *so much*.

He sometimes received his pupils and a few friends in the evening, at eight o'clock. Hahnemann was usually seated in his arm-chair, with a glass of light Leipzig white beer before him. "There sat the silver-haired old man," says Hartmann, "with his high, arched, thoughtful brow, his bright piercing eyes, and calm, searching countenance, in the midst of his pupils, friends and children. The serious exterior which he exhibited in his ordinary medical pursuits was laid aside, and the mirthful humor, familiarity, frankness and wit that he displayed are said to have been very engaging." Besides homœopathy, he descanted on chemistry, the natural sciences, the condition of foreign countries and people, about which he seems to have read much, and his remarks were very entertaining. Occasionally, he would criticize the proceedings of old-school physicians, then his countenance would become animated, he would shove his little skull-cap to and fro upon his head, and puff out clouds of tobacco-smoke, which enveloped him as in a fog. At times, he would revert to passages in his own eventful life, and often became so affected that he would forget his pipe, which then often went out, but was immediately lighted by one of his attentive daughters.

In these evenings of relaxation, Hahnemann did not like to be disturbed by patients. If they called, he would put them off until the next morning, if he could; he felt himself too much unbent, both bodily and mentally, to prescribe carefully—and he never would prescribe carelessly, or even in an off-hand manner.

As he was very anxious that his pupils and friends should assist him in proving drugs, he thought it right to give them a social supper now and then, to which only those young men were admitted who had distinguished themselves by their industry, intelligence, and strict morality. Hartmann says these festive suppers were not conducted altogether homœopathically, for the food was temptingly savory, and good wine made its appearance in the place of the usual thin, white beer. Still, they never exceeded the bounds of moderation, out of respect for their friend and master; cheerfulness, humor, and wit always reigned, for older and often highly intellectual men were generally invited. On these occasions, Hahnemann seemed the happiest of men, but, at eleven o'clock, they all took their leave of him, and banquetted long on the recollection of these delightful evenings.

During his business hours, Hahnemann devoted himself exclusively to his patients and studies—no idlers, or even ordinary friends were admitted. No person was permitted to enter the hall of his house who had not first passed "the review," as it was called; this duty was performed every week, alternately, by one of his daughters, for which purpose she placed herself at a little window, next the hall-door, like a warden, or house-porter. Occasionally, Hartmann would call, during his office hours, and usually found his apartment filled with patients, and a considerable time always elapsed before Hahnemann would attend to him, for he never allowed a friendly visit to prevent his giving the necessary attention and reflection to each patient. He examined each person accurately, and wrote down himself, in his journal, all the symptoms of which the patient complained, even those apparently insignificant, to which he successively referred, previous to furnishing the medicine required, which, as Hahnemann smoked in his consultation-room, was always kept and procured from another room. I have seen letters to Hahnemann, in which persons desirous merely of seeing and conversing with him, complained of having frequently been denied admittance to him during his hours of consultation.

It is needless to say that Hahnemann's fame and his practice increased from day to day; he soon was obliged to have two assistants constantly occupied in preparing the cruder portions of his medicines, the more delicate and higher dilutions and potencies he always prepared himself. Even when he was (January 5, 1843,) eighty-eight years of age, and at Paris, we find him writing to Lehmann, of Cœthen, who prepared all his medicines after he left Leipzig, to send him one or two grains of Mercurius-solubilis, of the third trituration, from which to prepare the higher dilutions himself.

Hahnemann is said to have always been kind and compassionate to his patients, and always ready, during his office-hours, to devote any necessary amount of time and labor in their behalf. He always listened patiently to their details, never put leading questions, and was always anxious to have them describe their ailments in their own language. His first examination of a new patient was always a long and careful one, for he always inquired, in addition to the ordinary routine of physicians, what his patients' circumstances were, how their household was arranged and conducted, how their table was supplied, what kind of food they ate and preferred, in what way and how much they worked, how they spent and divided their time, how much they slept, how much exercise they took, &c., &c. The numberless letters, which he received from abroad, were pasted in folios, each of which was numbered and had its date upon its back; but, previously, he had made such extracts from these letters as referred to the patient's case, and methodically arranged the symptoms in his case-books or journals. Every symptom of which his patients complained to him was carefully recorded, and every prescription made was noted. At proper periods, Hahnemann always indexed his journals, case-books, and letter-folios. All these painstaking processes are far removed from quackery.

Soon after his second arrival in Leipzig, he commenced a new manuscript materia medica, or record of symptoms and effects produced by different drugs, and also a repertory. He completed this in two large folio volumes; but, as he was not satisfied with it, he made another, a few years later, and, after his removal to Cœthen, he made a third. It is supposed that these manuscript materia medicas and repertories contained many marginal notes by Hahnemann; that they were not the bald and dry list of symptoms contained in his published materia medicas, but contained references to many cases treated by Hahnemann himself, many reflections and suppositions, practical hints, &c., &c.; in short, they contained an epitome, not only of the effects of drugs on the healthy, but of all his experience in the treatment of disease. These most valuable books have never been published. After he entered fully upon his homœopathic career, Hahnemann published few or none of his cases. His disciples were left to study and delve in the materia medica as best they could; they were obliged to build up practical guides in the treatment of disease, or works on therapeutics, slowly and painfully. Even when Hahnemann moved from Leipzig to Cœthen, and it was known that he had two copies of manuscript materia medica, he was urged. most earnestly, by Dr. Schweikert to give his older and less useful copy to the Leipzig Homœopathic Hospital and Dispensary, which had been established by his friends and followers, at their own expense, not only to benefit the poor, but to give fame to Hahnemann and stability to homœopathy. But Hahnemann refused; he presented the work to one of his daughters, as her own special property after his death, but it was taken away to Paris, and has never been restored by his widow to the rightful owner, much less published for the benefit of the world.

Hahnemann's residence in Leipzig was chequered with many literary controversies and polemical discussions, with Professor Hecker of Berlin, Dzondi of Halle, Jœrg of Leipzig, Heinroth, Wedekind, Puchelt, Sachs, and many others—most of them world-renowned professors, all of them learned men. Besides, Hahnemann had to endure a pamphlet, journal and newspaper-war, both from laymen and physicians; much of it was carried on with a bitterness contempt and sarcasm that would have crushed a man of less heroic mould. It is said that Hahnemann never noticed any of the personalities which were directed against him. His own person was ridiculed, his family life was slandered and calumniated; it was sought to cover his name with scorn, and to debase him in the eyes of the public. We are told that Hahnemann comported himself worthily; that he bore the calumnies which constantly irritated him with the greatest composure; he never answered abuse, but continued steadily and quietly to develop his system. Although Hahnemann seemed to treat all attacks upon his character and works with silent contempt, he could not be said to have viewed them with indifference; for his most intimate disciples suppose that there is every reason to believe that they rankled in his soul and communicated more bitterness to his disposition than naturally belonged to it. If he did not reply directly to these attacks, in each new edition of his works, he attacked the dominant school of medicine with increased acerbity and almost malignity.

He published the first volume of his "Materia Medica" in 1811, when he had scarcely been a year in Leipzig, and, consequently, when he was fifty-six years old, and published seven more volumes before 1821, or before his sixty-sixth year of age. He also published, from time to time, essays in the *Allgemeiner Anzeiger der Deutschen*, a popular journal; more particularly, one on a severe form of typhus fever, caused by the disorder and misery consequent upon the stupendous military operations of that period, and the disastrous and disorderly retreat of the French from the campaign of Russia. A second edition of the "Organon" was also published during this period.

Thus matters went on until the year 1820, when Hahnemann was sixty-five years old, and the celebrated Austrian Field Marshal, Prince Schwartzenberg, came from Vienna to Leipzig to place himself under Hahnemann's care. He was supposed to have an incurable organic disease of either the brain or heart, or both. It will be interesting to say a few words about Prince Schwartzenberg's career, in order to form a better idea of the extent of the compliment which was paid to the fame of Hahnemann by the placing of this noble patient under his care

SCHWARTZENBERG.—Passing over the earlier parts of Schwartzenberg's career, we find that, in August, 1813, just before the battles of Dresden and Leipzig, the grand army of the allies, consisting of one hundred and twenty thousand Austrians, and eighty thousand Russians and Prussians, were commanded in chief by Schwartzenberg, who had his headquarters at Prague. Blucher lay in Silesia, at the head of eighty thousand Russians and Prussians, and Bernadotte was at Berlin, with thirty thousand Swedes and sixty thousand Russians and Prussians. Thus Schwartzenberg was in command of two hundred thousand men, and Blucher and Bernadotte less than one hundred thousand each. On the fifteenth of August, 1813, when Napoleon left the city to attack Blucher, Schwartzenberg advanced upon Dresden, with the sovereigns of Russia and Prussia, in person, in his army. Had he attacked it at once with his vast host, while St. Cyr, with only twenty thousand men, was left to defend it, Dresden would have fallen before Napoleon's return, which soon took place with the two hundred thousand men he had accumulated from various sources, and Schwartzenberg had to retreat with great loss; yet he skirted around the hills to the west, for the purpose of joining Blucher and Bernadotte at Leipzig. Napoleon reached Leipzig on the thirteenth of October, 1813, and, almost immediately, the heads of Schwartzenberg's columns began to appear towards the south, having now with him in his army the Emperor of Austria, as well as Alexander of Russia, and Frederick William of Prussia. Blucher was ready to coöperate with Schwartzenberg. Napoleon had but one hundred and thirty-six thousand men, Blucher and Schwartzenberg had at least two hundred and thirty thousand. On the eighteenth of October, Bernadotte's corps joined Blucher's, and ten thousand Saxons deserted from Napoleon. During the three days through which the stupendous battle of Leipzig raged, the burghers of Leipzig surveyed from their towers and steeples one of the longest, sternest, and bloodiest of battles. Hahnemann was then, probably, working quietly in his studio, for not a word of this war experience is to be found in his writings, except his pamphlet on typhus fever. The disastrous retreat of the French through the city of Leipzig, probably did not disturb Hahnemann much, although fifty thousand French were left dead, wounded, or prisoners in and around Leipzig, and four sovereigns, each at the head of his own victorious army, and Schwartzenberg, with the Austrian, met at noon in the great market-place of Leipzig.

On the twentieth of December, of the same year, Schwartzenberg, with the Grand Allied Army, crossed the Rhine into France, at the head of nearly three hundred thousand men, in three mighty hosts, including representatives of every tongue and tribe, from the Germans of Westphalia, to the wildest barbarians of Tartary. The Emperor of Austria still accompanied his army and his general. At nearly the same time, Wellington had crossed the Pyrenees, from Spain, with the combined English and Spanish armies; Blucher, with the Prussians, had crossed the Rhine at Coblentz, and the Russians, under Bulow, were coming by the way of the Netherlands—all centering toward Paris. In March, 1814, the Allies were in Paris, and the bulletins were signed by Schwartzenberg, as commander-in-chief of the allied armies. He was the acknowledged head of those countless hordes, warlike bands, and well-drilled soldiers, which, lounging and parading about the streets and gardens of Paris gave it the semblance of some enormous masquerade.

Circassian noblemen in complete mail, and wild Bashkirs with bows and arrows were there; all ages, as well as countries, seemed to have sent their representatives, to stalk as victors amid the nation which but yesterday had claimed glory above the dreams of antiquity, and the undisputed mastery of the European world. We do not pretend that the chief command was given to Schwartzenberg on account of his transcendent military abilities, for he was the most cautious, if not the most timid of that galaxy of commanders that numbered Wellington and Blucher among its leaders. The command was given to the Austrian field-marshal, perhaps, somewhat in consequence of the numbers he led, and, still more, to mark the prominent adherence of the Emperor of Austria, Napoleon's own father-in-law, to the cause of the Allies.

This was the man who subsequently came expressly from Austria to Leipzig, to place himself under Hahnemann's care, as a last resource, for his disease was regarded as mortal by his usual medical attendants.

In consequence of Hahnemann's medical treatment of Prince Schwartzenberg, he was, for a time, elevated from the situation of a mere private physician. He was placed in daily communication with royal and imperial Austrian councillors, with Saxon dignitaries, and with the ministers of various foreign courts to Saxony. For a short time, calumny ceased and abuse was hushed; Hahnemann was at the very pinnacle of his career. But, in the short space of six months, all this was ended, when Schwartzenberg's disease proved incurable by homœopathic means, as well as allopathic, and his death took place; which it did on the fifteenth of October, 1820. By a somewhat wonderful coïncidence, Schwartzenberg's funeral-train passed out of Leipzig on the anniversary of the day, and almost to the hour, when, seven years before, he had made his victorious entry into the city. Hahnemann was courteously and solemnly invited to attend the funeral, and followed the mortal remains of his friend and patron beyond the walls of the town. It would seem as if he had carried his own peace of mind to be buried outside the gates of Leipzig. The opposition to him was now renewed, and, after being allowed to practice and dispense his own medicines for over ten years, and to lecture in the University, the most important of these privileges were withdrawn the very next month, viz., in December, 1820. Hahnemann was notified that a fine of twenty thalers (about fifteen dollars) would be imposed upon him for every dose of medicine which he gave or dispensed to his patients. He was watched very closely, but it was not necessary; Hahnemann did not attempt to evade the law. He had battled against it with all his energies; he had left no argument and endeavor untried to have the law altered; he had dispensed his own medicines as long as he was not pointedly and absolutely forbidden to do so—but, although he would not evade or break the law, he would not yield to it. He preferred retiring from the practice of medicine, and banishing himself, not only from Leipzig, but also from Saxony, his fatherland, rather than submit to it. We have seen that his practice was so extensive, that he required two assistants to prepare his medicines in his own house; he would not have them prepared and dispensed by apothecaries, however good and faithful—and good and faithful druggists could surely have been found in Leipzig. Hooker very innocently asks why Hahnemann did not get one of his friends to act as his apothecary, not knowing that apothecaries in Germany are only allowed to follow their art by special license, that only a certain number of apothecaries are allowed to each town, district, or population. A new one cannot get a license until the population increases up to the required mark; that it is quite as difficult to establish a new apothecary shop in Germany, as it is to admit a new State into our Union, or to introduce an additional representative into our Congress. Hahnemann might possibly have made interest to have one or both of his assistants placed in apothecary stores, to prepare his medicines there in proper rooms; but they, doubtless, were young students of medicine, who did not wish to become mere apothecaries. His devotion to infinitesimal doses, probably made him think it unsafe to have his delicate preparations exposed to such varied smells as abound in an ordinary drug store, and prepared in ordinary bottles, mortars, &c. But, throughout Saxony, so-called homœopathic "*Officinen*" are now attached to all the licensed apothecary establishments. Good drugs are furnished from them, and it is only too probable that one or several of the Leipzig apothecaries would have been glad to devote a separate room, separate utensils, and one or more special clerks to the preparation of Hahnemann's medicines. But he would not. Dudgeon even suggests that his antipathy to apothecaries was the main-spring in driving Hahnemann to infinitesimal doses. He says the persecution of the apothecaries commenced in 1799, at Wolfenbüttel. Previous to this time, Hahnemann had given material and palpable doses, as we learn from the cases published anterior to that date. In 1800, we first meet with anything like infinitesimals, and these only in certain cases. As the opposition of the apothecaries became more violent, and the injury inflicted on him, pecuniarily and otherwise, more severe, Hahnemann's doses became more and more refined and attenuated, until, at length, we find him stating that the mere smelling of a globule is not only sufficient, but the best of all methods of administering remedies, and he adds, with marked emphasis, "*this will enable us to dispense entirely with the apothecaries' services.*" When he got out of the sphere of the influence and annoyance of the apothecaries, he changed his doses, and adopted a method in Paris much nearer in approximation to the method of the dominant school. This may have had its influence, but I feel convinced that his attention to mesmerism was another controlling cause; for, from the year 1784 onward, the doctrines of Mesmer and Barbarini spread rapidly over Sweden and Germany, and their followers styled themselves *spiritualists*, to distinguish themselves from more material persons. It is well known that Hahnemann believed that succession and trituration produced a real *spiritualization* of the dynamic property of each drug; that these processes produced a change in the remedies, so incredibly great, and so inconceivably curative, that this development of the *spiritual* power of medicines, he thought, deserved incontestibly to be reckoned among the greatest discoveries of the age. All this is too much of the nature of mesmeric and spiritualistic procedures not to have been derived from them.

Hooker is surprised that Hahnemann, after having come so deliberately to the firm belief that he had discovered the true art of healing, should, at the first show of opposition from physicians and apothecaries, be frightened into a relinquishment of the practice of his art. He thinks that a higher courage, and more indomitable perseverence than this indicates, were to be looked for in a reformer. But he does not seem to know that Hahnemann had been fighting this battle with the apothecaries for nearly fifteen years; nor to have had any idea of the opposition and abuse against which Hahnemann had so long struggled —it was not the beginning, but the end of a long campaign. Besides, Hahnemann must have been greatly discouraged about this period by family misfortunes; especially those of his only son, Frederick, who had graduated, as a physician, at the University of Leipzig, in 1812. He, soon after, purchased an apothecary establishment, in Wolkenstein, in order to pursue his practice untrammelled by the apothecary laws, which bore so heavily on mere physicians. He is said to have been an excellent but eccentric young man. He not only understood, but spoke Latin, Greek, French, English, and Italian, and knew enough of Arabic to read it fluently; he was also a good musician, and played the guitar and piano well. He was the favorite of his parents, as he was an only son. In his new field of practice, his fame spread rapidly, as he took rather unusual means to get practice: he drove about, in a splendid carriage with four horses, from hotel to hotel, throughout the district in which he lived. He was quickly cited to appear before the Board of Health, for dispensing his own medicines, although he had an apothecary's license and the diploma of a physician. To the surprise of every one he left the country and abandoned his wife and children. He first went to Hamburg, then to Helder, in Holland, where he was in 1818; thence to England, in 1819, and, finally, all traces of him were lost, but not until several letters from him, to his sisters and parents, unequivocally proved him deranged. The last letter received from him was dated London, June 25th, 1820, and Hahnemann often expressed the opinion that his dear but unfortunate son had died in some lunatic asylum. Schwartzenberg, we have seen, died in October, 1820, hence, Hahnemann must have been greatly discouraged and depressed at this time, and more willing to yield to external pressure than he usually had been.

It was also more easy for Hahnemann to change his place of residence than most other physicians. His numerous publications, and the violent attacks upon them, had made his name known all over Germany, and even in distant countries. A large portion of his practice was carried on by letter, which the capital arrangements of the German post-office easily enabled him to do, and his small doses could easily be sent by mail. His belief that the symptoms of a case were all that were required to be known in order to treat it, and that the patient should give these in his or her own language, and the long period which the remedies were allowed to act, all rendered the presence of a physician much less necessary than in any other system of medicine. This was the largest and most lucrative part of his practice, and Hahnemann could carry it on as well in one city as another. He answered no letters in which his fee was not enclosed, and this course gave great offence to his opponents, and he has often been loaded with the most opprobrious epithets because he introduced this custom—then unusual in Germany—of making the patients, with whom he corresponded, pay him for each epistolary correspondence. His friends say that he was led to adopt this course from the fact that so many sought his advice from mere curiosity, or worse motives, without any intention of paying him, and that he was driven to the adoption of what may be, and was then an unusual plan for securing promptly the fees of his patients. His enemies doubtless compared him to the Hunters, Fitches, Sandborns, Goodales, physicians of our time, "whose sands of life have almost fled," &c., &c. The abuse was all the greater because he exacted unusually large fees; he did so because he had a very high idea of the dignity of his profession, and because he most faithfully and laboriously examined the cases of his patients, and selected his remedies, however erroneously, with unusual care and expenditure of time, and also because he had a very high idea of the value of the services his remedies would render to his patients.

Thus ended the third act in the drama of Hahnemann's career. Baffled, but not defeated, the persecution of his enemies, and the stringent laws of his country, forced him either to give up practice entirely, or, like Brown, the great medical theorist and systematist, who immediately preceded him, to change his place of residence and, in fact, his country, for he not only could not practice in Leipzig, but nowhere in Saxony. Under these discouraging circumstances, the Duke of Anhalt-Cœthen, who was a patient, correspondent, and ardent admirer of Hahnemann and homœopathy, offered him an asylum in the tiny capital of his tiny dominions, and accordingly he proceeded to Cœthen, in 1821, aged sixty-six years.

Hahnemann lived fourteen years in Cœthen, as active as ever in his literary labors and office-practice; for, after settling in Cœthen, he seldom (according to Dudgeon and the "Biographisches Denkmal of Hahnemann," composed from the papers of his family and letters of his friends,) crossed the threshold of his door, except to visit the Duke of Anhalt-Cœthen when he was sick—all other patients he saw at his own house. In Cœthen, he published the third, fourth, and fifth editions of his "Organon," and the second and third editions of his "Materia Medica." In 1828 he published his "Chronic Diseases." On the tenth of August, 1829, he celebrated the fiftieth anniversary of his graduation as Doctor of Medicine. His disciples assembled in Cœthen in great numbers, presented him with a large oil painting of himself, also a medallion likeness, engraved by Kruger, of Dresden; and the medical faculty of the University of Erlangen, where he had graduated fifty years before, renewed his diploma, or rather presented him with a new and honorary diploma. At this festival, the first collection of money was taken up, to establish a free dispensary or hospital in Leipzig. The Duke and Duchess of Anhalt-Cœthen not only sent Hahnemann congratulatory notes, but the one presented him with an antique goblet, and the other a golden snuff-box, set with brilliants. On the same day, the Central Homœopathic Society was founded, with Hahnemann for its first and perpetual president.

In 1834, Hahnemann's first wife died; she had borne him nine daughters and two sons. During the next year, 1835, he married Madame Melanie d'Herbilly Gohier, and moved to Paris, where he lived eight years more, or until the fourth of June, 1843, aged eighty-eight years. His practice, in Paris, is said to have yielded him upwards of two hundred thousand francs per year. He received the same honors and attentions in France, from his disciples and friends, that he had previously enjoyed in Germany. His birth-day and the anniversary of his graduation were always celebrated, he was presented with marble busts—one from the chisel of David—with medals, engravings of himself, and portraits without number. In short, he always possessed the faculty of obtaining warm and earnest friends and adherents and enthusiastic disciples.

Thus we have given an outline of the career of Hahnemann; we have endeavored to do justice to his industry and ability, and free him from the charge of being a mere quack.

THE

PRINCIPLES AND PRACTICE OF MEDICINE.

SECTION I.*

OF MEDICINE AS A SCIENCE AND AS AN ART; ITS OBJECTS AND ITS EXTENT.

THE study of Medicine is prosecuted under two relations, namely, as a *science* and as an *art*. Medicine, considered as a *science*, takes cognizance of all that relates to the existence and the general nature of diseases, their prevention and their general treatment; considered as an *art*, its object is to distinguish, prevent, and to cure particular diseases.

Many branches of human knowledge are combined in the constitution and elucidation of the *science;* and the practice of medicine, as an *art*, ought to be founded on principles and facts of universal, or, at least, of extensive applicability, such as the great law, "*similia similibus curantur*," and others equally well proven, if there be any.

The great object and aim of the art and the science is to alleviate human suffering and to lengthen out human existence, by warding off or by modifying disease, "as the greatest of mortal evils," and by restoring health and even, at times, reason itself, "as the greatest of mortal blessings."

A consideration of the different topics which together make up the science of medicine, suggests a division of the subject into the following departments, namely: 1. Physiology, which embraces the study of the healthy functions, of which the human body is the seat or instrument. 2. Pathology, subdivided into *special pathology* and *general pathology*, which together embrace a consideration of everything relative to the existence and nature of disease: special pathology being intended to comprehend the consideration of the essential nature and origin of *particular* diseases, as they occur in man and animals, and general pathology to include those more *general facts or principles* which result from the comparison of particular diseases with each other.

---

* From "Aitkins' Handbook of the Science and Practice of Medicine."

3. Therapeutics, which exhibits a general view of the various actions of remedies in the diseased economy, or the means by which nature may be aided in her return to health. 4. Hygiene, which embraces a consideration of the means of preventing disease, or, in other words, of preserving health.

Physiology, general pathology, therapeutics, and hygiene are sometimes designated indifferently by the titles of the "*institutes*," the "*institutions*," or the "*theory of medicine*." These departments of science are all preliminary subjects of study, and constitute a necessary and appropriate introduction to the practice of physic, in which special pathology and the treatment of special diseases are the leading topics of consideration.

Each of these departments has grown or expanded itself into a great branch of science, and any single section is sufficient of itself to occupy the lifetime of an individual, in working out and studying it in detail. It is, therefore, not possible for the human mind to embrace all of them, in their whole extent and their bearings or relations to each other; and, setting aside the consideration of theories and systems, it has been truly observed "that no man possesses all the pathological knowledge contained in the records of his art" (CHOMEL); and it is, therefore, far less possible to embrace, in any single treatise, an absolutely complete view of the science of medicine in all of these departments.

For the purpose of teaching the science of medicine, in its application to practice, its elementary principles, as developed in the departments of pathology, are the most useful guides to the allopathic student; while the study of the effects of remedies, upon the healthy and the sick, is the more prominent study of the homœopathist. Thus, the allopathist is apt to become better acquainted with the pathology and diagnosis of disease than with its successful treatment, while the homœopathist often cures diseases symptomatically, the essential nature of which he knows very little about.

Although special pathology comes first, in the order of nature, yet, wherever the arrangements for medical education are complete, general pathology is taught as an introduction to, or conjointly with the special study of diseases; just as in other sciences—for example, in chemistry—it is found convenient to give a general view of the principles which have been established by special experiment and observation, before entering upon the particular details of the science.

It is intended, however, in the introductory part of this handbook, merely to guide the student to notice: 1. How the nature of diseases have been and are now elucidated; 2. The means and instruments of investigation into their nature; 3. An account of some of the more elementary constituents of disease; 4. An account of some complex morbid states associated with individual diseases.

In the body of the work, it is intended to consider some of the details of the practice of medicine—to furnish the student with:

I. A system by which to classify and name diseases.

II. A detailed description of characteristic diseases, in their respective classes. Under this heading, a definition and a history of the nature of each disease will be given, the probable course and succession of events described, and the grounds on which an accurate diagnosis may be made, or a prognosis expected, together with a detailed account of those rational modes of treatment which are consistent with the established principles of the *institutes of medicine.*

How the Nature of Diseases may be elucidated.

The derangements to which the human body is liable may be studied under the three following aspects: 1. As they present themselves in individual cases, becoming thereby the subjects of clinical medicine; 2. As they constitute particular genera or species of disease, forming the topics of special pathology; 3. As they may be reduced to and studied in their primary elements, forming thereby the science of general pathology.

But, in whatever aspect we may view disease, there is invariably presented to the student the same subjects for investigation, namely: *First*, The *morbid phenomena* or *symptoms*, by which we become aware that derangements have taken place in the economy, and it is by a mental effort that either the student or the physician must convert these symptoms into signs of disease—hence arises the necessity of studying *symptomatology*, or *semeiology*. *Second*, The agents by which derangements and diseases are produced, generated, or brought about, constituting the department of *causation*, or *etiology*. *Third*, The seats or localities of disease, or of derangements, and the peculiar nature, general forms, and types of disease must be studied, together with varieties in their course, duration, and termination, constituting *diagnosis* and *pathogeny*. *Fourth*, The morbid alterations discoverable in the structure of the body, before, but more especially after death, constituting *morbid anatomy*, *must be studied in connection with the symptoms*, *the causes*, *and the course of the disease*. *Lastly*, The elementary constituents of diseased products, constituting *morbid histology*, must be recognized and contrasted with the analogous constituents of the healthy state.

Relative Nature of the Terms Life, Health, Disease.

The word *disease* is used in a general and also in a specific sense; as when it is said that a person is diseased, without stating the nature of the affection; or that he suffers from a particular disease, such as small-pox. The attempts to give a logical definition of the term *disease* have all been unsuccessful. The relation of the state to the condition of health, and of health to the performance of the vital functions, are of such a kind that their phenomena can merely be described in their relations to each other, but not not defined.

If *life* is understood to imply that active state resulting from the concurrent exercise of the functions of the body, then there are conditions of activity, and of mutual adaptability of states and of parts, both as regards body and mind, which are necessary to the state of health.

Our notions of *the conditions of health* have thus considerable latitude. "*Health*" is merely a name we give to that state or condition in which a person exists, fully able without suffering to perform all the duties of life. Many degrees of this state are, therefore, at first sight obvious, from the mere evidence of the possession of a feeble existence to the most robust condition of the body; and there are many degrees of feebleness and delicacy of health which we cannot call either disordered or diseased states of the frame.

So extremely indefinite is our notion of normal life, that it is only by a forced abstraction the normal can be separated from the abnormal. Hence, also, our idea of *disease* is very indefinite; it cannot be separated by any well-defined boundary from the idea of *normal life*, and the two conditions are connected by a kind of debatable border-land.

When we observe, therefore, the phenomena of the living state and the conditions of health, we can readily observe when and how *disease* is but "*a deviation from the state of health, and consisting, for the most part, in a change in the properties or structure of any tissue or organ which renders such tissue or organ unfit for the performance of its actions or functions, according to the laws of the healthy frame.*"

It is now a received pathological doctrine that "*disease*" does not consist in any single state or special existence, but is the natural expression of *a combination of phenomena*, whose instruments of vital action are impaired in function or altered in structure.

All attempts, therefore, to define disease by the use of such terms as "*derangement*," "*modification*," "*alteration*," "*change*," from the preëxistent state of health, show, in the first instance, that very various ideas are attached to the term or to the state; and, secondly, these terms point to a nosological division into structural and functional disease, rather than to a state common to all forms of disease.

A definition of any state of disease ought to include all the circumstances, whether functional or organic, which constitute the deviation from health; and, for very obvious reasons, such a definition can only be approximatively expressed.

Principles by which Diseases have been Distinguished and Classified, and their Nature Determined and Explained.

The associations or groups of morbid phenomena which constitute disease have been distinguished in a variety of ways, each of which has, at one period or another, been in common use.

Although diseases are named as if they were individual entities, yet they present such great varieties that they will not admit of that species of classification which can be made with objects of natural history. But, as in the healthy body, we can observe the properties of its functions and the structure of its parts, so, in disease, we can observe *the phenomena which constitute the morbid states*, and can also often recognize the constituent elements of disease or material changes which affect the organs and functions of the body. They become perceptible to the eye or the feelings; or, by instruments or other methods of research, these material changes become the subjects of pathological study in the department of morbid anatomy. But there are also many conditions of the vital phenomena which are obviously morbid, the nature of which cannot be determined during life, and, when death affords an opportunity for anatomical investigation, no material change is capable of being detected by the most zealous pathologist. Chemistry, however, in such cases, sometimes demonstrates that chemical changes, of a quantitative or qualitative kind, are connected with the morbid state.

The grounds on which diseases have been classified may be described under the following seven divisions, namely:

I. *The nature of the ascertained causes of disease.* On this principle two classes of diseases are recognized, namely: 1. Diseases arising from general causes; 2. Diseases arising from specific causes.

This classification would lead to the search for two great classes of remedies, viz.: First, such as act upon the system in general; and second, such as act upon particular parts by preference, or in a peculiar and *specific* manner.

II. *The pathological states or conditions which attend diseases.* The principle of this classification consists in determining alterations of structure or chemical composition of parts, from which names are given to the disease, *e. g.*, pleuritis, pneumonia, &c. The distinctions of Sauvages, 1768, were generally derived from symptomatic and pathological characters, or external symptoms alone. Cullen following, 1792, adopted similar grounds of classification.

This classification ought to have led to the search for remedies which modify the nutrition, exudations, structural and chemical changes in vital parts.

III. *When the properties, powers, or functions of an organ or system of organs are deranged.* By this principle of classification the most prominent effects or phenomena of morbid states are considered as the disease; *e. g.*, palpitation, diarrhœa.

When disease consists in perverted powers or functions, it is then denominated a *dynamic* affection or disorder. When it depends on change of structure, it is termed an *organic* lesion or disease.

This third basis of classification is physiological, and was adopted by Mason Good.

This classification led to the study of remedies which affected the functions and secretions, such as emetics, cathartics, diuretics, diaphoretics, &c

IV. The diseases comprehended under the two latter principles of classification are sometimes inaccurately and loosely brought together under the heads of *structural* and *functional* diseases. The diseases of function, for instance, being made to embrace the *neuroses*, *hæmorrhages*, and *dropsies;* while *inflammation*, *tubercle*, *cancer*, *melanosis*, *hypertrophy*, and *atrophy*, are the subordinate classes of the diseases of structure.

The diseases of function embrace all those diseases in which *the action, the secretion, or the sensation of a part* is impaired, without any primary alteration of structure of the organ or tissue affected, so far as our imperfect means of research can ascertain. Thus, *mania*, *catalepsy*, *neuralgia*, are sometimes called *neuroses* of the brain, or other portion of the nervous system. *Colic*, *vomiting*, *diarrhœa*, and *constipation*, are regarded by some as *neuroses* of the alimentary canal; and so on of other parts. *Hæmorrhage*, or the effusion of blood, and *dropsies*, or an effusion of water into the shut cavities of the body—as that of the head, chest, or abdomen—are also cited as instances of functional disease. Such are the grounds of classification adopted by the late Dr. Williams, of St. Thomas' Hospital, London.

This classification would lead to the search for and study of remedies which affect the functions and secretions of the various organs or parts, or such as alter the physiological actions of these parts; and also of remedies which influence the structural or chemical arrangements of the different organs, and which have been called *organic*, or *alterative* medicines.

V. A basis of classification has been adopted, founded on *the pathological nature of the different morbid processes*, but the arrangement of the orders and subdivisions are determined by the anatomical arrangement of the textures and organs of the animal body, as originally developed by Bichat and others.

Such is the principle and mode of classification adopted by Dr. Craigie, 1836.

This classification should have led to the discovery and study of remedies which act specifically upon the various textures and tissues of the body, such as the cellular, serous, mucous, parenchymatous, fibrous, gelatinous, &c.; but it did not, except in the most imperfect manner—so imperfect, in fact, that most pathologists, despairing of finding such remedies, at one time sank into all the peurilities of the "expectant mode" of the French, or the *nihilisms* of the Germans.

VI. A ground of classification exists, having reference to *the general nature and localization of the morbid states.* It comprehends three classes: 1. Diseases which occupy the whole system at the same time, and in which all the functions are simultaneously deranged; these have been named *general* diseases, such as *fevers.* 2. Constitutional affections, meaning thereby diseases which display themselves in local lesions in any part, or in several parts of the system, but not in all parts at the same time; *e. g., rheumatism, gout.* 3. Local morbid processes.

Such is the classification adopted by Dr. Wood, of Pennsylvania, 1847.

This method should have led to the study of remedies which affect the principal systems of the body specifically, such as the nervous, vascular, glandular, lymphatic, &c., &c., i. e., of *general* and *constitutional* remedies, and of those which affect local morbid processes, and hence act specifically upon certain organs and formative processes.

VII. Applying the principles of a *purely humoral pathology,* we have a classification consisting of:

a. Fevers.

b. Dyscrasiæ, *e. g., tabes, chlorosis, scorbutus, dropsy, diabetes, pyæmia, tuberculosis, carcinoma.*

c. Constitutional diseases, induced by: 1. Specific agents; 2. Vegetable substances.

Such is Wunderlich's arrangement of diseases, 1852.

None of these principles lead to a complete or perfect classification, because diseases are not yet sufficiently understood to permit us to see clearly their mutual relations. The tendency of modern investigations, by the varied instruments and methods of research, proves that many diseases, hitherto supposed to be altogether functional, are accompanied with changes of structure, either of an anatomical, physical, or chemical kind. It is, therefore, not unreasonable to anticipate that all, or, at least, many of the so-called functional maladies will be found to depend upon some concomitant alteration of structure; and when we are unable to detect an alteration either of the solid or fluid parts of the body, in cases where the existence of disease cannot be doubted, we must attribute our failure to the imperfection of our means and instruments of observation, or our modes of using them. In the present state of our knowledge, however, there are diseases which have baffled the attempts of the morbid anatomists to associate them with structural changes of a characteristic or constant kind. Some convulsive diseases of the nervous system are of this class.

In the present imperfect state of our knowledge, therefore, diseases cannot be philosophically classified; and their names must yet be derived from some constant and striking feature of the morbid state, whether structural or functional. When no change of structure can be detected, the definition of the disease should include the most prominent symptoms only. Most of the diseases of the nervous system are named in this way. The following considerations generally regulate the naming of a disease: The first alteration of the animal economy, upon which all the subsequent changes depend, is generally recognized as the essential element of the disease (*pleuritis*, *tuberculosis*); and, if such cannot be discovered, the first tangible link in the chain of causation is used instead (*typhous poison*); next to that, the most characteristic symptoms furnish the name (*palsy*, *diarrhœa*); and, if death at once follow the application of a cause, that cause generally names the disease (*lightning*, *Prussic-acid*, *Arsenic*).

It is obvious, from these statements, that the names of diseases must change as our knowledge changes and becomes more precise; and many diseases which were once named after their symptoms, are now called according to the lesion from which most of those symptoms proceed. An apt illustration of this is to be found in paralysis, which is no longer regarded as a disease *per se*, but is merely a symptom of several structural alterations of the brain and spinal marrow; and so also *diarrhœa*, which now ought to be excluded as a disease from tables of the causes of death.

SECTION II.*

MORBID ANATOMY AND PATHOLOGICAL HISTOLOGY—THE MEANS AND INSTRUMENTS BY WHICH THE NATURE OF DISEASES ARE INVESTIGATED.

Morbid, or as it is also sometimes called, pathological anatomy, is that department of medical science which treats of the changes produced by disease in the solids and fluids of the body; while morbid or pathological histology treats of the origin, development, growth, and decay of the *new products* or *new formations*, which are the elementary constituents of structural or organic diseases. They stand in the same relation to the development of morbid phenomena and conditions of disease that the anatomy of healthy structures and the histology of the textures do to the natural functions and process of development, growth, and nutrition in the healthy body.

The vestiges left by the prolonged existence of a morbid state, whether in the body of man or of the lower animals, have always claimed from the physician a large share of attention; and in proportion as a knowledge of healthy anatomy and physiology has become extended and prosecuted in all its bearings, so has pathological science been extended, and morbid anatomy has gradually but steadily acquired an important

---

* From "Aitkins' Handbook of the Science and Practice of Medicine."

and prominent position among those branches of study on which medicine rests its claims as a science.

It is a department of medical science which has gradually grown out of the accumulated experience and observation of ages. As a science, pathological histology is of modern origin. It is but yet in process of development, but its foundations may be traced in the works of the earliest medical writers of antiquity; for all of them refer to changes which they *merely supposed* to take place in the internal organs; and they were doubtless led to the assumption by observing the connection that existed between structural lesions of the external parts and their accompanying symptoms. Hippocrates describes the deposit of tubercles in the lungs, the symptoms occasioned by them in a crude state, and those which attend their softening and discharge.

The science of morbid anatomy is a record of facts concerning disease, quite as much so as common anatomy is a record of facts about the structure of the healthy body. In its relation to the progress of medicine, it is a history or living record, whose pages must be ever open to receive the observations which are constantly being made by those engaged in pathological pursuits, and a record from which one may ascertain, at any time, the conditions under which morbid changes or new formations in the body have taken place. The pages of this record show that, at the present day, the department of pathology is in a transition state; and the position of medicine, as a science, must now result from a re-arrangement of the innumerable details which the records of morbid anatomy and histology can disclose and unfold. It is necessary, therefore, and often advantageous to look back upon the past and see what has already been done, so that its venerable facts may not be lost sight of, but grouped in series with the extensively verified experiments and observations of the present day. In so doing, if we pause and contemplate the steps which have been taken to arrive at our present position, such a contemplation may stimulate the youthful student to the noblest exertions of his intellect, as he cannot fail, with extensive study, to see before him and on every side much unlabored but productive soil.

Such a retrospect will, at the same time, have the effect of placing in a prominent aspect the varied influences which morbid anatomy has had on the science of medicine, the conditions under which it has flourished, and the legitimate objects of its investigations.

The art of printing was not long invented when books on morbid anatomy began to be printed, and although the early period of the fifteenth century has left little enduring literature of any kind, but has been mainly distinguished by the number of colleges then founded, yet it is about that time that pathological anatomy, in the medical school of Florence, shows the earliest traces of its existence. The increase in the facilities of study soon stirred up ardent students; and the sixteenth and seventeenth centuries produced much that will ever remain famous in the annals of medical science. Eustachius, Tulpius, Ruysch, Harvey, Malpighi, and Leuwenhœck, are names familiar as household words to the student of medicine.

The earlier attempts of this period to form a system of pathological anatomy is characterized by abortive endeavors to explain all results upon some exclusive and general principle. A spirit of speculation marks the character of the age. The men of that period had observed but few facts, and on these facts they preferred to speculate and dogmatize, rather than prosecute the farther interpretation of nature, or record the observation of more. Accordingly, theories in abundance successively led captive the minds of the medical world, and disappearing, one after the other, demonstrated the unstable nature on which the science of medicine had been placed. The leader of each sect founded his so-called school or system, all of them distinguished by a due amount of arrogance and contempt for predecessors and cotemporaries—a feeling, unhappily, not yet quite extinct. The "*vital agency*," the "*influence of the humors*," and of the "*solid organs*," have each been considered, by turns, as the only orthodox belief; and each has had their school and sect, respectively designated as the *Vitalists*, the *Humoralists*, and the *Solidists*. The theories of Galen, of Paracelsus, and others, have all been famous in their time, but are now unheard of and almost unknown. The same fate awaits the false theories and absurd conceits of more recent origin, although, as in the case of Stahl, Cullen, Brown, and Broussais, they have had a wide prevalence in the schools of Europe, and made impressions on the sentiments of the profession which yet influence their motives of practice, and the reasons of their belief. Broussaisism, Hahnemannism, and some other systems, must all, like the others, descend the same inevitable slope to oblivion; but the vast collection of facts, which the founders of such systems accumulated, are as unchangeable as nature, and will continue to recur, in the daily experience of our profession, just as they appeared to the venerable fathers of medicine centuries before the Christian Era. The practice of medicine on rational principles, and a knowledge of the nature of diseases, has oscillated through all these systems and theories, and morbid anatomy throughout has been marked by unmistakable periods of *progress*, of *stationary existence*, or even of *retrogression*, according as one or other exclusive system had the ascendancy, or as each principle challenged for itself a supreme importance.

The modern doctrines, relative to the nature of disease and the practice of medicine, may be said to be guided by the dictates of physiology, and what is known regarding the development of the human body. Ordinary dissections alone, or *post-mortem examinations of the body, have long since ceased to furnish us with facts before unknown;*

and new modes of extending observation and research, by taking advantage of every physical aid to the senses, are diligently looked for by the modern anatomist, physiologist, and physician; and the means and instruments which advance the science of physiology are well able to advance our knowledge regarding the nature of disease-processes.

Organic chemistry and the *microscope* have opened up new fields of labor, which are being diligently cultivated; and, while alterations in the ultimate tissues and organs are more especially attended to, the first beginnings of disease and the development of new formations claim a large share of attention.

Histology, or the study of the development and arrangement of the tissues in the formation of normal and healthy organs, *is characteristic of the anatomical investigations of the present day;* while the histology of morbid products, and chemico-physiological investigation into the nature of morbid changes, is characteristic of the pursuits of the science of modern pathological anatomy.

It is also a very significant fact, that now, in the nineteenth century, the leading doctrines of the *humoral* pathology which prevailed in the seventeenth are again revived. The experience and learning of that erudite period are now being made available for modern uses. By the improved means, instruments, and methods of research of modern times, important truths may be sifted from the errors and theories with which they are mixed up in the ancient chronicles of medical science; and when we get analogous conditions of disease with which the phenomena described by the ancients may be compared, "not a few of the apparently modern beliefs will be daily found to have a time-honored reputation unappreciated before."

The chemist and the histologist now combine their researches, and work hand in hand, and we regard them as the most inquisitive anatomists of the time. They lend assistance, of the most important kind, in working out the foundation of our knowledge regarding the nature of diseases, the details of which can only be made more certain and perfect by taking advantage of every kind of scientific knowledge which can be brought to bear upon medical research, and, more especially:

1. By physical aids to the senses, in the use of the stethoscope and other instruments of auscultation, as well as in the use of the microscope, aided by a careful study of the writings and labors of the men who have more particularly devoted their attention to observations aided by such means: Laennec, Louis, Walshe, Skoda, Stokes, Hope, Bennett, Queckett, Vogel, Beale.

2. By the knowledge (gradually being made more extensive) of the textures, organs, and functions of the body, whose normal exercise constitutes a healthy existence: Longet, Muller, Sharpey, Valentin, Allen Thomson, Carpenter, Kirkes, Paget, Kölliker.

3. By an intimate knowledge of the normal development of the human textures, as well as those of plants and animals, from the fecundated ovum: Bischoff, Costa, Allen Thomson, Huxley, Newport.

4. Besides these kinds of investigations, the science of practical medicine is being advanced by what may appear to some as an objectionable means of research, namely, by operations (vivisections) and experiments upon the internal organs of living animals; and, at some of our great schools of medicine, such investigations are now being actively prosecuted and taught; as by Bernard, in Paris, Drs. G. Harley and Pavy, in London.

Successful inquiries into the nature of diseases cannot be said to have commenced till the middle of the eighteenth century, when the great work of the *life-time* of Morgagni issued from the press. In the eightieth year of his age, and not till then, did he consider himself warranted to publish his observations, "*De Sedibus et Causis Morborum*" (1761); a work whose material and circumstances of publication read us the practical lesson, that the more frequently a disease occurs the more necessary it is that its phenomena should be carefully investigated. And when we observe, also, the prudent reserve, the anxious and the conscientious delay exhibited by Harvey, Morgagni, and by Jenner, in the publication of their respective researches, we cannot but contrast the circumstances with those under which the exuberance of medical publications are now given to the world.

Morgagni modified and corrected many of the views entertained and promulgated by his predecessors, and the study of the nature of diseases was carried into the commencement of the present century by Cullen, William and John Hunter, Portal, and Bichat.

The knowledge of the physician, regarding the nature of disease-processes, may now be observed to have advanced simultaneously with that of *general anatomy;* and, when the component parts of an organ and of the human body came to be distinguished, it was soon observed, also, that membranes and tissues might be individually diseased, while neighboring membranes and tissues remained untouched. Bichat's idea, therefore, of decomposing the animal body into its elementary parts, must be regarded as the foundation of modern special pathology; and while he pointed out the necessity of studying diseases with reference to the different tissues, as separately and *specially* affected, it has been since shown, in a remarkable manner, how general anatomy, deduced from physical properties of parts and crude observation, may coïncide with more minute investigations of a chemical and microscopical kind. The membranes and tissues, composing organs roughly torn asunder by Bichat, are now themselves being daily subjected to a more inquisitive analysis of an anatomical and chemical nature, which have unravelled them into still more minute histological elements. The experiments of

Hahnemann and his best disciples have, and will still lead to the better cure of these diseases of tissues and minute parts.

Although, therefore, Bichat entertained the view that each tissue had its own *diathesis*, it is to Cullen and the Hunters, of England, more especially, that the application of the distinction of tissues was made to illustrate the nature of disease-processes. Cullen's descriptions of diseases are descriptions of groups of phenomena which comprise complex morbid states.

The written labors of the Hunters form but a small part of the memorials of what they did to elucidate the nature of diseases, and it is only those who, having an opportunity of carefully investigating their museums, preserved in London and in Glasgow, are able to form any conception of the comprehensive nature of their labors, or can assign to them a proper place among those who have successfully advanced the science of medicine. They hold a position at least one hundred years in advance of the age in which they lived. Bichat, Cullen, and the Hunters, in their respective countries, have thus reciprocally influenced and advanced the progress of our knowledge regarding the nature of diseases.

Although it was reserved for Bichat to complete a more perfect system of general anatomy, it must not be forgotten that Dr. Carmichael Smith, in 1790, applied his knowledge of textural anatomy to elucidate the nature of disease-processes, and that Pinel, after him, in his "*Nosographie Philosophique*," made the distinction between the membranous and other animal structures the foundation of his pathology. The classic work of Baillie, viz., his "Morbid Anatomy," published in 1793, closed the labors of the past century.

If we look now to the tendency of the studies and researches of those men we have now mentioned, including Bichat, we shall find the truth gradually being more fully appreciated, *that it was necessary to study alterations of structure, so as to connect morbid changes with the symptoms of diseases during life, and with the operations of ascertained causes of morbid action.*

Thus the progress of morbid anatomy is, in a great measure, a record of the history of modern medicine; and we can trace the science of special morbid anatomy, giving a character to the various systems of the healing art which have prevailed from time to time.

The nature of the morbid changes were now observed to be more apparent in the progress of external diseases; and, therefore, surgical experience was brought to bear upon the elucidation of internal disease-processes.

All the writers, up to the time of Bichat, Laennec, and Abercrombie, were pure morbid anatomists, who did not connect the effects of disease with their causes, and who recognized the changes of disease as important in proportion to their magnitude, as apparent to the senses. They are, therefore, to be regarded as pure solidists, whose researches contributed much towards a correct knowledge of the changes in the organization of the body, while, at the same time, the condition of the fluids of the body was neglected, as well as the relation of the textures, organs, and fluids, in their combined exercise of function. Simple functional disturbances were wholly overlooked, and the constitutional connection of local affections entirely lost sight of.

The cotemporaneous surgery of the period previous to Bichat, was marked by its unwillingness to recognize anything but material facts, mechanical processes, and contrivances. The surgeons of those days desired to know nothing but anatomy and mechanics; and, accordingly, it may be recognized as the period of pure anatomical and mechanical surgery, distinguished by the works of men whose every individual page bears ample testimony that the surgery of the period was founded on exact and even minute anatomical knowledge. No allusion is made, however, by them to *medicine*—they make no application of physiological truths, and they *encourage no therapeutic* tendency apart from mechanical or instrumental interference.

The purely solid, as well as the purely humoral principles by which the nature of diseases have been explained, may be said to have long ago died a natural death; but, as already noticed, the remembrance of what is valuable in the results of both are preserved in the modern pathology, which takes its stand upon anatomical and physiological facts, connected by simple methods of inductive observation with the symptoms and signs of disease, as seen and expounded to the student by the distinguished professors of clinical medicine at most of our celebrated metropolitan schools.

In this field of instruction it seems invidious to mention here the names of men still living. For their own sakes, as well as for science, may they be long deprived of being thus honorably and respectfully mentioned. As teachers, they are in our own country familiar to every student. As recorders of what they observe at the bedside and after death, they are not less celebrated abroad than appreciated at home.

Tested by extensive clinical observations, the character of the present period in the history of practical medicine is one of *probation* as well as of *progress*, marked by a close inductive examination of past generalization and classification of facts, however remote, which illustrate the nature of diseases and their treatment.

Side by side, since 1816 and 1819, the microscope and the stethoscope, under the influence of such men, have advanced our knowledge of the nature of diseases with a regular and accelerated velocity; but they have only done so as assistants and in subordination to laws and facts, whose knowledge we have acquired by a close observation of general symptoms. Such instruments have never been intended to take precedence of the close observation of general symptoms. They have never accomplished, nor can they ever accomplish, useful practical results to the exclusion of such other methods of observation as I have just noticed. We are not to confound *relative* smallness with *absolute* simplicity, and believe that because a simple organic cell is a small object, which, because we can see around it, through it, and on every side of it, the functions and conditions of its existence are less *complex* or less obscure on that account than are those of a more complex organ, or the functians and existence of a living body.

We are not to suppose that, because the stethoscope enables us to detect a mitral murmur, or a crepitation in a lung, we are justified at once in adopting one, and only one, method of treatment. It is this exclusive use of instruments, to the disregard of general symptoms and signs of disease, derived from close observation and knowledge of the living functions, which leads to the repudiation of the use of such instruments by the sagacious and experienced physician, who sees the numerous errors not unfrequently committed by his younger brethren, trusting too exclusively to these instruments in the diagnosis of disease.

Like the stethoscope, the microscope has been unjustly and unnecessarily burdened with labor, and has been equally unjustly blamed and brought into unmerited discredit when it has failed to elucidate the nature or even presence of a morbid state, the existence of which could not be doubted, but which the sense of sight could not appreciate, even when presented in small quantities greatly magnified. In such instances, the microscope has been applied to uses which it is not the nature or province of the instrument to detect. The gravimeter, or hydrostatic balance, the microscope, the stethoscope, the pleximeter, are merely instruments of pathological inquiry, each one adapted for the determination of particular classes of facts, and can only elucidate disease when they are brought to bear upon the physical properties of the textures, organs, and regions, the nature of which they are able to appreciate; and it is only from their *combined and appropriate* use, in connection with the general signs and symptoms, that our knowledge of the nature of diseases will be advanced.

In all the temperate regions of the world, histology, as applied to morbid products, has been cultivated, and has advanced our knowledge regarding disease ever since 1838. In warmer latitudes, our knowledge of practical medicine has been advanced by extensive observations on physical climate, medical topography, and by organic chemical analysis, applied to obtain therapeutic agents from the vegetable world. These may be said to be the characteristics of the researches of our own country, Germany, France, and America, as compared with the nature of the observations prosecuted in India.

No exclusive doctrine will now stand the test of well-directed pathological inquiry; the main object of which is to connect all organic changes (lesions) and functional derangements with their symptoms and causes, with the view of applying rational remedies and prophylactics.

The too exclusive study of pure organic pathology and morbid anatomy, leads to no distinction between the signs and causes of disease; and the obvious tendency of such exclusive study is to exaggerate the importance of the principles it may establish, *to hold out no hopes of cure, and to undervalue the power of remedies and remedial measures.* To obviate this tendency, it is necessary to have recourse to inductive reasoning, so as to connect all the morbid changes seen or appreciated after death with the signs and symptoms of disease observed during life. Thus it is that links in the chain of disease-processes which, from a one-sided or exclusive view, appear isolated and localized, are found to be connected with, it may be, a long, but intelligible series of processes developed during life throughout the metamorphosis of tissue, and going on in apparent health or obviously morbid exercise of function. The constitutional origin of many local diseases, otherwise inexplicable, then becomes apparent.

Among the more eminent exponents of this rational school of pathology, who, at an early period, in England, discerned and appreciated such doctrines, we find such names as Mr. Allen, Golding Bird, Sir Robert Carswell, Gregory, Hope, Hodgkin, Marshall Hall, Prout, William Stark, John Thomson, Tweedy Todd, and many others, who, although now no more, have left behind them imperishable evidence of their labors. The younger pathologists of the present day, "whose name is Legion," follow now in the footsteps of these men, extending the fields of observation and the boundaries of the science of medicine.

By them, the importance of morbid anatomy is now sufficiently appreciated, and its province distinctly defined and *limited*, as follows, namely: 1. To detect the changes which have taken place, during the course of diseases, in the structure of tissues and organs of the body; 2. To demonstrate the exact seat of local alterations established during the progress of disease.

The investigation and elucidation of the *nature*, *course*, and *causes* of those changes constitute the prominent objects of the science of pathology. By the aid of morbid anatomy and clinical observation, during life, pathology seeks to establish the relations of the changes which lead to the evidence of lesions, and so to connect the general progress of disease with its symptoms.

Morbid anatomy goes beyond its province when it attempts to point out the nature of the proximate cause of disease. It is only by the application of inductive reasoning that the connections of causes and morbid effects can be shown, and such constitutes the main object, and is the highest aim of the science of pathology.

The *morbid anatomist* finds a lesion or change for what ought to be the natural structure, appearance, or condition of a part. The *pathologist* seeks to connect such lesions with signs and symptoms during life, that the *practical physician may suggest a remedy to the disease;* and that the *nosologist* may give it a name, distinguishing characters, and a place, in his classification of diseases.

The foregoing chapter is taken from "Aitkins' Theory and Practice of Medicine." I subjoin the following, somewhat altered from an article published by me in 1842, seventeen years ago, after a patient study of homœopathy from the year 1837; after constant intercourse with some of the ablest homœopathists in this country, such as Gram, Gray, Hull, Channing, &c., and opportunities of seeing the practice of some of the most renowned homœopathic physicians abroad, such as Noack, Fleischmann, Hartmann, &c. It is reproduced here simply to prove that my course has been a consistent one through my whole medical life; that I have ever tried to be an earnest searcher after real *truth*, wherever it is to be found, and that I have always been anxious to foster, in myself and others, a spirit of conciliation between all honest and liberal-minded physicians of whatever school.

In the meantime, according to one of the most liberal and practical physicians of the age, "the partizans of both schools are under the strongest possible obligations to examine the rules of practice from which they habitually dissent, with an attentive and tolerant spirit; not only because such study produces greater circumspection in the care and cure of the sick, but because it promotes the progress of truth and sound conciliation.

"In the records and theoretic writings of both schools there is certainly much error, but assuredly also a great deal of truth, and the sooner a catholic eclecticism inspires both parties, the better for mankind at large and for the true honor of the profession. It is not true that the homœopathic method is inert, or quackery, as is gravely asserted by writers of the dominant school. On the other hand, it is not true that the thousand methods, pursued hitherto, are all totally depraved, void of good results, and to be instantly and wholly abandoned, as is affirmed by many of the new school. The adherents of both plans of cure do a great deal of positive good in society—at least those of them do, who are well educated, conscientious, and thoroughly stored with plain common sense. *The truth, so far as practice is concerned, must therefore lie in some yet unascertained middle-point between the two systems.*"

I have not the least hesitation in saying that this middle-point will be found in "the specific alterative method." Homœopathic remedies act similar to, yet somewhat *different* from the action of the disease, and hence exert an *alterative* action upon the disease; specific homœopathic remedies always have been, and always will be an important integral portion of the practice of medicine. Specific allopathic remedies—i. e. such as act specifically upon the seat of the disease, but simply different from its action—also exert purely *alterative* action, and may and must often effect many cures. The ordinary allopathic practice of the dominant school is rarely or never *specific*, in the above sense, but purely counter-irritative or revulsive; yet it often effects good cures, although, perhaps, in a harsh and circuitous manner. Still, if life can be saved in no other way, it must be enforced, however unscientific, and however painful to the patient, relatives, friends, and physician. The thorough-going advocates of the one school often do too much, and do it in an unpleasant, perhaps kindly cruel manner; the strict partizans of the other, at times, do too little—the one school often seems to be trying how much medicine they can give without killing their patients, the other would seem to be experimenting how little they can give without letting their client die. There is a vast difference in the doses of the two schools, but no absolute antagonism in the theories, laws, or principles of the opposing factions.

SECTION III.

A REVIEW OF THE LATE REFORMS IN PATHOLOGY AND THERAPEUTICS.

"Let us no longer catch at shadows, but endeavor to seize upon the spirit of science itself; let us now discriminate between the letter and the spirit, or, what is the same, between system and true art, in order that we may no longer lose the spirit by clinging to the letter, nor true art by blindly adhering to system."—HUFELAND.

§1. Pathology and therapeutics, or the study of disease, and the study of the cure of disease, collectively include the whole of the study of medicine. And, if we glance our eye at the present state of medicine, we notice that late, although not very recent reforms have taken place, and are still progressing in each of the two great divisions above mentioned; and mark, also, that neither of them has, as yet, exerted that influence upon the medical profession, as a whole, which they should and ultimately must.

Inasmuch as a considerable space of time has now elapsed since these two great reforms were first set in motion, we think the time has now arrived for physicians to regard them, neither with the eye of enthusiastic preference, nor yet of excessive aversion, but to canvass their merits with the eye of a critic, which should be as eager to detect truth as it is usually only keen to detect error. Before proceeding further, it is well to premise that it has been said, that "every one should endeavor to ascertain the truth on every separate subject of inquiry, instead of following the ordinary process of adopting whole bundles of opinions, as they are commonly found connected together;" and, it is added, that "whoever does this, is very sure to agree with one party on some points, and with another on others, and is equally certain to be called fidgetty and crotchety by all parties." But, as this is suffering in a good cause, "every good man and true," should be willing and firm enough to bear up under it. From this digression, we turn to make another, because we believe that the shortest and best method of truly estimating the perfections and imperfections of any system of pathology is to compare its results with the requisitions of a theoretically and practically perfect study of disease. We advance as axioms: 1. That disease only occurs in living organized beings; 2. That all organization is the result of power; 3. That all organization presupposes the existence of form, structure, and composition; 4. That all function is the result of a power, which, in living organized beings, is termed the vital power. Hence we draw the conclusions that disease consists (1) in an alteration or modification of the vital power, which (2) forthwith produces alterations of function, followed (3) by alterations of form, structure, or composition, either singly or collectively. And further conclude that the proper study of disease necessarily presupposes and forces, *a.* the study of the operations of the vital power, and of the healthy functions, which are investigated in a science called physiology; *b.* the study of the form and structure of living organized bodies, which is learned in a science called anatomy; and *c.* the study of the healthy composition of these bodies, which is learned in a third science, which has received the name of physiological chemistry. Hence, we conclude, in the second place, that the proper study of disease necessarily requires, *a.* the existence of a science which treats of altered or diseased functions, and which might be termed morbid physiology, although it is commonly termed pathology; *b.* another science, which busies itself with the diseased alterations of form and structure, and which should be and is called pathological anatomy; and *c.* a third, which investigates diseased alterations of composition, and which should and does bear the name of pathological chemistry. Again, alterations of function are made known to us, during life, by means of symptoms, or so-called rational signs; while alterations of form and structure can only be studied during life, by means of the so-called physical signs; and alterations from the normal composition can only be accurately learned by means of chemical signs or tests. Hence we draw the final conclusions that any system of pathology which does not absolutely force the study of all of the six accessory branches of medicine, viz.: anatomy, physiology, and physiological chemistry, and morbid anatomy, pathology, and pathological chemistry, and does not equally force the study of rational, physical, and chemical signs of disease, must, necessarily, if not entirely erroneous, at least be imperfect.

We now turn from all our digressions to a critical examination of the last reform in the study of disease. The publication of "*De Sedibus et Causis Morborum*," of Morgagni, in 1760, opened a new era in the study of disease. This work, it is well known, contains a prodigious collection of dissections of the bodies of diseased persons, made by the united exertions of Morgagni and Valsalva. It is true that others preceded Morgagni in his peculiar labors, and we are, in fact, obliged to make particular mention of Bonet, of Geneva, who is said to have been extremely zealous in the study of morbid anatomy, and his hearing having become impaired, in the latter part of his life, he was led to devote the remnant of his days to the arrangement and publication of the materials he had amassed, and labored with such success that his principal work, the "*Sepulchretum*," published in 1679, was very highly approved, and, with some show of reason, is even considered to have subsequently formed the foundation of Morgagni's great work. Other minor worthies preceded both Bonet and Morgagni, but still we think that none but the hypercritical will deny the claim of Morgagni to the title of the "father of pathological anatomy," which has been thrust upon him by almost universal acclaim.

The example of Morgagni soon engendered an enthusiastic and one-sided devotion to the study of morbid anatomy, and the "*Historia Anatomico Medica*," of Lieutaud, and the "Morbid Anatomy," of Baillie, followed, in quick succession, upon the publication of "*De Sedibus et Causis Morborum*;" while, in later times, the works of Bichat, Carswell, Laennec, Louis, Broussais, Andral, Bright, Rayer, Rokitansky, Hasse, Gross, &c., &c., all bear evidence of the devotion to morbid anatomy which has been perpetuated in the medical profession up to the present day.

The necessary consequence of an improved knowledge of the structural ravages of disease, as revealed after death by the morbid anatomist's scalpel, was to turn the attention of physicians strongly towards perfecting the means of detecting and marking the progress of these ravages in the sick man during life; and hence the study of symptomatology received a fresh impulse, especially that branch of it termed *diagnosis*, which teaches us the signs by which one disease may be distinguished from another. But it is evident that pathological anatomy throws light but on that class of diseases which are attended with evident objective, physical, or structural alterations; and it is equally certain that neither the subjective, or the so-called rational signs of disease, nor yet chemical signs, will serve to diagnose organic or structural alterations. Hence, when we find that it is the objective, or so-called physical diagnosis of disease, which was principally and almost exclusively developed by the pathologico-anatomical school, it not only excites in us no surprise, but we recognize it at once as a necessary consequence. In fact, so intimately connected with pathological anatomy is the study of physical diagnosis, that we almost expected, before comparing dates, to find that the first great step toward the development of physical diagnosis was taken by Avenbrugger, of Vienna, in 1761, just one year after the publication of Morgagni's great work on pathological anatomy. Thenceforward, under the auspices of Corvisart, Laennec, Andral, Louis, Stokes, Piorry, Skoda, &c., &c., the improvements in the study of physical diagnosis kept pace with those in pathological anatomy. Still, in like manner, as Bonet was but a pioneer in morbid anatomy before Morgagni, so were Avenbrugger and Corvisart but pioneers in physical diagnosis before Laennec, who has been styled the "father of physical diagnosis." He, however, did not carry auscultation and percussion to any high degree of perfection before the year 1816. The consequence of the example of Laennec, as a matter of course, was to induce a number of physicians to turn their attention, almost exclusively, to the study of physical signs of diseases, and this was soon carried to such a height, especially in France, that many physicians seemed entirely to have forgotten that some diseases are characterized only by alterations of function, and others principally by alteration of the chemical composition, and that such diseases necessarily cannot be attended with physical signs, but only by functional, or so-called rational, or by chemical signs. The consequence was that the fingers and ears of the physicians soon had more to do in the diagnosis than their brains. Perhaps it is better for some physicians to rely upon the former, in preference to the latter, and hence we will not allow ourselves to descend into invectives against this one-sided aberration, the more especially as it led to the discovery and great present perfection of auscultation and percussion. It is but justice, however, to state that Laennec never discouraged, but urged every one to excel in the study of rational signs, and that, at present, the authorities in physical diagnosis, viz.: Stokes, Graves, Louis, Andral, Chomel, Bouillaud, Schœnlein, Skoda, &c., also excel in rational diagnosis.

The perfections and imperfections of the pathologico-anatomical school are evident at a glance. In like manner, as one may be a brilliant anatomist and yet be no physiologist, so may one be a master in pathological anatomy and yet be no pathologist; but, on the other hand, in like manner as one can never become a competent physiologist without being an accurate anatomist, so can one never be an expert pathologist without an extensive and accurate knowledge of pathological anatomy. Again, one may be a master in physical diagnosis, but he will not the less be an ignoramus in those diseases which are not attended with local structural lesions, and which, hence, cannot be attended by physical signs.

The more the pathologico-anatomical school perfected the knowledge of the ravages of disease, and the more they perfected the physical diagnosis of structural alterations, the greater became the contrast between the advanced state of one part of the study of disease, when compared with the neglected and imperfect state of the study of the cure of disease. They soon found that the old Hippocratic dogma, "*cognito morbo facilis curatio*," only to be true when we possess an equally exact knowledge of the means of curing disease; they soon felt, to its full extent, that no possible amount of knowledge of disease, exclusive of all, or but imperfect knowledge of the means of curing disease, can possibly teach us to cure at all, much less in a speedy, certain, and safe manner. They had set one great section of the study of medicine rapidly rolling onward toward its ultimate perfection, and now they anxiously turned their attention to the other and more important section, viz.: the study of the cure of disease. But this school, and all of its discoveries, had risen out of the dissecting-room and charnel-house, and to these they naturally looked for the means of curing. Hence we are not at all surprised to find Magendie, Orfila, and others, poisoning hundreds of dogs, cats, rabbits, sheep, &c., with huge doses of powerful drugs and poisons, solely in order to dissect them after death, in order to learn the material, physical, or structural alterations and disorganizations thus produced. Now, it is well known that the pathologico-anatomical school had almost come to the conclusion that disease is synonymous with inflammation, hence it is quite natural that when they found almost every powerful drug and poison causes inflammation, of greater or less degree, that their astonishment should be so great as to make them forget that these very substances had previously cured many and very severe diseases. Having forgotten this, the next step—that of proscribing the use of almost all active drugs and poisons in the cure of disease—was easy, and it is all in keeping to find one portion of them casting reliance, with the tenacity of despair, upon blood-letting, and that *coup sur coup;* and another sinking into the imbecilities of the *methode expectante*, and resting their "forlorn hope" upon ptisans and gum-water. With all their accurate knowledge of the structural ravages of diseases, and their dazzling use of physical diagnosis, it soon became a proverb in the profession, that one must go to Paris—i. e., to the hot-bed of this school—in order to learn what disease he is afflicted with, but he must go away again if he wish to be cured. We detect but a single prophetic voice against the therapeutics of this school, and that proceeds from the very man who, perhaps, was mainly instrumental in plunging it into its grossest errors—it is the voice of Magendie, ascribing a specific and peculiar power to Tartar-emetic and Corrosive Mercury, in causing engorgement, inflammation, and hepatization of the lungs, and arguing that, as it is well known that Antimony and Mercury cure inflammation of these organs, we cannot well explain their beneficial effects unless we admit them to exert a specific action upon the lungs. (See "Pereira's Materia Medica." American edition. Vol. I; pp. 140 and 561.)

§ 2. In the foregoing section, we briefly traced the history and results of a great reform in the study of disease; we now turn our attention to the peculiarities of an equally great reform in the study of the cure of disease. The means of curing disease are generally said to be contained within the narrow limits of the materia medica, and hence any reform in the cure of disease, must be preceded by a reformation in the materia medica, which, in general, is made to embrace two great classes of substances, viz.:

1. *Materia alimentaria*, i. e., food and beverages, or such substances as are positively essential in order to keep up life and health in the healthy person. As we have already seen that there is a science called *physiology*, which treats exclusively of life and the healthy functions, we take the liberty of terming these *physiological means*.

2. *Materia medica* proper, i. e., drugs and poisons, or such substances as are injurious to the healthy person and cause disease. As we have a science called *pathology*, which treats solely of disease, we may term these *pathological*, or, more properly, *pathogenetic means*.

However paradoxical it may appear, it is no less true on that account, that the physiological or health-preserving means are generally utterly powerless to cure disease, and are even loathed in some affections, especially in acute fevers, inflammations, &c.; while the pathological, or pathogenetic, or disease-producing means, form the main reliance of physicians in the treatment of disease. As these means, i. e., drugs and poisons, are injurious to the healthy person, they must, necessarily, also, be injurious to the sick, unless properly applied, and it hence becomes a positive duty, on the part of physicians, to use all possible means of attaining knowledge of the action of drugs and poisons prior to attempting to cure diseases with them, and also to be earnest and constant in the search of true laws and principles of guidance in the administration of them. If humanity demands that we should experiment as little as possible upon the sick, we have no resource but to experiment upon the healthy, viz., men and animals. If physicians be too squeamish to experiment upon animals, and neither noble nor generous-minded enough to experiment upon themselves, we then can only rely upon accidental or suicidal cases of poisoning, and upon the pangs and sufferings which are wrung from the agonies of the sick in slovenly and rash attempts at cure, for our knowledge of the action of drugs and poisons. If we are limited to these latter means, such knowledge can only make accidental and occasional, and not regular, systematic, and constant advances. As all these methods of attaining knowledge of the action of drugs and poisons are necessarily attended with suffering, it is well here to compare the advantages of each and all of them, in order that we may learn whether any of them may be dispensed with, or whether, cost what suffering they may, they must be constantly and unflinchingly put in practice: 1. By experimenting on healthy animals, we may push our experiments to the extent of causing severe local lesions, tumultuous constitutional disturbances, and death; after which we may learn the pathologico-anatomical, or structural, and the chemical changes produced by drugs and poisons. But animals do not speak a language that we understand, and hence many pains, sensations, and functional derangements must escape cognizance, unless we experiment, 2. on healthy human beings, on whom, of course, we can only experiment within reasonable bounds—we dare not cause severe local lesions, tumultuous constitutional disturbances and death, but, at the most, may only bring on functional derangements, evidenced by sensations or symptoms, from which we can only dimly and indistinctly guess at the internal morbid conditions which drugs and poisons are capable of producing, and to which these symptoms point, and from which they proceed. But our knowledge of the action of drugs and poisons on healthy human beings may be very materially aided by a thorough study of the accidental or suicidal cases of poisoning which have been carefully collected and preserved in the various works on toxicology. There we may learn the symptoms during life, and note the structural and chemical changes after death, and further compare the former with the results of experiments on healthy men, and the latter with the severe effects of drugs and poisons on animals. It is evident, that by employing all these means, we must attain to a far more perfect knowledge of the action of drugs and poisons than by using only a part of them; hence, while we receive thankfully all new discoveries gained by the employment of one or the other of these means, we must deny that a one-sided and enthusiastic devotion to one method only, exhausts all our means of acquiring such knowledge, and peremptorily refuse it all claims to actual and ultimate perfection. Although Hahnemann experimented exclusively upon healthy human subjects, yet he made use of all the treatises on toxicology up to his time, and thus gave his labors a much greater completeness. Again, we cheerfully admit that humanity demands that such experiments should only be continued as long, and pushed as far as is absolutely necessary definitely to settle the peculiar action of each drug and poison. But Magendie, Orfila, and Wibmer have experimented largely on animals; Hahnemann, Stork, Joerg, and others, have experimented freely upon healthy human beings; and Orfila, Christison, Sobernheim, &c., have furnished admirable treatises on toxicology. Now humanity is certainly not so exacting as to demand from us not to study the details of these experiments; indolence and prejudice must be more potent in dissuading physicians from making a close and accurate acquaintance with them.

It is possible that results thus obtained may enable us to deduce laws for the application of drugs and poisons in the cure of disease; but the absolute truth of such laws can only be truly demonstrated at the bedside, by trials upon the sick. Now physicians have been making such for over two thousand years, the details of which are preserved in many huge folios; hence, before we should dare to experiment further, we should compare the results of the actions of drugs and poisons upon healthy men and animals with the effects which these same substances are known to have produced upon sick men and animals. By such comparison, laws and principles of guidance in the art of healing must flow easily, naturally, and certainly. We therefore draw the conclusion that a theoretically and practically correct materia medica should contain accurate and voluminous details and experiments with drugs and poisons on healthy men and animals, and the results of accidental or suicidal cases of poisoning; while an equally correct therapeutics should contain a comparison between the effects of drugs and poisons in health and disease; an elucidation of the principles according to which cures have followed; an establishment of laws and principles according to which future cures or injury of the sick may and must ensue.

We now turn to a critical examination of the late reform in the materia medica and therapeutics, or in the study of the cure of disease. We find that a favorite pupil of the celebrated Quarin, a pupil whom he so loved and respected that he often entrusted him with the care of part of his extensive and arduous practice, even before he had reached the years of manhood; a man well grounded in the study of medicine, as taught by Hippocrates, Galen, Paracelsus, Van Helmont, Hoffmann, Stahl, Boerhaave, Cullen, Brown, and Darwin, put forth, in 1796, a little "*Essay upon a new method of discovering the curative powers of drugs, with a criticism of the methods previously pursued.*" Starting with the position that all drugs are injurious to the healthy person, but exert positive and specific curative powers against many diseases, and that it is the special and only vocation of the physician to cure and relieve the sufferings of the sick, and not to experiment, much less heedlessly to inflict injury upon them, he generously set the example, and earnestly urged the whole medical profession to join with him in making experiments with drugs and poisons upon healthy persons, in the ardent hope of finding fixed and true laws of guidance for their correct administration to the sick, so that the medical world, at least, learn under what circumstances certain drugs must prove beneficial or injurious.

The intentions of Hahnemann were philanthropic and honest, and his aim was a truly noble one, but as he experimented upon the healthy human subject only, his "Materia Medica Pura" necessarily contains mainly the details of functional derangements and symptoms; and, in point of fact, does contain an unexampled host of isolated and often very trivial drug-symptoms, fewer connected groups of drug-effects, still fewer distinct and complete descriptions of drug-diseases, and comparatively scanty details of severe local structural disorganizations and chemical decompositions. As Hahnemann devoted himself, through a long series of years, with almost unparalleled industry, and with a devotion which could only have been excited by the most elevated and philanthropic desires, he necessarily reaped an unexampled harvest of drug-symptoms, but from what internal morbid functional, structural, or chemical changes they flowed, and to which they pointed, remained either nearly unknown to, or could only be darkly and uncertainly guessed at by him, because true pathology and physical diagnosis had been comparatively but little cultivated before his time. He was immensely in advance of his time in the study of the materia medica, and his followers, instead of rehashing over his materials, should labor in the same grandly progressive, and, if necessary, revolutionary spirit which actuated the great reformer.

It of course became necessary for him to arrange his vast materials, and, as isolated drug-symptoms formed the majority of these, the most natural ordination was to arrange them according to the localities or organs which they affected, and hence he classed them under effects upon the head, eyes, nose, &c., arms, legs, toes, &c., according as they influenced these parts. This certainly is a natural arrangement, and we would have no exception to take to it, if it had not been cited by unfair critics as the only proof that the Hahnemannian school are in possession of sound knowledge of anatomy and physiology. They admit that it is sound knowledge of anatomy and physiology to know that human beings have heads, eyes, noses, arms, legs, &c., but insist that every child knows thus far, and that they expect learned anatomists and physiologists to exhibit greater knowledge in their peculiar studies than every child is in possession of. They say they look in vain, in the "Materia Medica Pura," for an accurate diagnosis in which individual nerve, tissue, organ, system, &c., are seated, each particular pain, ache, swelling, and what not, produced by hundreds and by thousands by every drug, inert or active, with which he experimented. They must know full well the great difficulty with which far greater evils than isolated and apparently trivial drug-symptoms are at times diagnosed, and ought to be perfectly willing to admit, as a partial excuse for the non-performance of this, the extreme difficulty and often, perhaps, utter impossibility of such a procedure. But it is now very possible to diagnose the exact locality of many permanent and severe pains and lesions, and our knowledge of the effects of drugs and poisons must not be considered perfect until such diagnosis be made; besides the exact application of the Hahnemannian method demands that, in order to cure, *the drug must act specifically upon the locality of the disease*, and if we know not upon what locality the drug acts, how can we cause it to impinge upon the seat of any disease? There are very many of the Hahnemannian school who possess the most accurate knowledge of anatomy and physiology, and are also adepts in the diagnosis of natural disease—it remains for them to perfect the diagnosis of drug-diseases. We suggest, as another and, perhaps, a true reason why Hahnemann could not complete the diagnosis of drug-diseases, the fact that, from the time of Bonet and Morgagni onward, rational diagnosis was falling into disrepute, because it did not suffice to detect structural alterations; while, as we have seen, the discovery of physical diagnosis did not take place until 1816, and we know that Hahnemann published his first tract in 1796, his "Materia Medica" in 1811, and his "Organon" in 1810. Hahnemann's method was, perhaps, the best which could have been adopted in his time, more than sixty years ago; but the immense advances which have been made, since his time, in physiology, histology, microscopy, pathological anatomy, and pathological chemistry, have not been properly incorporated in his system by his followers. He was eminently progressive; many of them are eminently stationary.

The arrangement of the isolated drug-symptoms above-mentioned, sharp critics admit, was the best which could have been instituted with the least trouble; but, they say, it would certainly have been better to have pointed out not merely upon what organ a drug acted, and the manner of its action, but also the exact part, tissue, &c., of the organ it affected particularly. But, they assume, science was outraged when Hahnemann laid violent hands upon his groups of drug-effects and upon his drug-diseases, and scattered their component parts like to the twenty-four winds of heaven, by forcing them into the same arrangement which he had adopted for his isolated drug-symptoms; thus destroying every trace of the chronological, causal, or sympathetic relations which the individual parts of groups of drug-effects and diseases bore to one another. They say, as well might an artist, who is in possession of a large collection of fragments of statuary, and a smaller one of entire statues, commence by arranging all the fragmentary heads, arms, legs, &c., together, and then proceed to break off the heads, arms, legs, &c., of his perfect statues, and arrange their fragments in like manner as the first, in order to have unity of arrangement, and exact systematic order.

But they have thus far been acting on the supposition that the symptoms detailed in the "Materia Medica Pura" are truly the effects of drugs. It, however, has been proven incontestibly, say they, that Hahnemann and his aids noted down almost every abnormal sensation, &c., which accrued, from the commencement of their experiments to their termination, and hence think it is but fair to infer that some accidental catarrhs, rheumatisms, headaches, eruptions, &c., &c., are put down as the effects of drugs. They assume that Hahnemann no doubt possessed as ardent an impulse to collect drug-symptoms as a miser has to collect the goods of this earth; but suppose misers rarely collect worthless things, but only close their lean and skinny fingers upon jewels and gold—they would that Hahnemann had collected only very important, positively true, and practically useful effects of drugs. They cite the anecdote of Lessing, the celebrated philosopher and critic, in which it is said that, while a mere lad, he and a school-companion each began to form a collection of minerals, and labored with equal industry. They separated after a while, and did not meet again for years, when the first question was: "Do you still continue your collection of minerals?" Lessing responded by leading his friend to a choice, but small cabinet; the latter in astonishment exclaimed: "Why, you had more when a mere school-boy, and my collection is more extensive by an hundred-fold; in fact, I still have every mineral, worthless or priceless, that I ever was in possession of." Lessing, the critic, drily remarked, that he had early commenced to throw many of his away. Supercilious and impatient critics assume, that if Hahnemann had exerted a rigid criticism over his collection of drug-effects, if he had ever and constantly struggled to ascertain the exact value of each of his acquisitions, he would have employed some of his untiring industry and honest zeal in throwing away, and that part of the medical world would never have fallen into the belief, that Chamomile-flowers, charcoal, and chalk, produce thousands upon thousands of strange effects.

But this is a very one-sided, and, by far, by very far, the darkest side which can be given of the "Materia Medica Pura." With much irrelevant and badly-arranged matter, it contains, beyond all comparison, a much more extended account of the effects of drugs than is to be found in all other materia medicas, taken collectively, which have ever been published, and it must still be regarded as a great authority in therapeutics. It is true that its details are so voluminous, as to become, in some measure, confusing, and that it requires an immense amount of patient and laborious study to attain even to a respectable amount of knowledge of its contents, and even then one is very apt to overlook the peculiar and specific action of drugs, on account of the vast accumulation of secondary, accidental, or occasional effects which are there recorded. Yet, if physicians would be pains-taking enough to use several, or a dozen, or even more common materia medicas, as commentaries or grammars to this huge work, i. e., the "Materia Medica Pura," they would be astounded at the vast flood of knowledge which will thus be elicited by comparison and contrast.

If, to the legacy of symptoms contained in the "Materia Medica Pura," we add the knowledge of a great therapeutic law, for the correct application of drugs to the cure of disease, the advantages of the homœopathic materia medica and therapeutics may become forcibly evident to every one.

We forbear to enter more minutely here into the difficulties of treating disease with no other guide than the "Materia Medica Pura," and, although we honestly think that the homœopathic method offers, even in its present condition, an excellent means of curing many diseases, yet experience teaches us that its application is always laborious, frequently uncertain, and often utterly impracticable, and hence we must add that, although much has been done, yet much more remains to be effected. Still, when we call to mind what Hahnemann and the homœopathic school have done to increase our knowledge of the action of drugs, and what they have tried to do towards rendering the cure of disease more certain, quick, and gentle, we become disarmed of all reproach and invective, which we think due to the manifold errors and inconsistencies into which some of this school have plunged, and cheerfully take our stand as one of the upholders of some of the truths which we conceive to be contained in the doctrines of this as yet reviled and persecuted sect. We have no wish to detract from the merits of Hahnemann, but, on the contrary, have a sincere desire to see him elevated from the station of a reviled leader of a comparatively small and despised sect, to the rank of a universally-respected and great reformer in medicine; that he may be regarded, by the whole medical world, as a highly philanthropic and generous man, and a truly noble-minded and skilful physician. We cherish the ardent hope that his name, too, may soon be enrolled, by common consent, in that "invisible church of genuine physicians, who, faithful to nature, have been actuated by her spirit, and have always acted according to her intimations, and have preserved her holy word;" we earnestly wish that the time may not be far distant when his name will be honorably associated by all with those of Hippocrates, Sydenham, &c. But, in order that that time may soon, as it inevitably must come, homœopathy must not only be lifted from its present empirical basis into a science, but must be purged from numberless crudities, errors and absurdities, which have crept into and still defile it.

The physiology of many homœopathists commences with the vital powers, and ends in the consideration of a part only of the vital functions, particularly those of sensation; while those functions which tend to structure and composition are comparatively neglected; hence it dispenses almost entirely with anatomy and physiological chemistry. As their notions of pathology are based upon such physiology, they consist almost solely in a consideration of the aberrations of the vital power and of sensation, while alterations of structure and composition, or pathological anatomy and chemistry, find no place in them. Hence their theories of health and disease are one-sided vital theories. The consequence is, that dynamic and functional diseases are more within the control of their remedies than alterations of the structure and chemistry of the body.

The pathologico-anatomical school commenced at the opposite extreme. Their physiology was almost sunken into anatomy, while their pathology scarcely outstept the bounds of pathological anatomy. The vital functions, except those which preside over structure, were almost unheeded; of the vital powers they were so profoundly ignorant, that they thought them the result of organization; hence their notions or theories were one-sided, material, physical, or mechanical ones. One would suppose that this school cured structural alterations with the same readiness that the homœopathic cures functional diseases. But, until lately, the former, unlike the latter, were not in possession of a great therapeutic law; the knowledge of disease was the strong side of the one, the cure of disease is the bright side of the other, and we have no hesitation in adding that the homœopathic school often cure even structural lesions with far greater facility than the pathologico-anatomical, whose therapeutic means were mostly confined within the narrow, but sanguinary or puerile limits of blood-letting, cupping, leeching, Mercury, Antimony, Opium, starving, tsisans, and gum-water. But, if the pathology of the homœopathic school be extended, so as to embrace pathological anatomy and pathological chemistry, and if their knowledge of the action of drugs be enlarged, so as to include their pathologico-anatomical and pathologico-chemical effects, then we have not the least hesitancy in asserting that, by means of the homœopathic and other therapeutic laws, we may, in time, be able to cure some structural and chemico-vital diseases with the same certainty, if not with the same celerity that we are able to diagnose structural lesions by means of physical diagnosis. And the homœopathic school may place themselves *instanter* in position to effect this—the works of Andral, Louis, Gross, and Rokitansky, on pathological anatomy; those of Liebig, Simon, Lehman, Berzelius, and Dumas, on physiological and pathological chemistry; those of Laennec, Stokes, Raciborski, and Skoda, on physical diagnosis; those of Magendie, Orfila, and Wibmer, on the pathologico-anatomical effects of drugs; and those of Christison, Orfila, Sobernheim, &c., on toxicology, will enable us to take this giant stride as soon as their contents be mastered.

We here feel ourselves constrained to add a few remarks upon the well-known law, "*similia similibus curantur.*" It is self-evident that, in order to cure any disease, a *different* state or condition of things must ultimately be induced. It is well known that Hahnemann insists strongly that the action of the curative agent must not be identical, but only similar to that of the disease to be cured. He admits that the greatest similarity, i. e., identity, would certainly add so much more to the already existing disease, and, of course, aggravate it; while he asserts that a *lesser*, though still a great similarity of action, between that of the drug and disease, will be followed by a cure, in which the drug-action is first substituted for that of the disease, which is, as it were, driven out or dislocated; next, the drug-action, which is transient, gradually subsides, and a perfect freedom from all complaint is the result. *Of course, only something different can be substituted*, for, if it were identical, we have seen that it would be added to swell the amount of original suffering. In point of fact, all similarity presupposes and includes some *difference*, which is an essential element in every cure, and homœopathic remedies hence exert a differential or an alterative action.

But the question may be put, may we not dispense with the similarity, and cure with drugs which only act *different* or opposite to the action of the disease? We unhesitatingly reply in the affirmative, and assert that any drug, which acts specifically upon the locality of the disease, may reasonably be expected to effect a cure, act it similar, different, or opposite, for it is evident that two different actions cannot go on at the same time in the same place; one of the two, viz., the weakest, must cease. Hence, if the dose be well proportioned, and the drug be powerful enough, a time must arrive when the diseased action ceases, and the drug-action is about being substituted; at this juncture a cure of the disease is effected, but a drug-disease may supply its place, if the physician has not wit enough to withhold the further application of his drugs. It will now be seen that the dogmas, "*similia similibus*," and "*contraria contrariis curantur*," are only relative—the main law which Hahnemann's disciples wish to confine to, "*similia similibus*," exclusively, belongs neither to this nor to its opposite, but lies between, in a common centre, in which both laws unite and become one. This common centre is *difference*, for similarity, difference, and opposition all agree in being *greater or less degrees of difference.* We must, then, unconditionally deny that homœopathic remedies only are specifics. To render this more clear, we suggest that the homœopathic method might be extended, so as to embrace not only the exciting of a similar state in the very same locality, system, organ, tissue, or function which is affected by the disease, but also in similar parts and different. The confines of the antipathic method may be enlarged so as to include not only the production of an opposite condition in the very parts diseased, but also in similar and different systems, tissues, organs, and functions. The boundaries of the allopathic method, of course, admit of the same extension. Then we would say that the production of similar, different, or opposite states in the very parts, or of the very functions implicated by the disease, must all be regarded as *direct* and *specific* methods. The proper application of these methods demands the most accurate knowledge of the every action of remedies, both upon the sick and healthy, upon men and animals.

On the other hand the exciting of similar, different, or opposite states, not in the very parts diseased, but in similar, different, or remote parts, must be regarded as indirect or revulsive methods, which may occasionally prove useful. With the aid of all these methods, we need not be fearful of curing too many diseases, and, doubtless, a century hence we shall hear no longer of exclusive homœopathists, allopathists, or antipathists, but every physician will strive to apply all these various methods skilfully and accurately.

It is well known that it has long been insisted, by a small sect of medical men, that the homœopathic is the only true method, and that it is applicable to every variety of disease. I have labored long and zealously to prove that the homœopathic is a true, safe, and certain method of treating very many diseases; but I deny that there is any proof extant that diseases can be cured by no other method. Besides, homœopathic remedies have not yet been discovered for all varieties of disease, some of which we know, to our cost, are only cured slowly and unsatisfactorily; hence, even admitting, for the sake of argument, that the homœopathic is the only specific and direct method, no physician is, as yet, justified in rejecting the indirect and palliative methods.

On the other hand, many diseases have no opposites; what, for instance, is the opposite of a headache, a pustular eruption, a rheumatism, an erysipelas, &c., &c.? Hence, if it be absolutely necessary to create an opposite state, in order to cure any given disease, very many diseases must necessarily be absolutely incurable. *The antipathic method never can be an exclusive and universal one.*

Again, diseases are often so painful and dangerous that every expedient which the ingenuity of man can devise, for relief or cure, may be brought in play. No physician is justified in sacrificing the life or comfort of those who rely upon him with confidence, under their afflictions, to a system or a theory. In future ages, universal and exclusive systems may, perhaps, come to be regarded in the same light as universal panaceas for "all the ills that flesh are heir to."

We would merely add here, that, in like manner as we regard pathological anatomy and physical diagnosis as the greatest advances which have as yet been made in the study of disease, so do we regard the specific method as one of the greatest advances which has yet been made in the study of the cure of disease. But a century may tell a different tale; much has been done, but much more remains to be done. In like manner, as Morgagni, the father of pathological anatomy, has been far outstripped by Andral, Louis, Cruvelhier, Rokitansky, &c., and Laennec, the father of physical diagnosis, has been far surpassed by Piorry and Skoda, so should Hahnemann, the father of specific medicine, be far outstripped in the study of the cure of disease, or else the practice of medicine must remain comparatively stationary where he left it, almost a quarter of a century ago. The labors of those who came after them only served to reflect credit upon Morgagni and Laennec, so will the labors of those who come after him reflect more and more credit upon Hahnemann.

As the so-called homœopathic and allopathic methods now divide and alienate the medical world, I intend more particularly to apply the above modes, rules, and principles of examination to them, especially as the two methods are almost universally regarded as diametrically opposed to each other, and as incapable even of compromise, much less of union. But, if there be some truth in each, then there must be some principle common to both; if there be no such principle, then one or the other method must be absolutely and totally false, for every true theory or generalization must not only be a legitimate deduction from many facts, but, also, must not be opposed to other and equally well substantiated facts. A true theory, deduction, or generalization must not only help us to a complete view and explanation of all the hitherto discovered facts, but all pertinent facts which may be hereafter discovered must be in accordance with it, else it must be a mere fragment of some more general law, still to be sought for and discovered.

Hahnemann was the first to assume the theory or generalization, that there can be but *three* modes of medical treatment, viz.:

1. The *antipathic* or *antagonistic* mode—based upon the old Galenical law, "*contraria contrariis curantur*," and which he affirms to be simply a rule for palliation, never of cure.

2. The *allopathic* or *alterative* mode—characterized by the giving of remedies which act differently, i. e., neither similarly nor antagonistically to the action of the disease; in accordance with the axiom, that in order to cure any disease, a different state of things must be brought about. This, Hahnemann also declares to be merely palliative.

3. The *Homœopathic*—consisting in the administration of remedies which act similarly, i. e., neither identically nor widely different from the action of the disease. This he declares to be the only curative and truly specific mode.

Hahnemann and his followers could perceive that the antipathic and allopathic, i. e., the antagonistic and alterative methods, were allied to each other, for antagonism is merely the *greatest degree* of difference; but both he and they have repeatedly declared the homœopathic method to be as different from the two others as day and night, forgetting that there are degrees of similarity as well as of difference; that, although similar things resemble each other, they also differ; that similarity always includes and presupposes some difference; that, in fact, similarity is merely the least degree of difference, and that, therefore, the homœopathic method is only relatively different from, not absolutely opposed to the alterative method, and this, in its turn, we have seen, is only relatively different from the antagonistic method.

Although Hahnemann, in his reasoning, assumes the homœopathic method to be as different from the alterative as day is from night, yet, in his explanations, he is repeatedly forced to admit the contrary. Thus, he says, in one paragraph of his "Organon": "Without a natural *difference* between the action of the medicine and that of the disease no cure could possibly take place, but, surely, an addition to or aggravation of the evil." Again, (see German "Organon," p. 68,) he tells us, that, "If we apply continually to a frozen limb the same degree of cold which originally froze it, a cure will not take place isopathically, but the part will remain lifeless and dead; if, however, we apply a somewhat lesser degree of cold, [i. e., a somewhat greater degree of warmth,] we will gradually restore the limb to comfortable temperature, and effect a cure homœopathically. Thus, if the room in which the frosted patient is, be at the temperature of +10°, Reaumur, and the cold applications be at +1°, Reaumur, and the frozen part be at zero, then the cold application will supply one degree of warmth to the limb, and the surrounding atmosphere of the room will gradually supply nine degrees more." Hence, it is not the constant application of cold, but the gradual application of warmth which effects an alterato-antagonistic cure. To treat a frost-bite according to the antipathic or antagonistic mode, we should apply a sudden and extreme degree of warmth to the frozen limb—this is notoriously injurious. According to the allopathic mode, we should apply a medium degree of heat, persistently—this is well known to be dangerous; while, according to the homœopathic method, we should apply a slight degree of warmth, gradually increased—this is the only safe way, but it will be seen that in this instance the three methods differ in degree only, not in kind.

Again, Hahnemann tells us, that, "A hand scalded with boiling water will not be cured isopathically by the fresh application of scalding hot water, but we may cure it homœopathically by contact with a lesser degree of warmth, [i. e., by a somewhat greater degree of cold]; thus, if we place the scalded part in a vessel filled with warm water, at the temperature of 60°, Reaumur, the water will gradually become somewhat less hot, i. e., more cold, until, finally, it and the scalded part will very gradually have fallen to the temperature of the room." The antagonistic mode would require us to apply ice or ice-water to the scalded part, and this might, doubtless, bring on mortification. The alterative method would oblige us to use cold applications, which might or might not be dangerous; while the homœopathic method directs us to apply warm, or even moderately hot fomentations, gradually reducing the temperature. Still, the three methods again differ in degree only, not in kind.

To a starving person, we would first administer, homœopathically, such small quantities of food as would enhunger, if not almost starve a hearty person, but gradually the quantity must be increased until the patient is on full diet. The allopathic mode would oblige us to give much food at once, and the bad consequences which would follow are too well known to require mention; while the antipathic method would call for a surfeit.

All the above so-called homœopathic cures consist in the *gradual* bringing about of a different or even opposite state, and we have seen that Hahnemann admits, and, in fact, assumes, that without a natural difference between the action of the remedy and that of the disease no cure can take place. We would next inquire how great a natural difference Hahnemann regards as necessary or admissible. He says, in section 45, "Two diseases, which *differ greatly* in their species, but resemble each other strongly [i. e., differ slightly] in their symptoms, always mutually destroy each other." Here we have a great essential difference and a slight symptomatic difference between the action of the drug and the disease allowed. Again, on page 138, we are told that, "A homœopathic remedy is not necessarily improperly chosen, even if several of the drug-effects are antagonistic, opposite, or antipathic to several of the medical and less important symptoms of the disease, provided that it covers the other characteristic and important symptoms." Hence, to sum up, we have a partial symptomatic antagonism allowed, *plus* a slight symptomatic difference, *plus* a great essential difference. Here is latitude enough to effect a gradual alterative, or even antagonistic cure, as in the case of the frozen, scalded, and starving persons. But we are not obliged to confine ourselves to generalities, for Hahnemann has furnished us with examples whereby to regulate our practice. In his proofs of the truth of the homœopathic method, he cites a case of purulent discharge from the bladder, cured by Uva-ursi, which drug, he truly says, is apt to cause a mucous discharge from that viscus; but there is a difference between mucus and pus, and the Uva-ursi may cure by altering, changing, or reducing a purulent to a mucous flux, which latter may then subside of itself or be removed. He also tells us that the vaccine fever has cured two cases of intermittent fever homœopathically, which experience, he says, confirms the assertion of John Hunter, that two fevers, i. e., two similar diseases, cannot exist in the same subject at the same time. But it is evident that there is a great difference between fevers, and, especially, between the vaccine and intermittent fevers—one is the result of an animal infection, the other of vegetable decomposition; the one is always inflammatory in its nature, with a strong tendency to suppurative inflammation, while the other is generally merely congestive, very rarely inflammatory, and, perhaps, never suppurative. He also cites a case of dysentery, said to have been cured homœopathically by a purgative; but purgatives generally cause merely an artificial diarrhœa, and there is much difference between diarrhœa and dysentery. Thus far, we are utterly at a loss for any good reason why the homœopathic method only should be truly curative and specific, and the alterative and antagonistic modes merely palliative, for they all agree in producing a greater or less degree of difference or alteration in the action of the disease: for by diminishing the dose, we might bring about a safe, prompt, and durable cure by allopathic and antipathic remedies. It is true that Hahnemann assumes the preference for the homœopathic mode because dissimilar diseases may coëxist in the organism; for their dissimilitude will allow of their occupying different regions or localities, while a stronger similar disease may exercise an influence upon the very parts occupied by the disease to be cured, and even throw itself by preference upon them, so that the original disease, finding no other organ to be acted upon, is necessarily extinguished. Hahnemann here almost admits that a specific remedy should act primarily upon the seat of the disease. But there is more than one *non sequitur* here: 1. The same parts, localities, or organs may be differently affected, although not at the same time; hence, if we can bring a differential or alterative influence to bear upon the seat of the disease we may dislodge it. 2. A remedy, which acts differently from the action of the disease, may also act by preference, or specifically, upon the parts occupied by the disease. 3. Remedies which act similarly to the action of the disease do not necessarily act specifically upon the seat of the disease, much less do they occupy the organism so completely that, if they dislodge the disease from its original seat, it can find no other organ, system, or locality to act upon. In point of fact, there may and must be a specific and curative alterative method, and a specific and curative antagonistic method, as well as a curative homœopathic mode. But I must first explain what I understand by specific drugs and remedies, disclaim empirical specific, and uphold rational specific treatment.

1. By a *specific drug*, I merely mean one which acts by preference, and in a certain, peculiar and characteristic manner upon certain parts, organs, or systems. A drug is a disturbing, perturbating, disease-producing, or pathogenetic agent.

2. By a *specific remedy*, or medicine, I refer to a curative agent, or drug, which not only acts by preference upon certain parts, organs, or systems of the organism, but exerts a curative influence upon all or some of the diseases of those parts, and thus becomes a remedy or medicine.

3. By *specific treatment* of disease, I merely mean the exhibition of such drugs and medicines as act peculiarly and specifically upon certain organs, parts, or systems, against the diseases of those parts. And here I hope to have found that direction in which Forbes thinks homœopathy is destined to be the remote, if not the immediate cause of more important fundamental changes in the practice of medicine than have resulted from any system of medicine promulgated since the days of Galen. As we may have three or more remedies acting equally specifically upon a certain locality, and yet acting, the one similarly, the other differently, and the third oppositely to the action of a given disease of that locality, we may have three varieties of specific treatment, viz.:

1. The *specific antipathic*, or *specific antagonistic* treatment—i. e., the exhibition of such medicines or remedies as act by preference upon the locality of the disease, and quite or nearly oppositely or antagonistically to the action of the disease.

2. *Specific allopathic*, i. e., *specific alterative* treatment—consisting in the use of such remedies as act by preference upon the seat of the disease to be cured, and specifically different from, i. e., neither exactly opposite, nor yet identical or similar to the action of the disease; and,

3. *Specific homœopathic* treatment—characterized by the use of such medicines as act by preference upon the seat of the disease, and similar to, yet somewhat different from the action of the disease.

But I may be required to prove that there are specific drugs and remedies, and that their specific virtues have been and can be discovered. Christison (see "On Poisons," p. 15,) says: "Drugs and poisons are commonly, but, he conceives, erroneously supposed to affect the general system. A few of them, such as Arsenic and Mercury, affect a great number of organs, but not the whole system, and even they affect some parts by preference; but by far the larger portion of drugs and medicines act on one or more organs only, and not upon the general system. Thus, Arsenic, whatever way it be introduced into the system, inflames the stomach and rectum. It has such a peculiar elective affinity for these parts that it will produce these effects even when the fumes of it are inhaled, and Headland (see *London Lancet*, Oct. 21, 1843,) says, he is unacquainted with any other fume or gas which will produce like effects. The specific action of Mercury upon the gums is also a very familiar, but by no means the most striking instance, although it will "touch the gums," even if rubbed upon the soles of the feet, or upon the inside of the thighs. Christison (*ibid.*, p. 372,) tells us that the effects of Chromate of Potash, when introduced into a wound in the thigh of a dog, are equally, if not still more remarkable. For, when thus applied, it seems to cause inflammation of the mucous membrane of the air-passages, specifically, for even the wound, to which it was originally applied, does not become much inflamed; but the larynx, bronchi, and minute ramifications of the air-tubes are found inflamed and to contain fragments of fibrinous exudation, evidently the result of previous inflammation, (reminding one of the action of the specific diseases, measles, scarlatina, and varioloid,) while the nostrils are filled with similar matters, and even the conjunctiva of the eyes are covered with mucous and purulent effusion. Again, however intense the inflammation of the stomach and bowels produced by Arsenic, Oxalic-acid, and many other acrid drugs, this rarely extends to the peritoneum, causing true peritonitis, which Corrosive Mercury, Colocynth, and the mineral acids are very apt to produce, showing conclusively that these latter agents act specifically upon the peritoneum. Finally, Dr. Headland has seen Aconitine, when rubbed upon the skin of the arm or body, produce a remarkable state of the throat, amounting to distinct tonsillitis or quinsy; and this specific action of Aconite constrained Dr. Headland to endeavor to draw the attention of the medical profession to the little progress which medical men have made in the knowledge of the peculiar and *specific* action of drugs and medicines—they being, at the end of fourteen hundred years, acquainted, as Colton truly says, with only two specifics! These examples may suffice, for the present, to prove that specific drugs do exist. It now remains to be seen whether specific remedies or medicines are known, and whether specific treatment is practicable and desirable.

In the American reprint of the *London Lancet*, vol. ii, p. 823, we read, that "Many thoughtful men, who practice medicine, are unwilling to acknowledge that any of those medicines which are sometimes termed 'specific,' really possess any specific quality. There is, however, reason, on close inspection, to admit that the belief in specific remedies, for particular morbid tissues or actions, is in strict analogy with much that we know positively of the functions of life, both in health and disease. In health, various organs are subject to peculiar and appropriate stimuli, which excite in them actions that would not be excited by the same stimuli in other organs. Thus light stimulates the retina to vision; vibrations of the air excite the nerve of the ear to hearing; food elicits from the alimentary canal those secretions which are requisite for its digestion. The blood is called a universal stimulus, but each of its component parts stand in a *specific* relation to some particular tissue or organ; for, while the blood supplies every part, indiscriminately, with the materials of nutrition and renovation, each part, so supplied, exercises a peculiar and specific function, in selecting such of the constituents of the blood as are capable of ministering to that function. These are unquestionable facts in physiology; and what is the inference that may be directly derived from them, in relation to our present subject, namely, the specific treatment of disease? Simply that every healthy vital action results from the operation of a specific substance on a particular texture, function, organ, or system. What is proposed, in the administration of curative agents, but to reëxcite those normal actions, the departure from which produces and constitutes the morbid state? Why, then, should we reject the doctrine of operating, to restore health by means that are analagous to those which nature uses for the maintenance of health, i. e., by applying to the diseased parts, tissues, or organs such substances as are capable of exerting specific actions upon those tissues or organs? According to such experiments as have as yet been made, every substance which exerts a specific action on a part is found to excite that action, as well when injected into the circulation, introduced into a wound in the skin, or into the nostrils, rectum, vagina, &c., as when introduced directly into the stomach; thereby demonstrating that it acts specifically upon the part, or parts, and is more capable of being placed in relation to the vital endowments of those parts than to those of any other. That, in short, it is a "specific," which acts in a precisely parallel manner to that of the "natural specifics," by which all the healthy vital functions are excited and sustained. While this principle—which is one of the most important and universal in the philosophy of medicine—has hitherto been but little recognized and admitted, many specifics have been and are still used blindly and empirically. It is remarkable that, however little the above positions have been adopted into the theory of medicine, the ordinary language of medicine has always borne testimony to the specific action of drugs and medicines on particular parts or organs. The very names of the different classes of medicines imply a full recognition of the above fact. What do we mean by purgatives, emetics, emmenagogues, sudorifics, diuretics, &c., except that these articles exert a peculiar and characteristic, in short, specific action upon the stomach, bowels, uterus, skin, or kidneys, &c.? Aloes will purge, whether introduced into an ulcer upon the leg, an issue upon the arm or any other part of the body, when injected into a vein, &c., as well as when introduced into the stomach, and hence is a specific purgative. Tartar-emetic will cause vomiting when injected into a vein, and hence is a specific emetic, &c. All remedies which do not act specifically upon the locality of the disease, can only cure by setting up a new or more powerful action upon more or less distant and healthy parts; thus drawing off, by so-called counter-irritation or revulsion, the lesser irritation which is going on in the diseased part. There are also three varieties of revulsive treatment, namely:

1. *Antipathic revulsive treatment*—Consisting in the use of remedies which act opposite or antagonistic to the action of the disease, and upon parts more or less distant from the locality of the disease.

2. *Allopathic revulsive treatment*—Characterized by the use of remedies which act differently from, i. e., neither opposite, identical, nor very similar to the action of the disease, and upon parts more or less distant from the locality of the disease. These two modes of medical practice are so well known that it is, perhaps, unnecessary to cite examples of them; but it is well to add here, that all of Hahnemann's remarks against antipathic and allopathic treatment are leveled solely against the revulsive, and not against the specific methods. Thus, he inveighs, with some justice, against the indirect mode of applying stronger heterogeneous irritations to parts distant from the seat of the disease, thus exciting and keeping up irritations in, or evacuations from organs dissimilar in structure and tissue from the parts really diseased, in order to turn the course of the disease toward the new locality selected by the physician. Again, he says, the aim of old-school physicians is to direct, or draw toward the parts they irritate, that morbid action which the vital powers have developed in the parts primarily diseased, and thus they seek violently to dislodge or drag off the natural disease, by exciting and keeping up a stronger heterogeneous irritation or disease, in healthy, although less important parts; that is, they make use of violent, painful, and indirect or circuitous means.

3. *Homœopathic revulsive treatment*—Consisting in the use of remedies which act similar to, yet somewhat different from the action of the disease, and upon more or less distant parts. This variety of treatment has long been recognized and practiced upon by dominant-school physicians. Thus, Mac Cartney (see "Treatise on Inflammation,") says: "We would observe that, *a priori*, it appears reasonable, and experience, we think, bears out the presumption that the mode of counter-irritation or revulsion should have a sort of physiological [pathological?] relation to the primitive morbid action. Thus, in internal diseases, characterized by a tendency to effusion of serum and lymph, blisters, which excite serous inflammation, with effusion of serum and lymph from the external surface of the skin, are advantageous—inflammations of the serous and synovial membranes are examples of the fact. While, in chronic diseases, especially such as are disposed to end in the formation of pus, those counter-irritants which produce a purulent secretion from the surface generally answer best. Thus, in ulceration of the cartilages of the joints, with effusion of pus, and in caries of the vertebræ, with formation of abscess, issues and setons, which excite a secretion of pus, are preferable to blisters, which merely cause an effusion of serum. Also, in scrofulous ulceration of the lungs, i. e., in phthisis, frictions with Tartar-emetic ointment, which produces

suppurative or purulent inflammation of the skin, are preferable to any other mode of counter-irritation. In the slighter morbid actions, which consist of simple congestions or determinations of blood, rubefacients are often sufficient." The use of blisters, in pleurisy, is also an example of homœopathic *revulsive* treatment, although, if the physician be not careful, it may become truly homœopathic, or even isopathic; for we read, in the American reprint of the *London Lancet*, vol. i., p. 301, that "A respectable surgeon found, on opening the cranium of a patient who had died after a blister had been recently applied, an inflamed mark, exactly corresponding in size and form with the external mark of the blister, which penetrated through the scalp and cranium, and was distinctly visible upon the dura mater. Again, we learn, from the same source, that another surgeon has repeatedly seen marks on the pleura, covering the lungs, having the size and shape of the blister which had been applied to the chest; and the same on the intestinal peritoneum, of the size and shape of the blister which had been applied to the abdomen. Porter (see "Surgical Observations on Diseases of the Larynx,") gives a case, where, in an acute inflammation of the lungs, the application of a blister was followed by aggravation of the symptoms, and, after death, a portion of the surface of the lung, exactly corresponding to the size and shape of the blister, was found in a more advanced stage of inflammation than the remaining parts of the lungs. Hence, it will not do for those physicians who use blisters freely in inflammatory affections, to scoff at the internal administration of small doses of Cantharides, Phosphor., Rhus., &c.; for a portion of Cantharides is frequently absorbed into the general system when a blister is applied, for strangury and increase of fever is not an uncommon occurrence, and the homœopathist may well assume that some of the so-called efficacy of blisters, in inflammations, is owing to the homœopathic curative action of that portion of Cantharides which has been absorbed, although this may have been too small to affect the kidneys. Another example of homœopathic revulsive treatment will be recognized in the common practice of using diuretics, sudorifics, or hydragogue cathartics in dropsy, for it is evident that these remedies act by exciting a profuse watery or serous discharge from free surfaces, in order to draw off like accumulations from shut cavities.

The question now arises, are we to reject any of these modes of treatment? If one mode be, as a general rule, preferable to all the others, are we hence to neglect the others entirely? Need we be afraid, with the aid of them all, of curing or relieving too many sick persons? Experience gives the only solution to these queries, and to that Hahnemann himself appeals, in his twenty-second paragraph, where he says: "If experience prove that the drugs which produce symptoms similar to, but somewhat different from those of the disease to be cured, also cure it in the most certain and permanent manner, then ought we to select such remedies in preference. If, on the contrary, experience prove that the most certain and permanent cures are to be obtained by remedies that act different or directly opposite to those of the disease, then the latter ought to be selected."

1. In proof of the efficacy of *specific antipathic treatment*, I cite the use of Secale in atony of the uterus. According to Sobernheim, (see "Materia Medica," vol. i., p. 51,) in seven hundred and twenty cases where it was used, it acted favorably in six hundred cases of tardy delivery, from deficient contraction of the uterus; also in five cases of retention of placenta, from the same cause; in five cases of hæmorrhage, also from the same cause; in sixteen cases, it was used with partial good effects only; in eighty-two cases, it failed, from bad quality of the drug or some other cause, but without bad effect, either upon mother or child; while in twelve cases only it acted injuriously, either to mother or child, or both. Again, according to Dungleson, (see "New Remedies," p. 437,) Professor Von Busch, of Berlin, used the Secale in one hundred and seventy-five cases, on account of deficiency of labor-pains, and one hundred and seventy-seven children were born, two of them being twins. Of these, one hundred and forty-two were born alive and well, evidently not at all injured by the Ergot; eighteen were in a state of asphyxia, which was removed by appropriate treatment—hence, if we assume that the asphyxia was produced in every case by the Ergot, it did not proceed to a fatal extent in any case; finally, seventeen were still-born, and of these seven were evidently dead before labor set in, as they were more or less putrid; ten died during labor, from various accidents and operations, such as prolapsus of cord, turning, perforation of head, &c., so that there was only one case of death of the child which could be referred to the Ergot, and, even in that case, there was no reasonable ground for such an inference. Hence, I agree with Dr. Hempel, that true, direct, and specific antipathic remedies do exist, and may and should be used under certain circumstances, for the purpose of making the patient comfortable, of arresting immediate and threatening danger, and in cases where we are sure of the true antipathic action of the drug, and no other treatment is required than that of holding the disease in check, for a time, by an antagonizing influence. Hence, I also agree with Rau, (see "Organon," Hempel's translation, p. 26,) that: "Antipathic treatment should not be rejected generally, as has been done by some vehement advocates of the homœopathic system; peaceful, impartial, and experienced physicians will keep aloof from that blind zeal which denies that happy results have been and will again be obtained by antipathic or antagonistic treatment."

2. The *specific allopathic*, or *specific alterative treatment*, is often-

times more difficult of application than the antipathic, for, although it may suffice, at times, merely to select a remedy which acts specifically upon the locality of the disease, and specifically different from the action of the disease; yet, at other times, disease is such a strange compound or hybrid of injurious processes and salutary reactions that we are forced to select a remedy, which not only acts specifically upon the seat of the disease, but specifically different from the injurious, and specifically similar to the salutary tendencies or terminations of the disease. Thus, in the first stage of pneumonia, we have a viscid and extremely tenacious secretion from the walls of the air-cells, through which the passage of air, in inspiration, occasions the true crepitant rhonchus, heard only at the end of inspiration. In the second stage, we have the air-cells completely blocked up with this viscid secretion, and still more plastic and fibrinous products, so similar in character to the exudation of true croup that Rokitansky styles hepatization of the lungs a true, croupous, pulmonary inflammation. This is the climax or acme of pneumonia, and from thence, in favorable cases, commences the retrograde or resolving salutary process; for serum is exhaled from the walls of the air-cells, and in it the plastic, fibrinous, or croupous exudation is first partially, then completely dissolved and broken down into a sero-mucous and muco-purulent matter, through which air again begins to penetrate, causing sub-crepitant rhonchus, heard both during inspiration and expiration, and finally it is cast out by critical expectoration. The true curative indication is to select a remedy which acts differently from the first or progressive stage, and similarly to the second or retrograding and curative process. As the inflammation is eminently plastic, fibrinous, and adhesive in its nature, we should, according to the specific alterative method, avoid remedies like the Nitrate of Silver, which excite adhesive inflammation, and may select Tartar-emetic, which causes purulent or suppurative inflammation, or Hydriodate of Potash, which excites mucous inflammation, or Cantharides, which excites serous inflammation; for nature cures pneumonia by substituting a serous, mucous, or purulent inflammation in the place of the original plastic and fibrinous one. Finally, when the inflammation has subsided, and a mere blenorrhœa remains, the expectorant blenorrhœagogues, such as Phosphor., Senega, Sambucus, &c., which are powerless in the first stage, may complete the cure. Again, in true or membranous croup, large quantities of tough, leathery, plastic, and fibrinous false membranes are secreted from the walls of the larynx, trachea, and bronchi; while, according to Dr. Ware, the natural cure of the disease is accomplished by the setting in of suppurative inflammation upon the diseased surface of the air-passages, by which the false membranes are detached, and may finally be expelled by coughing, and the natural cure is attended with copious expectoration of pus, with or without the presence of pieces of the false membrane, which becomes more or less completely, or often perfectly dissolved in the pus. The true *specific alterative mode* would require us to select a remedy which specifically produces a suppurative process on the mucous surface of the air-passages; this, if given early enough, would effectually prevent the formation of tough, leathery, and fibrinous false membranes, or, if already formed, would hasten their detachment, solution, and expulsion. Again, there are numerous varieties of inflammation, viz.: the plastic, adhesive or so-called fibrinous, the ulcerative, the purulent or suppurative, the mucous, serous, rheumatic, erysipelatous, &c., &c. Now, if ulcerative inflammation were committing its ravages, this mode would render it proper and advisable to give remedies which excite adhesive inflammation; if suppurative inflammation were progressing, we would be required to give remedies which excite mucous inflammation, and this has been done successfully. Not to appeal, a second time, to Hahnemann's cure of suppurative inflammation of the bladder by Uva-ursi, which excites mucous irritation of that viscus, I will appeal to the experience of Ricord, (see *London Lancet*, vol. i., p. 365,) from which we learn that the Iodide of Potassium often produces a catarrh of the nose, but without any disposition to pass into the suppurative stage. The catarrhal mucus provoked by the Iodide does not ripen, and if, indeed, previously to the administration of the remedy, there had existed a purulent secretion from the nose, this secretion, unless it has its origin in a carious state of the bones of the nose, will probably diminish and disappear under the influence of the Iodide. Again, in the so-called dry inflammations, the rules of the specific alterative mode would render it manifestly proper to administer even irritating remedies, which specifically induce serous or mucous secretions; in affections attended with the discharge of thin, ill-conditioned, and ichorous pus, we would give remedies which naturally tend to produce the secretion of healthy, cream-colored, and benign pus. This specific alterative method, it will be seen, requires the most extensive and accurate knowledge of the nature, course, tendencies, and natural terminations of disease, and forces a most comprehensive knowledge of the peculiar actions of drugs and medicines.

3. *The specific homœopathic method* is equally sustained by facts. Thus, Lead and Alum are both astringents, both cause constipation and colic; yet Eberlee (see "Materia Medica,") says, Alum is one of the most effectual remedies we possess in lead-colic, and quotes Richter, who speaks in the most exalted terms of its good effects in this painful and often intractable complaint, and adds that the testimony of a great many eminent writers might be adduced in favor of its virtues in this respect. Sobernheim (see "Materia Medica,") says, Grashius, Gendrin, Sunderlin, and Remer, advise Alum in lead-colic, while Kopp recommends

it in habitual colic. Noack says it is advised, especially in the chronic lead-colic, by Quarin, Schlegel, Zurken, Gebel, Goetze, and Montanciex. Dierbach (see "Materia Medica,") advises it in flatulent colic, and thinks it may prove useful in lead-colic. Vogt, (see "Materia Medica,") and also Pereira (see "Materia Medica,") says, in the treatment of lead-colic Alum has been found more useful than any other agent, or even whole class of remedies, and informs us that it was first used in this disease by Grashius, in 1752, and was afterwards administered, in fifteen cases, by Dr. Percival, with great success; and, finally, its efficacy has been fully established by Kapeller, physician to the Hospital St. Antoine, in Paris, and by Gendrin and Dr. Copland, not to mention numerous other distinguished authorities. It allays vomiting, abates flatulence, mitigates pain, and *even opens the bowels* more certainly than any other remedy, and frequently succeeds in the latter result when other powerful drugs and even purgatives have failed.

I have purposely cited this example, as one in which no rational explanation can, as yet, be given how the homœopathic cure takes place; we must be contented with the fact, and should be willing to institute analogous treatment in other diseases. But many homœopathic cures can be explained rationally, for the organism, even in its healthy state, is constantly carrying on an incessant struggle for its existence and normal preservation against the numerous exciting causes of disease, and when disease has attained a lodgment in the system, this preservative endeavor is prolonged into a curative one. As this preservative and curative endeavor is essential to life, it is never entirely wanting in any sick person, and hence the symptoms or signs of the same, viz., the reactive or curative endeavors are always evident, although, at times, in very slight and scarcely perceptible degrees, and they cease only when death sets in. The reactive or curative symptoms must not be regarded as something entirely new and peculiar to the sick organism, for they also occur during health, the whole difference between the reactive symptoms of the healthy and sick organism is, that the former are the phenomena of a struggle with the causes of disease, the latter, those with the disease itself. Hence, a more or less partial homœopathic treatment must form an element in the management of every disease; a portion of the treatment, viz., that which corresponds with and aids the curative endeavor, must always be homœopathic in kind, but not always in degree. If the reactive or curative endeavor be too slight, we must give remedies which act similar to, but more powerfully than the feeble curative action; if the reaction be sufficient, we may give remedies which act similar to, and equally or somewhat less intense, in order fully to sustain and keep it up; if the reaction be too violent, it must be moderated.

It is well known that Hippocrates was the first who clearly taught that it is the most important duty of the physician to watch the operations of nature, with the view of promoting those actions which appear to be salutary, and of checking or suppressing those which appear to be hurtful. The tendency of such precepts is to induce great caution in the treatment of diseases. Much was left to the superintendence of nature, in the salutary and self-correcting operations of which the Hippocratists placed a too implicit credence. The Hippocratic method requires a knowledge of what actions are salutary, and which injurious.

We commence (1) with the consideration of *fever*, the very name of which is said, by some, to be derived from *februo*, to purify. Gregory (see "Practice," p. 50,) says, "The earliest opinion on the nature of fever was that of Hippocrates, who imagined it to be a salutary effort of nature to throw off some noxious influence or matter; and it is remarkable that this opinion was entertained before the class of eruptive fevers were known, the phenomena of which certainly afford the greatest countenance to it." Stahl supported the same view, but acknowledged that, when the morbific matter was too abundant, or the vital powers not sufficiently energetic, fevers were hurtful. When speaking of the treatment of fever, (page 54,) Gregory says, "The most important feature to the physician is the natural tendency, in all febrile diseases, to run a certain course and terminate in the restoration of health. This is very strikingly illustrated in continued and eruptive fevers. The latter will always, and the former very frequently, run their regular course, in spite of all the efforts of art. In ancient times, nay, even at no very distant period, it was made a question whether it was safe and proper to cut short a fever. It may be practicable to do this, but it never can become the foundation of our treatment of febrile diseases. The natural tendency, on the other hand, of them to come to a crisis, or to work their own cure, may be often kept in view with the best advantage, and, though the extravagancies of the expectant method are justly blamable, the spirit of the doctrine should never be disregarded." Again, Cullen taught that, in the cold stage of fever, the blood collected in the great vessels and heart, and thus was the efficient cause of exciting them to the increased action, which is the essence of the hot stage. Armstrong (see "On Fevers," p. 56,) says, in simple and in inflammatory fevers there is generally more or less rigor, but he has never met with a case of true congestive fever which set in with universal shivering. As congestive fevers are least apt, of all others, to effect their own cure, he says, "this might lead us to suppose that the cold shivering-fit was intimately connected with the production of the hot or febrile stage," which he, a few lines above, says, appears to be an endeavor of nature to restore the natural balance of the circulation. Hippocrates believed the same of the cold stage. Parry (see "Elements," p. 329,) says, "Shivering consists in short, quick, and frequently repeated convulsions of various muscles, and, being one variety of muscular exertion, may be regarded as a modification of exercise, often intended to restore circulation and heat to parts in which both are defective. He thinks, when shivering precedes suppuration, its purpose is to effect the effusion of the pus already formed and present in the vessels of the inflamed part. In cases of gall-stone, shivering assists the propulsion of the foreign body, &c." Galen, Frank, Stahl, Hoffmann, Boerhaave, &c., all entertained similar views of fever. It, hence, may prove a true method of treating fever, to give remedies which act similar to the curative endeavors of nature—not in one point only, as by exciting sweat, nor in two points only, as by increasing the fever and sweat; but in all points to the internal curative process, and to the critical evacuations which it brings about. This method is free from the dilatory and negative practice of the expectants, and, as it demands the most accurate knowledge of the action of remedies, it is free from the perverse methods of the rude empirics of giving drugs hap-hazard, or of the rational empirics. Finally, instead of being obliged to wait, like the Hippocratists, until critical discharges have commenced, we support and hasten the salutary processes, and end by carrying out the crisis and critical evacuations more perfectly and powerfully than unassisted nature might be able to accomplish. An example will, perhaps, render this position more clear. The periodical fits of gout were regarded by Sydenham as cardinal crises for purifying the blood and discharging the gouty salts. Colchicum has long been regarded as somewhat specific in this disease. Yet we read, in the *London Medical Gazette*, No. 24, that a woman, after drinking one ounce of Colchicum tincture, was seized with severe stitches of pain in the fingers and toes—all the hand and foot-joints became swollen and painful; subsequently, pains in the shoulder and hip-joints ensued. When these reached their acme, they were relieved by the occurrence of profuse sour-smelling sweat. The reporter adds, "The whole presented the appearance of a rheumatic fever." Again, in the *Med. Chir. Rev.*, Oct., 1835, p. 375, we learn, from Dr. Weatherhead, that uric-acid, or its base, urea, superabounds in the blood of gouty people; that gouty chalk-stones consist of uric-acid and lime, and that, in the decline of every fit of gout, uric-acid is always observed to abound in the urine of the patient. Whence, the Doctor says, the probable inference, from all the foregoing facts, is that gout is really occasioned by the superabundance of urea in the blood, and that the deposition of it in the form of chalk-stones, and its excretion by the kidneys, may be regarded as salutary, although, at times, painful and troublesome crises. Now, we are also informed that Chelius, of Heidelberg, has ascertained that the quantity of uric-acid excreted by the kidneys is nearly doubled in a person who takes Colchicum for twelve days; hence, Colchicum not only produces critical processes, but also critical discharges similar to the salutary processes and evacuations of gout.

2. If fever has generally been regarded as a salutary process, convulsions rarely have, and we do not yet adopt the opinion as our own; yet Stokes (see "Practice," p. 293,) says: "The occurrence of convulsions, in a child laboring under symptoms of inflammation of the brain, is always looked upon as formidable; and, indeed, it is natural that convulsions, to persons unacquainted with pathology, should seem to point out a great intensity of disease. I (Stokes) have, however, been long of the opinion that convulsions, occurring during the existence of dropsy of the brain in children, or meningitis in adults, are not so dangerous as persons generally think. I (Stokes) will even go so far as to say, that the worst cases I have seen, in which a cure was effected, were those in which there were the greatest and most violent convulsions; and that in the majority of those cases which appeared to go on without any benefit from the treatment, there were scarcely any convulsions. I (Stokes) am hence of the opinion that convulsions are often of benefit by giving relief to the brain. This statement must appear paradoxical to some, but I (Stokes) trust that I shall be able to prove that it has some foundation in truth. Nor am I alone in this opinion, for Broussais has taught that there appear to be two great modes of reaction in the human economy, for the purpose of obviating the effects of irritation of important organs, viz., fever and convulsions. The irritations which affect the brain and spinal marrow, may be relieved by convulsions; those which attack the lungs, liver, stomach, bowels, &c., may be relieved by fever and increased secretion. So says Broussais, but I (Stokes) think they may be relieved by an *increase*, with or without alteration of their secretions. A violent expenditure of nervous power may relieve the brain or spinal marrow, and delirium or convulsions may prevent organic changes, just as secretion from the lungs or bowels may prevent ulceration. Thus, the earlier phenomena of apoplexy and epilepsy are the same, and depend upon an active congestion to the brain. In epilepsy, we have this, followed by convulsions, more or less violent and protracted, after which the patient recovers. In apoplexy, there are no convulsions, and death or paralysis follows. It is plain that, if we admit the identity of the phenomena in the early stages of both these affections, we must then also admit that the only course of relief we can ascertain is convulsions. Hence, I (Stokes) think that we should generally look upon convulsions in the light of an attempt at a crisis made by nature itself. What is a crisis? An organ in state of irritation is suddenly relieved by a new process taking place, either in itself or in some other part, and, when we come to examine what these modes of relief are, we find them to consist in increase of secretion, hæmorrhage, eruptions upon the skin, or convulsions. I (Stokes) am convinced that

the practice of checking the convulsions with opiates is wrong and dangerous." Hence, we might infer that the opposite of giving spasmodic remedies would be justifiable; however this may be theoretically, it has been carried out practically.

If we admit this to be true, then, when convulsions are absent, the indication must be to administer epileptifacient, or convulsive remedies, such as Nux-vomica, Brucine, Ignatia, Strychnine, &c. However this may be, convulsions themselves have been treated successfully by eminent old-school physicians with these very drugs. Thus, we read, in the *Encyclographie des Sciences Medicales*, for August, 1843, p. 65, that Lejeune used Nux-vomica in the treatment of chorea with success; that Fouilloux gave by accident a large dose of Strychnine to a patient with St. Vitus' dance, the effects were severe, but they cured the chorea; that Trousseau, Professor of Therapeutics in the Ecole de Medecine, at Paris, has cured eleven cases of chorea with the same remedy. Trousseau says, that he had long cherished the idea that many medicines only act by *substituting a different and peculiar*, but spontaneously and rapidly curable disease, for one, the severity of which is often very great, the duration long, and their cure not spontaneous. This, he says, may be called *homœopathic substitutive treatment*, but it is very different from that which flows out of the reveries and singular errors of Hahnemann, but is in accordance with the experience of those soundly practical physicians who treat ophthalmia, blenorrhagia, chronic inflammation, &c., with irritating drugs. Hence, it seems to him conformable with analogy to treat chorea, an eminently convulsive malady, with Nux-vomica, which causes convulsions. In Dunglison's "New Remedies," p. 455, we read, that Pereira has seen it serviceable in that shaking or trembling action of the muscles, which is produced by habitual intoxication. On next page, that Romberg, Professor in the University of Berlin, saw good effects from it in chorea. There is a vast difference, however, between the half-paralytic trembling of chorea, and the tetanic rigidity produced by Nux-vomica; hence this treatment is specific alterative treatment. The usual treatment of chorea is with the mineral tonics, Iron and Arsenic; Nux-vomica must be regarded as the most powerful tonic of the muscular system.

In Eberlee's "Materia Medica," second edition, vol. i., p. 44, we read, that, "In the memoirs of the Copenhagen Medical Society, there are some very interesting remarks on the use of Ipecac., as an anti-emetic, by Dr. Schonheyder. Even ileus, with obstinate vomiting of fæcal matter, has been relieved by it." Eberlee also quotes Burdach, who states, that Ipecac is very useful in habitual vomiting from morbid irritability of the stomach, but it must be given in very small doses."

3. The peculiar effect of Digitalis in rendering the pulse feeble, slow, and intermitting is well known. Yet, we read, in Pereira's "Materia

Medica," vol. ii., p. 292, that Dr. Withering correctly observes, "That, when given in dropsy, it seldom succeeds in men of great natural strength, of tense fibre, warm skin, florid complexion, or in those with a tight and cordy pulse. But, on the contrary, if the pulse be feeble and intermitting, the countenance pale, the lips livid, the skin cold, &c., we may expect the diuretic effects to follow in a kindly manner." On page 293, Pereira says, "In simple dilatation of the heart, the curative indication is to strengthen its muscular fibres;" yet, a little lower down, we read, "The enlarged and flaccid heart, observes Dr. Holland, though on first view it might seem the least favorable for the use of Digitalis, is, perhaps, not so. At least, we have reason to believe that, in the dropsical affections which so often attend it, the action of Digitalis, as a diuretic, is peculiarly of avail." A little lower down, Pereira says: "In patients affected with an intermittent, or otherwise irregular pulse, he has several times observed this medicine produce regularity of pulsa tion—an effect also noticed by Dr. Holland."

The only way, perhaps, in which the homœopathic action of Digitalis, in dropsy, with feeble state of pulse, can be explained away is the following. In dropsy, the secretion of urine and sweat is generally checked, and fluids which should be excreted through the kidneys and skin, are poured out in internal cavities or beneath the skin. The specific effects of Digitalis are to produce a slow, feeble, intermitting pulse, followed by profuse flow of urine. Paris (see "Pharmacologia," vol. i., p. 128,) even says, "It may be remarked that it seldom or never produces its diuretic effects without a concomitant reduction of the frequency of the pulse." Hence, diuresis would be most readily induced by it in persons with a naturally feeble pulse, and the free flow of urine may relieve dropsy in such persons. The action of Digitalis is somewhat antagonistic to that of Opium, which also causes slow pulse, but suppression of urine, which is compensated by free sweat. But homœopathy alone can account for its beneficial effects in the flaccid heart and intermitting pulse.

4. What remedy is nearer similar in its action to Lead than Alum, which, Pereira says, (vol. i., p. 517,) checks the secretions of the bowels, and thereby diminishes the frequency and increases the consistency of the stools. Yet, on pages 518 and 519, we learn that, "In the treatment of lead-colic, Alum has been found more successful than any other agent, or even class of remedies; it opens the bowels more certainly than any other medicine, and frequently when powerful remedies have failed." As Pereira scorns homœopathy, he adds, "The *modus operandi* of Alum, in lead-colic, is not very clear." Cullen, (see "Materia Medica," Barbour's edition, vol. ii., p. 12,) however, says, he has known large doses of it to purge. Yet, why should it act so much better than the true purgatives?

5. Billing says that alkalies relieve acidity of the stomach, for a time; but, in order to cure it effectually, tonics, but, better still, an acid should be used, such as diluted Sulphuric-acid. It is said, however, by some, that when the acids avail, there is alkalinity, instead of acidity of the stomach. In fact, Dr. Johnson (see *Med. Chir. Rev.*, vol. xxxv., p. 379,) says, that water-brash "is nearly always alkaline, occasionally acid, sometimes insipid, at others hot and acrid."

But, in order that we may be quite fair towards the sincere homœopathists, we here institute the inquiry, are there any recorded instances of homœopathic cures, in which it cannot be shown that the remedy acted by sustaining the salutary processes of nature, or by inducing a peculiar different action?

1. Good (see "Study of Medicine," fourth American edition, vol. iii., p. 290,) says: "It has been proposed to overcome the night-sweats, in consumption, by exciting a sweat of a *different* kind; 'for it is as practicable,' says Watts, 'to cure sweating by sudorifics, as diarrhœa by cathartics.'" Good adds, "There is something plausible in this remark," and tells us, on page 296, that "Dr. Young has sometimes succeeded very decidedly in checking such sweats with Dover's powders."

2. Billing (see "Principles of Medicine,") says, although no homœopathist, he knows full well that emetics will allay vomiting, and that purges will cure diarrhœa; that Tartar-emetic, and almost any neutral purging salt, will cure the vomiting and purging of Asiatic cholera quicker than any other remedies. Again, that it will perhaps astonish many, to learn that Tartar-emetic relieves nausea and vomiting, in like manner as sedative remedies do, and that the nausea and vomiting, in inflammation of the stomach, can often be relieved without the aid of blood-letting, by means of repeated small doses of Tartar-emetic.

SECTION IV.

BENNETT'S EXAMINATION OF THE PATIENT.

It is absolutely necessary that an examination of patients should be conducted with order, and according to a well-understood plan. Some physicians put their questions, as it were, at random, without any apparent object, and wander from one system of the economy to another, in a vain search for a precise diagnosis, and a rational indication of cure. But continual practice, and the adoption of a certain method, will remove all difficulty. No doubt, questioning a patient, to arrive at a knowledge of his condition, requires as much skill in the medical practitioner, as examining a witness does in counsel at the bar. They make it an especial study, we must do so likewise. We should remember that, in proportion as this duty is performed well or ill, is the probability that our opinion of the case may be correct or incorrect; and that, not only will the reputation we hold among our colleagues greatly depend on our ability in this matter, but that the public itself will promptly give its confidence to him whose interrogations reveal sagacity and talent.

The method of examination differs greatly among practitioners, and must necessarily vary in particular cases. Men of experience gradually form a certain plan of their own, which enables them to arrive at their object more rapidly and securely than that adopted with, perhaps, an equally good result by another. However, the plan which appears to be the best, has for its object to arrive, as quickly as possible, at a knowledge of the existing condition of the patient, in a way that will insure the examiner that no important organ has been overlooked or escaped notice.

For this purpose, we ascertain, in the first instance, the organ principally affected, and the duration of the disease, by asking two questions: "Where do you feel pain?" and "How long have you been ill?" Let us suppose that the patient feels pain in the cardiac region, we immediately proceed to examine the heart, functionally and physically, and then the circulatory system generally. We next proceed to those organs which usually bear the nearest relation to the one principally affected —say, the respiratory system—and we then examine the lungs, functionally and physically. We subsequently interrogate the nervous, digestive, genito-urinary, and integumentary systems. It is a matter of little importance in what order these are examined—the chief point is, *not to neglect any of them.* Lastly, we inquire into the past history of the case, when we shall have arrived at all the information necessary for the formation of a diagnosis.

The following is the arrangement of symptoms and circumstances demanding attention, under each of the seven heads into which the examination is divided:

I. Circulatory System.—*Heart:* Uneasiness or pain; its action and rhythm; situation where the apex beats; extent of dulness determined by percussion; its impulse; murmurs—if abnormal, their character, and the position and direction in which they are heard loudest. *Arterial pulse:* Number of beats in a minute; large or small, strong or feeble, hard or soft, equal or unequal, regular or irregular, intermittent, confused, imperceptible, &c. If an aneurismal swelling exist, its situation, pulsations, symptoms, extent, and sounds must be carefully examined. *Venous pulse:* If perceptible, observe position, force, &c

II. Respiratory System.—*Nares:* Discharges; sneezing. *Larynx and Trachea:* Voice, natural or altered in quality, hoarse; difficulty of speech; aphonia, &c.; if affected, observe condition of epiglottis, tonsils, and pharynx, by means of a spatula. *Lungs:* State of respiration; easy or difficult, quick or slow, equal or unequal, labored, painful, spasmodic, dyspnœa, &c.; odor of breath. Expectoration, trifling or profuse, easy or difficult; its character, thin or inspissated, frothy, mucous, purulent or muco-purulent, rusty, bloody; microscopical examination. Hæmoptysis, color, appearance and amount of blood discharged. Cough, rare or frequent, short or long, painful or not, moist or dry. External form of the chest, unusually rounded or flattened, symmetrical or not, &c. Movements—regular, equal, their amount, &c. Resonance, as determined by percussion, increased or diminished, dulness, cracked-pot sound, &c. Sounds determined by auscultation, if abnormal, their character and position.

III. Nervous System.—*Brain:* Intelligence augmented, perverted, or diminished; cephalalgia; hallucinations; delirium, stupidity, monomania, idiocy; sleep, dreams, vertigo, stupor, coma. *Spinal cord and nerves:* Pain in back; general sensibility, increased, diminished, or absent; special sensibility—sight, hearing, smell, taste, touch, their increase, perversion, or diminution; spinal irritation, as determined by percussion, motion, natural or perverted, fatigue, pain on movement; trembling, convulsions, contractions, rigidity, paralysis.

IV. Digestive System.—*Mouth:* Lips, teeth, and gums; taste in the mouth. *Tongue:* Mode of protrusion, color, furred, coated, fissured, condition of papillæ, moist or dry. *Fauces, tonsils, pharynx and œsophagus:* Deglutition—if impeded, examine the pharynx with a spatula, the cervical glands, neck, &c.; regurgitation. *Stomach:* Appetite, thirst, epigastric uneasiness or pain, swelling, nausea, vomiting, character of matters vomited, flatulence, eructations. *Abdomen:* Its measurement and palpation; pain, distension or collapse, borborygmi, tumors, constipation, diarrhœa, character of dejections, hæmorrhoids. *Liver:* Size, as determined by percussion, pain, jaundice, results of palpation, &c. *Spleen:* Size, as determined by percussion. If enlarged, examine blood microscopically.

V. Genito-Urinary System.—*Uterus:* Condition of menstrual discharge, amenorrhœa, dysmenorrhœa, menorrhagia, leucorrhœa, &c. If pain, or much leucorrhœal discharge, examine os uteri and vagina with speculum; uterine or ovarian tumors; pain in back; difficulty in walking, or in defæcation; functions of mammæ. *Kidney:* Lumbar pain; micturition; quantity and quality of urine, color, specific gravity; precipitates, as determined by the microscope, and by chemical tests;

action of heat; nitric acid, &c.; action on test papers; stricture; discharges from urethra; spermatorhœa, &c.

VI. Integumentary System.—General posture; external surface; expression of countenance; obesity; emaciation; color; rough or smooth; dry or moist; perspiration; marks or cicatrices; eruptions (see diagnosis of skin diseases); temperature; morbid growths or swelling; anasarca; œdema; emphysema, &c.

VII. Antecedent History.—Age; parentage; constitution; hereditary disposition; trade or profession; place of residence; mode of living, as regards food and drink; habits; epidemics and endemics; contagion and infection; exposure to heat, cold, or moisture; irregularities in diet; excesses of any kind; fatigue; commencement and progress of the disease; date of rigor or seizure; mode of invasion; previous treatment; in female cases, whether married or single, have had children and miscarriages, previous diseases, &c.

Such are the principal points to which our attention should be directed during the examination of a case. A little practice will soon impress them on the memory, and in this manner habit will insure that no very important circumstance has been overlooked. At first, indeed, it may appear that such a minute examination is unnecessary; but we shall have abundant opportunities of proving that, whilst a little extra trouble never does harm, ignorance of a fact frequently leads to error. It is surprising, also, how rapidly one thoroughly conversant with the plan is able to examine a patient, so as to satisfy himself that all the organs and functions have been carefully interrogated. Remember that the importance of particular symptoms is not known to the patient, and that, consequently, it is not in his power voluntarily to inform us of the necessary particulars. It is always our duty to discover them.

It is well to make a few remarks about the nature and treatment of some of the symptoms contained in the above paragraphs.

REMARKS ON FIRST PARAGRAPH.

Uneasiness about the heart may arise from embarrassment of its action, or want of sufficient power, from debility, to unload itself promptly, when Nux-vomica often proves a useful remedy, even if there is obstruction of one or the other, or too great patency of the valves. If the uneasiness be nervous in its character, Ignatia or Spigelia is often useful; if congestive, Aconite, Veratrum-viride, or Digitalis may be thought of. *Pain* in the heart may be spasmodic, neuralgic, or inflammatory. For the first, Nux is also often useful, but sometimes full doses of Conium are required; for the second, Spigelia, Argentum-nitricum, and even small doses of Opium may be used; for inflammatory pains, Aconite and Mercurius may be used in the primary stages, Arsenicum and Cannabis in the later ones.

The *action* of the heart may be strong, or weak, or irregular, or intermitting. If it be so strong as to lift the walls of the chest, the heart is enlarged; without this, however violent the action, there is probably no hypertrophy. Excessively violent action may be moderated by Aconite, Veratrum-viride, &c. A weak action of the heart may sometimes be aroused by very small doses of Digitalis; sometimes more effectually by moderate stimulus, aided by Nux, Ignatia, Glonoine, or Carbonate of Ammonia. Irregular action is often better controlled by Digitalis than any other remedy, although Spigelia, Laurocerasus, or, in default of the latter, an infusion of Wild Cherry Bark, or Ferrum may be used.

As regards *the extent of dulness* on percussion, if that exceed two inches square, the heart is considerably enlarged, provided the impulse be felt distinctly. If no impulse be felt, and the extent of the dulness be great, there is effusion into the pericardium. Hypertrophy of the heart is best treated with Bromide, or Iodide, or Bichromate of Potash; while effusion into the pericardium may be met with Arsenicum, Hellebore, Digitalis, or the Bromide or Iodide of Potash, or Muriate of Ammonia.

Most *murmurs* of the heart, with the exception of the chlorotic and pericardial friction-sounds, arise from disease of the valves, more especially the aortic and mitral. Aortic valvular murmurs are heard loudest at the base of the heart, toward the sternum, and upward along the course of the aorta; while those of the mitral valve are heard most distinctly toward the apex of the heart, near the nipple. Disease of the valves, unless very recent, are scarcely ever removed, although Thuja, Mercurius, and Bromide of Potash may be tried.

The indications of the *arterial pulse* are almost the same as those of the heart; the two should often be compared together.

An aneurism may generally be detected by the thrill and heavy jog which attends it; palliative benefit, at least, has arisen from the use of Lycopodium, Carbo-vegetabilis, and Zinc.

A *venous pulse* arises from regurgitation through the right side of the heart. It is, of course, most distinct in the jugular veins, and always indicates great disease, generally enlargement with dilatation of the heart. Palliative means, of course, are the only ones to be relied upon; the Apocynum-cannabinum often moderates some of the attendant symptoms, especially the dropsy which so often accompanies it.

REMARKS ON SECOND PARAGRAPH.

Discharges from the nose are of various kinds; those of *blood* are best relieved by Hammamelis, Arnica, Kreosote, Carb.-ammon., &c.

Crusts and scabs may be prevented by Aurum, Kali-bichrom., Nitric-acid, Ranunculus, and Thuja. *Acrid discharges* by Arsenicum, Mezereum, or Muriatic-acid. *Fetid*, by Chlorate of Potash, or Soda, Carbo-animalis, or Nitric-acid. *Greenish*, by Cannabis, Thuja, or Manganese. *Purulent*, by a very weak preparation of Tartar-emetic, Hepar-sulphur, Ledum, Nitric-acid, or Staphysagria. *Chronic discharges* are sometimes removed by Anacardium, or Phosphorus.

Sneezing often arises from catarrhal, or nervous irritation; when it is excessive, Conium, Teucrium, or Sabadilla may be tried.

Hoarseness of voice may often be removed by Phosphorus, Spongia, Hepar-sulphur. Difficulty of speaking, from debility of the laryngeal muscles, may be relieved by Nux, or Ignatia. Loss of voice is often remedied by Carbonate of Ammonia.

Difficult and labored respiration may arise from pain, spasm, congestion, or obstruction. *Painful* respiration may often be relieved by Conium and Bryonia. *Spasmodic* breathing by Conium, Ipecac., Musk, Assafœtida, &c. *Congestion*, by Aconite, Veratrum-viride, or Phosphorus. *Quick* breathing may be relieved by Conium, Aconite, or Veratrum-viride. *Slow and unequal breathing* often points to pressure on the brain, and may be benefitted by Hellebore, or Digitalis.

Scanty expectoration may be treated with Dulcamara, Euphrasia, Pulsatilla, Senega, Tartar-emetic, or Scilla. *Too profuse*, by Cuprum, Zincum, Alumina, or Stannum. *Membranous*, by Kali-bichrom., Iodide of Mercury, or Potash, Bromine, or Iodine. *Frothy*, by Daphne-indica, Phosphor, or Arsenicum. *Gelatinous*, by Laurocerasus, Baryta-muriatica, or Digitalis. *Purulent*, by Anacardium, Drosera, Ferrum, Phos.-ferri, Ledum, Nitric-acid, Phosphoric-acid, Plumbum, or Ruta. *Rusty* expectoration, of course, denotes the presence of inflammation of the lungs, and requires Aconite, Veratrum-viride, Phosphorus, Bryonia, or Tartar-emetic. *Bloody*, by Hammamelis, Arnica, Terebinth, Aconite, Nitric-acid, Kreosote, Plumbum, &c.

Cough, occurring from excessive accumulation of phlegm, may be relieved by Kreosote; from excessive irritation, by Conium; when very frequent and severe, by Ipecac. and Morphine. Hooping-cough, by Belladonna and Ipecac.; hoarse and crowing coughs, by Sambucus, Spongia, Aconite, and Antimony, Phosphorus, Iodine, or Bromide of Potash. Dry coughs, by Belladonna and Ipecac.; painful coughs, by Aconite and Antimony, Morphine and Ipecac., Conium and Antimony.

When the external form of the chest is unusually rounded, it often points to emphysema of the lungs, especially if there be unusual clearness on percussion. If the chest be flattened, with great dulness on percussion, there is usually a pleuritic effusion, or a tumor in the chest. Pleuritic effusions may be treated with Mercurius and Antimony, or Digitalis, if some febrile symptoms remain; by Hydriodate or Bromide of Potash, or Iodide of Iron, if there be no fever, or by Hellebore and Sulphur in alternation.

Dulness on percussion, especially at the base of the lungs, with entire absence of respiratory murmur, especially if there be some fulness of the chest, points to pleuritic or dropsical effusion; with bronchial respiration, if the attack be recent and acute, to pneumonia. Dulness on percussion, especially at the tops of the lungs, without recent acute symptoms, but with prolonged expiration and crackling sounds just below the clavicles, or on the tops of the shoulders behind, generally points to tubercular disease; and, if there be no acute symptoms, Phosphate of Iron and Soda, in equal parts, with or without cod-liver oil, in alternation, may very often be given with great benefit. If there be a recent acute feverish state, Aconite, in small quantities, or Veratrum-viride, are useful, in alternation with Phosphorus and Hepar-sulphur. Pneumonia is best treated with Aconite and Antimony in the first stage; with Bromide or Iodide of Potash, or with small doses of Mercurius and Conium, or of Iodide of Mercury and Conium in the second stage, and with Phosphor and Hepar-sulphur in the third stage. I have treated at least twenty cases of pleuritic effusion successfully with a few doses of Mercurius and Antimony, if febrile symptoms were present, or with Antimony and Hydriodate of Potash, when the febrile symptoms were slight, or with Iodide of Mercury, Hydriodate or Bromide of Potash, when little or no fever existed. Bryonia and Hellebore are also useful remedies when the pains are obstinate. The urine is always scanty in dropsy of the chest and pleuritic effusions, and then Digitalis and Hydriodate of Potash will generally increase the quantity of urine very decidedly, and relieve the shortness of breath and difficulty of breathing, with great rapidity, to the great comfort of the patient.

REMARKS ON THIRD PARAGRAPH.

Augmented intelligence, if excessively acute, may be somewhat dulled by Conium or Agaricus; if diminished, from torpor of the brain, it may be aroused by Anacardium; if perverted, it may be regulated by Agaricus, Belladonna, or Stramonium, &c.

Headache, if congestive, may be relieved by Aconite or Veratrum-viride; if nervous, by Agaricus or Spigelia; if rheumatic, by Bryonia, Aconite, Colchicum, or Rhus; if from gastric derangement, by Nux or Pulsatilla. Sick headache may often be prevented by Iris-versicolor, or by taking Phosphoric-acid, Lemon-juice, or Vinegar, for a long time.

Hallucinations are often removed by Belladonna, Stramonium, Hyosciamus, or Conium.

Delirium, if nervous, is often removed by Agaricus or Cannabis-indica; if from congestion, by Aconite, Belladonna, Digitalis, or Conium.

Stupidity may be benefitted by Conium, especially if it occurs in typhous or scrofulous subjects, or by small doses of Opium.

Monomania is sometimes removed by Anacardium, Aurum, Cicuta, Ignatia, or Sabadilla.

Dreams often arise from a preponderance of the action of the ganglionic system upon the cerebrum, when the controlling influence of the brain is withdrawn.

Vertigo is often relieved by Cocculus.

Stupor and coma sometimes yield to small doses of Opium, Digitalis, or Belladonna.

Pain in the back is often relieved by Oxalic-acid better than any other remedy.

Increase of general sensibility is often lessened by Agaricus, Aconite, or Conium. A diminution, by Nux-vomica, Ignatia, or Plumbum.

Excessive sensitiveness of sight is sometimes moderated by Conium or Belladonna; of hearing, by Agaricus or Cannabis-indica; of smell, by Agaricus or Cocculus; of taste, by Cicuta or Rhododendron; of touch, by Agaricus. A *diminution* of sight, by Conium; of hearing, by Pulsatilla; of smell, by Oleander; of taste, by Kreosote; of touch, by Plumbum.

Spinal irritation is often relieved by Aconite, applied to the spine, or by Agaricus or Cannabis-indica, given internally. Tenderness of the numerous spinal muscles, and their tendinous attachments to the vertebræ, is often mistaken for spinal irritation, and may be relieved by Conium.

A sensation of *excessive fatigue* may often be relieved by Cannabis-sativa. Pain on movement is often allayed by Rhus, Stramonium, Belladonna, or Conium. Trembling, by Ferrum or Plumbum; convulsions, by Conium; rigidity, by Plumbum; paralysis, by Arsenicum, Ignatia, Angustura, or Nux.

As no allusion has been made by Bennett to the ganglionic system, it is important to direct attention to this most important division of the nervous system.

SECTION V.

GANGLIONIC OR SYMPATHETIC NERVOUS SYSTEM.

AUTHORITIES.—Draper's Physiology, Carpenter's Physiology, Davy on the Ganglionic Nervous System.

THE ganglionic, or nerve of organic life, consists of a series of reddish or grey ganglia, connected with each other by nervous strands, extending along each side of the visceral surface of the vertebral column, from the head to the coccyx, *communicating with all other nerves of the body* and distributing branches to all the internal viscera, *or organs of involuntary function.* The chain on each side of the vertebral column communicates with its colleague on the opposite side through plexuses. The *ganglion impar* is the common uniting point of all of them on the coccyx below; and, by some, it is supposed that the ganglion of Ribes, and by others, that the pituitary body has the same function in the cranium above.

The connection of the ganglionic, or sympathetic nervous system, with the spino-cerebral nerves are so numerous and intimate that some physiologists have supposed that it originates from the roots of the cerebro-spinal nerves and terminates in the viscera. Others suppose that its origin is in the internal viscera, and its termination in the cerebro-spinal system. This opinion being supported by the proven facts, that the sympathetic nerve, in its primary development, appears before the other parts of the nervous system, and simultaneously with the viscera, or splanchnic organs; and that it has been found in monsters, without a brain or spinal cord. The most complimentary and liberal view is, that it is a special system, much more important to the life, structure, and functions of the animal economy than either the intellectual, motor, or sensor nerves, with which it simply establishes incidental communications, while its ganglia are so many independent nervous centres.

Each spinal nerve is brought into relation with the sympathetic nerve by two nervous strands, or prolongations from the spinal marrow and ganglia themselves; one of these strands is tubular and white, the other gelatinous and grey. The *tubular, or white nervous strand*, may be regarded as actually arising from the spinal cord, and consists of both motor and sensory filaments; it makes its way to a ganglion of the sympathetic nerve, passes over and through it, its fibres conjoining themselves with grey ones, which they have gathered in the ganglion. *The grey, or gelatinous strand*, is to be viewed as having its origin in a ganglion of the great sympathetic, and sends its fibres chiefly to the ganglion on the posterior root of the spinal nerve, although a few of them communicate somewhat doubtfully with the anterior root of the spinal nerve. The few fibres which seem to enter the spinal cord itself, are probably intended for the supply of blood-vessels.

Each ganglion of the sympathetic nerve is, therefore, *a nervous centre*, sending forth strands in three directions: First, to join the spinal fibres; second, to the spinal cord itself, or chiefly to the ganglia on the posterior roots of its nerves; third, to the next sympathetic ganglion above, and thence to the brain. The innumerable sympathetic irritations of the brain and spinal marrow, arising from primary disorder of the viscera, or sympathetic nerves which supply, form, and control them, are thus easily explained.

The branches of the sympathetic nerve which go to the viscera constantly form plexuses, four of which are remarkable, viz., the *pharyngeal*, *cardiac*, *solar*, and *hypogastric*. The first and last of these are in symmetrical pairs; the other two are single, and placed on the median line. The arteries are also surrounded with such a net-work. All these plexuses receive supplies from the cerebro-spinal nerves.

From its construction, the sympathetic may readily be supposed to be a self-acting system, although it is not an isolated one, since all its branches contain fibres derived from the cerebro-spinal. Compared with some other nerve-trunks, it is said the sympathetic is much less active, as regards sensation and motion—a high irritation of the parts supplied by it being often required to cause pain, while its motor fibres are little under the influence of the will. In fact, the sympathetic transmits sensations so tardily that it has been supposed that one office of its ganglia is for the purpose of cutting off such impressions; although some hypochondriacs seem to cultivate the cognizance of the obscure sensations, in all their viscera, to such a degree that they almost become conscious of all the involuntary and insensitive processes. In like manner, when motor fibres of the cerebro-spinal system pass through the sympathetic ganglia, their conducting power appears to be impaired. Draper even thinks that there does not seem to be any decisive proof that any of the fibres of the sympathetic, properly speaking, are either motor or sensory; the influence which they exert, in these respects, on the muscular structure of the heart, blood-vessels, digestive, or urinary organs being, perhaps, due to the associated cerebro-spinal nerves. In this manner, he thinks, by its distribution to the arteries, the sympathetic, as a compound nerve, exerts a power over the passage of the blood through them, by influencing their contractility, and thereby their diameter; in virtue of this, it also affects the rapidity of secretion, and also regulates the rate of nutrition. I regard this matter in an entirely different point of view. It is so important to remove all the nutritive and formative processes as far as possible from the influence of a perverted will and morbid fancy, that a special, unconscious, non-intellectual, and involuntary system of nerves are supplied to the entire digestive tract and all its dependencies—the heart, and all its dependencies of arteries, veins, capillaries and lymphatics—the urinary and genital organs and most of their dependencies; voluntary nerves being only supplied to the outlets of these parts to aid in the ingestion of food and excretion of fæces, urine, semen, &c., when the wants of the system require some voluntary aid. All other cerebro-spinal communications with the sympathetic nerve are, as it were, toned down to the instinctive, mathematically, and inflexibly correct, but unconscious operations of the latter. If men were allowed to fool with their organic functions, as they do with their intellectual and muscular powers, we would soon be reduced to sad monsters. On the other hand, the intimate communications of the sympathetic system with the brain, quickly warn us of important abnormal changes going on in the parts controlled by the sympathetic system, and arouse all the intelligence or folly of mankind for their removal.

It is much more than probable that the sympathetic nerve presides over the circulation of the blood, the motion of every artery and bloodvessel, the form, structure, and nutrition of every tissue and organ, and the formation of every secretion and excretion. We would most earnestly advise every young physician to make himself familiar with the anatomy, physiology, and pathology of the great sympathetic nervous system; at least, frequently to refresh his memory with anatomical plates of the distribution of the great plexuses and branches of this most important system of nerves. Not only do the functions of all the great viscera depend upon its integrity, but almost all diseased processes are regulated by it; the large class of fevers, inflammations, exudations, tumors, and heterologous formations, such as cancer, tubercle, &c., &c., all arise either from its disorder, or from that of parts under its control.

We are almost inclined to agree with Davy, that the ganglionic nervous system is the special residence and organ of the vital powers; that the ganglionic system of nerves, with the solar ganglion for its central organ, perform all the vital or organic functions; that secretion, nutrition, exhalation, absorption, and calorification are under its immediate influence and control throughout the whole body, and that it presides equally over the nutrition of the brain and spinal cord, as it does over that of the liver or uterus; and that, if either of these organs or viscera were removed from the influence of the ganglionic nerves, entering so largely into its very composition, its specific vitality would cease, for the ganglionic nervous system seems to be the source or organ of the creative force, or organizing principle, or vital power, just as a galvanic battery, or electrical machine is the source or organ for the generation, but not creation of those mysterious, electrical, and galvanic powers which are distantly comparable to the vital power. In short, Davy infers that the "*nisus formativus*," or "the energy truly vital," depends for its integrity and continuance upon the ganglia of the sympathetic nerve, which exercise, in some marvellous way, that *architectural* power which is employed in man and animals, from man downward, through the whole of animated nature, to the very lowest link in the chain of being. And he cannot doubt, that to their peculiar and vital influence must be conceded the wonderful and successive metamorphoses or changes which characterize not only the intra- and extrauterine existence of the human form, but also that of animals, and under all the circumstances both of normal and *abnormal* action; and this, not merely for inferior organs and functions, but for superior ones, for if the ganglionic nervous system have the power or capacity to develop and mature a liver, a heart, and a spleen, &c., and to excite them to the exercise of their appropriate functions, there can be no reason why it should not so much, or the same, for a brain, or spinal marrow.

It may be well to give a few of the facts upon which these opinions are founded. Blumenbach says, that in fœtuses without brain or spinal marrow, the circulation, nutrition, secretion, &c., proceed equally well as in others, which, besides spinal marrow, nerves, and a ganglionic nervous system, possess a brain. The absence of a brain and spinal marrow is found in no way to affect the generation, growth, and maturity of that portion of the animal organism which remains to them; the remnant of the organism is perfectly developed, and, therefore, all the strictly vital functions have necessarily been in full operation during intra-uterine life. If we see the body nourished, the viscera perfected, and the bony fabric matured, we may rest assured that circulation, absorption, secretion, &c., have been in full action, in perfect operation, without either a brain or a spinal cord, *and with only a ganglionic nervous system.* Again, Davy says, if a careful and graduated pressure be made, through the abdomen of a rabbit, on the upper part of the lumbar region, so as to press upon certain of the smaller ganglia of the sympathetic, the hinder extremities of the animal will presently become completely paralyzed; the rabbit, when placed on the ground, will be seen to use its fore-legs well enough, and with these it will drag itself to and fro, evidently much puzzled at its own sudden and unusual incapacity. However, after a few minutes, the spinal functions are restored, and the animal is as lively as ever. Again, it is well known that injury of the superior cervical ganglion, in both man and in animals, is productive of blindness, by arresting the vital actions (nutrition) going on in the eye.

The dependence of the circulation upon the ganglionic system has lately been illustrated by Claude Bernard. He says it has been known, for a long time, that cutting the medulla spinalis through, or certain other nervous cords, such as the par vagum, the sciatic nerve, and others, will cause a general, or partial, but decided diminution of the warmth of the body; but the *reverse* of this is the case, when the great sympathetic is cut through. Bernard noticed, in cutting through the cervical branch of the sympathetic nerve, which unites the cervical ganglions, that there followed immediately *an increase of heat* in the corresponding side of the face, which could be very easily appreciated by the hand, and which was found to be from four to six degrees, centigrade, higher by the thermometer. When the superior cervical ganglion of the great sympathetic was entirely extirpated, Bernard found the same effect produced, with even greater intensity; and, at the same time that the heat was increased, the circulation of the blood became more active. This new phenomenon of increased calorification, continued for a long time; he found it to last, at times, for several successive months, without being attended with, or followed by any appearance of inflammation, or œdema, or any other pathological change. If all this be true, it is easy to understand why a feeble or paralytic state of certain portions of the sympathetic nerve may be followed by heat and congestion to the head, from the loss of control of the nerve over that portion of the vascular system, allowing the blood to be thrown in full force to the head, unmoderated by the contractility of the arteries; for, while the injection of blood into the capillaries of every part of the system is due to the action of the heart, its rate of passage through these vessels is greatly modified by the degree of contractile activity of the capillaries themselves—for the capillaries possess a distributive power over the blood, regulating the local circulation independently of the central organ, in obedience to their controlling nerves, and the vital necessities of the parts they supply. According to Carpenter, this very important use of this contractile coat of the capillaries has been generally overlooked by physiologists—viz., that of *regulating* the diameter of the tubes, in accordance with the quantity of blood to be conducted through them to any part, which will depend upon its peculiar circumstances at the time, owing to the various phases of normal life, as well as in diseased states; and they will be found to be constantly in harmony with the particular condition of the processes of nutrition, secretion, &c., to which the capillary circulation ministers. Of this kind are the enlargement of the uterine and mammary arteries, at the epochs of pregnancy and lactation; the enormous size to which the spermatic artery will attain, when the testicle is greatly increased in size by diseased action, and many other similar phenomena. In such cases, it cannot be the action of the heart that increases the calibre of the vessels, since this is commonly unaltered; it must, therefore, be by a power inherent in themselves, or their nerves, that this change in the capillaries is effected. To explain this, we must again call upon the sympathetic nerve. The minute distribution of this nerve upon the walls of the arteries, so often alluded to, the known power which this nerve has of producing contractions, alike in their contractile and fibrous coat and in the muscular tunic of the intestinal canal, and various phenomena which indicate the power of certain states of the mind over the dimensions of the arteries, in particular parts of the body, at least, as in the erectile tissues, render it highly probable that the calibre of the arteries and capillaries is regulated, in no inconsiderable degree, through its intervention.

All these facts go to prove that in affections of the vascular system, such as fevers, inflammations, &c., remedies which act specifically upon the heart and arteries, and upon the ganglionic nervous system, must be more efficacious than mere blood-letting.

Thus, *Digitalis* acts specifically upon the heart, arteries, and kidneys, hence, probably, upon the three great cardiac nerves and two great plexuses, which arise from the superior, middle, and inferior cervical ganglions; also upon the two large renal plexuses, and the third splanchnic or renal nerve which arises from the last thoracic ganglion.

Aconite acts as specifically upon the heart and arteries as Digitalis, but more upon the skin than upon the kidneys; thus, while both will control the action of the heart and arteries, the one will tend to produce crises through the skin, the other through the kidneys.

Tobacco also exerts a specific action upon the heart and arteries, but also upon the stomach and respiratory organs; and hence, doubtless, act sspecifically on the gastric, and phrenic, or diaphragmatic plexuses.

Veratrum-viride has lately been proven to exert a most regular and powerful specific action upon the heart and arteries, and seems to act upon no other known organ or system, neither upon the liver, bowels, kidneys, or skin, and hence causes no critical evacuations from any of these organs; therefore, we may conclude that it acts upon the cardiac nerves and plexuses, perhaps upon the aortic plexus, which is a continuation of the solar plexus, downward on the aortic, for the supply of the inferior branches of that great vascular trunk. In the dominant school, it is regarded as a most reliable *arterial sedative*, in most inflammatory affections, in fact, more reliable than any other medicine of its class. Headache, restlessness, and other attendants upon an excited circulation, will almost always yield to it. Some suppose that its controlling power is most manifest in inflammatory affections of the chest and uterus, and in febrile excitements attended with headache; others say, with it they can control and subdue arterial action, almost at will, and regard it, in common practice, as far superior to Digitalis.

Belladonna is supposed to act more especially upon those spinal nerves which communicate with the great sympathetic, especially those which go to the sphincter muscles; although it acts very prominently upon many of the involuntary muscles and their nerves. The pneumogastric nerve has been pointed out as a special favorite for its action, especially those motor fibres which intermix with the spinal accessory and vagi nerves.

Pulsatilla acts upon the eye and ear, and upon almost all the mucous membranes of the body. It is supposed to act upon the mucous membranes, and affect some of their functions and control some of its diseases, as specifically as Aconite acts upon the skin, Digitalis upon the kidneys, Belladonna upon the involuntary motor fibres, and Veratrum-viride upon the arterial plexuses and nerves.

Nux-vomica acts upon almost all the voluntary and involuntary motor nerves in the body. Although its action may primarily be evidenced upon the spinal motor nerves, yet some of its influence is reflected upon those spinal nerves which communicate with the great sympathetic. Its action is also very manifest upon some portions of the cranial portion of the spinal marrow, which, we have seen, includes the corpora striata, optic thalami, corpora quadrigemina, &c., &c.; in this way it becomes clear how a strictly spinal remedy may become useful in some gastric and cerebral affections. Thus, Budge found, that by irritating the corpora quadrigemina and corpus striatum, he could produce marked peristaltic action of the stomach and bowels; even when all peristaltic action of the bowels had entirely ceased, it could, at once, be reproduced by irritating the corpora quadrigemina; and motions of the stomach could always be excited by irritating the corpus striatum, especially on the right side. These experiments throw much light upon the reciprocal action of some affections of the stomach, bowels, and other viscera, upon the spinal portions of the brain, and *vice versa*.

These remarks may be regarded as unnecessary refinements by some, and as purely hypothetical by others—but they are not so; they simply trace a little further into the organism well-known actions of drugs; make us acquainted, not merely with the bare symptomatology of remedies, but the very tissues, nerves, &c., upon which they act by preference; and, if the materia medica be faithfully studied, with the light of physiology and anatomy—those great studies which usually become a dead letter to most medical men, soon after they leave college—would always remain living studies, not merely interesting, but practically useful.

The importance of the pathological relations of the ganglionic nervous system has lately been more fully recognized. Indeed, it is difficult to imagine how it could be otherwise, when we remember the singular manner in which the whole vitality of the system depends upon its steady, uninterrupted, and vigorous action. Dr. C. Hanfield Jones has lately made its relations to the different febrile conditions an especial study. His arguments are as follows:

The arteries of the abdominal, thoracic, and cranial viscera are supplied by the sympathetic plexuses exclusively, and paralysis of these plexuses dilates the arteries they accompany, and increases heat and tissue-change in the locality where they are distributed; it establishes active hyperæmia, which, in states of debility, may pass into inflammation. The arteries of the rest of the body receive vaso-motor nerves from the cerebro-spinal filaments which accompany them, but, as they always carry with them fibres derived from the ganglia of the sympathetic, their supply is probably identical in character. In fact, the structure of these vaso-motor nerves is known to be the same as those of the visceral vessels, and a lesion of those would probably produce similar effects. He has found these vaso-motor nerves most distinctly in the skin of the fingers and dorsum of the foot.

The phenomena of malarious disease may be regarded as the results of a poisonous influence, operating on the cerebro-spinal and sympathetic nervous systems. It acts eminently on the solar plexus, occasioning a sense of debility and distress about the epigastrium, paralyzes the various plexuses which are offshoots from the solar ganglion, as well as others which are formed by the abdominal sympathetic, from which result dilatation of arteries, increased heat of blood and local hyperæmia. At the same time, the cerebro-spinal system is affected, in some parts debilitated, in others irritated. The hemispheres of the brain are evidently enfeebled and weakened in their actings. The sensory nerves are irritated, giving rise to neuralgic pains, and the motors, being similarly affected, produce the rigors. The shrinking of the skin is produced by the contraction of some organic muscular fibres, in its corium, as well as by the occlusion of its arterioles. The arrest of the secretions shows that the vital powers of the organs producing them is impaired or in abeyance. The action of the heart is, in most cases, directly enfeebled, just as the contractile coat of the arteries is; sometimes, however, as described by Dr. Bell, in cholera, and as is sometimes seen in cardiac neuralgia, associated with ague, it is rather enchained and embarrassed in its workings, by an abnormal, irritating stimulus. The short and labored respiration depends, in part, on congestion taking place in the lungs, but still more probably on disordered innervation of the phrenic and other respiratory nerves. In the case of the cold stage being replaced by an attack of convulsions, or one of coma, it may be supposed that the morbid influence has operated with unusual force on the principal nervous centres devoted to voluntary motion, in the first place, and on the cortical substance of the hemispheres, in the second. The phenomena of the second stage are, increased action of the heart, relaxation of the cutaneous arteries, paralysis of their vasomotor nerves, the condition of other parts remaining about the same. The congestions commenced in the first stage are apt to be increased as the blood is driven with increased force, through relaxed arteries, by a powerfully-acting heart. Epistaxis, apoplectic effusion, intestinal hæmorrhage, rupture of the spleen, may thus be produced. The relaxation of the superficial arteries is only an extension of the condition of the rest of the arterial system, but the increased action of the heart is the reverse. This may arise from its sooner regaining its contractility, in consequence of the more vigorous life of its contractile tissue, or from the stimulus of the heated blood, or from paralysis of the vagus. In fevers of a low type, the muscular tissue of the heart may become so impaired in its quality that it answers but languidly to the stimulus of the hot blood. Authors mention the occurrence of paroxysms of a cold or a hot stage only. In the former case, it may be supposed that the poison has operated chiefly on the cerebro-spinal system; no febrile reaction takes place, because the temperature of the blood has not been increased by paralysis of the sympathetic. In the latter, the poison operates exclusively on the vaso-motor nerves, and, therefore, pyrexial phenomena alone are produced.

In *algide* fevers, the prominent phenomena are, ice-coldness of the surface, elevation of the temperature after death, smallness or suppression of the pulse, peculiar cerebral torpor, but without coma or loss of consciousness, debility and depression. These appear to be the results of an irritating, rather than a paralyzing influence. The brain is evidently enfeebled, but rather benumbed than otherwise. It appears more like the result of peculiar irritation than loss of power. A similar state prevails in the vaso-motor nerves, which appear to be irritated and excited, rather than paralyzed, as during pyrexia. It is reasonable to suppose that the icy coldness may be, at least in part, a result of this state; as it was found, in Bernard's experiment, that when the cut end of the sympathetic was galvanized, the temperature fell below the normal point. The elevation of the temperature, after death, shows that some power was acting to depress the heat that should have been normally developed. The livid color of the surface is to be regarded, like the leaden hue of cholera, as the result of tissue paralysis, in consequence of which, and of arterial occlusion, stagnation occurs in the capillaries.

This is merely a hint as to the influence which the sympathetic, and, in fact, the cerebro-spinal system may have in the induction and origination of disease. It will be further adverted to in the treatment of fevers.

REMARKS ON FOURTH PARAGRAPH.

The principal morbid appearances on the *lips* are, the palor of chlorosis; the redness and dryness which attend fevers and inflammations; the cracked, parched, and black appearance, in typhoid fevers and severe inflammations; the swollen look which attends scrofula and chronic erysipelas; the obstinate fissures which attend some gastric derangements and menstrual disorders; the herpes which follow fever and ague, and catarrhal affections; the occurrence of cancer, &c.

The *teeth* present but few morbid appearances, except caries.

The *gums* furnish many important indications, such as the sponginess, which attends scurvy and mercurial action; the blue line, which marks lead poisoning; the pink line, which occurs in phthisis, &c.

A *bitter taste*, of course, often arises from bilious derangement, still it is said to attend phlebitis, brain affections, and suppuration of the lungs. When it occurs suddenly, in the height of a fever, without other evident bilious disorder, it is said often to precede a severe brain complication, and to be of fatal omen. A persistent bitter taste, in apparently convalescent patients, is said to indicate danger of a relapse, and, in dropsical patients, an incurable condition. It often occurs in hysterical and catarrhal subjects, and then is of slight moment. The principal remedies are Aloes, Chamomilla, Dulcamara, Colchicum, Mercurius, Nux, and Veratrum.

An *insipid* taste often points to great debility of the gustatory nerves or digestive organs; is common after profuse perspiration, and attends almost all fevers and catarrhal affections. It sometimes precedes vomiting of blood, and, when it occurs in convalescents, denotes an imperfect recovery and danger of relapse. The principal remedies are China, Nux, Pulsatilla, Digitalis, Phosphor, or Platina.

A *putrid* taste often arises from diseases of the teeth, tonsils, or throat, or from such debility of the stomach, and deficiency of gastric juice, as allows the food to putrefy rather than digest, or from the putrefaction of mucous impurities about the gums, mouth, tongue, throat, or digestive organs, or from the suppression of stinking-foot, or axilla, or perineal sweats. It is a bad sign in phthisis and fevers; points sometimes to the death of the fœtus in pregnant women, and to the occurrence of gangrene in inflammations of the lungs and bowels.

Agaricus, Anacardium, Spigelia, and Sabadilla are the principal remedies, although a weak solution of Chloride of Soda or Chloride of of Potash are useful palliatives, or moderate doses of yeast, or Belloc's Charcoal.

An *alkaline* taste occurs from contact with the negative electrical pole, before the occurrence of apthæ, and in alkaline states of the secretions of the stomach and mouth. Dulcamara, Iodine, Zinc, and Nitric-acid are the principal remedies.

Loss of taste may arise from debility or paralysis of the gustatory nerve, from febrile or catarrhal states; if persistent, it denotes a relapse, in acute cases, and, in quartan intermittents, is said to be a precursor of dropsy. Anacardium, Belladonna, Nux, Secale, and Sepia are said to be the principal remedies.

A *salty* taste occurs in the first stage of all catarrhal affections, or may precede bleeding from the lungs; in acute febrile chest affections, it is a good sign, if attended with free expectoration, and may lead us to expect recovery when some other symptoms are unfavorable. Arsenicum, Carbo-vegetabilis, Rhus, and Zincum are the principal remedies.

A *sour* taste arises from contact with the positive electrical pole, from digestive derangement, tendency to gout, and in scrofula and rhachitis. Muriate of Ammonia, Cocculus, Cuprum, Nitrum, and Phosphoric-acid are useful remedies, while Borax and the alkalies may be used, occasionally and sparingly, as palliatives.

Increase of taste arises from excitement of the gustatory nerves or papillæ, and is common in nervous subjects. In fevers, it is a sign of a threatening nervous disorder, or a tendency to delirium. The principal remedies are Conium, Agaricus, or Rhododendron.

A *sweetish* taste is common in catarrhal and consumptive affections, and sugar has then, at times, been detected in the expectoration, or other excreta from the mouth and fauces. Plumbum and Sabadilla are useful remedies.

The affections and coatings of the tongue, the variations of the pulse, and the varying conditions of the urine will be treated of, collectively, in another place.

In the *fauces*, we often find simple redness, which may be relieved by small doses of Aconite or Belladonna; if the redness be obstinate and chronic, small doses of Cantharides and Mercurius are often useful. Sometimes the throat is roughened or granular, like that which occurs in granular lids. Local applications of Nitrate of Silver are sometimes useful, although, doubtless, they are applied twenty times as as often as they are indicated; a long-continued course of Thuja, or Hepar-sulphur, or Iodide of Mercury will often prove of avail. Sometimes we find the fauces, in chronic cases of throat-trouble, as dry and glazed as if a hot iron had been passed over it, or a coating of varnish had dried upon it; in these cases, the Chlorate of Potash, internally, and used as a gargle, will frequently render the mucous membrane much more pale and moist. We frequently find, in other cases, large quantities of thick and tenacious greenish mucus plastered on the back of the throat, and projecting downward from the posterior fauces. Pulsatilla is useful, while gargling the throat with a weak solution of Soda, or Hydriodate of Potash, will so change the action of the mucous membrane that Phosphoric-acid, or Sulphate of Alumina, will complete the cure. In erysipelatous swellings of the fauces, and veil of the palate, small doses of Antimony or Rhus will often act like a charm.

Affections of the tonsils are of various kinds, and occur with very unequal severity in different cases, depending upon the number and variety of the parts which it involves; for they often spread to the uvula, velum palati, salivary glands, pharynx, and even to the root of the tongue, and neighboring cellular tissue.

When the inflammation is superficial, (mucous pharyngitis and tonsillitis,) it does not produce any great distress; when it penetrates beyond the mucous membrane, (sub-mucous variety,) it is apt to end in suppuration, and harass the patient much, as the tonsils often swell to an enormous size. It is worst of all when the back part of the tongue, and the muscular and cellular tissues become implicated, for it may even reach the larynx, and then is always extremely perilous; when the muscular coat alone is affected, (muscular pharyngitis,) although swallowing is difficult and exceedingly painful, there is no appearance in the fauces which can account for these symptoms; when the mucous crypts are the principal seat of the disease, (follicular tonsillitis,) opaque whitish spots appear on the red tonsil, consisting of the discharged contents of the follicles, and are often mistaken for ulcerating or sloughing points. When the inflammation is violent, the submaxillary and parotid glands sometimes swell, and become tender to pressure, and the patient may be troubled with profuse ptyalism. In severe cases, the pain often shoots from the throat to the ear, along the eustachian tube, and suppuration occurs, in the majority of cases attended with this symptom. Sometimes both tonsils are attacked at once; very frequently, one only is affected at first, and the disease begins in the other, as it subsides in the first, just as it does in mumps. When the back of the tongue is involved, the patient is unable to open his mouth sufficiently to allow the fauces to be seen, and even the finger cannot be introduced into the mouth.

The milder and superficial cases often terminate by resolution, in about three days. The follicular cases frequently end in the formation of small abscesses, for we often notice a small yellow spot, or phlyctæna, which may burst unnoticed, on the fourth or fifth day, either during sleep or a fit of coughing, and the small quantity of matter which is discharged, is not noticed, or its nauseous taste and smell may attract attention; the patient at once feels essentially relieved, and the rest of the disorder subsides rapidly. When the abscess is deep-seated, the patient often passes four, or five, or seven, or ten sleepless days and nights, when, finally, it bursts, or is opened artificially.

Treatment.—A large proportion of the difference of symptoms depends as much or more upon the seat of the disease than its nature. The treatment can generally be commenced with a few doses of Aconite or Stibium, as the constitutional disturbance often runs higher than might have been expected, considering the limited extent of the local inflammation, and the comparatively small importance of the part inflamed, for smart inflammatory fever, severe headache, and pains in the limbs, with a rapid pulse, of 100 to 120, or more, are not uncommon.

When the difficulty of swallowing arises mainly from the soreness of the mucous membrane, especially if the mucous follicles are much affected, Mercurius and Hepar-sulph., or Ammon.-caust., are the most important remedies. When the muscular coat is much involved, the rheumatic remedies, such as Mercurius and Mezereum, come in play; although Belladonna often proves highly palliative and curative. When suppuration threatens to ensue, Hepar-sulph. and Stibium are most useful. When there is much œdematous or erysipelatous swelling, Rhus, Cantharides, or Apis.-mell. relieve more quickly than other remedies. When the salivary glands, both submaxillary and parotid, become involved, Mercurius and Stibium afford most relief.

As regards the local treatment, gargling with warm milk and water, every hour or two; currant-jelly water is often useful, or the inhalation of the vapor of hot water, with or without the addition of Vinegar or Nitric-acid, although Dr. Jeanes recommends Benzoic-acid.

Diseases of the œsophagus are less common than affections of many other organs. Still its mucous membrane may be inflamed, and the inflammation may sometimes bear a croupous character, with the formation of false membranes; then Bichromate of Potash and Aconite are useful remedies. Sometimes there is a *diffused inflammation of the cellular tissue* of the pharynx and œsophagus, leading to suppuration; at other times the disease commences in the bones and periosteum of the spine and extends to the œsophageal cellular tissue. This affection is frequently associated with pyæmia, or with erysipelas, and is either diffused, as is common in pyæmia or erysipelas, or a defined abscess is formed. When the inflammation is diffused, the patient rapidly passes into a typhoid condition, the dysphagia becomes extreme, the respiration impeded, and, on examining the neck, we find either the erysipelatous redness of the skin, or a fulness and tenseness among the intra-typhoid muscles, impeding the free movement of the parts concerned in deglutition. When a *defined abscess* is formed in the sub-mucous cellular tissue of the œsophagus, there is often sudden and urgent dyspnœa, with fever, and, on examining the throat, we see a projection from the posterior fauces, sometimes on the level with the soft palate, sometimes above or below it; puncturing the abscess will relieve the urgent symptoms. In the diffuse inflammation the prognosis is very unfavorable; Rhus, Cantharides, Apis, and Hepar-sulphur may be tried.

The two most common causes of *spasmodic stricture* of the œsophagus are hysteria and hydrophobia. In the former case, it is most common in young women of an excitable nervous system, with leucorrhœa, or painful menstruation or impaired digestion; in some cases of hysteria, the refusal to swallow seems to arise rather from a disordered will than from any disease of the œsophagus. Spasmodic stricture is also often superadded to obstruction arising from organic causes, so that the degree of dysphagia often differs exceedingly in the same case, at different times. Hot fomentations around the neck; the use of fluid, instead of solid food, for a time, are useful means. The simplest cases are relieved by a few doses of Ignatia or Nux, or by Musk or Assafœtida. Where the general health is involved, or the nervous system be excessively sensitive, Valerianate of Zinc, full doses of Conium and Ferrum, with abundance of fresh air, exercise, and cheerful occupation of the mind will often be required.

The most true and marked spasm of the pharynx and œsophagus is found in hydrophobia, probably from extreme irritability of the nerves supplying the pharynx; in fact, of all the branches of the fifth and pneumo-gastric nerves. In some cases, the pharynx seems more than twice its natural capacity, the constrictor muscles being retracted to the utmost, and the fauces exceedingly large, from the rigid contraction of the soft palate; every part may appear expanded to the utmost.

Paralysis of the muscles of deglutition sometimes exists in a slight degree; in some mental diseases, the same occurs in a greater degree. With feebleness of muscular power, we may find that the will is unable to excite muscular action, and that the muscles of the pharynx appear paralyzed, because they are not stimulated to healthy contraction. Nux, Ignatia, or Plumbum may prove useful.

Organic obstruction of the œsophagus may arise from: 1, annular constriction; 2, ulceration; 3, cancer; and 4, pressure, from aneurismal or other tumors. Annular constriction arises from effusion of fibrinous material into the sub-mucous cellular tissues; this tissue contracts and becomes exceedingly dense, forming a firm, constricting band, while the tube above dilates. A long-continued course of Muriate of Ammonia is likely to prove useful.

Ulceration, of a non-cancerous character, sometimes occurs in the œsophagus. Sometimes the abrasion of the mucous membrane, or slight ulceration, may not be greater than that we often see in the pharynx, yet may lead to a great deal of spasmodic stricture. Where the ulceration is greater, difficulty of deglutition is the most prominent symptom during life. The pain is situated at the sternum, or between the shoulders, and attempts at swallowing are often followed by urgent dyspnœa, and food may be forcibly ejected through the nares; the patient emaciates and life may be prolonged by nutrient enemata. Iodide of Potash and Arsenicum, alone or in alteration, will often accomplish much, or Nitric-acid and Thuja. Occasionally the ulceration opens from the œsophagus into the trachea. Cancerous affections of the œsophagus are, of course, incurable, although Muriate of Gold, Conium, and Arsenicum may be used.

The size of the *liver* may very accurately be determined by percussion. The superior border is generally found about two inches below the right nipple, or corresponding with the fifth rib; its lower border is continuous with the lower margin of the ribs. If the liver be enlarged, it generally projects below the lower margin of the ribs, and may be felt by pressure or detected by percussion; the inferior margin of the liver may sometimes be detected readily from the contrast which, on percussion, its dulness and density present, when contrasted with the tympanitic and elastic feel of the intestines and stomach. Still this is far from being always the case; too frequently the abdominal muscles are thick and rigid, or the patient is sensitive and the slightest touch throws them into a state of spasmodic contraction, when they will feel hard and board-like. It must be remembered, that the intestines lie directly under the lower margin of the liver, or rather that a thin layer of liver descends on the right side over the bowels. It is, therefore, necessary to be cautious in determining the inferior margins, for a tolerably strong blow with the finger may give rise to a sympathetic sound from the intestine, heard through the liver; hence, as we approach the lower margin of the liver, from above downward, in percussing, the force of the blow should be diminished, and one should percuss cautiously and gently. Again, as the upper margin of the liver is overlapped by a thin layer of lung, it will be necessary to determine where the lung-sound terminates, inferiorly, by striking gently with the finger, and where the liver-sound ceases, superiorly, by striking forcibly, so that vibrations may be communicated through the layer of the lung.

In cases of pleurisy, with effusion on the right side, the liver is often pushed far down into the abdomen, and may seem to be enlarged, although it is not. The dulness on percussion may extend far up into the chest, and low down into the abdomen, and a superficial examiner may suppose that he has to do with a very much enlarged liver solely. To the expert, careful examiner, when fluid exists in the cavity of the pleura, the increased density of the liver may still serve to distinguish it, through the humoral sound of the fluid. It sometimes happens that a loaded colon, passing under the lower margin of the liver, will increase the dulness on percussion, and lead to the inference that the liver is much enlarged; the best way to avoid this mistake is to have the bowels well unloaded before making the examination. When the liver is enlarged, its lower edge is generally thickened, and this may be indicated, on percussion, by the dulness on percussion passing into the resonance of the intestines more abruptly than in health. A good mode of feeling this thick edge is, after a full evacuation of the colon, to lay the hand flat on the surface below its supposed situation, and, after pressing rather deeply, to slide it upward, so as to bring the radial side of the index-finger in contact with it; sometimes the point of the finger, pressed down deeply upon the abdominal wall, will detect this thick edge, if it exists, better than any other way. When tumors are present in the liver, the inferior border often presents an irregular form; the cancerous tubercles are large, and are generally easily discoverable when present; sometimes even the nodules of granular liver may be felt, if the abdominal walls be thin.

Spleen.—If to mark out the precise limits of the heart, constitutes the first difficult lesson in the art of percussion, to do the same for the spleen is a still more difficult problem. Singularly enough, few or no anatomists describe the exact situation of the normal spleen in the healthy body. In health, the spleen never projects below the false ribs, even during a deep inspiration. Its general size is about four inches long and three inches wide, but the dulness on percussion is not so extensive. In percussing the spleen, it is necessary that the patient lie on the right side, and it is better that the examination be made before, rather than soon after a meal. Anteriorly, the sonoriety of the stomach and intestines causes the margin readily to be distinguished; posteriorly, however, where the organ approaches toward the kidneys, this is more difficult. Its superior and inferior margins may be made out, with difficulty, by strong percussion, as this organ offers great resistance on percussion. In percussing the spleen, the finger should first be applied as nearly over its centre as possible, where the dull sound and sense of resistance are most characteristic; from the centre we should percuss gradually toward the periphery, or margin of the organ, and strike—now forcibly, now lightly—until the characteristic sound of the next organ be elicited. Then we should percuss gradually back again, until the dull splenic sound is again heard. The *upper* boundary of the splenic dulness, when determined under favorable circumstances, reaches the level of the tenth rib, posteriorly; but deep percussion must be used, in order reach it through the intervening portion of the lung. All that part of the spleen which lies below the margin of the left lung, imparts dulness on superficial percussion, which becomes continuous below with that of the left kidney; a little resonance and diminished sense of resistance sometimes intervening. Thus, the vertical extent of the dulness may sometimes be made out to be three and one-half inches. The lateral extent of the dulness is anteriorly bounded by the resonance of the stomach; theoretically, it should measure about three inches, but a normal spleen will rarely exhibit so much. In short, the normal spleen lies somewhat back toward the spine, extending from the level of the tenth left rib, down to the upper margin of the left kidney.

When only enlarged to a small extent, the spleen produces no palpable tumor; but, as it increases, its lower margin is to be felt, on pressing upward beneath the edge of the ribs, a little posterior to a vertical line drawn down from the nipple. Its border is generally somewhat thick and rounded, and is perceived to be somewhat moveable. As the spleen is very apt to increase regularly in all directions, we may often infer, from the size of the portion felt, the whole bulk of the organ; still, percussion will give this much more accurately, as it is much easier to percuss a large spleen than a small or natural one.

It is often important to distinguish a splenic pain from the hysterical pain in the left side of young females; they are often confounded together, but the splenic pain is generally seated more posteriorly than the hysterical pain, which has its seat under the left breast, at a spot corresponding to the commencement of the sheath of the rectus muscle, or at a place corresponding with one of the digitations of the serratus magnus and external oblique muscles. Both pains, however, may occur in delicate females who have had obstinate fever and ague.

REMARKS ON FIFTH PARAGRAPH.

The most frequently useful remedies in amenorrhœa are, Sepia and Pulsatilla in lymphatic cases, or Ferrum and Stramonium in anæmic cases, or Aconite in plethoric cases.

In dysmenorrhœa, Conium, Belladonna, or Stramonium, singly, or in alternation with Opium, are often useful when the pain is very severe; while a course of Cocculus will often prevent the recurrence of the attacks.

Obstinate menorrhagia is often relieved by small doses of Secale or Sabina; where there is much enlargement of the uterus, a course of Muriate of Gold, or Iodide of Mercury, will often prove useful. In leucorrhœa, even when attended with ulceration, a long-continued course of Arsenicum or Cantharides, in quite small quantities, will often prevent the necessity for the use of the speculum or of caustics.

The pain in the back, which attends so many uterine complaints, may have its seat in the muscles of the hips or loins, or in the pelvic nerves, from pressure or sympathetic irritation; quite frequently, when it is low down in the sacrum, the pain is seated in the last of the gangliæ of the great sympathetic nerve, viz., in the ganglion-impar; this is especially the case in which the pain is said to be at the very extremity of the spine. On close questioning, many patients will describe the exact locality of the ganglion-impar—viz.: on the anterior surface of the sacrum, or deep in the pelvis, or the front of the back-bone. Ordinarily, this pain is mistaken for some rheumatic affection of the ligaments of the sacrum or coccyx, or for some strain or bruise of the coccyx, or for pressure from an enlarged or retroverted uterus. It is very difficult to relieve these pains with ordinary remedies.

Argentum-nitricum is indicated when there is heaviness and drawing in the loins, with debility, weariness, and trembling of the legs; when there is a sense of weight in the small of the back, impeding sitting; heaviness, stiffness, and lame sensation at the sacrum, extending down along the pelvis to the hips; heaviness and painful drawing in the sacrum and along the pelvis, as if the menses would appear; when the whole lumbar region feels rigid, with nocturnal pains in the small of the back, and intense pain in the sacral region.

Phosphorus is indicated when there is a burning pain in the small of the back, especially when the menses are delayed; weakness and numbness of the small of the back; pain at the coccyx, as if ulcerated; intolerable pains in the small of the back, preventing walking; pain in the back, after sitting rather too long; pain in the back, produced by standing, rising, or a very little walking.

Staphysagria, when there is pain in the small of the back, with feeling as if strained, even while at rest; pain in the small of the back, as if broken, followed by disturbance in the abdomen and pelvis; intense burning pain at the lower and outer parts of the sacrum.

Kreosote is useful when there is much leucorrhœa, and excoriation, or even ulceration of the os. It may be used as a vaginal injection, or taken internally, when there are pains in the loins, like those which precede menstruation; when there are frequent pains in the small of the back and loins, like those which precede labor-pains; when there are pains in the small of the back, extending to the rectum, or over the abdomen, and through the pudendum and thighs, with anxiety, trembling, &c., all increased by lying down; pains in the small of the back, as if it would break.

The best palliative remedies are, quite large doses of Chamomilla, Lactuca-virosa, or Ambra-grisea.

As regards *ulcerations* of the os-uteri, we feel almost inclined to agree with Barclay, that they are comparatively rare, and, as a substantive disease, rather unimportant than otherwise. They sometimes occur as an accidental and rather trivial complication of other constitutional diseases; but, in their uncomplicated form, they have merely an ephemeral notoriety, and will soon pass away. True pathology and useful practice have neither been advanced nor benefitted by those who have made them a special study. What has been called ulceration, is generally only an aphthous or granular condition of the mucous membrane, and depends upon constitutional, and not merely on local causes; very often a patch of adhering mucus has been mistaken for an ulcer; oftentimes it is only a creation of the fancy; occasionally it is the result of excessive leucorrhœa, and then is a consequence, not a cause—merely a symptom, and that a minor one. If scrofulous, cancerous, or syphilitic diseases are not present, we may safely regard the petty ulceration as of no consequence, in so far as it is a local malady.

Weak injections of dilute Nitric-acid will often prove more useful than applications of Lunar Caustic. A long-continued course of small doses of Arsenicum will often remove the leucorrhœa and so-called ulceration. If the aphthous character be predominant, injections of a solution of Chlorate of Potash will often accomplish a cure. The general treatment should be like that generally adopted for aphthæ and nursing sore mouth.

In order to *percuss the kidneys*, the patient should lie upon his face. These organs, of course, lie close to the spine, in the region of the loins; but rather higher up than they are usually supposed to be. Their upper extent of dullness cannot always be accurately determined, in consequence of its being easily confounded with that of the liver and spleen, which lie here in front of them. The lower extremity of the kidneys, however, is more favorably situated for examination—the dullness of the solid organ contrasting forcibly with the resonance of the intestine, which is found between it and the crest of the ileum· sometimes, on very careful percussion, however, a little resonance and a diminished sense of resistance will be found, between the upper edge of each kidney and the lower margin of the liver and spleen, on either side. The right kidney lies a little lower than the left, and, of course, the dullness on percussion will be found lower on that side, without there being any enlargement of the right kidney.

In minor degrees of enlargement of the kidney, we may sometimes discover the lower part of the organ broader and more prominent, and descending somewhat lower than in health. If the kidney be very large, it may produce visible enlargement of the abdomen, or a fullness or bulging in the flank, lumbar region, and iliac fossa. It may be distinguished from enlarged liver and spleen, on percussion, by the tympanitic sound of the colon, in front of the enlarged kidney, on either side; while an enlarged liver and spleen always have the colon behind them, and, consequently, there is more anterior dullness on percussion. Careful manual examination will sometimes enable one to trace the renal enlargement back to the spine, while the fingers can be insinuated between it and the ribs, and occasionally detect the overlapping margin of the liver.

Alterations of the urine will be treated of in connection with those of the tongue and pulse.

TONGUE.—The indications from the *tongue* are important and numerous, although less reliable than most physicians think. Some patients always have a clean tongue, however much disordered they may be; others never have one, however well they may seem; exceedingly bilious and almost jaundiced persons often have clean tongues; and a very dirty tongue often points to some merely local affection of the mouth or throat. The remarkable cohesive power possessed by the epithelium of the tongue, in cases of "furry coat," is so great, says Chambers, that the scales may be seen sticking so closely together as to form long threads, rough and scaly, like the filaments of wool, so that one can easily imagine their being matted together and felting, if dried; they may even become mouldy and putrid. Coatings of the tongue arise from disorder of the epithelium of the tongue, and may, or may not be simultaneous with similar disorders in distant mucous membranes. If the epithelium is formed in too great quantity, and is more adhesive than usual, we have "coated" tongues, of various colors. If it is, at the same time, tough and adherent, like a skin, it then retains the shape of the thread-like papillæ, and projects from their ends, lengthening them so as—instead of a pile-like velvet—to form regular hairs like a fur, and the tongue is then said to be "furred;" but, if it is less tough, it merely fills up the interstices between the papillæ, and is called a smooth, "creamy" tongue. If there is a too rapid throwing off of epithelium, or if it is not formed in sufficient quantity, the tongue is bare, and is seen to be red or raw. If there is a want of red blood in the mucous membrane, the natural elasticity and swelling are deficient, and we have what is denominated a "pasty or flabby" tongue, which takes and retains the marks of the teeth.

A white even layer on the tongue is generally indicative of a slight gastric, catarrhal, or constitutional disorder.

A thicker coating, from accumulation of epithelium, exists to its greatest extent in affections of the fauces, and in mucous states of the stomach and bowels; less remarkably in conditions of general debility; while it has a creamy look in delirium tremens.

A peculiar buff-leather appearance is present in some cases of enteritis and hepatitis.

A patchy tongue is often indicative of considerable local irritation of the mouth.

A yellow color is generally believed to be bilious; a dark brown color is most common in severe internal inflammations, in typhoid and malignant fevers, and in hæmorrhage from the mouth.

A shining and glazed appearance, especially when chapped, is very common in inflammation of the bowels.

The papillæ project remarkably in scarlet fever; a less degree of projection, through a thin white coating, often points to a marked nervous disorder, and is common in hysteria.

Coatings of the tongue generally commence at the base, and gradually spread over the body and edges to the tip, from whence it should as regularly recede; departures from this rule generally point to some irregularity in the course of the disease.

A very considerable coating of the tongue is generally a certain sign of decided implication of the mucous membranes, whatever the part may be that is originally affected, and denotes tediousness and obstinacy of the attack.

The appearance of a coating of the tongue, in the midst of a disease, in which the tongue has been cleaner than it might have been expected to be, is often of *favorable* import, as it sometimes points to the occurrence of a crisis, just as perspiration, a sediment in the urine, free expectoration, and slight diarrhœa, or discharge from the nose, often indicate the reëstablishment of the suppressed secretions. At times, however, it denotes the setting in of some new complication.

The persistence of a coated tongue during convalescence, denotes an imperfect resolution of the disease, a slumbering and smouldering of some of the elements of the disorder, a tendency to relapse, or the occurrence of some after-affection, or, perhaps, to local debility of the digestive organs, often caused by heroic doses of salines, antimonials, or mercurials.

Local or partial coatings of the tongue are rarely favorable, as they often indicate a tedious course of the disease, or the occurrence of local affections.

Unilateral coatings often attend one-sided affections of the body, such as migrane, tic-doloroux, paralysis, &c.; a thick white coating of one-half of the root of the tongue, while the other is clean and red, often points to chronic disease of one lung; a unilateral coating, in febrile affections, without evident disease of one-half of the body, is of unfavorable import, and any crisis which may take place is generally only partial. Coatings occurring in isolated patches are among the most common indications of gastric or abdominal phthisis, and when they attend lung-disorders generally point to a simultaneous affection of the stomach.

When the coating extends, in a narrow line, towards the middle of the tongue, from the root to the tip, it often indicates a turgescence of gastric impurities upwards.

When the centre of the tongue has a tendency to become dry, it points to an obstinate or typhoid febrile affection, or to a fastly-seated inflammatory trouble, with tendency towards suppuration.

A soft *brown* coating is often a sign of bilious derangement or fever, or obstinate bilious or gastric disorder. A dry brown tongue, which looks as if it were parched or burnt, often indicates the obstinate adhesion of acrid bilious sordes, or it may be a sign of violent inflammation of some internal organ; while, in children, it often accompanies a treacherous arachnitis, or some typhoid or adynamic affection.

A very adhesive coating of the tongue, which can only be partially removed by scraping, is a sign of great torpor of the exhalent vessels, or of obstinate gastric derangement.

A yellow coating of the tongue often attends mucous and bilious derangements, or is a sign of the bilious character of some fevers and inflammations; still, when a previous white coating becomes yellow, it sometimes is a sign of an approaching favorable crisis. In pleurisy, when the tongue is yellow from the beginning, we may hope for a crisis in seven days; if it only appears on the third or fourth day, recovery is sometimes postponed for nine days. The sudden appearance of a yellow coating on a previously clean tongue, in inflammatory fevers, if the heat increases and the urine becomes more turbid, sometimes indicates the approach of a typhoid state, or of a more malignant form of inflammation; but, if the other symptoms are more favorable, a crisis may occur.

A punctated coating of the tongue occurs in scarlet fever. When it occurs in children, in other diseases, they are often sicker than they seem. In fever and ague patients, it often indicates an inflammatory irritation of the intestinal glands, and Quinine is very apt to disagree.

A black coating of the tongue generally points to a typhoid condition, or is a sign of intense inflammation, which is penetrating deeply into some organ.

White coatings of the tongue are frequently removed by Muriate of Ammonia and Pulsatilla; yellow coatings by Mercurius and Colchicum; brown coatings by Chlorate of Potash and Arsenicum; black coatings by Arsenicum and Nitric-acid; a very dry tongue may often be rendered moist by drinking freely of a weak solution of Chlorate of Potash, and Terebinth is a useful internal remedy.

A *livid*, or *purple* color of the tongue is usually dependent upon an insufficient aëration of the blood, and is a valuable sign in connection with the same color of the lips; it often arises from disease of the heart, or from emphysema, or great congestion of the lungs. It denotes a venous or congestive state of the system, just as a morbidly bright *red* tongue, not dependent upon local irritation, points to an arterial or phlogistic condition; while a morbidly *pale* tongue is a sign of deficiency of the blood in general, or of its red corpuscules in particular, as in chlorosis, anemia, or scorbutus.

When the *fur* is white, thickish, tolerably uniform, and accompanied with moisture, in febrile affections, it usually indicates an open, active state of fever, in which, though the obvious symptoms may be violent, there is not apt to be any lurking mischief, nor any malignant tendency. Muriate of Ammonia and Pulsatilla are reliable remedies. When short, very adhesive, and rather scanty, permitting the redness of the tongue to appear through it, and attended with some disposition to dryness, it is often a sign of a protracted and obstinate form of fever, which is apt to assume a low, nervous, or typhoid form; or else it indicates a fixed and somewhat intractable form of inflammation, which yields sullenly to remedies, is very apt to relapse, or rather is rarely decidedly and promptly removed by any kind of treatment, but which requires close attention on the part of the physician, who must not mistake an apparent, but transient improvement for a permanent overcoming of the disorder. A *yellowish* hue of the fur is usually indicative of bilious disorder, and generally produced by direct secretion from the tongue, consequent upon deficient excretion from the liver, and excessive production of bilious matter in the blood.

A *brown* or *black tongue* is usually regarded as indicative of a low state of the system, and an impaired condition of the blood, especially marked by a deficiency of fibrin, as in typhus and typhoid fevers. This coating is said to be owing to the secretion of a dark matter, apparently identical with that which collects about the teeth and lips in typhus fevers, and probably consists of blood, modified in its passage out of the vessels; a similar secretion to that which takes place on the tongue, is supposed to occur in the liver, stomach, and bowels in some malignant fevers, causing the black discharges so common in these cases. This state of things is sometimes said to depend simply on a diseased or deteriorated condition of the blood; others suppose it to arise from a profound derangement of the true secretive, formative and natural plastic processes, or of these and of the blood combined. Thus, it is supposed that unhealthy blood is brought to the capillaries, that it stagnates and exudes through their walls,—not as a simple hæmorrhagic exudation, as in purpura and scurvy,—not as a truly plastic inflammato-hæmorrhagic exudation as in true arterial inflammation; but as an intermediate, partly depraved, partly venous-inflammatory condition. This view gathers strength from the fact that a black tongue occurs in purpura and scurvy as soon as fever, or inflammation be added thereto; this proves that the disease of the blood alone will not cause it, but must be aided by some feverish or inflammatory trouble. It is evident that simple hæmorrhagic remedies will not relieve this state; neither will the remedies for simple fever or inflammation. Hammamelis, Kreosote, Nitric and Phosphoric-acids will do much; Chlorate of Potash is a useful palliative; but often the remedies for an asthenic or typhoid inflammation will also be required, such as Rhus, Arsenicum, &c. Very frequently, this darkness of the tongue supervenes upon a previously white coating, and then indicates the occurrence of fresh inflammatory trouble, of an unhealthy type and intractable character, or a deteriorated state of the blood or vital forces; one which will require all the skill and watchfulness of the physician.

We have already referred to the gradual recession of the coating, from the tip and edges, in favorable cases. In another mode of cleaning, the fur loosens and separates in flakes, often beginning at the middle or near the root, sometimes in large patches, or over almost the whole tongue at once, leaving a smooth, red, glossy surface, as though the papillary structure had been lost. In such cases, if acute, and if the tongue remains moist, convalescence almost always takes place, though usually tedious and somewhat lingering. In threatening fevers, Wood says, it is very desirable to witness this phenomena, which is often preceded by a feeling of soreness in the throat. Sometimes the fur recurs, once and again, before it ultimately disappears; and weeks or even months are occasionally consumed in the struggling and apparently uncertain advance towards health, which ultimately, however, takes place.

In less favorable cases, the tongue, after having commenced the process of cleaning, or even after completing it, instead of continuing *moist*, becomes as dry as a chip, with an aggravation of all the symptoms, and no little increase of danger. The indications are still more unfavorable, when, in addition to its *dryness*, the surface becomes gashed, chapped, or fissured, or exhibits a rough, scaly appearance.

A similar smooth, red, and glossy state of the tongue, sometimes with moisture, and sometimes with dryness, is not uncommon in chronic diseases, in which it is generally a bad sign, and is supposed to indicate serious organic derangement.

A still worse condition, however, is an aphthous state of the tongue, which is apt to come on in advanced stages of chronic diseases; although often a fatal sign, I have seen it disappear in advanced cases of consumption and dropsy, and the patient live for months after. Borax and Chlorate of Potash are often useful palliatives; a very weak preparation of Iodide of Mercury, or of Arsenicum, or Sulphuric-acid are often useful; Cicuta has been used in some very bad cases with benefit. A full diet, with ale, porter, or some stimulus, is often indispensably necessary.

Pulse.—The indications derived from the pulse are very important, not merely as regards the condition of the heart, arteries, and blood, but as an index of the state of the great sympathetic nerve, upon which the amount of strength, debility, or irritation of the system at large mainly depend; as this nerve is the nerve of organic life, and also supplies the heart and arteries, the amount of irritation, strength, or depression, which it and the vital powers and functions over which it presides may often be accurately determined by the state of the pulse.

The standard pulse of a healthy adult is 72 per minute, or four beats of the pulse to one act of respiration, of which eighteen should occur per minute. Of course, there are many deviations from this standard, without any necessarily great departure from health; thus, there are a few adult persons who, when they are quite well, always have a pulse of 80 or 90, and others in whom it seldom rises above 60. In early life the pulse is more frequent, being from 130 to 140 soon after birth; from 100 to 120 in the first year; from 90 to 100 in the second year; between 80 and 90 up to the eighth year; from 75 to 80 at puberty; from 65 to 75, generally about 72, in persons of middle age; and from 55 to 65 in the healthy old. In many old persons, the pulse ranges from 71 to 78, between the sixty-fourth and seventieth year of age; but, in these cases, there is generally some irritation or dormant organic disorder in the system. Constitutional idiosyncrasies have occurred in which the pulse has habitually exceeded 100, or fallen short of 30 or 40, without apparent disease; while, in some new-born infants, the pulse may be as slow as in adults. In women, the pulse is apt to be from five to ten beats more frequent than in men. The ordinary precautions, in feeling the pulse, should always be observed; thus the family physician should certainly endeavor to have some idea of the natural state of his regular patient's pulse in health. On the first examination, the pulse should always be felt on both sides; for, from some irregular distribution of the arteries, the right pulse may vary very much from the left. A gentleman, whose pulse was naturally much weaker on the left side than the right, was accidentally poisoned by eating partridges: the prostration was great, and for hours he was pulseless on the left side, while the right radial artery was beating regularly and distinctly, but feebly. A physician, who was not aware of this peculiarity, supposed him in a critical state, for hours after he had rallied, from not taking the precaution to feel the pulse on both sides. In another instance, a gentleman suffering from organic disease was in the habit of testing the knowledge and prudence of a new physician, by offering one or the other arm only for his examination, and asking his opinion as to the amount of strength he possessed, as divined by the pulse. A physician, who did not of his own accord examine both pulses, was never allowed to pay a second visit. Of course, great caution should be observed, while examining the pulses of nervous, excitable, or timid persons, to do so quietly and without any display of anxiety; for, in persons of this character, the heart is often excited to increased frequency of action by the slightest causes, and it is impossible to draw any correct inferences about their disease without waiting until the first agitation occasioned by the visit has subsided. The pulse should always be felt more than once on the first visit, and occasionally afterwards; for the physician thus becomes acquainted with its diversities, and will often have occasion to correct, if not reverse, upon the second examination, the conclusions he may have formed from the first. With a little patience and acumen, a physician may thus obtain a correct notion of the nervous excitability and organic stamina of his patient, and may avoid many errors; thus, the skins of many patients feel hot to the rather cool hands of the physician, who has just come in from the fresh air, and, if the pulse also be found unusually excited, the inference may be made that the sick person has a very high fever. By waiting a few moments, until the hands have become warmer, and until the patient's nervous flurry has subsided, it will be found that both skin and pulse approach more nearly to the natural standard than was at first supposed.

It is usually advisable to apply two or three fingers to the artery at once; and in cases where special accuracy is requisite, it is better to apply three or four fingers, as the larger the surface of contact, the more accurate is the impression received. The physician's nails should not be so long as to dig into his patient's flesh, for the natural indignation at such culpable coarseness will flush the face and quicken the pulse of a gentlemanly or ladylike person, if absolute pain does not do the same thing. At first, sufficient pressure only should be made, with the bulbs of the fingers, to get a fair idea of the fullness and quickness of the pulse; then, the fingers may alternately press upon the artery, and relax the pressure, so as to appreciate its degree of force and resistance.

When great accuracy is required, it is better to count the number of pulsations, and in every fit of sickness it is essential to do this, occasionally at least; but, after some little experience has been gained, the physician should be able to make a very close approximate calculation of the quickness of the pulse, without always being obliged to count it; in fact, if he cannot do this reasonably well, it should be regarded as a sign of long-continued acts of carelessness and inattention.

Frequency of the pulse is one of the most common attendants of irritative, febrile, or inflammatory disease; but, as augmented irritability may be an attendant of sinking of the vital powers, as well as exaltation of them, so may a merely frequent pulse be a sign of debility as well as of strength; but it is not a sign of simple debility, but of the existence of some source of irritation in the midst of the depression or debility. Sthenic quickness of the pulse may be relieved by Aconite, Antimony, Veratrum-viride, or Digitalis; a purely asthenic quickness may be helped by China, Ferrum, Alcohol, Nux-vomica, or small doses of Opium. When simple irritation is combined with it, Conium and Opium may prove the most useful remedies; when evident febrile irritation is associated with it, Nitric-ether or Acetate of Ammonia may come in play; when an obstinate and malignant inflammatory irritation is in the back-ground, Arsenicum and Conium may be given in alternation, or Cantharides and Hyosciamus, or Rhus and Belladonna, or Phosphorus and Stramonium. These latter cases will often tax the acumen and fortitude of the physician to the utmost;—routine physicians will either stimulate them into a more severely and malignantly inflammatory state, or depress them into a hopeless state of exhaustion. Weak animal broths, and light stimulant drinks, such as cider and water, or claret and water, or weak ale- or port-sangaree, may be allowed at first, and increased carefully in strength, or be omitted temporarily, as the tongue, skin, pulse, &c., indicate; rightly-administered wine will often cool the skin, assuage the thirst and pulse, lessen the delirium, and relieve the pains; wrongly given, it will aggravate all these.

A full, strong, hard, and frequent pulse denotes the presence of a frank and open febrile or inflammatory state, free from malignancy, and hence not of very unfavorable omen, unless it lasts too long, and the frequency becomes too great.

A very remarkable frequency of the pulse is common and natural in scarlet fever, and almost all the varieties of erysipelas, and we may assume, as a general rule, that excessive frequency of the pulse in febrile and inflammatory fevers denotes a tendency towards erysipelatous and malignant, rather than to simple and benign fever or inflammation; so that, instead of giving Aconite, Antimony, Veratrum-viride, or Digitalis alone, or in large doses, they will have to be given with caution and in alternation, such as Antimony and Arsenicum, Aconite and Rhus, Digitalis and Cantharides, Veratrum-viride and Phosphorus. The principal exceptions to this rule are the occurrence of treacherous inflammations about the brain, or bowels, and occasionally in some other organs.

A weak, small, empty, and very frequent pulse is a sign of progressive general exhaustion, of great deficiency of blood, or of colliquative and exhausting discharges, and generally is of very unfavorable omen; still, it may occur in persons just convalescing from very depressing diseases, and may gradually, under judicious treatment, be changed into a moderately quick and resistant pulse, with every surety of ultimate recovery.

When the pulse rises to 130 or 140, in previously healthy adults, it is a very serious phenomenon, as it either points to very fixed local disease of some vital organ, or is a sign of a dangerous nervous complication. In the one case, the purely antiphlogistic remedies must be given, with great steadiness and boldness; in the other, they must be alternated with narcotic remedies, such as Conium, Hyosciamus, or even Opium.

The occurrence of a *hard and frequent* pulse, in chronic diseases, leads us to fear the establishment of some hectic or suppurative complication. Very small doses of Antimony, and larger ones of Hepar-sulphur, will then often prove useful.

A small, weak, and very frequent pulse, after inflammation has lasted some time, often denotes exhaustion, paralysis of the great sympathetic nerve, or gangrene;—as the inflammation has then run its course, the case may often be treated as one of simple debility; but, if, as is too frequently the case, only a portion of the inflammatory trouble has reached this stage, while another portion is not so far advanced, a too free use of stimulants will only force on the remaining inflammatory trouble into its last and most fatal stage.

A strong and frequent pulse, in feverish patients, is not at all an unfavorable phenomenon, although it is always more or less a sign of crudity, and hence, when it recurs afresh, denotes that a new explosion of the disease has, or will soon take place. A quite unusual degree of frequency of the pulse often points to an erysipelatous tendency of the disease, although it at times precedes the outbreak of a critical perspiration.

A *persistent frequency* of the pulse, after the resolution of a fever, denotes that a remnant of the disease is not yet overcome, which may lead to relapses or to unpleasant sequelæ; still, it may occur after convalescence from some severe diseases, as the natural consequence of the great exhaustion induced by them. China and Ferrum are required in the latter case; Conium and Colchicum are often useful in the former, as they frequently bring about those critical changes in the urine and perspiration which are required to remove the disease.

A *very quick pulse, early in the morning*, generally proves that the patient has passed an uneasy and restless night. Conium, Coffea, or Digitalis will often obviate this.

When the pulse becomes more frequent, in some hysterical and nervous affections, we may generally conclude that improvement will take place; Agaricus and Ambra are then often useful.

Even a moderately frequent pulse is a somewhat unfavorable occurrence during fainting-fits.

A very frequent pulse, in erysipelas and scarlet fever, is less unfavorable than in other diseases in which such frequency is more unusual.

A moderately frequent pulse, in apoplectic persons, is more favorable than either a slow or very quick one.

When there are signs of plethora, and the pulse is very quick and frequent, we may infer that the hyperæmia is more apparent than real.

A *strong* pulse strikes powerfully against the fingers which are placed upon it; in an extreme degree, it cannot be compressed at all, but gives a feeling of puffing, even under the strongest pressure. The strength of the pulse depends chiefly upon the force with which the left ventricle contracts, and in some measure also upon the tonicity of the artery and the volume of the blood. Wood justly says, into the idea of a strong pulse enter not only vigor of impulse, but a steady resistance to pressure and a certain degree of fullness. A *sharp forcible beat*, not sustained by a certain amount of subsequent firmness, indicates irritation rather than real energy. Again, a very contracted pulse, however tense, and however sharp the impulse, can scarcely be called a strong one—for real force is the product both of velocity and mass; hence the more voluminous the pulse, the velocity being the same, the greater is its strength. In this latter combination, we find all the conditions which indicate a general elevation of vital substance, power, and action, viz.: power in the heart's contractions, a high degree of general tonicity, and a large amount of blood. Hence, a really strong pulse is necessarily considered a sign of a sthenic and vigorous state of the system, except when there is hypertrophy of the left ventricle, which may give strength to the pulse, even though the general strength be failing.

If there really be too much blood in the system, and important vital parts be seriously implicated, or threatened by congestion or inflammation, then blood-letting, in sufficient quantity to reduce the mass of blood to the normal standard, is the only safe resource. But, if the absolute quantity of blood be not too great, but is merely circulated too frequently and vigorously, or too strongly attracted towards an irritated, congested, or inflamed part, then truly scientific treatment would require that the increased action of the heart and arteries be reduced, by remedies acting specifically upon the vascular system and its motor organs and powers, such as Antimony, Aconite, Digitalis, or Veratrum-viride; and the local irritation, congestion, or inflammation should also be allayed by remedies specific to the nature of the disorder, and exerting specific powers upon the localities occupied by the disease. Tartar-emetic is more of an irritant, and more homœopathic to true inflammatory irritation than any of the other remedies. Aconite, Veratrum-viride, and Digitalis do not produce inflammatory irritation when applied to the skin, nor in any internal organ, hence they are more homœopathic to congestion, perhaps febrile congestion, than to true inflammation or inflammatory irritation; they may lessen the force and frequency of the circulation, prevent an excessive quantity of blood from being thrown to a congested or irritated part, and thus put it in a more favorable condition to recover its natural state and action; besides, Aconite tends to produce critical discharges through the skin, and Digitalis from the kidneys, and thus may exert counter-irritant, or revulsive, and evacuant actions. Conium and Tobacco also exert a powerful depressing action upon the muscular structure of the heart.

A strong, hard, and frequent pulse, in the dominant school, is always regarded as an indication for blood-letting. Sydenham even says, with such a pulse, bleeding must be resorted to, although the disease is the plague.

A simply and equably strong pulse sometimes precedes a critical hæmorrhage, and renders the prognosis in delirium, convulsions, trembling, and other threatening disorders, less unfavorable than it otherwise would be.

A moderately strong pulse is also a good sign in some chronic diseases; it is also not so unfavorable in apoplectic attacks as some suppose, but then it must not be decidedly hard also. It occasionally happens that a pulse which has been persistently weak, becomes decidedly strong shortly before death, and thus occasions a deceptive improvement, which soon passes over into paralysis of the sympathetic-nervous, and vascular systems.

If the pulse remains strong, after due antiphlogistic treatment, it is a sign that the disease is firmly rooted in the affected organ. Still this remark applies with greater truth to a hard pulse than to a simply strong one.

A strong pulse, as long as it is not too hard and frequent, is a good sign in inflammatory affections of the chest.

A *hard* pulse generally indicates a union of considerable strength of action in the heart with sthenic contraction of the coats of the artery; hence implies considerable vigor of the heart and arteries, and a certain, rather great amount of irritation of the sympathetic nerves which supply them, or of inflammatory irritation in some important organ. There is one condition in which hardness of the pulse is deceptive, as far as the existence of acute disease is concerned—that is, when the coats of the arteries have become indurated, ætheromatous, or ossified, in aged persons; if there be also hypertrophy of the left ventricle, which throws the blood forward more forcibly, the deceptive appearance of general power, in the pulse and system at large, may be very great.

A hard, full, and frequent pulse, when attended with increased heat of the body, dryness of the skin, and scanty discharge of dark saturated urine, is a sign of irritation and increased activity, not only of the heart and arteries, but of some important system or organ. It is an almost constant accompaniment of all really inflammatory conditions, especially those of serous and fibrous tissues. It is most decided in actual inflammation of the internal coats of the arteries themselves, and then may become exceedingly hard, violently throbbing, or even vibrating.

Hardness of the pulse, in inflammatory affections, may generally be expected, except in inflammations of the brain or bowels. If it persists unusually long, and other signs of a favorable termination are wanting, we may fear the occurrence of suppuration, copious inflammatory exudation or effusion, or active disorganization of some important part. If some hardness of the pulse remains, after almost all signs of inflammation have subsided, we may infer the treacherous smouldering of some phlogistic disorder, and the occurrence of suppuration or exudation. If the hardness of a vibrating, jarring, throbbing pulse increases, after rather heroic antiphlogistic treatment, we may conclude that general arteritis is present.

If the pulse once becomes decidedly hard, in the febrile or inflammatory affections of young maidens, we may be almost certain that some inflammatory affection has taken an obstinate and deep hold; for the comparative laxity of the arterial coats, in these subjects, rarely allows the pulse to become hard.

Hardness of the pulse, in fever patients, generally points to the addition of some inflammatory condition, or some very acute irritation of the vascular system, or, at least, to a persistence of the crude stage of the disease. Continuous hardness of the pulse, in fever patients, denotes great obstinacy of the attack, or the presence of some local inflammation. If it occurs during the course of a fever, it indicates a recurrence of the crude stage, or of disturbance in the critical efforts which might have been hoped for, or a tendency to metastasis. Hardness of the pulse, remaining or occurring after signs of coction have progressed somewhat, at times indicates that critical vomiting will occur. Hardness of the pulse, in asthenic and malignant fever, is always of unfavorable augury, as it often points to a sympathetic affection of the nervous system, and leads us to fear delirium, convulsions, subsultus, or some other unpleasant nervous complication.

A hard pulse, in hypochondriacal or hysterical subjects, generally denotes an obstinate and deep-seated cause for the affection. In children, it is generally a sign of inflammation; when associated with severe colic-pains, inflammation of the bowels is generally present. It is not dangerous in chronic nervous affections, but points to great obstinacy of the disorder. A hard and full pulse is unfavorable in apoplexy, especially if not relieved by antiphlogistic treatment. A small, frequent, and hard pulse, in consumptive patients, points to a more than usually inflammatory complication.

The hardest pulse is met with in inflammation of the arteries themselves; the pulse is apt then to be violently throbbing and vibrating.

A *full* pulse may depend upon general plethora, or a prolonged and forcible contraction of the left ventricle, and, to a certain extent, on relaxation of the arterial coats, or an obstruction in the capillaries, without diminished power of the heart. Of course, it may be associated with strength or feebleness of pulsation; in the latter case, the pulse yields readily to the finger, and, in its extreme debility, is sometimes called a gaseous pulse, and is supposed to denote a serous or impoverished condition of the blood.

A *slow, full pulse* is an accompaniment of true plethora. A frequent, soft, and full pulse is generally a sign of apparent plethora, or of excessive expansion of the blood. A slow, soft, and full pulse denotes some obstruction to the influence of the brain and nervous system upon the circulation, and is not an uncommon, but somewhat unfavorable sign in brain-affections, apoplexy, dropsy of the brain, injuries of the head, and severe nervous fevers. A soft, full pulse sometimes occurs periodically in chlorotic subjects, and depends upon some transient orgasm of the blood. Fullness of the pulse, occurring after the outbreak of some eruptive disorder, is generally favorable; also after spasmodic attacks. The soft, full pulse of some phthisical patients, does not arise from true plethora, but from expansion of the blood. A slow, soft, but full pulse, in apoplexy, is unfavorable.

Quickness of the pulse differs from frequency; a frequent pulse is always rather quick, but a quick pulse is not necessarily also always frequent. A frequent pulse is one in which the number of beats is greater than usual in a given time; a quick pulse, one in which each beat occupies less than the usual time, though the whole number may not be increased. Simple quickness of the pulse denotes irritation, but little strength—the heart and arteries merely make a short, quick, nervous contraction, which differs widely from the somewhat prolonged and forcible contraction of real energy; the former is usually a sign of nervous disorder, the latter frequently of arterial, febrile, or inflammatory disorder. A quick pulse is produced by the heart contracting too quickly, so that no perfect distension of the arteries takes place.

Quickness is generally connected with frequency, but a quick pulse may also be infrequent; it often indicates a spasmodic state, associated with great weakness.

A *large* pulse occurs when the artery itself is naturally large, well filled with blood, consequently fully expanded, or even somewhat distended. It is most common in young persons, in the spring of the year, when there is naturally more turgor of the blood, after being overheated, &c. It is supposed to arise, sometimes, from a withdrawal of the influence of the brain and cerebro-spinal nervous system from the organs of circulation, as is seen in narcotic poisoning, and when there is pressure on the brain, as in soporose and apoplectic conditions.

A *full, large pulse*, in febrile diseases, is generally regarded as a favorable sign, as it indicates freedom of the organs of circulation, and a good amount of strength. When it is present, otherwise unfavorable signs, such as delirium, convulsions, or unconsciousness, lose some of their dangerous import. If it has been preceded by signs of coction, a favorable termination of the attack may be expected, especially if a copious sweat occurs; but, if it remains after critical discharges have occurred, we may fear relapses or after-diseases. If it succeeds a small, hard pulse, we may generally infer that a previous irritative or spasmodic disorder has subsided, or that an inflammation has been resolved; still, a too sudden transition from a small pulse to a large one, in febrile diseases, may excite a suspicion that a nervous affection will, or has arisen. A large, but empty and weak pulse, in febrile diseases, is apt to be attended with fainting-fits, as it often occurs after excessive blood-letting.

A large pulse, following after a small one, in comatose conditions, often indicates danger of a new attack of apoplexy. Largeness of the pulse, in apoplectic conditions, following upon a previous small one, if attended with invincible inclination to sleep, points to an approaching fatal termination. A large pulse, in febrile delirium, is rather favorable than otherwise; also, when fainting has occurred, and in spasms or convulsions.

Slow pulse (*pulsus tardus*) is marked by persistent distention of the artery at every beat, so that it remains perceptible under the finger for a long time. The slow pulse is generally, also, *infrequent*, and we may usually infer that anything which diminishes the frequency of the pulse will also make it slower. A slow pulse is common in phlegmatic, aged, and quite plethoric persons; in the latter, the pulse often becomes more frequent and quicker after blood-letting.

A not very inconsiderable retardation of the pulse occurs naturally during sleep, in the morning, a short time after waking, when lying down, from depressing mental emotions, from excessive pain, from the use of a warm bath, from taking acids, Digitalis, Squills, Colchicum, Lead, &c. It is also said to be somewhat slower in autumn and winter, and in moist weather than in dry.

A slow pulse is a sign of difficulty and disturbance of the circulation of the blood, and may arise from diminished irritability and tension of the circulatory organs, or from a deficiency of blood, or from the presence of a too thick, viscid, and not sufficiently oxydized mass of blood, or from considerable stagnations or infarctions of blood in large and sanguineous organs, from an imperfect influence of the brain and nervous system upon the motion of the blood, and, finally, from a true, general deficiency of vital power.

An unnaturally slow pulse is an attendant on organic diseases of the heart, obstruction of the circulation through the lungs, or of infarctions in the portal system, of scorbutic and typhoid conditions, of affections of the brain and nervous system; it also occurs from chronic lead-poisoning, from soporose and apoplectic conditions, exudations within the brain and skull, organic diseases of, or pressure upon the brain.

A full, soft, and slow pulse generally points to true plethora, and is not uncommon in pregnant women.

A full, but hard and slow pulse, indicates some obstruction to the free circulation of the blood, from impermeability of some large viscus; or it may arise from some pressure on the brain or medulla-oblongata. This pulse is not uncommon in aged persons, and is especially marked in chronic lead-poisoning.

The weak, empty, soft, and slow pulse always indicates exhaustion, at least of the circulatory organs, and often precedes an attack of syncope.

A partial, but very slow pulse, is sometimes noticed in paralyzed parts. An unusually slow pulse, in epileptic patients, indicates the presence of some brain-affection.

A remarkably slow pulse, in fever patients, is always a suspicious circumstance, as it may arise from great exhaustion, or some affection of the brain or nervous system, or a typhoid state.

The gradual slowing of a previously very quick pulse, is favorable in almost all diseases. A very slow pulse, in jaundice, is unfavorable, although a moderately slow pulse is common in that disease.

The occurrence of a very infrequent and slow pulse, in diseases of the heart, is unfavorable.

When the pulse becomes slow, in child-bed fever, it is very favorable. A small, unusually slow pulse, with dry or naturally warm skin, and normal stools, sometimes occurs in acute dropsy of the brain in children; still, it may be noticed in chronic affections of the heart and liver, infarctions of the abdominal organs, and in scrofula.

An excessively slow pulse, in comatose and apoplectic conditions, is very unfavorable.

The two great causes of slowness of the pulse, are debility of the heart, and pressure on the brain. Of the remedies which produce slowness of the pulse, the principal are Veratrum-viride, Aconite, Digitalis, and Nitrate of Potash. The *Veratrum-viride* has lately attained a great reputation in the dominant school, in cases attended with high arterial excitement—many think it superior to Digitalis, and more reliable; in repeated instances, the pulse has been reduced by it from one hundred to its normal standard. Almost every American country-practitioner regards it as his most reliable daily companion, for its ability to control the pulse is supposed, by many, to be far greater than any other article known in medicine; in appropriate cases, it is said to accomplish its work speedily and readily. In the threatened convulsions of children, where the pulse is one hundred and eighty, or more—as in the beginning of some violent eruptive fevers, or irritations in the alimentary canal—the pulse may be brought down to its natural standard, or even below it, at pleasure, and the convulsions generally prevented. In pneumonia, pleurisy, carditis, and pericarditis, in their acute form, it is said to be an agent of great power and efficacy.

Dose.—The common dominant school dose, for an adult, is three drops of the saturated tincture, repeated every two or three hours, in severe, but not immediately pressing cases, or every twenty or thirty minutes in very urgent attacks, but for two or three doses only; when the pulse is thus brought down to the point desired, it may be retained there by the maximum dose of five drops, repeated every three or four hours. In children, of course, the doses must correspond to the age and strength of the child. To a robust child of one year old, one drop is a maximum dose; of two years old, one and one-half drops; of three years, two drops, &c.—repeated more cautiously than in adults. Other physicians regard it as a diaphoretic, acting with a certainty which is characteristic of no other remedy; also as an alterative of great value, which may often be substituted, in ordinary practice, for Iodine and Mercury. It has also been used, with astonishing success, in epilepsy from spinal irritation; while its virtues as an expectorant are by no means small. About this I know nothing, but I have repeatedly seen it relieve the most violent coughs, when connected with organic disease of the heart. But the most important of all its properties, and that which gives it preëminence over all others, is, of course, its power to control excessive action of the heart and arteries; when the pulse is beating most tumultuously, it may almost be controlled *ad libitum*, without resort to the lancet or other means. In pneumonia, it controls the pulse, moderates the action of the heart and arteries, prevents an excess of blood being thrown to the inflamed lungs, in a rapid and tumultuous manner; thus relieves congestive oppression of the chest, while it promotes perspiration and expectoration. But it is not known whether it exerts any specific action over the local inflammatory disorder, although it has repeatedly reduced the heart's action from one hundred and fifty to seventy-five in less than twenty-four hours, and sometimes down to fifty; yet mere excessive action of the heart and arteries is not the sum of inflammation, on the contrary, it is merely the consequence of inflammatory irritation, propagated to the ganglionic nerves, and thence to the heart and arteries. Hence, it is probable that Veratrum-viride is a valuable adjunct in the treatment of inflammatory engorgements and congestions, and places the patient in a more favorable and comfortable condition in true inflammation, and also promotes some of those secretions and excretions which also relieve the system of some of its load of effete matters, and thus enables nature to accomplish a victory over many inflammations to which she would otherwise succumb; still, it may not be a true specific remedy against true plastic inflammation, but merely against vascular irritation, congestion, and activity.

From doses insufficient to cause nausea or vomiting, it generally produces feelings of chilliness and considerable diminution in the frequency and force of the pulse, with a sense of weakness in certain muscles, or want of due command over them, which are supposed to be the results of a direct sedative influence upon the nervous centres, both ganglionic and cerebro-spinal; the pulse may be reduced to thirty-five per minute without nausea or vomiting. It is evident, then, that a reduction of the circulation, and a semi-paralysis of sensation and motion, may be produced by this medicine, independently of nausea; but, when it is carried far enough to produce nausea and vomiting, its depressing effects on the circulation and nervous system are most striking. The pulse falls from seventy-five or eighty down to thirty-five or forty, and, at the same time, becomes small and feeble, and occasionally almost imperceptible; the surface is pale, and covered with a cool sweat, with chilliness and sometimes numbness and tingling, with vertigo, dimness of vision, dilated pupils, faintness, and headache, from emptiness of the brain of blood. These signs of prostration may be so great as to become alarming, but they are rarely or never fatal. Although the Veratrum-viride seldom or never purges, almost all who have experimented with it, say its general depressing effects on the nervous system and circulation are also frequently attended with an increase of many of the secretions, probably, also, from relaxation; thus the salivary, pulmonary, biliary, and urinary secretions are often increased by doses insufficient to occasion nausea or vomiting. Of course, in the dominant school, it has an extensive application to reduce the circulation when morbidly excited, and to calm nervous irritation, and, consequently, has been used chiefly in inflammations, fevers, and nervous diseases.

In inflammations, it is supposed to act only as a sedative to the heart and arteries, and not by changing the character of the inflammatory blood, nor by removing the local affection of the inflamed tissues.

Aconite, Antimony, and Nitrum are more powerful in this latter respect.

It has attained its greatest credit in the treatment of pneumonia, especially those typhoid or other varieties which do not bear depletion well. Dr. Norwood gives eight drops per dose, every three hours, with the addition of a drop to each successive dose, until the pulse is reduced sufficiently, or nausea or vomiting are caused, and afterwards the dose is to be so managed, as regards number of drops and interval of time, as to sustain the depressed state of the circulation with as little disturbance of the stomach as possible. The testimony in favor of the remedy is so strong, and comes from so many sources, that all impartial men will incline to admit that it is impossible to refuse it credence; it is asserted that the symptoms of inflammation decline with the reduction of the pulse, and the patient, in due time, enters into a very favorable convalescence. Still, it is a very dangerous remedy.

It cannot be too frequently impressed upon the judicious practitioner that *the slow pulse of debility* must be treated very differently from the slow pulse of compression of the brain. The former will bear, if it do not absolutely require, stimulants, tonics, wine, ale, spirits, China, Quinine, Ferrum, &c.; the latter requires remedies which will produce absorption of serum, blood, plastic lymph, &c., &c. Arnica, Hydriodate of Potash, Bromide of Potash, Iodide of Mercury, and even Digitalis may come in play.

The *frequent pulse of debility* also requires very careful discrimination. If some nervous irritation be present, Chamomilla, Asafœtida, Musk, Conium, or even Opium may be admissible, aided by the milder kinds of sustaining food, drink, and medicines. If the irritation be inflammatory, the highest skill of the physician will often have to be called in play; very small doses of Aconite and Antimony, not sufficient to depress, may be used, although Lactuca-virosa, or Lactucarium, or Laurocerasus, or infusion of Wild Cherry Bark may be given in alternation. Lately, the *Gilseminum-sempervirens*, or Yellow Jessamine, has been strongly recommended in these states. It is said to possess an almost perfect control over the nervous system, while it is also an unrivalled febrifuge; it is said to produce gentle diaphoresis, and suspend and hold in control muscular irritability and nervous excitement with more force and power than any known remedy, and perform its wonder-working cures, in many febrile diseases, without exciting either nausea, vomiting, or purging. As a sedative to the heart and arteries, it is deemed superior to either Aconite, Digitalis, or Veratrum-viride; for, although not so powerful as the latter, it is more safe and manageable, as it neither excites nausea or diarrhœa. It reduces the circulation and frequency of the respirations, promotes perspiration, relaxes wonderfully all the muscles, and relieves all sense of pain and uneasiness, while it leaves the intellectual faculties entirely unaffected. It is said, by some, to be the only agent ever yet discovered capable of subduing—in from two to twenty hours, and without the least possible injury to the patient—the most formidable and most complicated, as well as the most simple fevers incident to our country and climate: quieting all nervous irritability and excitement, equalizing the circulation, promoting perspiration, without exciting nausea, vomiting, or purging. All the primary symptoms of typhoid fever are said to be rapidly removed by it. In typhoid pneumonia, it is said quickly to remove the typhoid symptoms, leaving only a simple pneumonia, which may be quickly cured by Aconite or Veratrum-viride. In asthenic fevers, when the pulse runs up to one hundred and thirty, it may often be reduced to seventy-five, in eight or twelve hours, with profuse perspiration; the pulse has also been reduced from one hundred and forty, or one hundred and sixty, to one hundred and two in twelve hours. It is a direct remedial agent, of no inconsiderable value, in a very large number of dangerous and painful inflammatory diseases, including inflammations of the brain, lungs, pleura, viscera, rheumatism, &c.

It is in this class of cases that Phosphorus, Rhus-toxicodendron, Arsenicum, &c., are often used with great benefit, in quite small doses, i. e., when the pulse is frequent, from some inflammatory irritation existing in the midst of depression or debility.

Of course, *Phosphorus* is homœopathic to some forms of inflammatory irritation; it is said to be a powerful stimulant to the system, especially to the circulation. It also stimulates the nervous centres, and promotes the secretions, especially those of the skin and kidneys; it increases the frequency and fullness of the pulse, the heat of the skin, invigorates the mental functions and muscular power. It has proved useful in some febrile diseases of a low or malignant form, and even in some of the obstinate and malignant phlegmasiæ, such as typhoid pneumonia, catarrhal croup, chronic pleurisy, and malignant chronic bronchitis; also against the collapse which takes place in the early stage of certain fevers, and great prostration occurring in the course of febrile diseases generally, the alarming depression sometimes attendant on the retrocession of scarlatina, erysipelas, &c. Where there is an under-current of smouldering inflammation, the doses should be small; but, in some low states of the system, which require prompt and powerful stimulation, and in which ordinary stimulants fail, larger doses should be given of this energetic remedy.—Wood.

According to Trinks, Phosphorus is almost indispensable in all acute affections, during the course of which the cerebro-spinal and sympathetic nervous systems have undergone an extensive and deep-seated consumption of their vital activities, and they, as well as the vascular system, are threatened with complete exhaustion, or a neuro-paralytic condition, although there may be turbulent disturbances and confusions in the actions of all these systems. Such dangerous conditions are apt to arise in the course of pleurisies, pneumonia, typhoid fever, and some acute exanthems, and are frequently removed, as if from magic, by Phosphorus, and the apparently hopeless patient is saved. In some dangerous and malignant fevers—where there has been hiccough, when fluids fell from the mouth into the stomach as into a lifeless vessel, a very small and frequent pulse, coldness of the extremities, rattling respiration, and rapid sinking of the vital powers—Phosphorus has saved the life of the sick person: the hiccough having ceased after the third two-hourly dose of a few drops of a solution of four grains of Phosphor. in one drachm of Sulphuric-ether. Also, in putrid fevers, when gangrenous bed-sores have formed, the stools have been offensively putrid, and there was an almost perfect prostration of the vital powers. It has also been used successfully in febris-nervosa-torpida; in febris-hectica, in abdominal typhus, with rapid prostration, nocturnal delirium, and dryness of the tongue, and in other cases; in the second and third stages of typhus, where congestions, obstructions, or infarctions of the lungs have occurred, attended with oppression of the chest and anxiety, expectoration of bloody mucus and sputa, stitches in the side, and rattling in the air-tubes and trachea. Also, when, in addi tion to the pneumonic complication, there has been diarrhœa and tenderness in the cœcal region, so that it has seemed to stay the progress of typhoid ulceration of the bowels. It has even proved serviceable in typhus-putridis, when the patient lay comatose, with open mouth, relaxed jaws, dry black lips and tongue. In pneumonias, it has proved most useful in those which bear a neuro-paralytic character, with tendency to purulent infiltration of the lungs, and in those tedious, obstinate, and dangerous cases of pneumonia in which there is a great loss of strength and deficient critical efforts and excretions; and in asthenic pneumonias with hepatization. Phosphorus should be regarded as a normal and most genial vital stimulant in these cases.

The action of Rhus, Anacardium, Arsenicum, Ammonia, and Cantharides is somewhat similar to that of Phosphorus in similar attacks.

An *intermitting pulse* often occurs naturally in some healthy persons, especially aged or adult ones, and then generally becomes regular when the patient is taken sick. Occasionally, it occurs as a sign of plethora, in very full-blooded persons, and after the suppression of some hæmorrhages; still more frequently, it is a sign, in chronic cases, of debility of the heart, or of a fatty and flabby condition of that organ, or of disease of the valves of the heart, or dilatation of its walls and cavities. In acute attacks, it often attends inflammation of the heart or pericardium, or dropsy of the pericardium.

An intermitting pulse also occurs in consequence of compression of the brain, or of exhaustion of the cerebral or ganglionic nervous system, and after the use of some narcotic remedies, like Digitalis, Veratrum-album, and Aconite; also in inflammations or organic diseases of the brain, effusions or exudations within the cranium, in hæmorrhagic apoplexy, and paralysis.

It was supposed, by the ancients, to be a frequent attendant upon disturbances of the chylo-poetic viscera, collections of gastric or intestinal impurities, venous congestions or infarctions of the portal system, &c., and was conjectured to precede, at times, a tendency to diarrhœa and vomiting.

Frequently it is a sign of general exhaustion, and hence occurs previous to and during fainting-fits, in typhoid and putrid affections, after excessive loss of blood, &c.

Intermitting pulse, on one side, generally arises from disease of the heart, but may indicate disorder of the liver or spleen.

A regular intermittence, always occurring after a certain number of pulse-beats, is said to point to greater danger than irregular intermittence, although Behrends supposed just the contrary.

The omission of a single beat of the pulse, at long intervals, generally is not of serious import; but intermissions are apt to occur frequently, shortly before death, and in states of great exhaustion. The failure of several pulse-beats, directly after one another, is almost always a serious sign. Intermission of the pulse, corresponding with the diastole of the heart, was once supposed to point to disease of the aorta, and that synchronous with the systole, to disease of the heart or valves.

If an intermitting pulse is very large, full, and soft, it was once supposed to point to disorder of the abdominal organs; but a very large, soft, and, at the same time, remarkably rarely intermitting pulse, is said to indicate disease of the brain.

A remarkably small, weak, and very frequent pulse, with intermittence, or the same kind of pulse, with only occasional irregularity and intermittence, is said to be a sign fraught with danger, as it denotes great exhaustion of the vaso-motor nerves, and of the heart and arteries.

A hard and jarring pulse, varying much in rhythm, force, and frequency, being, at the same time, irregular and intermitting, is one of the most common attendants of disease of the heart, valves, and arteries.

An intermitting pulse, in abdominal dropsy, was once supposed to arise from pressure on the large blood-vessels. But, at times, it occurs soon after the operation of tapping, and was then supposed to indicate the withdrawal of much blood into internal vessels, which had previously been compressed. But, in both cases, it often arises from some attending disease of the heart, or tendency to syncope or exhaustion. If it passes away soon, of course it points to some temporary disturbance only; but, if it remains obstinately, it of course points to some organic disease, generally of the heart.

Intermitting pulse, occurring after the suppression of hæmorrhage, is not of serious import.

An intermitting pulse, in pericarditis, was often mistaken for pleurisy, and supposed to arise from the disturbance of respiration from the acute pain; still, it was not regarded as a contra-indication for bleeding and other antiphlogistic treatment.

An intermitting pulse, after the slightest exertion, in dropsy of the chest, was once supposed to point to the simultaneous presence of hydro-pericardium.

An intermitting pulse, in chronic affections, was not formerly regarded as a very serious phenomenon, or, at least, not as one importing immediate danger, yet it too often proceeds from disease of the heart; still it was always regarded as indicating an obstinate cause of disease, which it was difficult, if not impossible to remove.

An intermitting pulse, in inflammatory affections, if it be at the same time frequent, small, weak, and associated with other unfavorable symptoms, often points to the occurrence of a fatal neuro-paralytic state, which is frequently mistaken for mortification, and generally indicates a near approach of death. When associated with less threatening symptoms, it is often a sign of the great severity of the attack, or of a complication with inflammation of the heart or arteries.

An intermitting pulse, in febrile diseases, was generally, in olden times, regarded as arising from gastric impurities, and tendency to nausea, vomiting, worms, &c. A soft, large, moderately frequent, and intermitting pulse, in some febrile diseases, was often regarded as a precursor of some eruptive disorder, or of some critical discharge, by sweat, urination, diarrhœa, or vomiting. It will be much more safe to assure one's self that there is no disease of the heart present.

When an intermitting pulse is associated with jaundice, in the commencement, or at the height of some febrile diseases, great danger is to be apprehended. A very frequent, hard, small, and weak pulse, which intermits every few beats, is a very dangerous sign in malignant fevers. An intermitting pulse, when attended with signs of exhaustion, in fever patients, generally indicates a fatal termination.

An intermitting pulse, in inflammation of the uterus, was thought to be frequently noticed by the ancients, and was not regarded as a very unfavorable sign. In gouty persons, it was supposed to point to the speedy occurrence of a new attack, but more frequently arises from some concomitant heart-affection. An intermitting pulse, in aged persons, sometimes arises from ossification or rigidity of the arterial coats, but more frequently from a like condition of the valves of the heart.

As persons often live a long time with heart-affections, it was not regarded as immediately or particularly unfavorable, not as much so as when the pulse suddenly became regular.

An intermitting pulse, in heart-affections, is a common occurrence, and always an unfavorable one, although a fatal termination may be long postponed; but, if it becomes very small, weak, jarring, and very irregular, a near approach of death may be expected.

An intermitting pulse, in inflammations of the brain, and in brain-affections generally, belongs among the more dangerous phenomena.

An intermitting pulse, in hypochondriacal and hysterical, or nervous subjects, is a frequent and not dangerous occurrence, as it may be produced by mental emotions and strong odors.

An intermitting pulse, in children, was formerly supposed to arise from gastric derangements or worms; but it is much more frequently a sign of disease of the head, or of the paralytic stage of dropsy of the brain.

An intermitting pulse, in injuries of the head, is a bad sign. In consumptive patients, it points to extensive disease of the lungs, or implication of the heart; if it becomes very sunken, small, extremely frequent and intermitting, sudden and great exhaustion is apt to occur. In rhachitic subjects, it may arise from pressure of the distorted spine upon the aorta or heart, and is sometimes associated with great enlargement of the liver. In rheumatic affections, it generally points to some disease of the heart, either endo- or peri-carditis.

An unusually unfrequent and intermitting pulse, in comatose subjects, indicates much danger; in apoplectic patients, it is a very common, and always an unfavorable occurrence; in tetanus, it is also unfavorable. A large, slow, and intermitting pulse, in intermittent fevers, often points to the occurrence of apoplexy, or at least a comatose febrile attack. An intermitting pulse is not an unusually dangerous sign during violent spasmodic attacks.

To sum up, intermittence of the pulse may arise from debility of the heart or vaso-motor nerves, from acute inflammatory disease of the heart, or disease of the mitral valve, or fatty degeneration of the heart, and, finally, from concussion or compression of the brain, from dropsy, apoplexy, or some other brain-affection.

A dicrotic, or double-beating pulse (*pulsus dicrotus* and *bisferiens*) is when two dilatations of the artery follow quite rapidly, one upon the other, to one beat of the pulse. It always points to a violent irritation and exertion of the heart and arteries, and hence is usually a sign of a relatively too great quantity of blood, or of a very much increased determination of blood towards certain parts, such as would occur in powerful and well-nourished persons, and in violent inflammations; it sometimes fortunately denotes a tendency towards a beneficial and critical hæmorrhage, or to a critical nose-bleed or perspiration. It sometimes occurs in healthy, plethoric persons in one arm only. It, at times, arises in consequence of considerable disturbance of the circulation, from obstruction of the lungs, and, in chronic lung-cases, is not an uncommon accompaniment of consumption.

Disharmony of the pulse is a term applied to differences in the pulse in various parts of the body, or with reference to the beats of the heart. Want of proportion or harmony in the size and strength of the pulse in different arteries is often a natural occurrence, depending upon accidental differences in the size, distribution, and situation of should-be symmetrical arteries; or it may arise from some pressure upon, or disease of the coats of one artery. It may also arise—when there is a great difference in the frequency and rhythm of the paired arteries—from some irritation or inflammation in parts supplied by one or the other of them. Thus, a very considerable disharmony has been noticed in the carotid and radial pulses of many insane persons; in felons on the fingers, the artery supplying the inflamed part generally beats more rapidly and forcibly than either the heart itself or the artery of the sound side.

A general want of harmony between the beats of the heart and that of the arteries usually arises from disease of the heart.

In contraction of the mitral orifice of the heart, there is often a want of proportion between the force of the impulse of the heart and that of the pulse in the arteries; the latter being often small and indistinct, while the former is strong and manifest; and also a want of proportion between the rate of the manifest pulsations of the heart and of the pulse at the wrist—the former being often apparently more rapid than the latter. In contraction of the mitral valve, both auricles are enlarged, and also the right ventricle; while the left ventricle is diminished in size and vigor, the right ventricle is actively enlarged and pushed forward towards the sternum by the dilated auricles above and behind it, and these three cavities have a resistance to overcome at the mitral or left auriculo-ventricular aperture;—hence, we have no reason to be surprised at the vigorous impulse of the heart, to which the diminished left ventricle can contribute but little, as it is placed so much behind its usual position. Secondly, the pulse in the arteries is small, weak, and irregular, and less frequent than that of the heart, because the pulse of the former is the indication of the state of the left ventricle, which, as has already been mentioned, is reduced in size. And we can account for the irregularity of the pulse in the arteries when we bring to mind that the left ventricle derives from the left auricle above it a very precarious supply of blood, owing to the contraction of the mitral valve—a diminished supply, which is probably often inadequate to fill its cavity. Under such circumstances, the left ventricle may contract in unison with the right; but the stream it has to transmit will not be sufficient to distend the arteries, or make the pulsation sensible. At such a moment, there is a total failure of the arterial pulse, while that of the heart (caused by the action of the right ventricle, mainly,) is strong and vigorous. Hence, the phenomenon characteristic of this disease—the occasional double pulse of the heart, for the single pulse in the arteries.

A *thread-like* pulse (*pulsus filiformis*) occurs when there is unusual hardness of the pulse, combined with great smallness of it, so that it feels like a thin thread. A thread-like pulse is generally regarded as a sign of great debility of the heart, or of a very considerable diminution of the whole quantity of blood. Hence it occurs after excessive losses of blood, and other profuse evacuations, when there is a complete prostration of the nutritive processes, and in the colliquative stage of hectic disorders.

On the other hand, it often associates itself with violent inflammations of internal parts, viz., of the lungs, heart, and brain, and then is a sign of urgent proclivity towards a neuro-paralytic condition, or to gangrene. Finally, it also occurs in connection with extensive disorganizations, especially of the organs of the chest and abdomen, and is then often a precursor of extreme exhaustion and speedy death.

Pulselessness, (*pulsus nullis*,) of course, means an entire absence of the beats of the pulse. General pulselessness is often mistaken for excessively weak and scarcely evident pulsations, and, in a very few rare instances, is not an absolutely fatal sign, unless connected with entire stoppage of the heart. It is a common attendant of the higher degrees of syncope and apparent death, of dead-drunkenness, (in which the pupil may also be perfectly insensible and dilated,) and poisoning with Aconite; it may not be followed by death for some little time. This condition sometimes occurs in Asiatic cholera, in which the pulse may fail in the arms and legs, and yet the patient may be able to sit up and move a little.

Autenreith supposed that he had seen a patient with dropsy of the chest, pulseless, and yet recover.

A transient general pulselessness sometimes occurs in violent suffocative attacks, and from carditis.

Pulselessness, in single portions of the body, points to disease or compression, or unusual distribution, or obstruction of the corresponding arteries. The pulse is occasionally wanting in paralyzed parts. Pulselessness of the radial arteries, with violent throbbing of the carotids, has occasionally been observed without a fatal termination. Pulselessness of one side of the body has occasionally been observed in hysteric paroxysms and in nervous fevers. Absence of pulse, in the lower half of the body, often indicates the presence of aneurism of the abdominal aorta, or of compression of it by tumors. Stokes records a case, in which a gentleman, with fatty and other disease of the heart, lived for six weeks, with difficult respiration and declining strength; yet, during the whole of this time, the most careful examination failed to discover any pulse in any artery of the body; the action of the heart being not sensible to the hand, and, on the application of the ear, an obscured undulating sensation was all that could be observed.

In attacks of angina-pectoris, the pulse is almost imperceptible.

A *jumping* pulse (*pulsus caprizans*) refers to a more powerful action of a single beat of the pulse, followed immediately by a weaker one; it is, in general, a rare phenomenon, and frequently is an indication of some deep-seated nervous affection, and may precede violent attacks of nervous spasms; still, it has also been observed during the active febrile commotions which precede a critical turn in a disease, and, finally, it sometimes occurs during the death-agony, especially in apoplectic attacks.

A small pulse (*pulsus parvus*) arises from deficient dilatation of the artery, so that its calibre always seems too slight under the finger. It is normal in persons who have small, deep-seated arteries, or covered with an unusual amount of adipose or cellular tissue; hence it is common in women, delicate men, and in all fat persons. According to Baglivi, those persons who naturally have a small pulse are more apt to live long, and are less liable to disease than those who have strong and large pulses; the ancients also supposed that the pulse of most persons became rather smaller in the autumn.

If the pulse is small, and at the same time weak, it is a sign of deficiency of blood, loss of vital tone, or of inability of the heart to propel the blood onward with sufficient power; hence it attends excessive losses of blood or other evacuations, profuse formations of pus, or dropsical accumulations, hectic and other adynamic fevers, and all colliquative affections.

It often occurs in consequence of nervous exhaustion, as after great loss of sleep, during and after excessive pain, previous to fainting attacks, after exhausting spasmodic affections, long abstinence from food, and many organic affections.

Sometimes, however, it is a sign of sham debility, as in the higher degrees of plethora, when the power of the circulatory organs is not great enough to propel the excessive quantity of blood with sufficient force and vigor; it may attend very violent inflammations of the heart, lungs, or gastro-intestinal canal; it also precedes attacks of nausea, saburral conditions, and the development of bilious and other gastric fevers; also wind-colic, mucous conditions, worm-affections, obstructions and infarctions of the abdominal organs, and more especially affections of the kidneys.

A remarkably weak, soft, and empty small pulse often indicates true deficiency of blood and absolute exhaustion; but the ancients also thought that a soft, small pulse, especially on the affected side, sometimes attended a very violent attack of inflammation of the lungs.

An intermitting, weak, and empty pulse is often a precursor of death.

A hardish and somewhat frequent small pulse, sometimes discloses the presence of an obscure inflammatory or spasmodic affection, and generally indicates merely a suppression, and not an actual exhaustion of the powers of the circulatory organs.

A one-sided small pulse arises from an unusual bifurcation or distribution of an artery, or an unusually small size of the artery, or a deeper location of the same, or a compression, or partial obliteration of the same, or the presence of an aneurism higher up, or a neuro-paralytic affection of the vaso-motor nerve of the affected artery. The ancients supposed that it attended unilateral affections, such as pneumonia, or pleurisy of one side.

Smallness of the pulse, with redness of the face, is regarded as unfavorable; a small pulse, attending large and deep ulcerations, is unfavorable.

A weak, small pulse, in pleurisy, was supposed to denote the simultaneous existence of a rather extensive pneumonia; if the respiration be almost entirely abdominal, if the pulse becomes at once fuller and larger, on deep inspiration or coughing, then the smallness was supposed to arise from a suppression of respiration from pain.

A weak, small pulse is generally less unfavorable in chronic diseases than in acute; but it usually indicates an obstinate disease, depending upon some disturbance of the nutritive processes, or upon imperfect and deficient formation of blood, and a tendency to colliquation and exhaustion.

A hard, frequent, and small pulse, in inflammatory affections, is a sign of the great intensity of the attack, and consequent suppression of the powers and activities of the circulatory organs, such as occurs in inflammations of the heart and blood-vessels, the lungs, intestinal canal, and serous membranes. If this state of the pulse persists for many days, we may fear an unfavorable termination, or at least the occurrence of exudations or hepatizations. A soft, empty, weak, and unusually frequent small pulse, in inflammatory affections, is often a sign of a neuro-paralytic or gangrenous condition.

A small pulse, in febrile diseases, sometimes depends on the gastric nature of the affection, and a tendency to nausea, or else arises from an intense internal inflammatory condition, or from the non-development of some exanthem. But, if none of these conditions are present, and a previously large pulse changes to a small one, it denotes malignancy of the affection, or a smouldering internal inflammation, which may easily lead to disorganization; or it may depend upon great debility, which may lead to repeated fainting-fits, spasms, silent delirium, coma, or to a typhoid state in general.

When jaundice attends smallness of the pulse, at the commencement or height of a febrile affection, it is a sign of great danger.

An unusually weak, small pulse, at the period of a crisis, if the other signs are favorable, would lead one to expect a crisis through the urine. A small pulse, during, and for a short time after very profuse critical evacuations, is not unfavorable, and generally disappears spontaneously; but, if it persists, and also becomes unusually frequent, and the crisis seems imperfect, then there is danger of a relapse, or of some subse quent disease, especially in eruptive fevers.

A frequent small pulse, with signs of dropsy of the brain, occurring after neglected rheumatic attacks, denotes a fatal termination; an intermitting, or very depressed small pulse, in organic affections of the heart, is a sign of approaching death.

A small pulse, in children, which becomes larger and fuller after feeling it some time, is a sign of some internal inflammation.

A frequent, soft, small pulse, in pneumonia, after it has been large and hard, points to a termination in suppuration. As a general rule, we may infer that the softer and smaller the pulse becomes, in inflammations of the lungs, the more extensive the disease is. An intermitting, empty, weak, and small pulse, in consumptive subjects, denotes the approach of a fatal termination.

Persistent smallness of the pulse, after severe operations, is an unfavorable sign. The occurrence of a very frequent, weak, small pulse, in dysentery, leads us to fear a neuro-paralytic or gangrenous affection An intermitting, very depressed, and small pulse, in dropsical affections, is very unfavorable.

A frequent, small pulse, during the apyrexia of intermittent fever, points, at times, to danger of a soporose condition, and is generally a sign of malignancy of the attack.

An *empty* pulse (*pulsus inanis*) is marked by slightly perceptible dilatation of the easily compressible artery, which also seems only partially filled under the finger. An empty, small, and weak pulse indicates either actual deficiency of blood, or too thin a condition of the same, hence it is common after profuse hæmorrhages, extensive suppurations, and colliquative conditions. Sometimes it occurs from the accumulation of much blood in internal organs, as when there has been a great exposure to cold, after violent mental emotions, such as fright, fear, or hysteric attacks, in violent and extensive inflammations of very sanguineous organs, such as the lungs; in the latter case it is a dangerous sign.

The *creeping* pulse (*pulsus formicans*) is described as a frequent, unequal pulse, constantly becoming weaker, and even intermitting. It is a sign of excessive debility, and hence observed in dangerous fainting-fits, profuse and exhausting hæmorrhages, in the colliquative stage of consumption, in treacherous and dangerous nervous fevers, &c. It is, of course, of most unfavorable import; it often follows upon the worm-like pulse, but is, of course, more dangerous.

A weak pulse (*pulsus debilis*) is marked by a feeble dilatation and contraction of an easily compressible artery. A remarkably small and weak pulse is found in persons with small, deep-seated arteries, which are also surrounded with much cellular and adipose tissue. This is most common in rather stout women, and in corpulent, lymphatic, and melancholic subjects. Under other circumstances, it is frequently a sign of debility of the heart, of general prostration of the vital powers, of deficiency of blood, or a thin and watery composition of the same. Hence, it is common after very profuse and exhausting discharges, after violent exertions of body or mind, excessive loss of sleep, deprivation of a sufficiency of nourishing food, after depressing mental emotions, racking pains; also in chlorotic, leuco-phlegmatic, scorbutic, dropsical, consumptive, and otherwise cachectic individuals, also in those predisposed to fainting-fits or spasms, and, in fact, in all delicate persons in general. As a matter of course, it is common in diseases of the heart, especially in fatty disease of that organ. It is also supposed to be common in all saburral and verminal affections, in all non-inflammatory lymphatic disorders, and transiently in very violent spasmodic affections.

A very frequent and weak pulse, irregular in rhythm and strength, is of very unfavorable import, as it generally indicates a very great degree of exhaustion. An unusually weak pulse, which feels, however, like a tense wire under stronger pressure, is often a characteristic sign of abdominal inflammation, although occasionally it precedes the resolution of abdominal infarctions. A remarkable increase of weakness of the pulse, after every deep inspiration, is a characteristic sign of true debility of the lungs. A weak pulse, in chronic diseases, even if a favorable termination is possible, points to obstinacy of the attack. A weak pulse, in inflammatory affections, is of unfavorable import, as it points to great violence of the disorder, or to an asthenic character of the same. If the pulse, in inflammatory affections, becomes remarkably weak, without being preceded by the signs of a true crisis, and, at the same time, all the inflammatory symptoms subside in a sudden and unaccountable manner, we may fear the occurrence of a neuro-paralytic state or of gangrene. An unusually weak pulse, in the commencement of febrile affections, indicates a threatening adynamic character of the attack, or one arising from an inflammato-gastric, or acute cerebral or pulmonary disorganization. A weak, unsteady pulse, in fever patients, sometimes excites suspicion of the existence of effusions into the cavity of the cranium. A weak pulse, in the crude stage of fevers, especially if associated with jaundice, always indicates danger.

URINE.

AUTHORITIES.—Gross on the Urinary Organs, (1). Bennett's Clinical Lectures, (2). Thudichum on the Pathology of the Urine, (3). Dalton's Physiology, (4).

There is no fluid which, within the limits of health, is liable to so many variations in its physical and chemical properties as the urine. Its quantity, also, is extremely uncertain. On an average, a healthy person voids about forty ounces in the twenty-four hours. It may range, consistently with health, from twenty to fifty ounces. Its normal color is a pale amber—transparent, saline in its taste, and of a slightly aromatic odor. Its specific gravity may be stated to be, at an average, 1.020. In health, it is acid, imparting a red tint to litmus paper. On standing, it deposits a minute quantity of mucus, mixed with epithelial cells. The solid matters excreted by means of the urine, vary from one and a half to two and a half ounces. (1.)

Healthy urine has been divided, by modern writers, into *potous*, *chylous*, and *sanguineous* urine; or, the *urine of fluids*, *urine of food*, and *fasting* or *morning urine*. (1.)

Potous urine is of a pale color and low specific gravity, rarely exceeding 1.009. (1.)

Chylous urine ranges between 1.020 and 1.030, the latter of which, however, it rarely attains.

Sanguineous, or fasting urine, is of the average density of 1.015 to 1.025, and exhibits all the essential qualities of this important fluid.

The analysis of healthy urine may be stated to be as follows:

Water,	933.00
Urea,	30.10
Uric Acid,	1.00
Sulphate of Potash,	3.71
" " Soda,	3.16
Phosphate of Soda,	2.94
Phosphate of Ammonia,	1.65
Muriate of Soda,	4.45
" " Ammonia,	1.50
Phosphate of Lime and Magnesia,	1.00
Siliceous earth,	.03
Vesical mucus,	.32
Free Lactic Acid, Lactate of Ammonia, and animal matter not separable from them,	17.47

Besides these, the urine also contains a small amount of sulphur, phosphorus, and a yellow coloring matter (*urœmatine*) not yet obtained in a separate state. In the urine of infants, there is said to be some benzoic acid. (1.)

Mucus.—Urine always contains, even in the healthy state, a small quantity of mucus, which only becomes visible on standing. It is not coagulated by boiling water, is soluble in caustic potash, and forms, on the addition of acetic acid, a characteristic pellicle. Under the microscope, it has the same globular appearance as pus, but the particles are less numerous, and less distinctly granular. When in excess, the mucus is suspended in a glairy fluid, more or less albuminous, and the urine is generally alkaline and remarkably prone to decomposition, which renders the fluid excessively offensive and disagreeable. It generally adheres tenaciously to the bottom and sides of the vessel. (1.)

The process of secretion, constantly going forward, sometimes proceeds to a morbid extent, in consequence of which substances are generated which do not occur naturally in the urine, such as albumen, fibrin, and the coloring matter of the blood, (hæmatin). And such substances as the yellow coloring matter of the bile, asparagus, oil of turpentine, and the like, may occasionally find their way into it. (1.)

Practically, the rule holds good, that, *as long as a patient secretes the normal amber-colored urine, or pale urine, he is not affected by any severe illness of a febrile and acute nature.*—VOGEL. (2.)

When a disease, acute or chronic, takes a fatal turn the quantity of urine frequently becomes very small, or remains in a fluctuating low state. This is the case in all diseases ending with or by exhaustion of the material of the component parts of the body. In some cases, however, the fatal termination of which is due to a more sudden interference with the powers of the nervous system, or with the mechanical action of the lungs and heart, the quantity of the urine is not usually much diminished. (2.)

The quantity of urine is materially diminished in dropsical diseases, with or without diseased kidneys, and greatly increased in diabetes. (2.)

When there is great scantiness of the urine, Apocynum often deserves the name which Rush gave it, viz.: "The vegetable trocar;" its promptitude and copiousness of action is often little short of marvellous.

Urea.—Urea may be looked upon as the principal product of the metamorphosis of the nitrogenized food and tissues. It is essentially an excretory matter, incapable of any longer serving the purposes of the economy, because it cannot be more highly oxydized; and, when retained, it becomes a poison to the system, both directly, and perhaps by the products of its decomposition. Its regular occurrence in healthy blood, and in the juice of flesh of man and animals, has established the opinion that it is formed in the tissues, and carried by the blood to the kidneys to be discharged. (1.)

Urea is colorless, of a bitterish. cooling taste, like saltpetre. When dry, it is not changed by exposure to the air, and then attracts very little moisture. It may be decomposed by the influence of heat, acids, alkalies, salts, putrid animal matter, and yeast. (1.)

A healthy man, who lives well, is said to discharge, on an average, from thirty to forty grammes of urea (about six hundred grains) in twenty-four hours. Wherever, or however the urea may arise, one great fact is undoubtedly established, that urea is the product of the disintegration of the tissues and of nitrogenized food, and, consequently, the quantity of urea must stand in direct relation to the quantity of food taken, or to the nitrogenized tissues disintegrated in the place of food. More urea is produced during waking than during sleep, more during mental and bodily exertion than during inactivity. A large amount of nitrogenized food will increase it; a small amount of vegetable food diminishes it. (2.)

An excess of urea is common to the *stadium incrementi* of all acute febrile diseases. This becomes an important feature when the ingestion of nitrogenized food is also at its minimum. As the fever abates, however, so does the production of urea. (2.)

In diseases which are chronic, and accompanied by impaired nutrition, the amount of urea sinks below the average. So low an amount of urea as seventy-five or ninety grains in twenty-four hours generally occurs towards the fatal end of diseases, when not only the production of urea is very limited, but also the excretory activity of the kidneys becomes languid. The diminution of the quantity of urea may, however, be due to the failure of the excretory activity of the kidneys alone, and then the phenomenon of uræmia or blood-poisoning arises. (2.)

Urea is sparingly furnished in chronic inflammation of the liver, in Bright's disease, phthisis, gout, and intermittent fevers. (2.)

Uric Acid.—This is supposed, by Dr. Prout, never to be present in healthy urine; but Thudichum unequivocally says that it is a constant ingredient in urine. It generally predominates in arthritic affections, as is shown by the formation of earthy concretions, so frequently seen in joints, apparently composed of urate of soda or lime. Gravel commonly consists of uric acid, and forms one of the worst bases of urinary calculi. In most instances, uric acid appears in combination with an alkali, and, so long as this is the case, it does not yield a crystalline deposit. (1.)

Its undue secretion is caused by errors in diet, &c. It most commonly prevails in dyspeptics, gouty, and irritable persons. (2.)

It is a light white powder, of a satin lustre, and consists of small, delicate scales, with irregular outline, the rhombic plate sometimes defined. To the unassisted eye it is not detectable. (2.)

Uric acid forms the basis of most of the gravels and sand found in and passed from the urinary bladder, and, in this case, the deposit is formed *in* the bladder, instead of precipitating after its passage. There seems but little reason for drawing any particular distinction between common uric-acid deposits, on the one hand, and sand and gravel on the other. Indeed, the common deposits of pulverulent uric acid are frequently called gravel and sand, by laymen, and even medical men. This, however, is not quite correct. What we call the common pulverulent deposit of uric acid, is made up of single crystals of that substance; whereas, sand or gravel is an agglomeration of crystals of uric acid, of a roundish form. By sand, therefore, should be understood those masses from the fortieth to the twentieth part of an inch, and by gravel, all above the twentieth part of an inch in diameter. These last are chiefly remarkable for the great number in which they are formed, and nephritic attacks are due to their accumulation in the pelvis of the kidneys or ureters. (3.)

The number of calculi, of which uric acid forms either the nucleus or the entire substance, is very great, standing to the number of all other calculi as one to two or three. (3.)

Colchicum often favors the excretion of uric acid more than any other remedy.

Urate of Ammonia.—This salt is always produced when uric acid and ammonia are allowed to act upon each other. When pure and dry, it is a white amorphous mass, perfectly soluble in water, one part, however, requiring 1.608 of water, at 77°, Fahrenheit.

It has, in a few instances of albuminous urine, in dropsy after scarlatina, been observed in the form of spherules, with crystals of uric acid adhering to their exterior. As a general rule, urate of ammonia, when occurring as a deposit, forms a dark, granular, perfectly amorphous precipitate. To the naked eye, these deposits of urate of ammonia appear as a subtle powder, varying in color from absolute whiteness, through rose-color, pink, brick-red, purple, and brownish red.

The Chlorides.—Simon and Redtenbacher first stated that chloride of sodium—a salt always present in healthy urine—was absent from that fluid during the onward progress of pneumonia, and returned to it when absorption of the exudation was about to commence. This statement was confirmed by Dr. Beale, of London, who published a paper upon the subject. Dr. Bennett's attention was called to it by being informed that Prof. Oppolzer, at Vienna, found it of great diagnostic value. It so happened that a man was admitted, just at this time, into Dr. Bennett's wards, laboring under well-marked simple pneumonia at the apex of the right lung. He was a laborer, who had enjoyed perfect health until two days before admission, when, on being exposed to wet and cold, working at drains, he was seized with shivering, followed by fever, and the usual concomitants of pneumonia. On adding a drop of Nitric-acid to some of his urine, in a test-tube, and then dropping into it a little of a solution of Nitrate of Silver, the fluid remained clear, although so great is the delicacy of this test that a white cloudy precipitate is at once formed if a very minute quantity of the chloride of sodium be present. It was on the fourth day of the disease that the observation was first made, and the chlorides remained absent during the fifth and sixth days, during which the disease extended from above downwards, until it occupied the upper two-thirds of the right lung. On the seventh day, a slight haze was observed in the urine, indicating that the salt was returning to that fluid, and the man expressed himself as being much better. On this day, there was great dullness on percussion, all crepitation had ceased, the breathing was tubular, with bronchophony. On the eighth day, slight returning crepitation was audible, the dullness had diminished, but the urine, owing to some accident, had been thrown away before the visit. On the ninth day, however, the chlorides were abundant in the urine, together with lithates; loud crepitation was now universal throughout the lung, and the dullness had nearly disappeared. From this time, the man made a rapid recovery, never having been bled, and was discharged quite well on the sixteenth day.

Uræmatine.—It is very probable that a number of blood-corpuscles are constantly undergoing the process of disintegration in the blood, and that the hæmatine which is thus set free, however changed from its original character, finds its way out of the body in the form of coloring matter of bile (cholæmatine) and uræmatine. We know the indestructible nature of hæmatine, how obstinately it retains its color under the most varied circumstances, whether in extravasations within the body, or during decomposition out of the body. We know, moreover, that the changes of color which hæmatine undergoes, under certain circumstances, in the body—for example, when effused into a bruise—correspond with the destructive changes in the blood; so that hæmatine, thus effused, will go through all the stages of color, from red to green, yellow and pale yellow—i. e., the colors which are found in the *cholæmatine* and *hæmatine.* Thus tenacious of its color, it is highly improbable that hæmatine should leave the body as a colorless principle. And if, therefore, it be probable that it *be* discharged as a colored substance, the only excreta which are colored—viz., fæces and urine—probably owe their color to this; and, as the purest uræmatine always contains some iron, its origin may be still more distinctly traced to the blood-corpuscles.

The amount of uræmatine discharged during acute febrile diseases is considerably increased, and, notwithstanding a large decrease in the total quantity of urine, it amounts to sixteen, twenty, and even more. This amount becomes even much higher in typhoid and septical fevers which are combined with a dissolution of the blood.

Phosphoric Acid.—A deficiency of Phosphoric acid is not less injurious than an excess of uric acid. Prout supposes that, in certain cases, the earthy materials of which it is the base are converted into neutral salts, which, on being deposited in the bladder, give rise to calculous concretions. This is especially the case with lime and ammonia, the soda and potash producing little or no inconvenience. (1.)

Lactic Acid.—The lactic acid, which, according to Berzelius, naturally exists in the urine, is seldom or never altered in quantity.

Bile.—In severe cases of jaundice, the bile is sometimes found in the urine; it may result from duodenitis, inflammation of the liver, or obstruction of its natural outlets. The most delicate test of its presence is muriatic acid, which gives a green or brownish tint to the urine. The muriate of iron and acetate of lead produce a yellow precipitate, and the sulphate of copper a dirty-green one.

Mercurius, Colchicum, and Digitalis favor the excretion of bile from the urine.

Albumen.—Albumen is said, by some, to be always contained in very minute quantity in healthy urine; but its presence, in detectable quantities, always indicates disease. In Bright's disease, it almost always exists in large quantities, and is generally, though perhaps not entirely pathognomonic of that disease. It has also been occasionally observed in pneumonia, ascites, tubercles, prurigo, and typhoid fever, which are then generally complicated with some congestion of the kidneys. Bouillaud and Piorry declare that they have frequently noticed the transient appearance of this substance in diseases which had no apparent connection with urinary troubles.

Albuminous urine is generally of low specific gravity, from deficient quantity of urea and salts, of a pale, opaline color, and readily coagulable on exposure to heat. The ferro-cyanate of potassium, corrosive mercury, alum, and nitric acid also coagulate it. If present in any considerable quantity, it often gives a smoky appearance to the urine. It is very common in dropsy and convulsions occurring after scarlet fever, and in that œdematous state which precedes the occurrence of puerperal convulsions. Mercurius-corrosivus, Phosphorus, Arsenicum, Nitric-acid, Terebinth, and other remedies have a specific relation to albuminous urine.

Bloody Urine.—This may be owing to various causes, the most common of which are external violence, eventuating in a laceration of some of the vessels of the genito-urinary apparatus, the passage of a renal calculus, ulceration of the mucous surfaces, cancer of the kidney, and encephaloid, fungous, or erectile tumors.

It may be in so small quantity as barely to tint the urine, or so much as to impart a dark-red claret or blackish aspect. In the former case, a pinkish or tawny sediment is deposited; and, when abundant, some of it is usually presented as black, half-dissolved clots, or short, cylindrical pieces, resembling leeches. The readiest mode of detecting blood is by its examination under the microscope; but its presence may be pretty certainly predicated from the peculiar color which it imparts to the urine, its alkalinity, and its tendency to subside to the bottom of the vessel.

When it exists in large quantity, it is commonly to be regarded as denotive of serious mischief. When mixed with pus or mucus, or both, and voided with pain, it indicates ulceration of the bladder, kidney, or prostate gland. When passed along with particles of soft, jelly-like matter, it denotes the existence of encephaloid disease or of fungous hæmatodes. Voided in a pure state, and in large quantity, without pain, it is probably merely an exudation from the mucous membrane of some portion of the urinary tract. It commonly occurs when there is great congestion of the kidneys. Hammamelis and Terebinth have been used successfully against bloody urine.

Pus.—Pus is a very frequent ingredient of urine, and is generally denotive of organic lesion. Its admixture may exceptionally be purely accidental, as when an abscess bursts into the bladder. The urine with which the pus is combined always contains albumen, is indisposed to putrefy, and is generally acid or neutral; when first voided, it is more or less turbid, but it soon assumes a pale appearance.

By repose, the pus falls to the bottom of the receiver, forming a dense homogeneous stratum of a yellowish-white, or greenish-yellow tint. Under the microscope, it exhibits the appearance of spherical corpuscles, floating in an albuminous fluid, opaque, white, rough on the surface, and more than one-third larger than the red corpuscles of the blood. By agitation, it readily mixes with the urine, imparting to it its peculiar color, but not dissolving in it. If a portion of the pus be mixed with an equal quantity of a solution of Potash, it will form a dense translucent, viscid compound, frequently so solid that the tube containing it may be inverted without any escaping.

When putrefaction and alkalescence have commenced, the globules disappear, and the whole fluid is transformed into a ropy, glairy substance, of a dirty turbid aspect. Its best test is its coagulability by Potash. Its fatty matter may be extracted by Ether. The albumen, which purulent matter always contains, is easily detected by heat and Nitric-acid.

Kiesteine.—This substance was supposed, until lately, to be peculiar to pregnant women; but it has since been ascertained to be generally present in the early months of lactation, and rarely or never in the virgin state. When first observed, it is usually present in the form of little isolated patches, which gradually coalesce, and form a pellicle from half a line to a line in thickness, of a whitish, opaline tint, not unlike the greasy scum upon the surface of fat broth. Dr. Kane states that it sometimes appears in striated, irregular lines, as of a spider's web, and in rings, circles, trapeziums, &c. It consists of a filamentous, flakey tissue, and is so coherent that it may occasionally be lifted off entire from the fluid which it covers. Its chemical nature has not been determined, although it is supposed to arise from the presence of some of the elements of milk in the urine. In the early stages of pregnancy, a small quantity of milk is formed in the breasts, is reabsorbed, and cast out by the kidneys; so that lactation is not a sudden effort of the breasts soon after parturition, but has been going on, in a slight degree, during the greater part of pregnancy.

Pale, thin urine (*urina aquosa, pallida, tenuis*) denotes an excess of water, or the suppression of other aqueous excretions, as those of the skin, or the absorption of fluids already poured out in other parts of the body. The urine of drunkards is often pale. Profuse, pale, and thin urine often accompanies violent mental emotions, such as fright or anger. Profuse watery urine is often a precedent and attendant of spasmodic and nervous affections, such as hysteria, hypochondria, epilepsy, migraine, spasmodic colic, &c.; the urine only becomes colored after these affections have ceased. When such pale, or so-called nervous or spasmodic urine is attended with pain in the kidneys, it is sometimes a sign of gravel and spasm of the kidneys and ureters. The urine is clear and watery in the cold stage of fevers, and the crude state of many diseases. Patients with nervous fever often discharge such a thin, crude urine for several weeks. Inflammations of the bowels, and even of the liver and spleen, in very irritable subjects, are occasionally attended with pale, watery urine, but it more frequently happens that these attacks are pseudo-inflammatory. Sprengel and Troga even affirm that the most intense form of nephritis is attended with the discharge of thin, watery, and pale urine, with great difficulty and much burning; the same happens, at times, in inflammations of the bladder, especially those excited by the presence of a stone, although the urine then sometimes assumes a pale, green color. Pale, thin, often odorless urine, containing much mucus, and occasionally a little blood, sometimes arises from induration of the kidneys and general debility; although it may precede an attack of mental derangement. An extremely bad-smelling, profuse, and pale urine often accompanies phosphatic deposits. Unusually heavy and pale urine generally denotes the presence of sugar. Pale urine, in dropsical persons, generally occurs in intractable cases; while a yellowish, watery urine is more common in those cases of ascites which admit of cure. Pale urine, in cases of hydrothorax, points to a threatening or already present aggravation. Persistent paleness of the urine, in chronic cases, is often a sign of debility, spasm, or obstruction of some of the viscera, and leads one to expect an obstinate resistance to remedies, even in favorable cases. Pale urine, in inflammatory diseases, is often a precursor of convulsions, fainting-fits, gangrene, or rapid and profuse internal effusions or exudations; still, it occasionally happens that the sudden occurrence of pale urine, if the other symptoms are favorable, is followed by resolution, but more frequently by suppuration.

In epileptic patients, when the urine becomes pale, and is passed for several days in large quantities, in proportion to the amount of drink, we may expect a more early and frequent occurrence of the attacks: the patients should then be encouraged to drink a good deal. Pale urine, in fever patients, points to a crude state of the disease, and, if it persists for a long time, and the heat and restlessness is great, we may expect attacks of sleeplessness, delirium, or convulsions, or, at least, a difficult and protracted convalescence. A sudden change, from thick urine to thin and pale, has the same signification in a still greater degree. Pale urine, when the other symptoms are favorable, points to the occurrence of critical abscesses, especially on the lower extremities. Pale urine, during the critical period of diseases, is generally a fatal sign, unless the crisis takes place in some other way, such as the outbreak of an exanthem, abscesses, or other metastasis. Profuse pale urine, after the irruption of miliaria, is often a fatal omen, if the urine was previously turbid and thick. Crude, pale urine, during the decrease of a bilious fever, is sometimes followed by an erysipelatous swelling of the legs. Pale urine, occurring suddenly in jaundiced patients, is generally followed by dropsy, unless it be prevented by proper remedies. Pale urine, in convalescent patients, often points to an imperfect recovery and threatening relapse. Pale urine, in brain-affections, is generally followed by a dangerous aggravation. Very pale urine, in delirious patients, is often followed by a fatal termination. Very pale urine, in children, is often followed by brain-affections and convulsions. A scanty and peculiarly glistening pale urine often attends rhachialgic muscular affections. Pale urine, after injuries of the head, is always a serious sign. Pale urine, in lung-diseases, is always unfavorable. A scanty, watery, and pale urine, in nephritis, denotes great severity of the attack and tedious recovery, and, when it persists after an abatement of the disease, it is often followed by induration of the kidneys. Quite watery, pale urine, with severe pain in the kidneys, denotes spasm of the kidneys, which may be excited by the presence of gravel, or by a violent cold, or the abuse of diuretic remedies. Frothy, pale urine, which was at first profuse and afterwards scanty, when attended with great dryness and coldness of the skin, after an attack of rheumatism, is often followed by dropsy. Pale urine, in apoplectic patients, is of unfavorable omen. Very pale urine, in intermittent fevers, the intervals between the paroxysms of which become shorter and shorter, the pulse being small and quick, denotes a threatening coma, or some nervous attack or delirium.

Brown urine (*urina fusca*) may occur from the use of Rhubarb, Balsam of Peru, Cassia, or from an admixture of blood or bile. A very saturated brown urine, somewhat resembling brown beer, may arise from the internal use of Phosphorus. Dark urine, verging upon brown, is common in plethoric subjects, and those suffering with atra-bile, abdominal infarctions, melancholy, and hæmorrhoids. An offensive, beer or coffee-like, thick, brown urine, when attended with pains in the kidneys, often points to the presence of nephritis, gravel, or medullary cancer of the kidneys. In inflammations of the veins, the urine is apt to be of a dark brownish-red color. Offensive brown urine often attends serious disturbances in the reproductive organs, inclination to scurvy or putrid fever, profuse suppuration of internal organs, or hectic fever, although it may arise from disease of the prostate gland or bladder. It is an unfavorable sign in whooping-cough, when previously clear and light urine becomes brown.

Thick urine (*urina crassa*) is never of favorable import in the commencement of febrile diseases; but if, in the latter stages of these disorders, the previously thin and pale urine becomes thicker and darker colored, especially if it deposits a sediment when it cools, we may expect a favorable crisis. Critical urine is, as a rule, thick, saturated, and abundant. Whitish, thick urine often depends upon the admixture of mucus, pus, or gravel. Light, gelatinous, thick urine often contains albumen or fibrin. Red, thick urine often depends upon the presence of uric acid or blood. Brownish or blackish thick urine often contains blood. Turbid, thick urine often arises from indigestion, infarctions, chronic congestion of the viscera, or disease of the urinary organs. Clear, honey-like, transparent, thick urine often attends colliquative diseases. A scanty, reddish-brown, thick urine is common in hectic fever. Thick urine, in apoplectic subjects, sometimes has a critical import. Reddish-brown, very hot, and thick urine, in dropsical subjects, often points to the disorganization of some important organ.

Filamentous, flocculent, or polypous urine (*urina polyposa*) sometimes occurs in leucorrhœa, and some local diseases of the urinary organs. Small, hair-like bodies, and branny scales in the urine were regarded by the ancients as indicative of the presence of scabies of the bladder. A brownish effusion and filamentous urine sometimes attends cancer of the kidneys. Small membranes and evidently tubular particles, swimming in a beer-like urine, are sometimes indicative of medullary cancer of the kidneys. Tubular, worm-like, and polypus-like masses of blood, which may be coated with a white membrane, are often passed after hæmorrhage from the kidneys or ureters. The occasional discharge of small polypus-like bodies, with excessive pain, is regarded as pathognomonic of hæmorrhoids of the bladder. The appearance as of spider-webs floating in the urine, or attaching themselves to the sides of the glass, is a reliable sign of larvate gout.

Yellow urine (*urina aurantica*, *crocea*) is natural when it is lemon-colored. A remarkably dark yellow color of the urine may arise from the use of Rhubarb, Saffron, excessive indulgence in meat or fat, or from admixture with bile; in the latter case, if a little Nitric-acid be added to the urine, a greenish deposit will occur. Bitter-tasting, dark yellow urine, with a tinge of reddish-brown or green, points to disturbance in the excretion of bile, and hence may be observed in bilious fevers, in acute and chronic disorders of the liver, and before and after jaundice. A thick, turbid, dark yellow urine, often indicates disorder of the digestive organs, and the gastric nature of the fever, if any is present. Saffron-yellow urine is common in hepatitis, tertian fevers, &c. The urine is apt to be of an orange-yellow color, during the exacerbations of rheumatic and hectic fevers. A very profuse, shining, golden-yellow urine, which becomes lighter and whiter about three hours after it is passed, is often a sign of diabetes. Yellow urine, in severe inflammations, not unfrequently points to a termination in suppuration or induration.

Inodorous urine (*urina inodora*) is often a sign of excessive spasm, or great debility, or perfectly prostrate digestion, imperfect assimilation, and absorptions, and hence is often not only of unfavorable, but fatal import. An entirely inodorous urine is sometimes noticed in severe attacks of gout.

Clear or transparent urine is, of course, natural in healthy people, but it is a suspicious phenomenon in sick people, especially in those with fever, for it is only in rare instances that a favorable termination occurs without being preceded by some sediment in the urine; in a few cases, however, recovery takes place after a profuse discharge of clear urine.

Furfuraceous urine (*urina furfuracea*) is marked by the presence of bran-like particles or scales in the freshly-passed urine, and is said to point to the presence of disease of the bladder, erysipelatous cystitis, obstinate ulceration of the bladder, arising from internal or repelled itch; but it may occur in colliquative, or treacherous nervous, or typhoid fevers, and in malignant inflammations, especially of the chest. When there are glimmering or glittering mica-like particles in the urine, in jaundice, we may infer that the attack will be obstinate. Bran-like particles in the urine of aged people, occurring after the suppression of eruptions, often points to the development of the so-called psora of the bladder. Turbid and whey-like urine, with mica-like glittering particles, often occur in the acute hydrocephalus of young children. Bran-like particles in the urine are often seen after the disappearance of the eruption on the face in small-pox and is not an unfavorable symptom.

Natural or normal urine is not of favorable import in febrile diseases; it shows that recovery is still far off. A scanty, but otherwise natural looking urine, in dropsy of the chest, is more unfavorable than it seems, although such cases admit of recovery.

Profuse urination (*urina copiosa, larga*) may arise from copious drinking, from diminution of the excretions from the skin and lungs, from a sojourn in a cool place without proper exercise, or from mental emotions, such as anger, fright, or it may be a nervous symptom. Profuse flow of urine, with violent gastric pains and loss of appetite, has been noticed in those who use sugar to excess. Profuse urine may arise from irritation or slight inflammation of the kidneys or bladder, which may be followed by scantiness or suppression. A profuse discharge of acrid urine, attended with great relief, generally proves that there has been either a voluntary or involuntary retention of this fluid. A turbid, or unusually pale and very copious urine is not an uncommon antecedent of many diseases, during the crude stage of which it generally persists. A saturated, copious urine, which deposits a sediment when it cools, is often of favorable and critical import in the latter stages of many diseases. Copious, turbid, bad-colored, and bad-smelling urine, or pale, curdy, and profuse urine, if attended with deranged digestion and loss of strength, points to debility of the urinary organs, or to general relaxation of the system, considerable disturbances in the reproductive organs, or commencing dissolution of the fluids, or colliquative discharges. Remarkably sour and profuse urine frequently attends rhachitis in children and adults. A quite unusually profuse discharge of light yellow, somewhat turbid, sweetish-smelling and tasting urine, attended with insatiable thirst, general emaciation, and exhaustion, are characteristic of true diabetes.

Profuse urination, unless it is transient, and attended with marked alleviation, deserves attention, as it may easily be followed by constipation and its consequences, dryness of the skin, emaciation, thickness of the blood and fluids and its consequences, such as obstructions of some of the viscera, &c. Profuse urination, in anginas, is usually favorable; this is also the case, in a more marked degree, in pleurisy, and when there have been signs of dropsy of the chest; diarrhœas also generally cease soon after free discharges of urine occur. Pale or turbid, and copious urine, in the early stages of fever, are among the signs of crudity, and, if they persist in the later stages of the disease, we may fear the occurrence of exhaustion, delirium, or convulsions. A saturated, rather dark, and copious urine, which deposits a sediment when it cools, may be regarded as favorably critical, especially when attended with marked alleviation of the symptoms; this holds true especially in gastric, bilious, catarrhal, rheumatic, and inflammatory fevers.

Profuse discharge of pale urine, in miliary fevers, leads us to fear the retrocession of the eruption, and increase of fever, and speedy death. In such cases, it might be allowable to give Rhus or Cantharides, to render the urine thicker, darker, and scantier. Profuse discharges of pale urine, in convalescent persons, must often be regarded as a sign of debility, and, if the patient is not carefully strengthened, emaciation and dropsy may occur. Profuse discharges of pale urine, in the commencement of eruptive diseases, are generally of quite unfavorable import. Free discharges of saturated, dark urine, in chronic eruptive diseases, are often very beneficial. Profuse excretion of pale urine is very common in hysterical and hypochondriacal subjects, especially just before and during the aggravation of the disease. The periodical, more profuse urinations, in hypochondriacal subjects, sometimes arises from decomposition of the blood.

Profuse urination is natural to teething children, and many disorders are brought on by its partial cessation, although convulsions, in young children, are often preceded by excessively profuse discharges of quite pale urine. Copious urination, with tendency to coma, often precedes the outbreak of aphthæ, while a peculiar-smelling and very profuse urine sometimes occurs in the exudative stage of acute hydrocephalus.

Turbid urine, which deposits a yellow sediment, is a very favorable sign in hepatitis; but, if the urine is profuse and pale, suppuration of the liver may be feared. Nearly the same holds true in inflammations of the lungs.

Pale and profuse urine is unfavorable in the commencement of measles; but, during the stage of desquamation, it is favorable.

Profuse urination at night, according to Hippocrates, occasions constipation.

Pale and profuse urine, in nervous and typhoid fevers, indicates great danger. Profuse urination, in mumps, is often more favorable than copious perspiration. Clear, watery, and abundant urine, previous to and during the outbreak of small-pox, is unfavorable, as it denotes a spasmodic state, and leads us to fear disturbances in the development of the eruption. Thick and copious urine, which deposits a sediment, in the latter stages of small-pox, after the salivation and swelling of the face have lessened, is a very salutary occurrence. Dark and profuse urine, in rheumatism, often removes the disease entirely. Thick and copious urine, in congestion of the brain, will sometimes obviate the tendency to apoplexy. Profuse, slimy urine, in mucous phthisis, occurring after the use of lime-water, sometimes gives hopes of recovery. Profuse urination, followed by relief, in dropsy, is the most favorable of all phenomena; but those dropsies which are habitually attended with copious urination are generally incurable. Crude and copious urine, in fever and ague, is generally a sign of tediousness and obstinacy of the disease. Very pale and profuse urine is generally observed in malignant intermittents. Profuse urination, in senile gangrene, is generally followed by death.

Red or reddish-brown urine (*urina rubra, flammea,*) is common in many feverish and inflammatory affections. A turbid, dark-red urine, resembling badly-fermented beer, is characteristic of the various forms of erysipelas and scarlet fever, although it sometimes occurs previous to attacks of gout. A remarkably thick and scanty red urine is a common attendant in dropsy of the pericardium. Thick, turbid, scanty, brick-red or rather brownish urine is common in ascites. Hectic fever is accompanied by scanty, red urine, upon which a fatty or whitish cream-like layer floats. Remarkably turbid and scanty red urine, in many chronic diseases, was thought to indicate some abdominal complication which was apt to be followed by dropsy or hectic fever. A scanty, clear, and very red urine, in febrile diseases, generally denotes great violence and obstinacy of the fever, or an inflammatory character of the same, or the occurrence of some local inflammation. An unusually long persistence of a clear, red urine, which forms no cloud and deposits no sediment, is generally to be regarded as unfavorable, as it indicates great violence of the disease and a remote convalescence. An abundant, thick, red urine, which deposits a sediment as the disease abates, is to be regarded as favorable and critical. Rose-red urine, in catarrhal fevers, denotes obstinacy, if not malignancy of the attack. Very red urine, in children, often points to some severe internal inflammation. A transparent, fiery urine, in consumptive patients, indicates inflammatory irritation of the lungs. Scanty, reddish-brown urine, in scarlet fever patients, sometimes precedes an attack of dropsy; during the dropsy, the urine is apt to be blood-red in color. Thick, red urine, in apoplectic congestion of the brain, is often of favorable import. Thick, hot, scanty, and turbid red urine, in dropsical patients, sometimes denotes decided disorder of some important viscus. Transparent, fiery-red urine, in dropsical patients, should make us suspicious of some inflammatory complication. Turbid, red urine, in obstinate quartan fevers, is often followed by dropsy.

Frothy urine (*urina spumosa*) occurs sometimes in the crude stage of many diseases. Very frothy urine is often seen in intermittent and bilious fevers, and in jaundice, ascites, suppurations, emaciations, and colliquative diseases. Dark, turbid, frothy urine often precedes an attack of ascites. A very decided froth, upon turbid, whitish urine, sometimes indicates the presence of much mucus, and is common in scrofulous, mucous, and verminous affections. A quite pale and very frothy urine is sometimes passed several hours before an attack of epilepsy. Very frothy urine, in fever patients, sometimes precedes an attack of convulsions or delirium, although it at times is a forerunner of favorable urinary crises. Watery and profuse urine, followed by scanty and frothy discharges, after an attack of rheumatism, if attended with coldness and dryness of the skin, some fever and swelling of the feet, is apt to be followed by anasarca.

Black urine (*urina nigra, nigricans,*) is apt to occur in scurvy, putrid fever, and other severe diseases; it was formerly supposed to arise from infarction of black bile, inflammations of the veins or spleen, malignant inflammations of the lungs, suppression of menses or lochia, or disease of the kidneys. The thinner and more offensive the black urine is, and the more decidedly it precipitates a sooty deposit, the more unfavorable the prognosis. Black urine, in lead-colic, is not unfavorable. The occurrence of black urine, in acute fevers, when attended with sleeplessness and frightful dreams, is often a precursor of delirium. Black urine, during the increase of malignant fevers, is a fatal sign; but, in the decline of a disease, if the symptoms are alternated, and a salutary nose-bleed and benign sweat occur, it may be regarded as favorable; but, if unfavorable phenomena are associated with it, death is apt to occur. When the previously saffron-yellow urine, in jaundice, becomes scanty and black, we may fear the setting in of dropsy. Black urine, in hæmorrhoids of the bladder, is not dangerous, nor in hysterical subjects; in abdominal infarctions it is often favorable. Black urine, in child-bed fever, especially if it alternates with fatty urine, is very dangerous. Black urine, in children, often precedes epilepsy or dropsy, which the use of Rhubarb may prevent. Excessively offensive black urine, intermixed with blackish lumps, in nephritis, if followed by entire cessation of pain, is very dangerous; but sometimes simple black urine relieves congestion of the kidneys. Black urine, in calculus of the kidney, is not always unfavorable. Black urine, produced by visceral remedies, is often favorable. Black urine, in quartan fevers, according to De Haen, is generally not only not dangerous, but often favorable and critical. And black urine, after suppression of the lochia, is often not of dangerous import.

Heavy urine (*urina ponderosa*) is apt to occur in persons who drink but little water and much spirits, who perspire profusely, and take active exercise; it is also common in fevers. Gravel and stone are attended with very heavy urine. Turbid, heavy urine is common in mercurial salivation, in inflammatory dropsies, diabetes, putrid fevers, and hectic colliquations. When pale urine is over 1.030, we may be pretty certain that diabetes is present. The urine is very heavy during urinary crises.

Scanty urine (*urina parca*) is common during profuse diarrhœas, sweats, or salivations. Scanty urine, if attended with œdema of the ankles, is a pretty constant precursor of dropsy of some internal cavity. Very dark, acrid, hot, and scanty urine is common in the commencement of feverish, inflammatory, bilious, gastric, and other fevers and inflammations of internal organs. In nephritis, the urine is darker, more fiery, hotter, and more scanty than in any other disease; it may even become entirely suppressed. Saturated, turbid, scanty urine often arises from congestions or stagnations in the kidneys. In gravel, the urine is commonly very turbid and scanty. The urine is apt to be very offensive, saturated, turbid, and scanty in persons with digestive troubles, abdominal obstructions and infarctions, lead-colic, and mucous piles. Acrid, exceedingly offensive, and scanty urine is common in maniacal persons, consumptives, and those affected with tabes. Whitish, turbid, scanty urine sometimes attends organic disease of the liver. Pale, thin, and unusually scanty urine may occur in severe attacks of nephritis, paralysis or spasm of the kidneys, and in some affections of the spinal marrow. Saturated, scanty urine, when discharged with great difficulty, although there is much urging thereto, with fullness of the bladder, as evident from percussion, denotes retention of much urine in the bladder. Scanty urine, remaining after inflammations of the chest, especially if there is difficulty of breathing and much debility, leads us to fear dropsy of the chest. Very scanty urine, after taking cold, is unfavorable. Saturated, scanty urine, in the commencement of febrile affections, is natural. Diminution of the urine, at the critical periods, should lead us to expect critical sweats, diarrhœa, or dropsy, or a urinary taste in the mouth may occur, followed by drowsiness, spasmodic trembling, and apoplexy. Scanty urine, in gouty subjects, threatens a new paroxysm, or the development of stone or gravel. Scanty urine, which deposits a chalk-like sediment, in children, when attended with great restlessness, constant screaming, disturbance of sleep, and constipation, belongs among the precursors and attendants of the first stage of dropsy of the brain. A light yellow, peculiarly glittering scanty urine is observed in rhachialgic muscular restlessness. Pale, scanty, watery urine, after nephritis, is sometimes followed by induration of the kidneys. Scanty urine, after scarlet fever, especially if attended with difficulty of breathing and heaviness of the whole body, is often a precursor of dropsy. Scanty urine, in dropsical subjects, which cannot be increased by remedies, is unfavorable, for discharges by stool and sweat are not so reliable as relief from the kidneys. Pale, scanty urine is observed in malignant intermittents. If the urine becomes very scanty, in the latter stages of fever and ague, we may fear dropsy. Scanty urine, in females, is often associated with derangement of menstruation.

Turbid urine (*urina turbida*) attends many different diseases. Whitish, offensive, turbid urine, which quickly putrefies, is common in some derangements of digestion, in crudities and impurities of the bowels, in mucous and verminous conditions, especially when these occur in persons with delicate muscles and sensitive nerves. Turbid urine, which resembles that of cattle, (*urina jumentosa,*) is said to arise from infarctions and congestions of the abdominal viscera, such as the liver, spleen, portal system, mesenteric glands, or kidneys; occasionally, chronic inflammation is present in some one of these organs. There is a class of persons who become indisposed almost every four weeks, and are relieved after the discharge of jumentous urine. It is, however, sometimes a precursor of gout or hæmorrhoids, especially of the kidneys or bladder, or a sign of tendency to gravel or dropsy. Habitual, offensive, slimy, and turbid urine, when attended with pain in the kidneys or bladder, is often a sign of chronic disease of the urinary organs.

Habitually offensive, slimy, turbid urine, attended with pain in the region of the kidneys and bladder, is frequently indicative of chronic disease of the urinary organs. In tubercular disease of the kidneys, the urine is of a straw-yellow color, and curdy. It is thick, slimy, and, perhaps, tinged with blood, in cases of stone in the bladder or kidneys, and occasionally in phosphatic gravel. It is pale, flocculent, and turbid, in catarrh and hæmorrhoids of the bladder. It is actually ichorous in some examples of cancer of the kidneys.

Arthritic nephritic colic is apt to be attended with the painful discharge of curdy, turbid urine. Attacks of hæmorrhoidal colic are apt to be preceded by the discharge of jumentous turbid urine in the morning and evening. Scanty, offensive, and jumentous urine is often passed by dropsical, consumptive, and cachectic subjects. Very dark-colored, acrid, turbid urine, with or without a sediment, is often indicative of an inflammatory affection of some abdominal organ, such as the liver, spleen, or kidneys. Similar urine, but scanty, and without sediment, is commonly observed in inflammations of the heart, and other heart-affections. The urine is often dark red, thick, and turbid in bilious fevers and other bilious affections. It is often of a clayey or loamy appearance in pneumonia-notha and false pneumonia. Reddish turbid urine, in chronic affections, is sometimes followed by dropsy.

Jumentous urine is often of favorable import in chronic abdominal affections. Thick, turbid urine, in the commencement of febrile affections, often denotes gravity and malignancy of the attack, or the violent implication of the digestive organs. If jumentous urine is associated with a small, weak pulse, stupor or wakefulness, heaviness or painfulness of the head, violent thirst, or dryness of the tongue, then we may fear delirium, convulsions, or lethargy. Baglivi erroneously supposed that jumentous urine was always a sign of brain-disease in acute affections. A favorable termination may be expected when the urine becomes turbid, at the acme of a fever, but begins to grow clear as it cools, and even deposits a white, thick sediment. Thick, blackish, and turbid urine, in jaundice, is generally followed by a speedy resolution of the disease. Gouty patients may fear a new paroxysm when their urine becomes turbid; but, if the urine deposits a sediment during an attack, we may hope for a more rapid recovery. In abdominal infarctions, the occurrence of a thick, turbid urine is often beneficial. In children, whitish and turbid urine is often a sign of worms, but may also arise from disease of the mesenteric glands, general atrophy, or dropsy of the brain. Turbid urine, after overloading the stomach, is favorable. Turbid urine, in dysentery, without the occurrence of a sediment, is unfavorable. Heavy, turbid urine, in visceral affections, is beneficial.

Offensive urine is of various import. An unusual degree of the natural urinary odor is indicative of energetic assimilation, plethora, an active life with much corporeal exertion, of a strongly nourishing animal diet. The urine of aged persons is stronger than that of younger persons; also in febrile diseases, and when the urine is scanty. A nauseous, offensive, thick, and turbid urine, which putrefies rapidly, often arises from an excess of mucus or pus in the urine, although it occasionally depends upon decided disorder of the digestive organs. Obstinate and insupportable headaches, of plethoric females, are sometimes followed by the excretion of thick, nauseous urine, owing to deep-seated disease of the lymphatic and chyliferous systems. A similar smell is common to the thick saturated urine of deranged persons. A quite peculiar nauseous smell of the urine sometimes arises from the suppression of habitual foot-sweats, or the cure of old profusely-secreting ulcers or eruptions. The urine is apt to smell like that of mice or cats after eating asparagus, pansy, or heart's-ease, and is often noticed in rhachitic children, and those with scald-head and chronic affections of the brain. An absolutely cadaverous smell is associated with the turbid, curdy, or dark brown and flocculent urine, which occurs in suppuration of the kidneys or bladder. An acrid, ammoniacal, penetrating smell of the urine may occur in chronic abdominal affections. A nauseous sour odor is noticed when there is acidity of the primæ-viæ, in scrofulous and many abdominal rhachitic affections, before the outbreak or during the decline of gout, in gravel, miliary fevers, and sometimes in the urinary crises of catarrhal and rheumatic affections. A disagreeably sweetish odor of the urine is noticed in mucous fevers and diabetes. A sulphurous smell is often noticed in croup, and after the long-continued use of Phosphorus. A garlicky smell has often been noticed after the use of Phosphorus. A characteristic fish-like odor is unfavorable in adynamic fevers and some other diseases. Offensive urine, as a general rule, is not of favorable import, especially if noticed in the early stages of disease, although there are persons who feel well as long as their urine is strong and offensive, and while the disappearance of this is a pretty certain sign of threatening disease; in like manner, the occurrence of offensive urine, in the latter stage of some diseases, if the other signs are favorable, is remarkably salutary. The profuse discharge of offensive urine, in epileptic patients, frequently precedes a new paroxysm. Offensive urine, in gastric diseases, is often salutary. Dark, offensive urine, in nephritis, is unfavorable.

Variable urine (*urina variabilis*). Frequent variations in the color, quantity, thickness, transparency, and smell of the urine is not generally favorable, as it indicates either obstinacy of the attack, or else a threatening nervous affection. A very decided fickleness and variability of the appearance of the urine is observed in hypochondriacal or hysterical subjects, and also in nervous, putrid, and malignant fevers, in heart-affections, mucous phthisis, worm and other affections. Remarkable variations in the urine of dropsical persons is often a sign of approaching death. Very variable urine, in intermittent fevers, indicates either obstinacy of the attack, or a tendency towards continued fever.

White urine (*urina alba*) must not be confounded with pale or watery urine; on the contrary, it is more often milky and curdy. The muddy, whitish color of urine often arises from copious admixture with pus or mucus, albumen or phosphatic deposits; generally, the admixed substances are precipitated after a while, and the superincumbent urine then presents its natural yellow color. Whitish urine is often observed in impurities of the first passages, in mucous conditions, worm-affections, gout, scrofula, hæmorrhoids of the bladder, catarrhs, and during convalescence from severe diseases. Curdy urine, attended with pain in the kidneys or bladder, often attends tubercular disease, ulceration, &c., of these organs. An unusually heavy milky urine is sometimes observed in mercurial salivation. White urine, depositing a chalk-like sediment, has been noticed in verminal and arthritic affections. Some persons habitually pass a white, turbid, slimy urine, depositing a chalk-like sediment, which all disappears when they are regularly attacked with gout. Urine which becomes white and thick on standing is often observed in gastric, nervous, and hectic fevers. The urine may be white in inflammatory, gastric, and rheumatic affections, in rheumatic tetanus and pneumonia-notha. Arthritic blenorrhœa of the urethra is apt to be attended with turbid milky urine, in which clouds or mucous fibres float, but which soon clears up after it is passed, and then presents a pale yellow color after it has deposited a whitish, mucous, and chalk-like sediment. Blisters are then said to afford speedy relief. White urine, in children, is said to be indicative of mucous derangement, worm-affections, scrofula, or atrophy. The urine may also be white in inflammations of the chest and bowels; it is often milky white in acute hydrocephalus. Children who pass white urine for a long time, often die of softening of the stomach. Milky urine, in puerperal women, often indicates a threatening puerperal fever, or metastasis of milk.

Pleasant smelling urine (*urina suaveolens*) is often noticed after the use of Turpentine, Violet-roots, and Juniper-berries; it has also been noticed in the commencement of hectic fever.

Urinary deposits or sediments (*hypostasis sedimentum urinæ*) arise from the precipitation of insoluble solid substances from the urine; they are often important in forming a diagnosis or prognosis. A moderately large, white, or reddish sediment, which is flocculent, or as if composed of a fine powder, floating on the bottom of the vessel and easily disturbed, is of favorable import, especially if flat at the edges and rather conical in the middle. A flat, immovable, solidly lying, and too copious sediment, or a too scanty, unequal deposit, the different particles of which frequently alter their position or float about, are, if not of unfavorable import, at least rarely salutary and critical. A dark yellow urine, which is passed frequently, but in small quantities, and deposits a sediment at the commencement of the disease, is indicative of gastric or bilious impurities. A bluish sediment (*s. cæruleum*) has been observed in gouty and cachectic subjects. A lead-colored deposit (*s. lividum*) is always unfavorable, and most frequently noticed in putrid diseases. A brown sediment (*s. fuscum*) is often noticed in bilious and erysipelatous affections, and in scarlet fever, and then is not an entirely unfavorable appearance. Absence of sediment, in diseases in which we should expect one, always indicates a distant resolution, or a tendency to an unfavorable termination; in fevers, we may expect a nervous complication, and, in inflammations, a termination in suppuration or induration; in inflammations of the lungs, we may fear tubercles. A flat sediment (*s. planum*) is favorable when it is loose, light, and even. A solid, heavy, and quite flat sediment is rarely salutary and critical.

A gelatinous sediment (*s. gelatinosum*) sometimes occurs in dropsy of the brain, in adults, and in hydatids of the kidneys. A heavy, gelatinous sediment, resembling frog-spawn or vitreous slime, is often a sign of chronic catarrh of the bladder. In persons who have a tendency to gravel, we sometimes notice a gelatinous mass, which sinks to the bottom of the vessel, and soon assumes an amorphous or imperfectly crystalline appearance, evident at first on the top of the sediment, but afterwards pervading it through and through.

Yellow sediments (*s. aurantiacum*, *croceum*, *flavum*,) often arise from an excess of bile; orange yellow sediments have been observed in gastric and bilious fevers, especially when complicated with a nervous or intermittent fever. This kind of sediment is also not unusual in rheumatic affections. An isabel yellow deposit has been observed in simple rheumatism and in erysipelas, although, generally, the sediments in these two diseases differ widely from each other. A thick, heavy, pale yellow sediment, which gives the urine a milky appearance when it is shaken up, but which soon settles to the bottom again, has been noticed when there is pus in the urine.

A grey sediment (*s. cinereum*) has been observed after the free use of gold. A grey sediment, which is easily mixed with the scanty red urine upon which it forms, and which redissolves, in whole or in greater part, on the application of warmth, is a sign of a favorable crisis in inflammatory, catarrhal, gastric, mucous, bilious, intermittent, and nervous fevers.

A green sediment (*s. viride*) has been occasionally noticed in bilious diseases. A dark green deposit is cast down when nitric acid is added to urine containing bile.

A furfuraceous or bran-like sediment (*s. furfuraceum*) is rarely salutary and critical, but is generally a sign of postponement of a resolution or crisis, or else arises from local disease of the urinary organs. It has been observed in nervous fevers and cachexias, in weakness of digestion, hæmorrhoids, and infarctions; it may also occur in gravel, mucous fluxes, hæmorrhoids or ulcerations of the bladder, and in so-called psora of the bladder.

A reddish, glistening, crystalline deposit, resembling glittering sand, has been observed as salutary and critical in inflammations of the lungs, provided the urine has been turbid previously.

A red sediment, (*s. rubrum,*) from scanty and saturated urine, denotes great violence of the existing fever, and an imperfect resolution of the disease, but is not otherwise unfavorable. Something similar has been observed when acids are first used freely. A partially fluid, clear, red, somewhat lumpy or gruel-like, thick, dark, or almost blackish red sediment, which is not soluble by heat or by the addition of more fluid, and which, when shaken, renders the superincumbent clear urine of a dark red color, but soon settles again, arises from the admixture of blood in the urine. A rose-red sediment (*s. roseum*) occurs in rheumatic affections, and at times in dropsies, hectic fevers, and chronic infarctions of the viscera, especially of the liver. A sediment which resembles dissolved red clay, but which, when shaken, seems composed of mucous flocculi, that, however, soon disappear, is said often to precede attacks of hæmorrhoidal colic. A sediment which resembles brick-dust in color and appearance (*s. lateritium*) is a common attendant of catarrhal, rheumatic, and intermittent fevers, acute and chronic rheumatism, gout, jaundice occasionally, and many dropsies. It not uncommonly indicates the presence of larvate fever and ague, or is a precursor of abdominal dropsy, or an attack of gout. Brick dust-like sediment, in putrid fevers, is often of fatal omen. Lateritious sediment, in previously watery and clear urine, is a favorable sign in whooping cough. When attended with vomiting of bile, in injuries of the head, it sometimes indicates the occurrence of abscess of the liver; in cancerous diseases, it leaves little hope of a favorable termination; in apoplectic, it is rather favorable than otherwise.

Black sediments (*s. nigrum*) occur when blood is mixed with the urine. A coffee ground-like, black sediment, has been witnessed in bilious fevers, scarlet fever with marked bilious complication, in liver affections, jaundice, black jaundice, melancholy, and many dropsies. A soot-like sediment, in black urine, was supposed to indicate internal mortification. Black sediment, in pleurisy, is often of fatal omen, although sometimes it may arise from hæmorrhage from the kidneys, and then be less unfavorable.

An uneven sediment, (*s. asperum*,) in which the upper surface of the deposit is irregular, and the separate parts of which vacillate or float about, is unfavorable, or, at least, is not often salutary and critical.

A transient sediment (*s. evanescens*) is unfavorable when it disappears of itself, or when the urine is lightly shaken. A sediment which resembles red clay, but disappears when shaken violently, is a precursor of hæmorrhoidal colic.

A white sediment, (*s. album*,) if loose, flocculent, easily deposited when the urine is in repose, but easily intermixed with it again when shaken, but quickly settling down again, is a sign of the presence of much mucus in the urine, especially if its color is of a dirty white. It is always a sign of a tedious or obstinate disease, and occurs in mucous conditions, verminal affections, rhachitis, scrofula, indigestion, &c., &c. In measles, a heavy white sediment is often noticed below yellow urine. A sediment consisting of irregular flocculi, which swim about in turbid red urine, has been observed in catarrhal, gastric, rheumatic, and intermittent fevers, and in inflammatory dropsies. A very heavy white sediment, which cannot be intermixed with the urine, is often indicative of catarrh of the bladder. A slimy sediment, which looks like melted tallow, has been noticed in the suppurative stage of small-pox. In tubercles of the kidneys, we often observe a meal-like, light sediment precipitated from a straw-yellow, curdy urine. A solid, crystalline, or granular white sediment is often composed of phosphatic salts. A scaly, white deposit occurs in infarctions of the abdomen, in hæmorrhoidal affections, hypochondria, chlorosis, intermittent fever, and hydrocephalus. A solid, chalk-like sediment (*s. cretaceum*) may often occur, for years, in gastric affections, worms, scrofula, or gout, but is a special diagnostic sign of the first stage of acute hydrocephalus in children; it also occurs in chronic hydrocephalus as soon as inflammation is superadded. It also occurs in cachectic softening of the bones, when there are violent bone-pains, and becomes more and more evident the more progress the bone-disease makes. A pyramidal or acuminated sediment (*s. acuminatum*) is the most favorable, salutary, and critical.

The chemical tests and analyses of urinary deposits will be treated of more particularly under the head of urinary diseases. In the present place, although we may have been prolix, we have only aimed to record the more evident, diagnostic, and prognostic significance of such alterations of the urine as are readily observed by the eye of the practitioner.

SECTION VI.

NOSOLOGY; OR, THE CLASSIFICATION OF DISEASES.

"Nosology is that branch of the science of medicine, the objects of which are, *first*, to distribute or arrange diseases into classes, orders, genera, or species; and, *second*, to distinguish each disease by an appropriate name. These two divisions of nosology are respectively known as the *classification* and nomenclature of diseases."

To further this portion of medical science, a statistical congress of the European powers was held at Paris, on the tenth of September, 1855, for the purpose of devising and adopting, among other matters, a uniform system of nomenclature, for recording diseases, and the causes of death from them. Its importance was fully estimated by them, and a definite nomenclature of the causes of death was determined upon; the same, in point of fact, as that used in England and Geneva. Subsequent arrangements were made, at a second congress, held at Brussels, to hold a third congress at Vienna, when it is expected that a system of nosology will be adopted which shall be similarly uniform, and applicable to the requirements of all countries; certainly, until the demands of new developments and discoveries shall necessitate a new revision.

By classifying diseases, and recording the causes of death, the most valuable information is obtained, relative to the health of the people, or of the unwholesomeness and pestilential agencies which surround them. We can take this or that disease and measure, not only its destructiveness, but its favorite times of visitation. We can identify its haunts and classify its victims. We are able to trace diseases also as they perceptibly get weaker and weaker, as some have done of late. We know, from the valuable returns of the Registrar-General of England, prepared by Dr. Farr, that scarlatina is, or rather was decreasing, and that it has been growing less and less destructive since 1851; that, until quite lately, the whooping cough has likewise declined, in some measure, and that measles alone, out of these severe diseases, has exhibited any tendency to increase. The advantages, therefore, of adopting some system of classifying diseases, which can be put to such useful practical purposes, must be obvious to every one. In former times, we were indebted to Linnæus, Vogel, Sauvage, Macbride, Sagar, Cullen; more recently, to Cooper, Copeland, Mason Good, Craigie, Bright, Addison, Watson, and Wood, of Pennsylvania. The system of Cullen is now too old to serve a very useful purpose, and it is preferred to adopt some system which, while it meets the requirements of science, will illustrate, by its use, the practical questions of the day, relative to diseases, and their bearing upon the public health; and which will show those causes which are injurious or fatal to the life of man, and so contribute to remove those causes which tend to shorten life.

As classification is only a mode of generalization, there are, of course, several modes which may be followed for special purposes. The physician, the pathologist, the jurist, the hospital statist, may each make a classification from his own point of view;—the physician divides diseases according to their treatment, as medical or surgical; the pathologist on the nature of the morbid action or product; the anatomist or physiologist on the organs or tissues implicated;—and all of these may give useful and interesting results. Dr. Farr, of England, has completed a system of nosology, which is to be submitted to the members of the approaching congress for their consideration; and, being eminently useful and scientific, a tabular view of it is appended. It is supposed that it will soon be adopted, both in Europe and America.

TABULAR VIEW OF THE CLASSES AND ORDERS OF DISEASE IN THE PROPOSED NOSOLOGY OF DR. FARR.

CLASS I.—Zymotic Diseases. *Zymotici* (ζύμη, leaven).—Diseases that are either epidemic, endemic, or contagious; induced by some specific substance, or by the want of food, or by its bad quality. In this class there are four orders of diseases, namely:

ORDER 1. MIASMATIC DISEASES—*Miasmatici* (μίασμα, stain, defilement).

ORDER 2. ENTHETIC DISEASES—*Enthetici* (ἔνθετος, put in, implanted).

ORDER 3. DIETIC DISEASES—*Dietici* (δίαιτα, way of life, diet).

ORDER 4. PARASITIC DISEASES—*Parasitici* (παράσιτος, parasite).

CLASS II.—Constitutional Diseases. *Cahetici* (καχεξία, bad habit of body), sporadic diseases; affecting several organs in which new morbid products are often deposited; sometimes hereditary.

ORDER 1. DIATHETIC DISEASES—*Diathetici* (διάθεσις, condition, diathesis).

ORDER 2. TUBERCULAR DISEASES—*Phthisici* (φθìσìς, wasting away).

CLASS III.—Local Diseases. *Monorganici* (μόνος, alone, without others; ὄργανον, organ), sporadic diseases, in which the functions of particular organs or systems are disturbed or obliterated, with or without inflammation; sometimes hereditary.

ORDER 1. HEAD DISEASES—*Cephalici* (κεφαλή, head).
ORDER 2. HEART DISEASES—*Cardiaci* (καρδία, heart).
ORDER 3. LUNG DISEASES—*Pneumonici* (πνεύμων, lung).
ORDER 4. BOWEL DISEASES—*Enterici* (ἔντερον, intestine).
ORDER 5. KIDNEY DISEASES—*Nephritici* (νεφρὸς, kidney).
ORDER 6. GENNETIC DISEASES—*Aidoici* (αἰδοῖα, pudenda).
ORDER 7. BONE AND MUSCLE DISEASES—*Myostici* (μῦς, muscle; ὀζέον, bone).
ORDER 8. SKIN DISEASES—*Chrotici* (χρὼς, skin).

CLASS IV.—Developmental Diseases. *Metamorphici* (μεταμόρφωσις, change of form); special diseases, the incidental result of the formative, reproductive, and nutritive processes.

ORDER 1. DEVELOPMENTAL DISEASES OF CHILDREN—*Paidici* (παιδία, youth).

ORDER 2. DEVELOPMENTAL DISEASES OF WOMEN—*Gyniaci* (γυνή, woman).

ORDER 3. DEVELOPMENTAL DISEASES OF OLD PEOPLE—*Geratici* (γῆρας, old age).

ORDER 4. DISEASES OF NUTRITION—*Atrophici* (ἀτροφια, atrophy).

TABULAR VIEW OF THE CLASSES, ORDERS, AND NOMENCLATURE OF DISEASES.

CLASS I.—Zymotic Diseases. *Zymotici.*

ORDER 1. MIASMATIC DISEASES—*Miasmatici.*

ENGLISH NAMES.	LATIN NAMES.
Small-Pox,	*Variola.*
Varioloid,	*Varioloides.*
Chicken-Pox,	*Varicella.*
Miliaria,	*Miliaria.*
Measles,	*Morbilli.*
Scarlet Fever,	*Scarlatina.*
Hybrid of Measles, and Scarlet fever,	*Rubeola.*
Dengue,	*Scarlatina Rheumatica.*
Quinsy,	*Tonsilia.*
Diphtheria,	*Diphtheria.*
Mumps,	*Parotia.*
Croup,	*Trachealia.*
Whooping Cough,	*Pertussis.*
Typhoid Fever.	*Febris Typhoides.*
Relapsing Fever,	*Febris Recurrens.*
Typhus Fever,	*Typhus.*
Erysipelas,	*Erysipelas.*
Erythema,	*Erythema.*
Hospital Gangrene,	*Gangræna Nosocomialis.*

CLASS I. ORDER 1.—Continued.

ENGLISH NAMES.	LATIN NAMES.
Purulent Infection,	*Pyemia.*
Childbed Fever,	*Febris Puerperarum.*
The Plague,	*Pestis.*
Carbuncle,	*Anthrax.*
Boil,	*Furunculus.*
Influenza,	*Influenza.*
Dysentery,	*Dysenteria.*
Diarrhœa,	*Diarrhœa.*
Cholera,	*Cholera.*
Yellow Fever,	*Typhus Icterodes.*
Remittent Fever, Crimean Fever,	*Febris Remittens.*
Hong-Kong Fever, &c., &c.,	*Febris Tropicorum.*
Ague,	*Febris Intermittens.*

ORDER 2. ENTHETIC DISEASES—*Enthetici.*

ENGLISH NAMES.	LATIN NAMES.
Syphilis (primary),	*Syphilis (primarius).*
Syphilis (secondary),	*Syphilis (secundarius).*
Gonorrhœa,	*Gonorrhœa.*
Leprosy, (Including Greek Elephantiasis, or the Leprosy of Moses)	*Lepra.*
Yaws,	*Frambœsia.*
Pellagra,	*Pellagra.*
Radesyge,	*Radesyge.*
Purulent Ophthalmia,	*Ophthalmia Purulenta.*
Glanders,	*Equinia.*
Hydrophobia,	*Rabies.*
Necusia,	*Necusia.*
Malignant Pustule,	*Pustula Maligna.*

ORDER 3. DIETIC DISEASES—*Dietici.*

ENGLISH NAMES.	LATIN NAMES.
Famine Fever,	*Febris à Fame.*
Scurvy,	*Scorbutus.*
Purpura,	*Purpura.*
Rickets,	*Rachitis.*
Bronchocele,	*Bronchocele.*
Cretinism,	*Cretinismus.*
Alcoholism, including Intemperance, Delirium Tremens, and Catacausis,	*Alcoholismus.*

ORDER 4. PARASITIC DISEASES—*Parasitici.*

ENGLISH NAMES.	LATIN NAMES.
Thrush,	*Aphtha.*
Porrigo,	*Porrigo.*
Itch,	*Scabies.*
Phthiriasis,	*Morbus Pedicularis.*
Worms,	*Vermes.*
(*a*) Hydatids,	*Acephalocystis, echinococcus hominis.*
(*b*) Tape Worm,	*Tænia Solium.*
(*c*) Strongulus Gigas,	*Strongulus Gigas.*
(*d*) Round Worm,	*Ascaris Lumbricoides.*
(*e*) Thread Worm,	*Ascaris Vermicularis.*
(*f*) Guinea Worm,	*Dracunculus.*

CLASS II.—Constitutional Diseases. *Cachetici.*

ORDER 1. DIATHETIC DISEASES—*Diathetici.*

ENGLISH NAMES.	LATIN NAMES.
Rheumatism,	*Rheumatismus Acutus* vel *Febris Rheumatica.*
Gout,	*Podagra.*
Anæmia,	*Anæmia.*
Dropsy,	*Hydrops.*
Cancer,	*Carcinoma.*
(*a*) " Soft,	" *Encephaloides.*
(*b*) " Colloid,	" *Alveolare.*
(*c*) Cancer, Osteoid,	*Carcinoma Osteoides.*
(*d*) " Scirrhus,	" *Scirrhoma.*
(*e*) " Epithelial and Sweeps',	" *Epitheliomata.*
Melanosis,	*Melanosis.*
Lupus,	*Lupus.*
Canker,	*Noma.*
Mortification,	*Gangrena.*
Dry Gangrene,	*Gangrena Senilis.*

ORDER 2. TUBERCULAR DISEASES—*Phthisici.*

ENGLISH NAMES.	LATIN NAMES.
Scrofula,	*Scrofula.*
Tuberculosis, Mesenteric,	*Tuberculosis Mesenterica.*
Tubercular Peritonitis,	*Peritonitis Tuberculosa.*
Consumption,	*Phthisis.*
Hydrocephalus,	*Hydrocephalus.*
(with tubercular deposit,	*Meningia Tuberculosa.*

CLASS III.—Local Diseases. *Monorganici.*

Order 1. Brain Diseases—*Cephalici.*

English Names.	Latin Names.
Meningitis	*Meningitis.*
Encephalitis	*Encephalitis.*
Cephalitis	*Cephalitis.*
Myelitis	*Myelitis.*
Apoplexy	*Apoplexia.*
Paralysis	*Paralysis.*
Shaking Palsy	*Paralysis Agitans.*
Chorea	*Chorea.*
Delirium Tremens	*Delirium Tremens.*
Mania	*Mania.*
Monomania	*Monomania.*
Dementia	*Dementia.*
Epilepsy	*Epilepsia.*
Hysteria	*Hysteria.*
Tetanus	*Tetanus.*
Convulsions	*Convulsio.*
Laryngismus	*Laryngismus.*
Neuralgia, Tic Douleureux	*Neuralgia.*
Neuroma	*Neuroma.*

Order 2. Heart Diseases—*Cardiaci.*

English Names.	Latin Names.
Carditis	*Carditis.*
Pericarditis	*Pericarditis.*
Endocarditis	*Endocarditis.*
Disease of Heart Valves	*Morbus Cordis Valvularum.*
Heart Hypertrophy	*Hypertrophia Cordis.*
" Atrophy	*Atrophia Cordis.*
" Fatty Degeneration	*Cordis Degeneratio.*
Aneurism of the Heart	*Aneurisma Cordis.*
Aneurism of the Aorta, &c.	
Angina Pectoris	*Angina Pectoris.*
Fainting	*Syncope.*
Arteritis	*Arteritis.*
Atheroma	*Atheroma.*
Phlebitis	*Phlebitis.*
Varicose Veins	*Varix.*

Order 3. Lung Diseases—*Pneumonici.*

English Names.	Latin Names.
Hæmoptysis	*Hæmoptysis.*
Laryngitis	*Laryngitis.*
(Œdema of the Glottis)	*Œdema Glottidis.*
Laryngismus Stridulus	*Laryngismus Stridulus.*
Bronchitis	*Bronchitis.*
Pleurisy	*Pleuritis.*
Hydrothorax	*Hydrothorax.*
Empyema	*Empyema.*
Pneumothorax	*Pneumothorax.*
Congestion of Lungs	*Apoplexia Pulmonalis.*
Pneumonia	*Pneumonia.*
Pleuri-Pneumonitis	*Pleuri-Pneumonitis.*
Asthma	*Asthma.*
Emphysema of Lungs	*Emphysema.*
Grinders' Asthma	*Asthma.*
Miners' Asthma, Colliers' Phthisis, Spurious Melanosis	*Asthma Metallicorum.*

Order 4. Bowel Diseases—*Enterici.*

English Names.	Latin Names.
Glossitis	*Glossitis.*
Stomatitis	*Stomatitis.*
Pharyngitis	*Pharyngitis.*
Œsophagitis	*Œsophagitis.*
Gastritis	*Gastritis.*
Enteritis	*Enteritis.*
Peritonitis	*Peritonitis.*
Ileus	*Ileus.*
(Constipation)	(*Constipatio*).
Intussusception	*Intussusceptio.*
Dyspepsia	*Dyspepsia.*
Pyrosis	*Pyrosis.*
Gastralgia	*Gastralgia.*
Hæmatemesis	*Hæmatemesis.*
Melæna	*Melæna.*
Supra Renal Melasma	*Morbus Addisonii.*
Pancreatic Disease	*Morbus Pancreatici.*
Splenitis	*Splenitis.*
Hepatitis	*Hepatitis.*
Jaundice	*Icterus.*
Gall-Stones	*Chololithus.*
Cirrhosis	*Cirrhosis.*
Ascites	*Ascites.*

Order 5. Kidney Diseases—*Nephritici.*

English Names.	Latin Names.
Nephritis	*Nephritis.*
Ischuria	*Ischuria.*
Diuresis	*Diuresis.*
Nephria, (Bright's Disease), Albuminuria	*Nephria.*
Diabetes	*Diabetes.*
Stone, Gravel	*Calculus Vesicæ* vel *Renalis.*
Hæmaturia	*Hæmaturia.*
Cystitis	*Cystitis.*

ORDER 6. GENNETIC DISEASES—*Gennetici.*

ENGLISH NAMES.	LATIN NAMES.	ENGLISH NAMES.	LATIN NAMES.
Varicocele,..........	*Varicocele.*	(Uterine Tumor),...	(*Tumor Uteri*).
Orchitis,..........	*Orchitis.*	Ovarian Dropsy,....	*Hydrops Ovarii.*
Hydrocele,..........	*Hydrocele.*	(Ovarian Tumor),...	(*Tumor Ovarii*).
Hysteritis,..........	*Hysteritis.*		

ORDER 7. BONE AND MUSCLE DISEASES—*Myostici.*

Synovitis,..........	*Synovitis.*	Curvature of Spine, .	*Curvatura Spinæ.*
Ostitis,..........	*Ostitis.*	Caries, ...	*Caries.*
Exostosis,..........	*Exostosis.*	Necrosis, ...	*Necrosis.*
Brittle Bones,......	*Fragilitas Ossium.*	Muscular Atrophy or Degeneration,	*Atrophia* vel *Degeneratio Musculorum.*
Soft Bones, ...	*Mollities Ossium.*		

ORDER 8. SKIN DISEASES—*Chrotici.*

Roseola,..........	*Roseola.*	Mentagra,..........	*Mentagra.*
Urticaria,..........	*Urticaria.*	Lichen,..........	*Lichen.*
Eczema,..........	*Eczema.*	Prurigo,..........	*Prurigo.*
Herpes,..........	*Herpes.*	Psoriasis, ...	*Psoriasis.*
Pemphigus,........	*Pemphigus.*	Pityriasis,..........	*Pityriasis.*
Rupia,..........	*Rupia.*	Ichthyosis,..........	*Ichthyosis.*
Ecthyma, ...	*Ecthyma.*	Phlegmon,..........	*Phlegmon.*
Impetigo, ...	*Impetigo.*	Whitlow,..........	*Whitlow.*
Acne, ...	*Acne.*		

CLASS IV.—Developmental Diseases. *Metamorphici.*

ORDER 1. DEVELOPMENTAL DISEASES OF CHILDREN—*Paidiaci.*

Stillborn,..........	*Natus Mortuus.*	Imperforate Anus, ..	*Anus Imperforatus.*
Premature Birth,...	*Prematurus Natus.*	Idiocy, ...	*Fatuitas.*
Atelectasis,..........	*Atelectasis Pulmonum.*	Congenital Deaf-Dumbness, ...	*Mutitas.*
Malformations, ...	*Vitia Conformationis.*	Teething,..........	*Dentitio.*
Cyanosis,..........	*Cyanosis.*		
Spina Bifida,.......	*Spina Bifida.*		

ORDER 2. DEVELOPMENTAL DISEASES OF WOMEN, CHIEFLY IN THE REPRODUCTIVE AGE—*Gyniaci.*

ENGLISH NAMES.	LATIN NAMES.
Chlorosis,..........	*Chlorosis.*
Childbirth, Miscarriage, Abortion,..........	*Partus, Abortus.*

(including death from "pelvis deformed, rupture of uterus, extra-uterine fœtation, flooding, puerperal mania, puerperal convulsions, syncope, hysteritis, breast-abscess.") See also "Metria," Class I., 1.

Paramenia, (including "amenorrhœa, leucorrhœa,")......	*Paramenia.*
Climacteria, (turn of life),..........	*Climacteria.*

ORDER 3. DEVELOPMENTAL DISEASES OF OLD PEOPLE—*Gyratici.*

Old Age,.......... *Senectus.*

ORDER 4. DISEASES OF NUTRITION—*Atrophici.*

Atrophy, Debility, (includes premature old age), ... *Atrophia, Asthenia.*

The preceding classification of diseases into four groups is not given as a perfect system, but as a convenient grouping of diseases.

By its use, the student will be able to preserve uniformity in the recording of his cases; it furnishes him with a table of reference, to aid him in naming diseases, and a system, to guide him in acquiring a knowledge of his profession. It will not be necessary to describe all the diseases mentioned under the various classes—some of them are more properly treated of in systematic works on surgery. Those diseases, however, will be described at length which mostly influence the health of the community, or which contribute to increase and maintain the causes of death.

THE NATURE OF DISEASES; SPECIAL PATHOLOGY AND THERAPEUTICS.

It is the object of this part to treat of diseases in groups or classes, which possess certain characters or types in common; describing, first, the common properties or characters peculiar to the respective classes mentioned in the previous part on systematic medicine; and describing, second, the several orders into which these classes of diseases may be subdivided; and, third, describing in detail the several diseases individually, their *general nature*, *symptoms*, *course*, and *complications; causes*, *diagnosis*, *prognosis*, and *treatment.*

CLASS I.

ZYMOTIC DISEASES.

CHAPTER I.

GENERAL REMARKS ON THE PATHOLOGY OF ZYMOTIC DISEASES.

This class comprises diseases which have been observed to be either *epidemic*, *endemic*, or *contagious;* and includes *fevers*, *small-pox*, *the plague*, *influenza*, *cholera*, and such other diseases as possess the peculiar character, in common, of suddenly attacking great numbers of people, at intervals, in unfavorable sanitary conditions. In the language of Dr. Farr, the diseases of this class distinguish one country from another—one year from another; they have formed epochs in chronology; and, as Niebuhr has shown, have influenced not only the fall of cities, such as Athens and Florence, but of empires; they decimate armies, disable fleets; they take the lives of criminals that justice has not condemned; they redouble the dangers of crowded hospitals; they infest the habitations of the poor, and strike down the artizan in his strength, from comfort into helpless poverty; they carry away the infant from its mother's breast, and the old man at the end of life; but their direst eruptions are excessively fatal to men in the prime and vigor of age. They are emphatically the *morbi populares*.

The name *zymotic*—first suggested by Dr. William Farr, to designate this class—is not to be understood as implying the hypothesis that these diseases are fermentations, which the derivation of the term would lead one to believe. It has become extensively used, of late, as applied to the diseases whose characters, as a class, are already indicated, and for which some convenient term is required. The class, then, to which the term ZYMOTIC has been applied, is intended to comprehend many of the principal diseases which have prevailed as *epidemics* or *endemics;* and all those which are *communicable, either by human contact or by animals in a state of disease;* as well as the diseases that result from the *scarcity and the deterioration of the necessary kinds of food*, or from *parasitic animals.* The diseases of this class are thus conveniently arranged into four orders or groups, of which *fever*, *syphilis*, *scurvy*, *worms*, are the common names typical of the respective groups.

In the greater number of the diseases of this class, the blood is more or less changed, and, by some, is presumed to be the primary seat of diseases which result from *specific* poisons of organic origin, either derived from without or generated within the body. These specific poisons tend to produce, in the blood, an excess of those decomposing organic compounds which physiology teaches us are always present in the circulating current.

PHYSIOLOGICAL MODES IN WHICH POISONS ACT ILLUSTRATE, BY ANALOGY, THE ZYMOTIC DISEASES.—If the reader will now consider the following statements, as to the modes in which mineral and vegetable poisons act physiologically, he will be prepared to appreciate the effects of those conditions which, like poisons, induce diseases of the class termed zymotic. The actions of poisons are subject to certain general laws—the most important of which are, *first*, that they have all certain definite and SPECIFIC actions; *second*, that they all lie latent in the system, a certain but varying period of time, before those actions are set up; and *third*, that the phenomena resulting from their action vary in some degree, according to the dose and to the receptivity of the patient. These laws are common to all poisons, but there are also many others which are peculiar to individual poisons or classes of poisons, and it may be necessary to notice a few of them.

The *first* law, or that of the *definite* and SPECIFIC actions of poisons, cannot be doubted; for, if it be supposed that agents acting on the human body do not produce their effects according to certain definite laws, we can neither determine the seat or cause of any disease, nor direct nor judge of the operation of remedies. No physician, for instance, has seen Castor-oil produce tetanus, or Colchicum intoxicate the brain, or Opium inflame the spleen; he knows perfectly well that the first of these substances acts on the intestines, the second on the ligaments, and the third on the nervous system generally. The action of poisons, therefore, is not accidental, but determined by certain definite laws.

The action of poisons, though definite, is variously limited. Some poisons, for instance, act on one membrane, or on one organ, or on one system of organs; while other poisons extend their action over two or more membranes, or organs, or system of organs, or even over the whole animal frame. We have examples, in Aloes and Jalap, of substances that act upon one membrane only, namely, the mucous membrane of the alimentary canal. In Digitalis, we have an instance of a medicine that acts principally on one organ, namely, the heart—greatly reducing or even stopping its action; while Strychnine is an example of a medicine acting on one system of organs, namely, the parts supplied by the spinal cord, producing powerful and sometimes fatal tetanic action of every voluntary muscle in the body.

It is seldom, however, that the action of poisons is limited to one membrane, or organ, or system of organs. The greater number of these noxious agents more usually act on two or more membranes, or organs, or systems of organs. Elaterium, for instance, acts on the mucous membrane of the intestinal canal and on the kidneys. Tobacco nauseates the stomach, intoxicates the brain, and affects the action of the heart. Antimony has an equally extensive range; it induces cutaneous perspiration, acts cathartically and emetically, and, in large doses, appears to cause gangrene of the lungs. Alcohol and Opium are examples of substances acting still more generally, affecting not only the action or secretion of every organ or tissue of the body, but even, in some instances, altering their structure. Thus, Alcohol, in its most limited action, has been shown to cause structural disease of the liver, of the stomach, and of the coats of the arteries, while Opium tends to produce apoplexy and structural disorganization of the brain and its membranes. From the circumstance of these two substances acting not only generally but locally on a given number of tissues, they resemble, in their effects, those of many morbid poisons, as that of typhus fever, of scarlet fever, or of the small-pox.

The *second* important law of poisons is, that they lie latent in the system for a period of time, which varies in different individuals, before they set up their specific actions. Rhubarb, for instance, produces no immediate result, but lies dormant in the system six or eight hours before its action is sensible on the bowels; Opium, in the usual dose, is generally thirty minutes before it subdues the brain to its influence. The convulsions from Strychnine do not follow till twenty minutes after its exhibition, and perhaps every substance, except Hydrocyanic-acid, has a greater or less sensible period of latency.

When a medicine, however, acts on more parts than one, a considerable space of time may elapse, after it has affected one organ, before it affects another: thus, Digitalis frequently occasions emesis before it acts on the heart, and the action of Mercury on the bowels is frequently sensible for many weeks before the gums and salivary glands are affected. The doctrine of the latency of poisons is, indeed, so generally admitted, that the actual period has been a point on which the condemnation or acquittal of a prisoner tried for murder has turned, in our courts of justice, when certain poisons have been supposed to have been given.

The *third* great law of poisons is, that their effects are modified by the dose, the temperament, and the existing state of the constitution, mentally and bodily, of the recipient. The effect of dose, in modifying the pathological phenomena of disease, may be exemplified in the actions of Oxalic-acid and of Arsenic. The specific action of Oxalic-acid is to inflame the mucous membrane of the stomach; but, to insure this effect, the dose must be limited, so that this poison may lie in the system many hours. On the contrary, if the dose be excessive and rapidly absorbed, the poison so disorders all the functions of the three great nervous centres that life is destroyed in a few minutes. Arsenic, likewise, is a poison which inflames and ulcerates the mucous membrane of the alimentary canal, but it requires some hours to set up its specific actions; for, when the dose is large, it, in like manner, destroys by general irritation, and before traces of morbid change of structure can be appreciated after death. It follows, from this law, that the larger the dose, or the greater the intensity of the poison, the more rapid its action and the less the probability of finding any trace of specific lesion induced by it.

In studying the effects of dose on the constitution, we find some poisons are absorbed and are *cumulative*, while others are not absorbed into the system, or else are so rapidly removed that no cumulative effect is produced. Thus, in persons predisposed to the effects of Digitalis, a dose so small as to produce no sensible effect whatever, will, if frequently repeated, at last destroy the heart's action. In cases, likewise, in which it is desirable to produce vomiting, at the least expense to the constitution, the means employed are *cumulative* —namely, a repetition of small doses of Ipecacuanha. This cumulative property of poisons, however, is by no means universal. There is no instance of Jalap or of Castor-oil proving cumulative, and if a frequent repetition of either of them produces an increased effect, it is, perhaps, in consequence of the nervous papillæ, with which they are brought in contact, being more easily irritated by each application, and hence they induce a more violent result. That the habitual ingestion of small quantities of decomposing matter in the water used as drink, is capable, by cumulation, of inducing conditions favorable to the development of zymotic diseases, admits of no doubt. Cogent instances of this are to be found recorded in the bitter experience of epidemics of cholera.

Temperament is also a circumstance which greatly influences the action of poisons. There are a few persons altogether insensible to the action of Mercury, so that no quantity will affect their gums or increase the secretion of the salivary glands. There are others, in like manner, the action of whose heart no quantity of Digitalis will control. On the contrary, there are some constitutions so morbidly susceptible to these remedies that it is scarcely possible to exhibit even a fractional dose without giving rise to their specific effects.

Besides natural temperament, *habit*, which may be termed an artificial temperament, has a powerful influence in reconciling us to particular classes of poisons, and of making them even sources of enjoyment. Thus, Tobacco, Alcohol, Opium, are all substances which are productive, in the first instance, to many persons of great discomfort; but, by frequent repetition, they cease to have any unpleasant effects, and their stimulus at length becomes a necessary indulgence. Still, there are many poisons to which no repetition can habituate us, as Arsenic, Corrosive Sublimate, or the preparations of Copper. On the contrary, each repetition only the more debilitates the constitution, and renders it more susceptible of the action of the poison.

A peculiar existing state of the constitution has also a powerful influence on the action of poisons; and it would seem proved, with some exceptions, that these agents act with an intensity proportioned to the debilitated state of the patient. There is, indeed, no duty more imperative on the physician than that of adjusting the dose to the strength of the patient, and nothing is more common than to forbear administering a dose of ordinary medicine, because the patient's strength will not admit of it. As a general principle, therefore, medicines or poisons may be said to act with a power proportionate to the debility of the patient.

Still, there are states of disease which render the constitution of the patient, though greatly debilitated, insusceptible to the action of even powerful remedies. Thus, in typhus fever, the patient will often bear a considerable quantity of vinous stimuli, without being affected by it. In tetanus, or hydrophobia, no quantity of Opium will tranquillize the symptoms or procure sleep. Fallopius mentions a singular instance of the constitution being armed against the action of a poison. He states that, in his day, a criminal was given up to himself, and other anatomists, to be put to death in any manner they might think proper. To this man, therefore, they exhibited two drachms of Opium; but, laboring under a quartan ague, and the fit just coming on, the "Opium was hindered of its effect." The man, therefore, having survived this dose, begged that he might take a similar quantity, earnestly entreating, if he escaped, he might be pardoned. The same dose was exhibited, but it was in the intervalof the attacks, and the man now died.

The experiments of Majendie may be referred to, as affording many curious proofs of the state of the constitution in accelerating or retarding the actions of poisons. He has shown, that if a poison be introduced into the system, of such potency as will usually destroy life in two minutes, on bleeding the animal, the same result will follow in half a minute, or in one-fourth of the time; and this experiment has often been repeated. Majendie has also brought to light the curious fact, that if, after having poisoned the animal, and even after the poison has begun to act, we inject an aqueous fluid into its veins, in such quantity as to cause an artificial plethora, as long as this artificial plethora can be maintained, the action of the poison is superseded. No sooner, however, does the plethora cease, from the general effusion of fluid into every cavity of the body, than the poison acts in the usual time, and with perhaps even more than its accustomed severity.

Mr. Hunter thought that no two poisons could *coëxist* in the same system together, or that, coëxisting, they could not set up their specific actions at the same time. This hypothesis, however, is unquestionably erroneous; for we constantly see Opium and Digitalis, Jalap and Mercury, as well as many other combinations of medicines producing their respective effects in the system, and at the same time, accelerating or retarding each other's actions. There is no truth better established in ordinary medicine than that a combination of Salts and Senna produces a much more efficient and pleasant action than the exhibition of either remedy separately; and Opium is an agent possessing a modifying or controlling power over every organ or tissue, without which it would be impossible for dominant physicians, on many occasions, to reconcile the system to the introduction of many necessary and essential remedies. Poisons, therefore, are capable of coëxisting together, and of so influencing the system that they reciprocally accelerate or retard each other's actions.

The general laws observable in the actions of medicinal substances are, for the most part, precisely similar to those which govern morbid poisons or zymotic diseases, or only differ in a few minor points; for these latter poisons have their *specific* actions and their periods of latency, while their phenomena equally vary according to the dose, the state of the constitution, the predisposition of the patient, or the receptivity of his blood to respond to the influence of the poison.

SPECIFIC ACTION OF POISONS WHICH PRODUCE ZYMOTIC DISEASES.—The *specific* actions of poisons which produce the zymotici are distinctly proved, by the fact that we are enabled to determine, within certain limits, the course, symptoms, and pathological phenomena which result from the presence of any given morbid poison. No man, for instance, can confound the phenomena of *small-pox* with those of *intermittent fever*, or those of *intermittent fever* with *syphilis*, or those of *syphilis* with *cholera;* each of these poisons has its separate and peculiar laws, and, consequently, its actions are definite and SPECIFIC.

The actions of morbid poisons, also, like those of medicinal substances, are variously limited, some affecting only one membrane or organ, or system of organs, while others involve two or more membranes or organs, or system of organs. Thus, *Tinea* is an example of a poison acting on one tissue of the body, and even then partially. In some parts of the world—for instance, in Switzerland—a poison exists, whose action is limited entirely to the thyroid gland. The contagion of *whooping-cough* and the virus of *hydrophobia* affect all the organs supplied by the eighth pair, or pneumogastric system. Instances of morbid poisons acting on two membranes or organs, or system of organs, are still more common, and form the great body of this class of disease. The poison of *measles*, for instance, acts no less on the mucous membrane of the eye, nose, fauces, and, perhaps, on the mucous membranes generally, than on the skin. That of *scarlatina*, acts not only on the mucous membrane of the fauces, and on the skin, but also on the serous membranes of the joints and of the abdomen. The *paludal poison* has still a more extensive range, hardly any organ or tissue of the body being exempt from its destructive ravages.

Morbid poisons, also, like other poisons, have their period of latency; and, generally speaking, a much longer time elapses before their specific actions come into operation than takes place with medicinal substances. The virus of the *natural small-pox* lies dormant from sixteen to twenty days before it produces any constitutional disturbance; and a still further period elapses, of three or four days, before the specific eruption appears on the skin. The poison of *scarlatina* lies latent from seven to ten days after exposure to the contagion; that of the *measles* from ten to fourteen; while the poison of *paludal fever* has been known to lie dormant for a twelvemonth, and that of *hydrophobia* for a still longer time. These are examples of periods of latency far beyond anything that has been observed in the action of medicinal substances; and *syphilis*, in its tertiary action, is still more remarkable.

When morbid poisons act on more tissues or organs than one, their actions are sometimes simultaneous; but, more commonly, they are consecutive, and frequently long intervals of time elapse between each successive attack. Thus, the poison of *typhus* may attack the lungs, the membranes of the brain, and the mucous membrane of the alimentary canal, and all these may be attacked cotemporaneously; but it is more common that their attacks take place consecutively—or, first on the alimentary canal, then on the brain, and lastly on the lungs, several days elapsing between each successive attack. In *syphilis*, the poison acts on the part to which it is first applied—as the skin, throat, bones, and ligaments; and cases have been met with in which the throat, the skin, and the bones have been affected at the same time with the primary sore. It is more common, however, for them to occur *seriatim*, and at very remote periods from the primary affection, so that many years frequently elapse before the poison has exhausted itself. In scarlatina, also, the peritoneum is not affected till many days after the eruption of the skin and the ulceration of the throat have altogether disappeared.

It occasionally happens that morbid poisons, which usually act on a plurality of membranes, exhaust themselves on one or more without affecting the whole series. In the disease termed *scarlatina simplex*, the poison sometimes exhausts itself entirely on the skin, without affecting either the mucous or serous membranes of the body. The *rubeola sine catarrho* is a similar example of the poison exhausting itself on the same tissue, the skin. In *intermittent fever*, when the dose of the poison is limited, and the disease properly treated, it is seldom that any organ or tissue is involved; yet, left to run its course, scarcely any organ or tissue would escape destruction.

Sometimes, when the morbid poison acts on many membranes, the usual order of attack is inverted. It is the general law of *syphilis* that the bones are the last that suffer, in the order of the secondary symptoms, but sometimes they are the first to be affected. In *scarlet fever*, the affection of the skin may precede that of the throat, or the reverse may take place; and, in *fevers*, the affection of the head may precede that of the intestines, though the latter is the most common.

It has been seen that the period of latency of medicinal substances being passed, and their actions set up, their effects vary in a considerable degree, according to the dose, temperament, or present state of the constitution of the patient. With respect to the dose of a morbid poison, we rarely possess any direct measure of its strength. The *paludal poison*, however, of tropical climates, to which *malarious fevers* are due, unquestionably greatly exceeds in intensity that of more temperate climates, and its effects are proportionally marked. Thus, in the West Indies, we have the *yellow fever*, with hardly a trace of organic diseases after death; while, in Holland, we have a fever of less severity, but followed by enlarged livers or spleen, or else by dropsy; while, in England, the same fever is comparatively mild, and, if properly treated, for the most part terminates without any visceral affection. With respect to the influence of temperament in modifying disease, *small-pox* offers very striking instances; for different persons, inoculated or poisoned from the same source, have suffered in every varying degree from this formidable malady—from the horn, the distinct, the confluent, and the bloody small-pox; while, in the worst cases, children have died in the primary fever, and before the specific action on the skin has been induced. It may, therefore, be laid down, as a general law, that the more intense the dose of the morbid poison the more severe the form of disease; and, also, that fewer traces of organic alteration will be found after death than when the poison, or the disorder it produces, has been of a milder character. Thus, enlarged livers, disorganized spleens, and dropsy, marked every case that died of the Walcheren fever; while, in the more intense West Indian and African fevers, though resulting from the same poison, scarcely a trace of disease was to be found.

The existing state of the constitution also influences the event. Thus, persons of a good constitution, but ignorant of their danger, are often seen to pass through a mild form of typhus fever, while the nurses and others contaminated by the same poison, but more alive to their critical state, have sunk without a struggle. A presentiment of death is a very unfavorable circumstance in the progress of *remittent* fever, especially in tropical climates. A soldier will say, "You have been very kind to me, sir, but this time I shall not get over it." There may be no appearance of absolute or immediate danger at the time, yet the man generally dies.—Martin. As a general principle, therefore, it may be stated that morbid poisons act with an intensity proportioned to the enfeebled or depressed state of the constitution; but this law is not universal. Want of a sufficient amount of food, is most powerful among the conditions which bring about zymotic diseases, and most constant in operation. It is a popular belief that the lowering of all the vital forces, by deficiency of food, constitutes the particular condition which renders a starved population so peculiarly open to the invasion of zymotic diseases; but it is also a curious phenomenon of starvation that a state of general putrescence supervenes during life, as if the want of material for the generation of new tissue were an obstacle to the deportation of that which has become effete.—Carpenter. The hardy mountaineer is a surer victim, whether he visits the low countries of the tropics or the marshes of a more temperate climate, than the feebler native of those countries. The immunity the latter enjoys is probably owing to his habit of living in the noxious atmosphere; for, let him remove to a more healthy climate, and then return to those regions of pestilence, and he will be found as susceptible of the poison as the hardier stranger.

Another law of morbid poisons is, that two may *coëxist* in the same system; thus, scald-head and fever, small-pox and cow-pox, have often been seen at the same time in the same person. In this case, the respective diseases sometimes appear simultaneously, and each runs its course, unaffected by the presence of the other; but the more usual law of febrile poisons perhaps is, that when two coëxist, the one lies latent while the other runs its course, or they interrupt each other's progress, the active one becoming latent while the latent one becomes active, and occasionally they modify each other's actions. A case of intermittent fever may suddenly subside, and the small-pox appear in its stead. The small-pox having run its course, and the patient being recovered from that disorder, the intermittent fever may return. A child, having been exposed to the infection of the small-pox, was vaccinated; in a few days, however, the small-pox appeared, and ran a very mild and modified course. When the small-pox had entirely subsided, some action was seen in the punctured part of the vaccinated arm, and the cow-pox vesicle formed, but not till three or four weeks after the time it usually appears, and then exceedingly small.

Peculiarities in the Action of Poisons which Induce Zymotic Diseases.—The principal points in which the effects of poisons which induce zymotic diseases agree with those of vegetable and mineral poisons generally having been stated, it will now be necessary to state those circumstances in which they principally differ. Many medicinal poisons have the property of accumulating in the system, and acting with an intensity proportioned, not to the last dose, but to the aggregate of the whole quantity that has been administered. Thus the last few minims of Digitalis may stop the action of the heart, or the last few grains of Mercury salivate the patient, or the last minute dose of Strychnine become fatal. There is, however, no well authenticated fact which can be arranged under this law in the whole circle of morbid poisons. The actual quantity, according to the experiments of Dr. Fordyce, is perhaps extremely small; for that physician, in hopes of mitigating the small-pox, inoculated with virus greatly diluted. The disease was not always produced; but, when produced, it assumed every form, character, and degree of severity, according to the temperament or constitution of the patient.

The puerperal female is not only highly susceptible of poisons of the zymotic kind, but is proved to favor their further development; and various forms of puerperal fever are also generated by *materies morbi* of a kind other than that which might be considered peculiar to it. It is a well-known fact, unhappily not of rare occurrence, that a medical practitioner or a nurse goes from a case of puerperal fever to attend on other cases of labor, and the chances are that these will be attacked with the disease. Further, the practitioner or nurse may go to cases of labor from attendance on a case of scarlatina, typhus, erysipelas, or small-pox, and his parturient patients become the victims of puerperal fever. Their system is peculiarly receptive of the zymotic poisons.

In the Vienna Lying-in Hospital, it is recorded that a mortality of four hundred to five hundred, in an average of three thousand deliveries per annum, appeared traceable to the introduction of cadaveric matters through the uncleanliness of the attending students; these matters being especially potent when derived from the bodies of those who had died from the adynamic forms of zymotic disease. Students of practical midwifery should bear in mind this fact. They ought not to attend cases of labor while they are also engaged with practical anatomy in the dissecting-room, and physicians should be very careful after making post-mortem examinations.

Another peculiar law of morbid poisons, and one wholly unknown in medicinal substances, is the faculty, which the human body possesses, of generating, to an immense extent, a poison of the same nature as that by which the disease was originally produced. A quantity of small-pox matter not so big as a pin's head will produce many thousand pustules, each containing fifty times as much pestilent matter as was originally inserted; and, moreover, the blood and all the secretions of the body are supposed to be also equally infected with the matter of the pustules. The miasmata secreted by one child, laboring under whooping-cough, are sufficient to infect a whole city.

There is still, perhaps, a more remarkable law of morbid poisons, which is that many of them possess the extraordinary property of exhausting the constitution of all susceptibility to a second action of the same poison. This is the case with scarlatina, measles, the small-pox, the whooping-cough, and, indeed, with a considerable number of others. Still, it would seem that a temporary protective influence is imparted by most morbid poisons; for it is certain that few persons suffer a second attack of the same epidemic disease; and, consequently, it follows that the previous action of the poison must, for a time, impair the susceptibility of the constitution to its attacks. This beneficent law is of great importance in social life: it enables those that have recovered to attend on those that are sick, and allows a mother fearlessly to nurse her child in a dangerous and contagious distemper she has herself passed through, if such an inducement is necessary to strengthen the moral courage of a mother.

It only remains to mention one other law, which is but little shared by poisons of the vegetable or mineral kingdoms. It is well known that the actions of vegetable or mineral poisons are not influenced by the climate in which they are administered. Climate, however, has the property of greatly modifying the intensity of morbid poisons. The severe forms of typhus, so common in the north latitudes, are hardly known in more southern latitudes, and the cholera has been infinitely more fatal in Europe and in America than in the country which gave it origin; but, besides influencing the intensity of the disease, climate or season, or both, greatly modify the specific nature of morbid poisons. In one season, for instance, typhus fever will attack only the glandular structure of the intestinal canal; in another, only the mucous tissue of the same part, the glands or follicles being healthy; while, in another season, no disease whatever of the intestinal canal can be traced. Again, in one paludal district, the liver will be inflamed and the spleen healthy, and, in another, the liver will be unaffected but the spleen disorganized. In both cases, the generic character of the disease remains the same, but its *specific* character varies. It will have been seen that this variety of pathological phenomena is also caused by peculiarity of idiosyncrasy, and that nothing can be more different than the distinct, the confluent, and the horn small-pox from each other; and yet all these different varieties may arise in different persons inoculated with the same poison. The character of the vaccine pustule is equally various, so that that which insures exemption from the small-pox has not yet been determined; neither have pathologists determined the primary forms of syphilitic ulcers. It is important, therefore, to remember, in the study of morbid poisons, that absolute uniformity of pathological phenomena is not to be expected in different persons and in different seasons. There is a limit, however, within which their variations oscillate, and within which nature has bounded her deviations.

The laws of poisons are more important than their *modus operandi;* and this part of the subject has been deeply investigated by modern physiologists, and deserves some consideration. The great and striking alterations which often take place in the blood, led, from a very remote period, to the doctrine of humoralism, or, that a morbid state of the fluids was the great and primary cause of disease. On the contrary, when anatomy began to be cultivated, and nerves traced into every organ and tissue, it was supposed that disordered actions of these prime agents of motion, and of the great phenomena of animal life, were the great causes of disease—the morbid state of the fluids being secondary. Fontana determined to prove this latter theory, and found, to his surprise, on laying bare the sciatic nerve, in a great number of rabbits, that neither the venom of the viper, nor the poison of the Ticunas, nor Hydrocyanic-acid, when applied to it, produced the phenomena of poisoning, and that no other consequence resulted, beyond what would have been produced by a similar mechanical injury.

Fontana, having shown that the phenomena of poisoning do not result from the application of the deleterious agent to the trunk of the nerve or to the *solids*, determined to ascertain whether they followed after absorption, and consequently contamination of the *fluids*. He therefore injected the venom of the viper, Hydrocyanic-acid, and other poisonous substances, directly into the veins of different animals; and he found that although the nerves of a part may be steeped in these poisons with impunity, yet, no sooner did the substance enter the veins than the animal, after uttering a few horrible shrieks, struggled and almost instantly died, and thus demonstrated a morbid state of the fluids, as well as the existence of a tissue of extreme sensibility, with which the poison being brought into contact accounted for the death of the animal. Fontana pursued this subject one step further, and showed, if poisons acted by absorption, that this absorption was, in many instances, extremely rapid. He submitted a number of pigeons to be bitten in the leg by the viper, and chopped the wounded limb off at different intervals after the introduction of the venom, and found, as the result of an extensive series of experiments, on several dozens of pigeons, that none recovered when the poisoned leg was removed at a later period than twenty-five seconds, though the phenomena of poisoning did not occur till several minutes later.

The experiments of Fontana had shown, supposing a poison to be introduced into the veins, that all the phenomena of poisoning were accounted for; but still it might be said that, to prove the fact of absorption, something was wanting in strict demonstration. And, for the further prosecution of this subject, we are indebted to Segalas, who showed, if the arteries and veins of the mesentery of a dog be tied, that a quick acting poison would lie in harmless contact with the corresponding portion of the intestine for many hours; but no sooner were these ligatures removed than poisoning took place in a few minutes. Majendie even has carried this proof of the veins absorbing still further, for he amputated the leg of a dog, having first introduced a portion of quill into the femoral artery and vein, in such a manner that, on dividing these vessels, the leg hung connected with the trunk solely by means of the quill, all continuity by means of the solids being cut off. The poison was now introduced into the paw, and in four minutes the animal was under its influence.

By these experiments, it is supposed that Fontana, Segalas, and Majendie have completely demonstrated the absorption of poisons by the veins, and consequently of their circulating with the blood; and that no doubt may remain on the subject, modern chemistry has demonstrated the actual presence of many medicinal substances, either in the blood itself or else in the secretions from it. Thus, after a treatment by Soda, large quantities of uncombined alkali have been found in the serum. Alcohol has been obtained by distillation from the blood; while Iodine, Rhubarb, the Nitrate of Potash, and a large number of other substances, taken into the stomach, have been found in the urine. It follows, then, that mineral and vegetable poisons are absorbed and mingled with the blood, *and are conveyed directly to the parts on which they act, passing with impunity over others for which they have no affinity.*

The fact of morbid matters, in like manner, being absorbed, and mingling with the blood, has been shown by many continental writers; but perhaps the experiment made by Professor Coleman is the most satisfactory: "I have produced the disease (the glanders) by first removing the healthy blood from an ass, until the animal was nearly exhausted, and then tranfusing, from a glandered horse, blood from the carotid artery into the jugular vein. The glanders, in the ass, was rapid in its progress, violent in degree, and from this animal I afterwards produced both glanders and farcy." Both scarlatina and measles have also been produced by inoculation from the blood of patients laboring under those diseases.

The circumstance of the presence of a poison in the blood is supposed, by Andral, to produce, besides its toxicological states, certain alterations in its physical condition. Thus, he conceives a specific cause has a tendency to destroy or reduce the quantity of fibrine in the blood, which he has found, in some instances, to be only one part in a thousand. Hence, he adds, whatever may be the nature of the pyrexia, the blood, whether it be taken from a vein or collected from the heart and arteries after death, always exhibits the following characters: namely, that the serum and clot are incompletely separated the one from the other, so that the clot is consequently large, and often appears to fill almost entirely the bleeding-basin. Its edges, also, are never raised, and its consistence is inconsiderable, so that it is easily torn, broken down, and reduced to a state of diffluence; in this state, it becomes grumous, and discolors the serum. It is also remarkable for the absence of all buff, which is rarely met with in typhus, in measles, in scarlatina, or in small-pox, unless there has been some inflammatory complication; and, even when it does exist, as in confluent small-pox with large collections of pus, the buff is soft and gelatinous, and, by expression of the serum, is easily reduced to a thin pellicle. This defect of fibrine he conceives to be the cause of the great tendency to hæmorrhage, and to that stasis or congestion so remarkable in typhus, scarlatina, and other diseases dependent on morbid poisons.

The facts and arguments which have been adduced, have, it is apprehended, distinctly proved that morbid poisons act, in all instances, not capriciously, but according to certain definite and *specific laws*, modified by the influence of climate, temperament, or the magnitude of the dose; also, that they mingle with the blood, with which they continue in latent combination a certain but varying period of time; and likewise that many of them are capable of coëxisting together in the same system. Two other remarkable laws result from the study of morbid poisons; or, that these singular agents are not acted upon by medicinal substances as long as they continue latent. And, again, *that when they act on more tissues than one, the remedy which is an antidote to the action on one is often absolutely powerless when it affects another tissue;* so that many different remedies are frequently necessary to combat the varying phenomena of the same disease. A knowledge of these laws is necessary for understanding this class of diseases, and it is hoped that by their application many of the difficulties which have hitherto obscured the doctrines of fever, of syphilis, of hydrophobia, and of many other diseases incident to this class of morbid poisons, may be removed, and that this portion of medical science may be placed on a surer foundation, if not a permanent basis.

Conditions Favorable to the Development of Zymotic Diseases.—The following observations are condensed from an interesting paper, by Dr. Carpenter, on the "Predisposing Causes of Epidemics." He shows that the conditions which bring about the diseases of the zymotic class, are referrible to three categories: 1. Conditions which tend to introduce into the system *decomposing* matter that has been generated in some external source. 2. Conditions which occasion an *increased production of decomposing matter* in the system itself. 3. Conditions which *obstruct the elimination* of the decomposing matter normally or excessively generated within the system, or abnormally introduced into it from without.

Of these in their order: 1. The decomposing matters, generated in external sources, may be enumerated as putrescent food, water contaminated by sewerage or other decomposing matter, and air charged with miasmatic emanations. These constitute poisons of a specific kind. 2. Poisons of a specific kind are also developed *by the degeneration of the tissues within the body*, such as are formed in the puerperal state, after severe injuries, and as a consequence of excessive muscular exertion. 3. Poisons are also engendered by an insufficient supply of air, a high external temperature, and the ingestion of alcoholic drinks. Each and all of these causes produce one and the same condition of the blood: namely, *surcharging it with decomposing organic compounds*, which should be neutralized or evacuated. By any of these conditions, a certain receptivity or disposition of the blood is produced, which makes it liable to undergo the morbid changes peculiarly characteristic of this class of zymotic diseases.

The practical questions immediately involved in this exposition of the nature of zymotic diseases is contained in the following statement: namely, that it is possible to extinguish the greater number of epidemic diseases, however intense or abundant may be the atmospheric or other agencies which constitute their potential causes, by preserving the blood of every individual in that state which shall prevent these poisons from finding the conditions of their development within the body. This end is to be attained, on the one hand, by preventing every unusual production of fermentible matter in or out of the body; and, on the other hand, by promoting its removal, when it is inevitably generated (as in the puerperal state) through the respiratory process, which ought to be favored as much as possible—not merely by a free supply of pure air, but by the reduction of that air to the lowest temperature at which the condition of the patient will allow it to be safely inhaled.

The specific nature of morbid poisons, and their similarity of action with that of vegetable and mineral poisons, as detailed by Aitkin, was first suggested by Williams, and more fully developed by later writers. This similarity extends not only to zymotic diseases, but to many others. Pereira (see "Materia Medica," American edition, vol. i., p. 177,) even divides the cerebro-spinal remedies into:

"ORDER 1.—*Convulsives or tetanifacients;* or, agents which augment the irritability of the muscular fibre, and, in large doses, occasion convulsions or tetanus. This order includes Strychnia, Brucia, and all substances which contain one or both of these alkalies; or, Nux-vomica, Ignatia, Snake-wood (*Lignum-colubrinum*), the Upas-tieuti, False Angustura Bark, &c.

"ORDER 2.—*Paralysers or paralysifacients;* or, agents which cause paralysis of voluntary motion, and lessen the irritability of the muscular fibres. This order contains Conia, an alkali obtained from Hemlock, which causes swiftly spreading paralysis; also Lead, which notoriously causes painter's paralysis. These remedies are the antipathic antidotes to Nux-vomica, Strychnine, Ignatia, &c., and the true antipathic remedies for tetanus, epilepsy, convulsions, &c.

"ORDER 3.—*Benumbers or anæsthetics;* or, agents which cause paralysis of the sentient nerves. Monkshood, and its alkali, Aconitine, occasion numbness in the parts to which they are applied. They are antipathic to neuralgia.

"ORDER 4.—*Epileptifacients or convulsive stupefacients;* or, agents which act rapidly and suddenly, to cause loss of consciousness, sensation, and volition, with convulsions and stupefaction. This order includes Hydrocyanic-acid, the Cyanides of Potassium and Zinc, Bitter Almonds and their volatile oil, Cherry Laurel and its volatile oil, and distilled water; the narcotic gases, namely, the Carbonic-acid Gas, and Sulphuretted Hydrogen Gas. The sudden loss of sensation and of consciousness, with violent convulsions, which are the characteristic effects of this order, constitute also the essential symptoms of an epileptic paroxysm." Again, Ammoniacal Gas, and all the Salts of Ammonia, excite convulsions; and we have somewhere read that, when the corrosive alkalies are applied to a bare nerve, convulsions will be excited, which is not the case when the corrosive acids are similarly applied.

"ORDER 5.—*Apoplectifacients;* or, agents which lessen feeling and the irritability of the muscles, cause contraction of the pupils, paralysis of voluntary motion, with deep sleep or stupor. Opium, and its alkali,

Morphia, constitute the type of this order, to which Lactuarium also belongs. In large doses, they produce an apoplectic condition." According to Christison, Opium rarely or never produces true apoplexy, or effusion of blood into the brain; Stramonium is more apt to do this than any other narcotic drug.

"Order 6.—*Cataleptifacients.* Cannabis-indica causes a very agreeable kind of delirium, augmented appetite, venereal excitement, and impaired vision, followed by insensibility, during which the patient retains any position in which he may be placed. Its effects, therefore, simulate the symptoms of catalepsy." According to Christison, Hydrochlorate of Tin, produces similar results.

"Order 7.—*Deliriafacients;* or, agents which cause dilatation of the pupil, obscurity of vision, and delirium, ending in stupor. Belladonna, Stramonium, Hyosciamus, and others, belong to this order." The effects of Agaricus-muscarius have often been compared to those of Belladonna.

"Order 8.—*Choreafacients.* By long-continued use, in small doses, mercurials occasion paralytic tremor or *tremor mercurialis*, and, ultimately, convulsive agitation of the limbs." Among our loose notes, we find the following upon mercurial trembling: "Many of the symptoms of mercurial tremor indicate a very marked resemblance between this disease and the chorea of young people: the agitation of the hands, the shuffling, dragging gait, the confusion of speech, the occasional imbecility of the mental powers, are common to both; perhaps, too, if the etiology of the two diseases were correctly known, an intimate alliance might be found to exist between them. The mercurial trembling, it has been proven, depends upon neuritis of the motor nerves and their sheaths. It is said that it usually creeps on gradually: at first, the patient finds his arms and hands are unsteady and trembling, and that he cannot keep them quiet for any length of time; he can with difficulty hold a cup in his hand, or direct his food to his mouth. Next, the legs become weak and tottering, they bend under when he attempts to walk, and he would fall if not supported. The speech may become affected, and *stammering* ensue. Sometimes, even the act of chewing is attended with a convulsive agitation of the muscles of the cheeks and throat. The head may be in a constant see-saw motion. Any attempt to obtain control over the muscles invariably renders the spasms more violent; mental emotions also increase them. There is no headache, the pulse is usually slow, bowels regular, salivary glands are but little, if at all engaged. An Iodine chorea has also been described.

"Order 9.—*Paraplegiafacients.* According to Dr. Coupar, Manganese causes paraplegia, without colic or tremor."

In the "Treatise on Poisons," by R. Christison, M. D., we find, on page 84, a chapter which treats "*Of the Symptoms of the Irritant Class of*

Poisons, compared with those of various Natural Diseases." We, following the example of Pereira, have taken the liberty of adding names to the drug-diseases described by Christison.

On page 86, we read: "At present, an important subject remains for consideration—namely, the *natural diseases* whose effects are apt to be mistaken for the effects of poison."

Arsenical Paralysis.—"Professor Berndt gives a well-marked case. The paralytic affection consisted of loss of sensation and power of motion in the hands, and of loss of motion in the feet, with contraction of the knee-joints." "Dr. Falconer, in his 'Essay on Palsy,' observes, that he has repeatedly witnessed local palsy, after poisoning with Arsenic. In one instance, the hands only were affected; in two others, the palsy spread gradually, from the fingers upward, till the whole of the arms were involved. On the whole, local palsy appears to be the most frequent of the secondary effects of Arsenic. It is sometimes very obstinate, and sometimes appears to be incurable; for, in one instance, it caused perfect palsy of the limbs, which persisted during the whole of a long life."

Arsenical Gastritis.—Page 245: "It is singular that, however severe the inflammation of the inner membrane of the stomach, caused by Arsenic, may be, inflammatory redness of the peritoneal coat is seldom found." This contrasts strongly with the almost specific action of the mineral acids upon the peritoneum.

Arsenical Proctitis.—Page 251: "The signs of inflammation, from poisoning with Arsenic, are seldom well-marked in the small intestines, much lower down than the extremity of the duodenum, and the colon is still more rarely affected. But it is a very curious fact that the rectum is often much inflamed, though the colon and the small intestines are not. Dr. Male even mentions that, in a man, he has found the rectum abraded, ulcerated, and even redder than the stomach itself. Baillie mentions two cases, in which the lower end of the rectum was ulcerated." Christison adds, "A common appearance, in lingering cases, is excoriation or ulceration of the rectum." The action of Colchicum upon the stomach and bowels is equally singular and specific; Orfila found that, when put into a wound in the thigh, or injected into a vein, it would always cause acute inflammation of the stomach and duodenum, then skip over or avoid the jejunum and ileum, and cause severe inflammation of the colon.

Corrosive Mercury-Dysentery.—Page 228: "Corrosive Mercury generally produces dysentery. This poison, like Arsenic, has the singular property of inflaming the stomach and intestines, even when it is introduced into the system through a wound." According to Murray, when five to thirty grains of Calomel are given to dogs, it occasions an afflux of blood to the minute arteries and capillaries, more particularly of the gastric and colic mucous membranes, imparting to them a capilliform, punctiform, or uniform red tinge, and attended with more or less sanguineous effusion, either in dots, like bleeding points, or in small streaks and patches. In doses of one, two, or three drachms, it produces, in addition, a dark, grumous, or sanious, or sero-albuminous effusion on the mucous surface of the bowels, *particularly of the colon.* All the appearances of acute dysentery are present.

Corrosive Mercury-Pneumonia.—"But this is not its only property under such circumstances. According to Smith and Orfila, it also possesses the power of inflaming both the heart and lungs. Orfila found the lungs unusually compact and œdematous in some parts." Christison adds, "The production of inflammation of the lungs by Corrosive Sublimate, when applied to a wound, appears to be well established."

Corrosive Mercury-Endo-carditis.—"As to the heart, Orfila invariably found, in one or the other part of its lining membrane, most commonly on the valves, little spots of a cherry-red or almost black color; nay, on one occasion, he observed these spots so soft that slight friction made little cavities." Schönlein says, (see "Allgemeine und Specielle Pathologie und Therapie," vol. i., p. 166), "It is well known that, when the stronger preparations of Mercury are given, for a long time, and in excessive doses, that the blood-vessels become fragile and friable. It is just as well established a fact that the heart may become similarly affected. The disease of the heart, which arises from the abuse of Mercury, has been called *hydrargyria;* but, on account of the peculiar eruption which attends it, it has always been classed among the cutaneous diseases. But the inflammation of the heart is, doubtless, the primitive, and the eruption a secondary affection." Page 289: "In whatever way Corrosive Mercury obtains entrance into the body, it causes irritation of the stomach and rectum, inflammation of the lungs; perhaps, also, inflammation of the heart, and of the salivary glands."

Mercurial Mumps.—Page 311: "Persons working in quicksilver mines, are subject to swellings of the parotids, aphthous sore throat, salivation, pustular eruptions, and shaking palsy or *tremblement mercuriel.*"

Mercurial Inflammations.—Page 312: "Many inflammatory diseases, not easily excited under ordinary circumstances, arise very readily from improper exposure during salivation; for example, dropsy, inflammation of the lungs and iris, erysipelas, and chronic eruptions."

Of the Morbid Appearances caused by Mercury.—Page 323: "The mouth and throat are more frequently affected than by Arsenic. Great enlargement of the papillæ, at the root of the tongue, is peculiar to Mercury." Page 326: "Corrosive Sublimate is more apt to cause peritoneal inflammation than Arsenic."

Corrosive Mercury-Nephritis.—"Dr. Henry, of Manchester, found an abscess in the left kidney; in all Valentine's cases, the kidneys were inflamed; in Olivier's case, they were a third larger than natural." In a case of poisoning with Corrosive Sublimate, in which we had an opportunity of witnessing the post-mortem appearances, the kidneys were much enlarged—at least half again as large as natural; they were very lax, loose, and soft instead of presenting the natural firmness; the whole cortical substance was of a pale reddish white, instead of the natural dark reddish brown; the external surface was mostly white, but dotted with minute reddish points; there was no appearance of granulation; *the urine was albuminous.* The observations of Drs. Wells and Blackall, go to prove that Mercury induces an albuminous state of the urine. In the *London Med. Gazette*, for March, 1843, p. 941, there is detailed a case of albuminous urine, after poisoning with Corrosive Mercury. For several days, *a considerable quantity of albumen was found in the urine*, which was turbid, and of a pale brown color; it was abundantly coagulated by heat and by Nitric-acid. It is added that albumen has frequently been detected in the urine in similar cases; so that it is evident that Mercury causes Bright's disease of the kidneys.

Copper-Jaundice.—Page 349: "Another symptom, which occasionally occurs in poisoning with Copper, is jaundice." Christison details a well-marked case.

Antimony Pneumonia.—Page 359: "Majendie's experiments go to prove that Antimony causes death by exciting inflammation of the lungs; for, in cases of poisoning with Antimony, he found the lungs of an orange-red or violet color throughout, destitute of crepitation, gorged with blood, dense like the spleen, and here and there even hepatized—the lungs were always more or less affected. It is a fact, too, worthy of notice, that, in whatever way Antimony is introduced into the system, its effects are nearly the same. Majendie infers, from his experiments, that Tartar-emetic causes death when swallowed, not by inflaming the stomach, but in consequence of causing a general inflammatory state of the whole system subsequent to its absorption, of which general inflammatory condition the inflammation of the stomach and bowels, and even that of the lungs, are merely parts or symptoms."—Page 360.

Hydrochlorate of Tin Catalepsy.—Page 367: "This drug may cause catalepsy or fixedness of position."

Chrome Bronchitis.—Page 372: "The effects of Chrome, when introduced into a wound in the skin, are still more remarkable. Thus applied, it seems to cause general inflammation of the lining membrane of the air-passages. The wound in the skin, to which it is applied, is not found much inflamed, but the larynx, bronchi, and minute ramifications of the air-tubes, are found to contain fragments of fibrinous effusion. The nostrils are found filled with similar matter, and the conjunctiva of the eyes are covered with mucus and purulent effusion.

Lead Palsy.—Page 416. This is too well known to need description.

Colocynth Peritonitis.—Page 447: "In cases of poisoning with Colocynth, the abdomen is tense and excessively tender to the touch. After death, the intestines are found red and matted together, with fibrinous exudations, while the usual fluid of peritonitis is effused into the cavity of the peritoneum."

Marsh Marigold Œdema and Pemphigus.—Page 448: "Five persons, having partaken of the Marsh Marigold, were all seized, in half an hour afterwards, with sickness, pain in the abdomen, vomiting, headache, and tinnitus-aurium; subsequently, with dysuria and diarrhœa; and, next day, with œdema of the whole body, particularly of the face; and, on the third day, with an eruption of pemphigus vesicles, as large as almonds: they dried up in forty-eight hours."

Mezereon Hæmoptysis.—Page 450: "Linnæus says he once saw a girl die from excessive vomiting and hæmoptysis, in consequence of taking twelve Mezereon berries."

Jalap Dysentery.—Page 451: "Jalap, when rubbed daily into the skin of the abdomen and thighs, excites severe dysentery in a few days." On page 493: Christison says, "Some remarks must be here premised, on the principal diseases which resemble the effects of the narcotic poisons in their symptoms and morbid appearances. Of these, the only diseases of consequence are: *Apoplexy, epilepsy, inflammation of the brain and spinal cord, hypertrophy of the brain, and syncopal asphyxia.*"

Of the Distinction between Apoplexy and Narcotic Poisoning.—"The symptoms of apoplexy are almost exactly the same as those of the narcotic poisons—viz.: more or less complete abolition of sense and power of motion, frequently combined with convulsions."

Of the Distinction between Epilepsy and Narcotic Poisoning.—Page 501: "Epilepsy closely resembles the symptoms caused by Prussic-acid and some of the narcotic gases. It also bears the same resemblance to the effects of many of the narcotico-acrid poisons, such as Belladonna, Stramonium, Hemlock, also Camphor, Cocculus-indicus, and the poisonous fungi."

Of the Distinction between Meningitis and Narcotic Poisoning.—Page 506: "Abercrombie has described a form of meningitis occurring among children. Its symptoms are delirium, convulsions, and coma intermingled. The only morbid appearance is congestion of the vessels, on the surface and in the substance of the brain. This affection imitates very closely, both in its progress and signs after death, some varieties of poisoning with the vegetable narcotico-acrid poisons, such as Belladonna, Stramonium, and Hemlock." Page 507: "Inflammation of the brain itself, occasionally excites symptoms not unlike those produced by some narcotic poisons; and, in a few instances, its course has appeared equally short." Page 510: "Extravasation of blood into the spinal canal, inflammation of the membranes, and *ramollisement* of the cord, occasionally approach closely to the characters of some of the slow cases of narcotic poisoning." We have notes of two cases of softening of the spinal marrow, caused by Strychnine; and of one case, in which softening of the cerebellum and spinal marrow was caused by Iodide of Barium. Lead, it is well known, causes induration of the brain.

Of the Morbid Appearances Caused by Opium.—Page 540: "Turgescence of the vessels of the brain; watery effusion into the ventricles, and upon the surface of the brain, are generally met with. Extravasation of blood is a very rare effect of Opium."

Hyosciamus-Typhomania.—Page 551: "This drug causes that singular union of delirium and coma which is usually termed typhomania."

Belladonna-Somnambulism.—Page 611: "It sometimes produces a state of mind which resembles somnambulism."

Stramonium-Nymphomania.—Page 616: "It is apt to cause nymphomania."

Stramonium-Apoplexy.—"It is more apt to cause extravasation of blood into the ventricles of the brain than any other narcotic drug."

Cicuta-Tetanus.—Page 622: "Cicuta-virosa appears to cause true tetanic convulsions, in frequent paroxysms. In one case, the convulsions were severe, the jaws locked, the eyes rolled, and the head and spine were bent backwards into so high an arch that a child might have crept between the body and the bed-clothes."

Enanthe-crocata Convulsions.—Page 623. "The Hemlock-dropwort seems to be the most energetic of the umbelliferous vegetables; it is particularly apt to excite convulsions, without any previous symptom or warning," i. e., true epilepsy.

The above examples are sufficient to prove that drugs and poisons possess the property of producing certain artificial diseases of a distinct and determinate character, and that they exert specific powers upon, and have strong elective affinities for certain organs or systems. Every one of these facts will subsequently be found to have a positive and practical therapeutic value, and they could be multiplied *ad infinitum.* Pulsatilla causes an affection of the eyes, mucous membrane, and skin, resembling that of measles. Belladonna and Stramonium cause a throat and skin affection, similar to those of scarlet fever. Baryta-muriatica and Iodide of Potash excite disorders of the eyes, nose, and ears, similar to those caused by catarrhal affections and influenza. Ipecac. causes asthma, &c., &c.

We shall now proceed to consider the zymotic diseases in detail, commencing with

SMALL-POX.

DEFINITION.—Small-pox is the product, and is productive of a morbid poison, which, after a period, develops a remittent fever, followed by an eruption on the skin, and sometimes on the mucous surfaces, with other concomitant and occasionally succeeding affections. The eruption on the skin passes through the stages of pimple, vesicle, pustule, scab; and leaves marks or cicatrices on the site of exudation. The disease runs a definite course, and generally exhausts the susceptibility of the constitution to another attack.

PATHOLOGY.—The theory, regarding the development of small-pox, is, that a poison is absorbed and infects the blood, and, after a given period of latency, gives rise to a "primary fever," which lasts from two to four days, till the eruption appears, when it for the most part *remits.* The secondary, or specific action of this poison, makes itself obvious by an exudation, in the form of an eruption on the skin, and also sometimes on the mucous membrane of the eyes, nose, the mouth, and of the fauces and great intestine. The eruption runs a given course—namely, of *pimple*, vesicle, and pustule—and, when fully out, or at its height, the febrile phenomena, which had remitted, return, and give rise to what is termed the *secondary fever.* The occasionally succeeding affections are, inflammation of the various tissues of the lungs, disorders of the urinary organs, and, lastly, of the cellular tissue of the body generally, which often becomes the seat of an endless number of abscesses.

VARIETIES OF SMALL-POX.—There are several varieties of this disease: 1. The *natural* small-pox, in which the disease occurs from natural causes—contagion or infection—in non-vaccinated and non-innoculated persons; 2. The *inoculated* variety, the phenomena of which differ, in many respects, from those that occur in natural small-pox, the most remarkable of which are the general singular mildness of the fever, the diminished number of the pustules of the secondary eruption; although, occasionally, the disease is extremely severe, and the danger to exposed and unprotected persons is always very great; 3. The *modified* small-pox, or varioloid; or, small-pox occurring in previously vaccinated persons.

There are also several varieties of natural small-pox, viz.: 1. The small-pox without eruption (*variolæ sine eruptione*); 2. The distinct, or discrete small-pox (*variolæ discretæ*), in which the pustules remain separate, or do not touch or run together; 3. The confluent small-pox (*variolæ confluentis*), in which the pustules are so numerous that they coälesce; 4. The blood small-pox of Dr. Mead, in which the pustules are filled with bloody ichor or fluid, instead of pus; 5. The black small-pox of Sydenham, which is very similar to the fourth variety; 6. The siliquous small-pox of Friend, in which the pustule resembles a small hollow bladder, but contains no fluid; 7. The horn small-pox, which is by much the mildest form of the disease, as the pustules, instead of maturating, shrivel on the fifth or sixth day of the eruption, and the disease terminates favorably three or four days earlier than in the natural course of the affection; 8. The crystalline or pearl-pock (*variolæ crystallinæ*), in which the vesicle contains transparent fluid, seldom maturates, and has a tendency to become confluent.

SMALL-POX WITHOUT ERUPTION.—(*Variolæ Sine Eruptione.*)

Sydenham and Frank observed, in every variolous epidemic, that some few persons were seized with all the symptoms of primary variolous fever, and, this having subsided, they have afterwards been found insusceptible of the disease. I have repeatedly noticed the same thing. In one family, in which an unvaccinated person had an attack of discrete, but severe small-pox, and a vaccinated person had the varioloid, two members were attacked with fever, severe headache, intense backache, and vomiting; on the fourth day, when the appearance of some eruption was confidently expected, none made its appearance—not even a single pimple—and the patients rapidly convalesced.

STONE-POCK, OR HORN-POCK.

This has also been called the five-day pock, and is sometimes confounded with the mild, mitigated, or modified form of variola, now so familiar to us as occurring in those who, in early life, had been well vaccinated. Still, it was known before vaccination was introduced, though formerly less frequent than now. Van Swieten described it under the title of *variola verrucosa* and *cornea*, or the so-called stone-pock, horn-pock, and wart-pock. It is, to all intents and purposes, identical with varioloid, although it may occur in unvaccinated persons who, however, have but little susceptibility to a severe form of small-pox. In this variety, the primary fever is little more than a febricula; the pustules, or rather vesicles, do not exceed from a half-dozen to two or three hundred, and, having passed through the stages of pimple and vesicle, they, on the fifth or eighth day, or about the usual time of maturation, shrivel, desiccate, and crust. The secondary fever does not occur—as pus does not form, the fluid in the pimples always remaining serous—so that convalescence usually commences on the eighth day, at latest, and the disease terminates on the eleventh. It is probably in this variety that Thuja has been supposed to be so useful.

ORDINARY SMALL-POX.

The progress of the disease may be divided into *four stages.* Of these, the *first stage* comprises the period of latency: the variolous poison having infected the blood, lies in latent combination with that fluid from ten to sixteen days. Gregory says, "At the moment of receiving the miasm, the patient may experience a feeling of sickness, giddiness, or inward alarm; while in attendance upon cases of confluent and malignant small-pox, I have repeatedly experienced decided nausea." A large accumulation of facts enabled Gregory to fix this period of incubation at fourteen days in all, viz., twelve days of apyrexia, and two of fever. As the incubation advances, the patient's nights become restless, and his spirits low; he is oppressed with languor and lassitude. The *second stage* comprises the *primary fever*, which commences with the onset of the disease, and terminates with the appearance of the eruption, on about the fourth day. The *third stage* begins with the appearance of the eruption, and terminates with the appearance of the *secondary fever*, or from the fourth to the eighth day. The *fourth stage* commences with the secondary fever, and lasts from the eighth to the eleventh day. Some writers admit a fifth stage, commencing with the subsidence of the secondary fever, on the eleventh day, and lasting to the falling off of the scabs, on the fourteenth or fifteenth day.

The ordinary duration of the *primary fever* is four days, and its most characteristic symptoms, in the adult, are, severe muscular pains, simulating rheumatism, especially in the small of the back, and the frequent occurrence of obstinate vomiting.

On the fourth day, the eruption appears, and the third stage commences; the great characteristics of this are those of a calm succeeding a storm; for, on the appearance of the eruption, the fever abates, the heat lessens, the head-affection subsides, the vomiting ceases, and the pulse returns to its natural standard. The blood is unloaded of its peccant matter, the whole internal system is relieved, the febrile phenomena have altogether disappeared, and the external surfaces, both cutaneous and mucous, are now to bear the brunt of the affection. The eruption now passes through the various changes, from pimple to vesicle and pustule, and, about the eighth day, when the eruption is fully out over the body, and the pustules on the face begin to suppurate or maturate, the *secondary fever* arises, marked by considerable increase of heat, frequent pulse, and often by slight delirium, from which the patient is easily aroused; the whole face, head, and neck swell, particularly the eyelids, which often close and blind the patient; the swollen parts often throb, and are painful when touched. The inflammatory tumefaction of these parts lasts three days, during which the spaces between the pustules inflame, and are of a deep red, or damask rose color, and the more nearly the interstices approach these colors the milder will be the subsequent affections. This secondary fever arises from the irritation, inflammation, and suppuration, caused by the acrid deposit from the blood-vessels upon the cutaneous and mucous surfaces. In favorable cases, the swelling of the face, redness of the intervening spaces, and secondary fever last from the eighth to the eleventh day, and then subside; the pustules, now fully ripe, burst, and discharge a yellow matter, which, concreting into scabs, fall off on the fourteenth or fifteenth day, and the disease is at an end.

DISCRETE SMALL-POX.—(*Variola Discretæ.*)

Second Stage, that of Primary Fever.—After the period of incubation is passed, the disease is ushered in with the ordinary prodromata of fever, sometimes in a severe degree. There are rigors, followed by heat and dryness of the skin, furred tongue, loss of appetite, *pain in the back* and across the loins, headache, nausea, and generally *vomiting*, sometimes pain in the epigastrium, with a hard and frequent pulse. We occasionally find delirium, and even convulsions, attending its invasion, especially in young and nervous subjects.

As far as these symptoms go, it is hardly to be distinguished from many other diseases ushered in by similar phenomena, and we must be mainly guided in our diagnosis, at this stage, by the presence or absence of the disease in the community, and by the fact of the patient having been exposed to the contagion. When the eruption is fully formed, however, its appearance is perfectly unmistakable, the presence of "*umbilicated vesicle*" being considered entirely conclusive. But, as small-pox may sometimes be very much mitigated by appropriate treatment at its outset, it is desirable to recognize it as early as possible; and especially to warn others of their danger from exposure to it. There are some minor points in which the early symptoms differ from those of the other pyrexiæ. The *peculiar pain in the back* is one of these symptoms, and *vomiting* is another; and these, taken in connection with the prevalence of the disease in the neighborhood, or with the fact of the patient having been exposed to it—still more, if he should never have been vaccinated, or only a long time ago—may generally lead to a pretty correct estimation of the significance of the symptoms. There are other occasional symptoms, which need only be mentioned in order to put the practitioner upon his guard. Thus, there is sometimes, during the first few days before the appearance of the eruption, an unusual tendency to perspiration, and, what may be still more deceptive, sore throat, inflammation of the mucous membranes, coryza, and an excess of tears are not uncommon. Some cases, too, may be attended with stupor, while, in others, there may be wakefulness, restlessness, or complete insomnia. Scarlet fever may be preceded by equally severe vomiting, but not by the distressing pain in the back. Measles is generally preceded by neither. The disease, in its first and second stages, is most frequently mistaken for measles. But, Gregory says, febrile lichen is the disease from which small-pox, at its onset, is with most difficulty distinguished, for the aspect of the eruption, in both cases, is nearly alike; but, in febrile lichen, the eruption comes out in twenty-four hours, in small-pox, not under forty-eight. Small-pox almost always appears on the face; lichen is developed, from the first, uniformly over the head and trunk; the itching is also more marked at first, and there is no backache, nor so much vomiting in lichen.

When *the pains in the back* or the *vomitings* are severe, they are usually the precursors of a severe form of the disease; more especially, if the vomiting continue after the appearance of the eruption, on the third day of the fever; it is then regarded as an unfavorable symptom. If the pain in the back be low down across the loins, it is generally regarded as a more unfavorable sign than if it be high up between the shoulders. Heberden, according to Dr. Watson, "noticed that acute pain in the loins was almost always followed by a severe disorder;" that it was less grave if higher up, and a very good sign if there were no pain in the back at all. Delirium or coma is regarded also as an unfavorable sign if it occur in the early stage of the disease; but exceptions to this may occur in the case of children. They both disappear when the eruption comes fully out, and the blood is unloaded of its acrid and peccant matters.

Third Stage, that of Primary Eruption.—The eruption has a strong tendency to show itself on the third day, but this is a point upon which the physician must be upon his guard. It is very easy for the eruption to be entirely overlooked by the nurse or attendants, for a while, as the papules are at first so small as to escape detection, unless carefully searched for; and the date of the eruption is thus often erroneously stated. The earlier the eruption appears the more severe is the disease apt to be. When the eruption is distinct, it consists, on its first appearance, of a number of small red pimples, about the size of a pin's head, more or less numerous, but separate and distinct from one another, and scarcely salient. The eruption of small-pox runs a given course of about eleven days, and in its progress undergoes many mutations. It is at first a pimple, then a vesicle, then a pustule, and lastly forms a crust or scab. The first, or stage of pimple, lasts from twenty-four to forty-eight hours; the second, or vesicular stage, four days; the pustular stage three days; while the stage of scabbing lasts three days more, making the whole duration of the normal pustule ten or eleven days.

It generally first invades the upper part of the body, the face, neck, and wrists; and, inasmuch as it makes its first appearance there, there also it first arrives at maturity. Making its appearance thus upon the face and upper extremities, it next invades the trunk and lower extremities, occupying five days or thereabouts in its course from head to foot, or, rather, it does not *cease to come out* until the fifth day. A few pustules may sometimes make their appearance after this time, but, as a rule, they do not arrive at the same state of maturity as the rest, but run a less complete course. Sometimes the eruption takes a reverse course, and makes its appearance first upon the extremities, and occasionally is found first upon the chest or about the arm-pits.

The papulæ, or pimples, which are the first appearance of the eruption, generally appear first on the face, in the shape of minute bright red specks; or, very often, especially in the confluent form of the disease, a general erythematous blush is at first perceived covering the body, greatly resembling the rash of scarlatina, but called variolous roseolæ. This gradually assumes a papular form, and these again progress to the stage of pustules; but the suppuration is not complete until the eighth day. This period may vary one day either way: thus, in children, the pustules may be ripe on the seventh day, and, again, in some adults, when the disease is severe, not until the ninth. Some writers fancy that they have observed a disposition of the papules to arrange themselves in groups of three or five, and often to assume a crescentric or circular arrangement. Upon the second or third day of the eruption, a little lymph is observed making its appearance upon the summit of each papule, and, on the third or fourth day, these vesicles have become fully formed pocks. Thus, about five days is consumed in the *coming out* of the eruption. At this period, the pocks are distinctly formed, round, flattened at the top, the cuticle for a while seeming to be bound down to the cutis-vera, giving a peculiar *umbilicated* appearance to the top of each vesicle. The contents of each pock gradually becomes more and more opaque, until, at length, it is truly purulent. As they approach maturity, this umbilicated appearance is lost, and they become fully distended, and round upon the top. The structure of the pock is quite peculiar. The inflammation commences at a certain point in the corium or true skin, whence it radiates, forming an areola; this point has been called the "phlyctidium," and, occupying it, in a great measure, beneath the cuticle, is found a peculiar, moist, and spongy substance, said to be exuded by the vessels, known as the "variolous slough." When the suppuration is at its height, this substance is swollen and moist like a sponge. Each pock is divided into a number of separate compartments—*multilocular*, in fact—and a thread of connective tissue binds down the cuticle, for a time, to the floor of the phlyctidium. The fluids, which distend the pock, at length destroy this connection, and the pustule becomes full, round, and plump. Dr. Watson describes a peculiar appearance, at about the fifth or sixth day, which is worthy of notice. He says,

"Without going minutely into the anatomy of the pustules, we may see, in many of them, two colors, viz.: a central whitish disc of lymph, set in or surrounded by a circle of yellower puriform matter. In truth, there is, in the centre, a *vesicle*, which is distinct from the pus—we may puncture the one without evacuating the other. The vesicles have even, by careful dissection, been taken out entire, and are said to consist of several little cells. It is most probable that the lymph contained in this separate vesicle is the purest part of the variolous poison.

Upon the eighth day of the eruption, or it may be a little sooner or later, the pocks upon the face, or those which were the first to make their appearance, are found to have turned—their apices have broken, and the pustules are discharging their contents. The matter exuded soon dries, and forms a hard brownish scab, which, in due time, desquamates, leaving a reddish-brown spot. In determining the exact period of scabbing or incrustation, however, we are not to regard the pustules which may have become broken by the patient's movements or restlessness, or by scratching, but only those which have run their true course.

The full coming out of the eruption may be looked upon as the commencement of the third stage; and then it is that the fever shows a marked disposition to abate, and, indeed, often to leave the patient entirely, and, by the time the eruption is complete, it is gone. This subsidence of the fever is often both marked and sudden.

During the progress of the eruption, a number of minor symptoms occur. Itching of the skin is one of the most formidable of these; for upon the patient's self-command often depends the amount of pitting. The mucous membranes appear to sympathize with the disturbance of the skin, and a whitish eruption makes its appearance upon the fauces, eyelids, prepuce, labia-pudendi, &c., but which contains neither pus nor lymph. Towards the end of the eruption, also, sore-throat, swelling of the tonsils, uvula, &c., may arise, and the secretions prove very annoying. Most authors place too little stress upon the throat-affection. The first pustules are often found upon the velum-palati sooner than on any other part; hence, it is always important to examine the inside of the mouth and throat, when small-pox is suspected, to aid in the diagnosis. Sometimes the parts are inflamed without any perceptible eruption; at other times, both inflammation and papulæ can be plainly seen. Along with this, there may be more or less tumefaction of the skin, of the face especially, which often extends to the scalp; but these symptoms all subside as soon as the pustules have reached their greatest height. The patient also exhales a peculiarly disagreeable odor, which, in confluent cases, becomes perfectly unbearable.

The number of the pustules is always in direct relation with the severity of the disease; the more copious the eruption may be, so will the disease be more severe. Dr. Watson says that the number of the pustules indicates the quantity of the variolous poison in the system. Thus, the system suffers from the amount of the poison in the blood, of which the number of the pustules is the distinct sign, and again the system may also be laboring under the great extent to which the skin may be interrupted in its functions. The peril, in almost all the worst cases of confluent small-pox, arises from the amount of suppuration going on, and the immense drain upon the enfeebled and debilitated system. Stimulants here demonstrate the nature of the difficulty, for their judicious administration is always attended with benefit.

It may be advisable to bear in mind the peculiar mode of appearance of the eruption, in order that no error may be made in an early diagnosis. It may commence as a scarlet efflorescence (*variolous roseolæ*), punctate in character, becoming, in time, papular, and then pustular, or it may be distinctly papular from the beginning. Watson saw one case, in hospital-practice, which bore so strong a resemblance to urticaria that he, for twenty-four hours, hesitated in his diagnosis. But, so soon as the papules begin to pustulate, the doubt is nearly at an end, especially when the peculiar umbilication can be made out. Watson's account of the stage of formation is exceedingly clear. "In the discrete variety," he says, "in which the disorder may be presumed to run its most natural course, the eruption is at first, according to the phraseology of Willan, *papular*. The pimples gradually increase in magnitude, but it is not till the third day of their appearance that they begin to contain a little fluid on their summits. For two days after this, they increase in breadth only, and a *depression* is observable in the centre of many of them. The cuticle is bound down somehow, for a time, to the cutis-vera. It is the eighth day *of the disease*, or the *fifth* day *of the eruption*, before the pustules become perfectly turgid and hemispheroidal. During the time in which they are thus filling up, the face swells—often to so great a degree that the eyelids are closed, and the natural aspect suffers a complete and hideous change. In favorable cases, the skin between the pustules on the face assumes a rose-red, damask-red color. About the eighth day of the eruption, a dark spot makes its appearance upon the top of each pustule, and, at that spot, the cuticle breaks, a portion of the matter oozes out, and the pustule dries into a scab. When this crust at length falls off, it leaves behind it either a purplish red stain—which is still very characteristic of the disease, and which very slowly fades—or a depressed scar, which is indelible. In the latter case, the patient, or, more properly, his skin, is said to be *pitted* with the small-pox, or *pock-marked*.

The eruption pursues the same course upon the extremities and trunk as upon the body, with the exception that it is two or three days later.

In this, the discrete variety of the disorder, the symptoms all undergo a vast mitigation upon the coming out of the eruption. The fever, headache, nausea, delirium, pain in the back, and all other unpleasant sensations may pass away from the patient completely, and, but for the eruption, which alone challenges the eye, he might be regarded as, in fact, well; proving that these symptoms depended upon vascular distention, which is relieved by the coming out of the eruption.

About the eighth or ninth day of the disease, or when the pustules are at their height, a second febrile disturbance—the "fever of maturation," as it is called—frequently takes place. It is dependent upon the sympathy of the system at large with the general irritation of the skin, and, of course, is apt to be worse in those cases attended with a very copious eruption. But it differs from the primary fever, in being symptomatic instead of idiopathic, and generally declines along with the pustules.

The *fourth stage* Dr. Wood regards as nothing more than a period of convalescence. About the eleventh or twelfth day, he says, the pustules on the cheeks begin to turn brownish, and dry upon the top, and from this time forward the process of desiccation goes on rapidly, the tumefaction of the face subsides, and at length only the scabs remain. During this time, however, the eruption still stands well out upon the extremities, and they still remain considerably swollen and enlarged. It is not until three or four days after the scabs have formed upon the face, that the desiccation is complete upon the ankles and wrists. Upon the extremities, the pustules will often dry up and disappear without the formation of a scab, though to the eye they may have seemed as perfect pustules as those upon the face. Eruption upon the mucous membranes almost always terminates in resolution, without the formation of any ulcer or scar. The scabs fall off entirely between the fourteenth and twenty-first day.

When the scabs begin to form, the fever declines, the tongue cleans, the appetite returns, and, by the time the skin has been relieved of its burden, the patient may be regarded as restored to health. The whole course of the disease is from two to three weeks.

Mortality in Discrete Cases.—In three hundred and seventy-three cases of distinct and varicelloid small-pox, under Gregory's treatment, only three died; of thirty-nine other cases, none died; and of one hundred and fifteen additional examples, only one died. When there is no tumefaction of the face and eyelids, death is apt to take place on the ninth or tenth day, in discrete cases, although, as a general rule, distinct small-pox is a disease of little or no danger.

CONFLUENT SMALL-POX.

But the malady, as thus described, is very different from the terrible disease with which we have to cope under its confluent form. In the one, the slight symptoms of disturbance which arise may be followed by so small an epanastasis as "a single pock upon the breast;" while, in the other, so completely is the body beset with pustules that it would seem almost a continuous mass of oozing and sickening corruption. Between these two extremes, however, we may have every degree of severity. We take the face as the index of the amount of disease, and, if the eruption be confluent there, whether or not it be so elsewhere, it takes the *name* of confluent, and should be so treated. Sometimes it is not strictly either confluent or discrete, but the pustules stand just thick enough to touch, without coälescing; and it is then termed *cohering*.

In all cases where the pustules show a tendency to run together upon the face, the initiatory fever is apt to be more violent and severe, the disturbance of the brain and nervous system more marked, and, in fact, all the premonitory symptoms are more severe and distressing. The eruption also makes its appearance sooner and more confusedly; the pimples are at first very minute, and accumulated together in patches, and often accompanied with a rash, not unlike that of erysipelas or scarlet fever (*variolous roseolæ*). This appearance may render the diagnosis, for a time, uncertain. The pustules, as they advance to maturity, do not seem to fill up so completely with fluid as do the pustules of the discrete variety.

It is apt to be accompanied with delirium at the outset, which, in some cases, may be caused by cerebral congestion; but, in other cases, is undoubtedly due to nervous irritation alone. Cough, oppressed breathing, and pains in the chest are not uncommon.

The variolous papulæ appear thickly upon the face, in some cases, so that scarcely any portion of healthy skin is left between them; but more frequently there are left intervals of sound skin. They are, in general, more separate and distinct upon the trunk and limbs than upon the face; but it occasionally occurs that, while discrete upon the face, they may have become confluent upon some portion of the body below, and, in this case, the disorder is more generally mild.

The eruption does not seem to run so regular a course as in the discrete variety. The pustules are less regularly formed, they are less full, their outline less circumscribed and round, nor do they rise so much above the surrounding surface. In many cases, the pustules appear to be fused into one undistinguishable mass, the cuticle covering what appears to be one uniform layer of pus investing the face. This may also occur, but less frequently, upon other parts of the body

In these cases, the inflammation often extends to the subcutaneous cellular tissue, and great destruction is made by ulceration.

The mouth and fauces are more apt to become implicated in this variety than in the discrete, and the consequent pain, swelling, &c., much more likely to be distressing. Wood says, that not unfrequently the eruption and inflammation extend into the larynx and trachea, and to the larger divisions of the bronchi, and this constitutes one of the most dangerous complications of this form of the disease. Consequent upon this condition, in its advanced stages, and arising from a want of arterialization of the blood, is a dark discoloration of the surface, a livid or purplish hue of the eruption, feebleness of the pulse, coolness of the surface, and universal prostration. The deglutition, which is painful, from the inflamed state of the fauces, becomes, in some of these cases, still more difficult, in consequence of the thickening of the epiglottis, and the want of proper adaptation between it and the orifice of the glottis. The nostrils are often stuffed with the tough secretion, or closed by the swelling of the schneiderian membrane.

The surface also, he says, often swells greatly, especially the face and scalp. Such is the tumefaction, that the eyes are frequently closed, almost every feature obliterated, and the whole head enormously enlarged. The patient is occasionally troubled with phymosis or paraphymosis, buboes form in the groin, and parts of the surface where there is little eruption become affected by an erythematous inflammation. He thinks the eruption usually begins to dry upon the face, about the tenth day of the disease, and, in place of the broad masses of suppuration, with its cuticular covering, the whole face is often invested with a mask of dark-colored scabs, beneath which matter still exists, giving a soft, mush-like feeling to the parts. Frequently the matter oozes from beneath the scabs, and sometimes, when they are torn off or scratched, as they are apt to be, in consequence of the insupportable itchiness which attends their formation, a bloody or ichorous discharge takes place from the raw surface.

The fetor, which had *remitted* upon the occurrence of the eruption, increases again on the eighth or ninth day, and the new accession is often marked by the occurrence of rigors. This *secondary fever* may still have more or less of the sthenic character about it, which, in some vigorous constitutions, it never loses; but very often it assumes a low form, consequent partly upon the exhausted strength of the patient, and partly, also, in all probability, upon the deteriorating effects of the absorbed pus and putrid secretions upon the blood. There may now be frequent and feeble pulse, a dark and dry tongue, low delirium, tremors, subsultus-tendinum, great muscular weakness, occasionally involuntary discharges, or perhaps retention of urine; and the patient, if no favorable change takes place, dies from exhaustion, or some local accident of the disease.

If the patient surmounts the period of maturation, and passes into the stage of decline of the eruption, he still has great dangers to encounter. It is then that various internal inflammations are to be feared. There may arise pseudo-membranous inflammation of the fauces, pneumonia or pleurisy, diarrhœa, dysentery, and occasionally inflammations of the brain. Virulent ophthalmia, often destroys one or both eyes; the eyeball may be completely disorganized, and the whole eye be converted into an abscess, or sloughing of the cornea may allow of the protrusion of the contents of the eye. Opacity may alone result, however, which sometimes is incurable.

Abscesses of the ear are by no means uncommon, and, indeed, abscesses in different parts of the head, neck, and face. Erysipelas may arise, of the head and face, and boils and various eruptions frequently break out all over the body, frequently giving rise to intractable sores, and adding greatly to the distress of the patient. Extraordinary disposition may remain to suppuration beneath the skin and among the muscles, and gangrene is by no means uncommon; portions of the surface may be attacked by it, and the skin slough.

The convalescence is necessarily slow—the skin is slow in getting rid of its burden of scabious crusts, slow in regaining its functions, and necessarily the system slow to resume its normal state of activity. As the scabs fall, they leave behind them deep pits, often running together and forming large scars and seams upon the face; and, long after the crusts may have fallen, and the furfuraceous desquamation of the cuticle following them may have ceased, an unsightly and repulsive spotted redness of the face remains, sometimes for a long time. By degrees, however, the skin recovers its fairness; but, though the cicatrices of the pocks may measurably diminish, their indelible and unmistakeable imprint is never totally obliterated from the face. In the *modified confluent* small-pox these severe effects do not occur; for, in most cases, the efficacy of an old vaccination is shown just at the time when the eruption is about running into the most destructive stage. It may have lain dormant during the whole period of the sickness—the disease appearing to run an unmodified course—but, at about the time when the pustules, in the ordinary course, should pass into the most extensive disorganization of the skin and subjacent tissues, they seem to turn and quickly disappear, leaving hardly a trace of their presence.

Desquamation is seldom complete before the end of four or five weeks, and, after a severe attack, the health may for a time remain indifferent and weak, and any latent tendency to scrofula or other constitutional disorder is apt to be aroused.

But there are many degrees of severity, which the confluent form may assume, some of them frightful, indeed, others scarcely more severe than the ordinary discrete variety. Occasionally, however, the disease appears, from the first, to strike at the very life of the patient. The precursory symptoms are severe, the period of incubation short, the eruption appears early, and, though confluent, makes no progress, and the patient sinks without a struggle; or a peculiarly asthenic state of system may appear, to impress *any* of the different types of the disorder, and conduct it to an unfavorable termination, though it is much more apt to accompany the confluent. Wood characterizes it as marked by an utter prostration of nervous power, inducing inefficient reaction, with coma, delirium, or excessive restlessness and anxiety, and sometimes an imperfect development of the eruption, or a sudden retrocession of it, when formed; or secondly, by those symptoms which characterize a depraved condition of the blood, such as petechiæ, vibices, oozing of dark blood from the mucous membranes or abraded surfaces, a purplish, or bloody and badly-developed eruption, which fills partially, and rises but little above the surface, paleness or lividity of the intervening skin, a disposition to gangrene, oppressed breathing, an anxious countenance, and great feebleness of the circulation. The signs of malignancy do not always manifest themselves in the initiatory fever, but, in other instances, the patients seem to sink from the beginning. This is the *black small-pox* of Sydenham, or the *bloody small-pox* of Mead; the pustules, instead of presenting their normal characteristics, are flat, red, purple, or blue, and contain, in place of pus, blood, or a sanious ichor. These appearances almost always augur death.

Hæmorrhage from the uterus is not uncommon, and in pregnant women abortion. The latter is almost always followed by death. It has been a vexed question as to whether the eruption ever appeared on surfaces not exposed to the air—the fact that they never appeared on hæmorrhoidal tumors, except when they projected beyond the verge of the anus,—nor upon the inner surfaces of the eyelids, except in *ectropium*,—nor upon that portion of the glans-penis covered by the prepuce, being held to prove that they did not. But the fœtuses, parted with by women with small-pox at term, have been found covered with variolous pustules, which puts at rest the theory that the contact of *air* is necessary to their production; but certainly parts exposed to the air are generally more heavily visited by the eruption than those more protected.

Dr. Watson argues that the fœtus in utero may have the disease, and safely pass through it during its intra-uterine life. He cites an example, where a fœtus at birth was found pitted with the small-pox, and another, where a woman was inoculated at the sixth month of gestation, and had the disease severely, and her child, on subsequent repeated inoculation, appeared to be insusceptible to the contagion.

Varieties of Confluent Small-Pox.—Besides the true confluent small-pox, we have to distinguish the *semi*-confluent, *corymbose*, the *confluent-superficial*, and the *confluent-modified* small-pox. In the corymbose, or partially confluent form, the vesicles are grouped into clusters, leaving intermediate spaces of unoccupied skin; it is always accompanied with severe and irregular fever. In the confluent-superficial variety, the eruption passes through all its regular stages, but the inflammatory action never extends beyond the outer layer of the corion; this is sometimes confounded with the confluent-modified small-pox, but the origin and progress of the eruption is very different in the two cases, for the confluent-superficial appears in the *un*-vaccinated, and the pustules mature equally and regularly; while the confluent-modified small-pox never appears except in the *vaccinated*, and the advance of the pustules is not only imperfect but *unequal* on the same portion of the skin. On the arm, for instance, at one and the same time, we may, or rather will observe some pustules fully maturated, and others of smaller size desiccating after the escape of a minute portion of pus, while part of the eruption has become tuberculated, without purulent formation, and with little or no surrounding inflammation. This *inequality* of aspect is the great characteristic of confluent variola, modified by previous, imperfect, or almost worn-out vaccination. I have witnessed several cases of this latter form of small-pox, viz., the *confluent-modified:* most of the patients had very distinct, although not perfect vaccination marks; the premonitory symptoms were decidedly severe; the vomiting almost incessant; the back-ache almost excruciating; the fever and headache intense; the primary eruption so copious over the body that it could easily be mistaken for roseola, febrile lichen, or very acute and extensive eczema; the eruption appeared on the chest and about the arm-pits before it became visible upon the face. Subsequently, the disease progressed as a decided and often very severe case of confluent small-pox, up to the eighth day of the eruption, or the eleventh day of the fever; but, when the secondary fever should commence, the whole disease faded away like a case of varioloid, and the patient was comparatively convalescent; only very small, scarcely visible pits are left, and the patient is but little disfigured. In these cases, the physician gains great credit, not only for saving his patient, but for preventing disfigurement of the face. It is needless to say that the credit mainly belongs to nature. I have seen cases which terminated in this satisfactory way, although the patient had been comatose before the eruption appeared, and all the other symptoms had been severe, the eruption being most copious and confluent, the eyelids closed, nose greatly swollen, and throat very sore, with great difficulty of swallowing and some difficulty of breathing. The prognosis of *un*-modified confluent small-pox is very much more grave than the modified-confluent. Under the celebrated Gregory's treatment, in Edinburgh, of six hundred and thirty-seven cases of *un-*

modified confluent, three hundred and four died, or nearly one half; of fifty-six other cases, which, although vaccinated, were scarcely or not at all protected, twenty-one died, also nearly one half; while of thirty-eight confluent cases, modified by vaccination, only four died. Again, of seventy-eight semi-confluent, unmodified, or unvaccinated cases, eight died, or one in nine; and of forty-two additional vaccinated, but unmodified and unprotected semi-confluent cases, four died; or one in ten. While of thirty-eight confluent cases, modified by vaccination, only four died, or one in nine; and of twenty-eight cases of semi-confluent, modified by vaccination, only one died, or one in twenty-eight. Hence, vaccination reduced the mortality of confluent cases to nearly the same low ratio of semi-confluent *un*-modified cases.

VARIOLOID, OR SMALL-POX MODIFIED BY VACCINATION.

The *varioloid*, or modified small-pox, is that occurring in an individual previously protected by vaccination. This protection may be at the minimum, allowing the patient to suffer an attack of corymbose, or indeed confluent small-pox; or it may, at the maximum, and ward off all but the sympathetic fever, known during variolous epidemics as *variolæ sine variola*.

Many persons, protected by vaccination, have noticed during an epidemic (and occasionally physicians, on some occasion, while attending a small-pox patient) that they have suffered from anorexia, headache, pain in the back, and disturbed sleep, for two or three days, which then passes off, leaving them well; this, probably, is nothing more or less than the variolous fever, occurring without eruption in a constitution all but insusceptible through vaccination; or, in other words, they have all they *can* have of the small-pox. It may also occur in those who have passed through the disease on some former occasion.

The vast majority of the cases, however, are attended with eruption, and may be ushered in by the ordinary symptoms of headache, fever, pain in the back, and vomiting. In most instances, according to Wood, the initiatory fever bears a much stronger resemblance to the fever of unmodified small-pox than does the subsequent eruption to that of the genuine disease. One of the most striking peculiarities, he says, of the varioloid disease, is the very small amount of eruption often succeeding a severe initiatory fever.

The eruption is, occasionally, as in the confluent variety, preceded by a scarlet efflorescence, which, however, by no means portends a severe eruption—it may be, in fact, quite insignificant.

Sometimes, however, it is copious, and even confluent, in rare instances; but it shows a tendency to appear first upon the body, and runs a less regular course than in the genuine disease. The pustules upon a part are not all in the same condition at the same time; we may find papule, vesicle, and pustule coëxisting upon the same part. They have a tendency, too, to stop short at an earlier stage; not to progress beyond the stage of papule, perhaps, or to desiccate at the vesicular stage, or again to undergo but a partial suppuration. All these are marks of distinction between it and the genuine disease. Sometimes the whole eruption will stop one or two days short of its appointed time, and this is regarded as a very favorable sign for the patient. The absence of all odor, and the rarity of secondary fever, are also prominent characteristics of varioloid.

BLOOD OR BLACK SMALL-POX.—(*Variolæ Nigræ.*)

According to Gregory, it happens occasionally, though happily not often, that the miasm of small-pox poisons the blood, alters its crasis or coagulating properties, and leads to hæmorrhages from every open surface. The evidences of this condition of the fluids are often perceptible from the first hour of initiatory fever; at other times, they are not noticed until the eruption has begun to develop itself, or even later in the maturative stage. The eruption has a livid or dingy aspect, and the expression of the countenance is highly anxious. Hæmorrhage takes place from the nose, mouth, lungs, stomach, bowels, and kidneys; petechiæ and patches of ecchymosis (called vibices) appear, intermixed with the variolous papulæ, and the variolous vesicles are filled with blood, instead of serum. Death may take place, in consequence of this remarkable condition of the blood, before any unequivocal signs of small-pox are developed. More commonly, the eruption, confluent in character, displays itself, but never makes much advance, and nature apparently gives up the struggle as hopeless—the patient being carried off, perhaps, on the fourth, or from that to the sixth day. Gregory saw one case, in a lady, in which the whole body was of the color of indigo, and whom he at first believed to be a Negro; she conversed in the most tranquil manner, and died a few hours afterward. I have seen three cases of this disease, under the care of other physicians, all of which terminated fatally. One case, in a young man, aged about nineteen, was mistaken, by the attending physician, for acute inflammation of the kidney; for the urine was excessively scanty and bloody, the pain in the back exceedingly severe, and the vomiting frequent and obstinate. When I was called in counsel, the eruption of small-pox was abundant, and confluent over the whole body; the papulæ and pustules being very small and indistinct, as a variolous affection, except on close examination, when the umbilicated character of them was very evident. Hæmorrhage took place from the nose and mouth; frequent bloody stools occurred, sometimes from four to ten per day, and the urine was very bloody; many of the sanguineous vesicles ruptured spontaneously, and the patient's bed was covered with blood; he was drowsy at times, but easily roused; at others, exceedingly restless and delirious. The two other cases occurred in the persons of exceedingly robust young adults, and hæmorrhage occurred from almost every organ and pore. In no other disease is the discharge of blood from so many organs and surfaces observed, except in malignant yellow fever. Gregory says, if the vesicles on the extremities and trunk be flat, with a clarety areola, while the eruption on the face is white and pasty, no reasonable hope of recovery can be entertained; and everything which indicates putrescency and a dissolved state of the blood, is highly unfavorable. Petechiæ, mucous hæmorrhages, menorrhagia, and vesicles filled with blood, if occurring simultaneously, preclude the hope of benefit, even from the most judicious treatment.

COMPLICATIONS OF SMALL-POX.

1. About the eighth day in the distinct, and the eleventh day in the confluent, a secondary fever is established, and, at the same time, a new series of phenomena present themselves, in a few severe cases, as affections of the lungs, urinary organs, or cellular tissue of the body generally.

2. The most frequent affection of the lungs is *hæmoptysis*, but occasionally inflammation takes place. In cases of active congestive hæmoptysis, Aconite, Ipecac., and Antimony are the most useful remedies. In passive cases, Arnica is much relied upon, in homœopathic practice, and Acetate of Lead in the allopathic. Watson says, the latter is certainly a very serviceable remedy, and Dr. Paris speaks of it as one of the most valuable resources of physic, that there is nothing like it, or even second to it, and that its use is equally safe and manageable. Of the use of Tartar-emetic, in hæmorrhages, Wood says it is most useful in those dependant on local irritation or active congestion in the part affected, and attended with an excited state of the circulation. It is supposed to be peculiarly adapted to the hæmoptysis of small-pox, but I have seen quite severe cases which recovered, under little or no treatment especially directed to it, although the bleeding had recurred for days.

3. According to Gregory, in a large proportion of confluent, and in some semi-confluent cases, the mucous membrane of all those parts to which the atmospheric air gets access, viz., the nose, mouth, and trachea, is occupied with the *variolous* eruption—sometimes distinct, more generally confluent. The early symptoms occasioned by this mucous complication are: Numerous white points on the tongue, palate, and rectum; hoarseness and alteration of voice, which indicate that the same condition extends to the mucous membrane of the larynx and trachea; there is great pain in swallowing, and, in bad cases, cough and dyspnœa; the cough is at first dry and tearing, but, as the disease progresses, there is expectoration, and, about the eighth day, a copious viscid se-

cretion takes place from all the affected structures. In these affections, Tartar-emetic, Phosphorus, Spongia, and Iodine are useful.

The ulterior effects of this mucous implication are far more important than any local mischief which it occasions; for the œdematous thickening of the larynx, and the swollen condition of the tracheal membrane, have, by the eighth day, materially impeded the free access of air to the lungs, and the consequences appear in every part of the circulating system. There is no crimson areola around the pustules, for the blood is not well arterialized; the vesicles on the extremities never acquire any inflammatory areola, by which alone the surface can be cicatrized. On the body, the areolæ are dark or claret colored; the vesicles do not accuminate, they lie flat. Sometimes the superficial inflammation takes on an erysipelatous character, and the results are large, watery blebs, from which flows out a thin ichor, and consequences still more serious happen in the next twenty-four hours; for the brain becomes affected, a low muttering delirium is observed, as the waves of ill-oxygenated blood begin to circulate; the tongue swells, and turns purple; restlessness and great anxiety succeed; the patient tries to get out of bed; the bladder loses its contractile power, and becomes distended; the limbs grow cold; dyspnœa increases, and the patient dies.

In such cases, the inhalation of oxygen is more useful than stimulants. According to Louis, fifteen-twentieths of all that die of small-pox perish from asphyxia, consequent upon affections of the larynx and air-passages generally. Œdema-glottidis is common, and may sometimes be relieved by an operation. According to Gregory, bronchial inflammation is occasionally present during the whole course of the complaint, especially in the winter season, and sometimes pneumonia occurs; but the great peculiarity is the frequency of *variolous pleurisy*, which often occurs from the seventeenth to the twentieth day. It is a peracute form of inflammation, remarkable for its sudden invasion, rapid progress, and invariable termination by empyema. The symptoms are very unequivocal—viz.: Intense pain, a hard, wiry, and incompressible pulse, *shortness* of breathing, and a dry state of the skin. Gregory says, blood-letting is almost powerless in this complication, and death usually happens on the third or fourth day, from the invasion of the chest-symptoms. The treatment of purulent pleurisy is, of course, very difficult; the usual remedies, such as Aconite and Bryonia, so useful in simple pleurisy, are of little or no avail here. Sulphur, Hepar-sulph., and Arnica have been used, with how little prospect of success may be gathered from the following:

Post-Mortem Appearances.—The lungs sometimes display the usual evidences of inflammation—viz.: Vascular engorgement, purulent infiltration, and hepatization; the chest, on one side, may be filled with a sero-purulent fluid, resembling a mixture of cream and water, the result of acute pleurisy, and the pleura itself may be seen injected with blood and covered with a dense layer of coagulable lymph. The condition of the larynx and trachea is unique; for the mucous membrane appears covered with a copious, viscid, puriform secretion, of a gray or brownish color; on detaching this, the mucous membrane is seen deeply congested with blood, thickened, pulpy, and, in the worst cases, black and sloughy, exhaling a most offensive odor. These appearances may be traced to the third division of the bronchial tubes.

4. According to Gregory, the *cellular tissue* is very apt to become involved, in the progress of small-pox. In the discrete variety, the skin continues movable, on the subjacent textures, but, in all bad cases, both confluent, semi-confluent, and corymbose, the inflammatory action dips deeper and invades the cellular tissue. These are the only varieties in which scars are left. The skin becomes swollen and tense, and, when the scalp is affected, enormous intumescence may take place, followed by profuse pustulation, or a succession of small and most troublesome abscesses. The cellular tissue of the throat is peculiarly liable to take on this action; the salivary glands participate in the inflammation, and salivation, with great turgescence of the neck follows. Occasionally, the tongue becomes involved, and glossitis is superadded to other evils, and few, if any, survive when matters have proceeded to this extremity.

The face always suffers severely in this aggravated form of cellular small-pox, except in that form called confluent-superficial. As regards

TREATMENT.—When profuse suppuration occurs, the diet must be changed, from light and cooling to decidedly nourishing and strengthening. Hepar-sulphur is regarded as a useful remedy.

M. Ozanam has lately presented to the French Academy of Sciences, through M. Cloquet, a paper upon a new effect of Chamomile, (Anthemis-nobilis, or Roman Chamomile,) in which he stated that it is capable of *preventing and of arresting suppuration* when it has already commenced. If this be a fact, it will render the medicine a most invaluable aid to us in the treatment of many inflammatory affections. He says, that "Chamomile is described, in all treatises on materia medica, as emollient, digestive, tonic, &c., but makes no mention of this most important property, which he has discovered, of preventing suppuration when the local disease is not too far advanced, and gradually stopping it when it has existed for a long time. For this purpose, it is administered in powerful doses, one-half or one ounce of the flowers, in one and a half or two pints of water, and this amount of the infusion to be drunk in the course of the day, and to be continued until a cure is effected. Compresses, moistened with the infusion, may be locally applied: they aid in the cure, but are not necessary—the infusion alone, taken internally, being quite sufficient." In support of his assertion, M. Ozanam quotes several extraordinary cases in which cures have been effected. When the remedy produces an apparent aggravation, it is a sign that the dose is too strong for the patient, and may require diminution.

5. The *secondary fever* sets in with rigors, followed by a hot and dry state of the surface, and an unquenchable thirst; and, in the progress of this fever, we must be prepared for all sorts of troubles. The skin is sure to suffer first; the elbows, legs, scrotum, knees, back, and hips may take on a mixed erysipelatous and phlegmonous action; the result is either boils, or abscesses, or large imposthumes, or carbuncles, or even gangrenous destruction of large portions of the skin.

Sydenham says, the confluent small-pox does not in the least endanger life in the first days of illness, unless there happens a flux of blood from the urinary passages or lungs; yet, in the decline of the disease, or on the eleventh, fourteenth, seventeenth, or twenty-first days, the patient is often brought to such a state that it is equally uncertain whether he will live or die. He is first endangered on the eleventh day, by a high fever, attended with great restlessness, and, from the fourteenth or seventeenth days, a very vehoment fit of restlessness comes on every day, towards evening, and there is the greatest difficulty in saving him.

Aconite, Veratrum-viride, or Tartar-emetic are often required on the eleventh day, for the secondary fever; while Opium, Coffea, or Hyoscíamus are said to be especially useful from the fourteenth to the seventeenth days, when there is delirium, with restlessness, wakefulness, and a frequent pulse. These remedies are also often given in alternation with Tartar-emetic.

6. The *brain and nervous system* are apt to become involved in bad cases of small-pox; children grind their teeth and squint, cereoral inflammation may supervene, and the child die either in an epileptic fit, or with evident signs of hydrocephalus. Adults may become delirious; but, generally speaking, the variolous delirium depends more on some peculiarity of temperament, or some highly irritable condition of the nervous system, than upon inflammation; and delirium, coma, and convulsions are all less dangerous during the primary fever, before the eruption has come out, than afterwards.

Gregory says, a peculiar nervous affection often supervenes on the tenth day, when the skin is extensively occupied by the confluent eruption, without nervous complication; it is thought to be identical with that which is familiar to surgeons as the consequence of extensive burns and scalds. General tremors, low delirium, a quick, tremulous pulse, a dry tongue, collapse of the features, cold extremities, and subsultus-tendinum are the precursors of a fatal event.

In ordinary practice, beef-tea, brandy, and Opium are used for the latter symptoms; in the homœopathic practice, Muriatic-acid, Arsenicum, or Rhus are often relied upon. In healthy and rather robust subjects, when there is delirium, violent screaming, intolerance of light and sound, and heat of the head, all of which indicate a tendency to meningeal congestion or inflammation, Aconite, Veratrum-viride, or Tartar-emetic are often more useful than Belladonna, Stramonium, or other remedies of that class, excepting Cuprum or Hellebore.

7. Small-pox is often accompanied by *ophthalmia.* This does not arise from pustules on the cornea and conjunctiva, but from simple conjunctival inflammation and iritis, or still deeper seated inflammation. It generally occurs only in its worst form when there is simultaneous great destruction of the skin, in distant parts or upon the face; then variolous ophthalmia may set in, on the tenth day, and advance so rapidly that, in forty-eight hours, the whole eyeball is irremediably injured. More frequently, an ulcer forms at the outer edge of the cornea, by which the aqueous humor escapes, or protrusion of the iris occurs; or the aqueous humor becomes clouded, or specks form on the cornea, from which blindness more or less complete and permanent results.

According to Mackenzie, the eyes are not safe, even after the small-pox pustules over the body have blackened, and the scabs fallen off; on the contrary, it is then that the chief danger is to be feared; it is then that secondary variolous ophthalmia, or *corneitis post-variolosa*, is apt to occur. A dull whitish point is first observed a little below the centre of the cornea, with surrounding haziness; the whiteness becomes slightly elevated and more extensive, and then the part becomes yellow, and is almost certain to fall into a state of ulceration. If two or more such points form, the whole cornea is rendered nebulous; or this effect may be produced even by one large central abscess. An onyx, or collection of pus in the anterior chamber, may also appear at the lower edge of the cornea, the sclerotica is apt to be reddened, pain and lachrymation are excited by exposure to light, and, in adults, the iris may become discolored, and the pupil more or less contracted, irregular, and more or less filled with lymph.

Mackenzie says, secondary variolous ophthalmia seldom leads to destruction of the cornea, unless the case is altogether neglected. By proper treatment, the matter of the abscess or onyx is generally absorbed; in other cases, ulceration takes place, leaving, after cicatrization, a leucoma, which is apt to be permanent; but the surrounding haziness of the cornea is gradually dissipated, and vision is injured only according to the size and situation of the leucoma. Belladonna, Mercury, and Tartar-emetic are thought to be the most useful remedies.

8. Gregory says that *variolous gangrene* is not necessarily connected with the petechial state, nor with debility; it may occur where the

fever is of a truly inflammatory type, and where no previous symptom gave evidence of unusual danger. He says it is more common in the irregular and corymbose small-pox than in purely confluent cases; its chief seats are the scrotum, feet, back, or even upon the breast. He cannot doubt that, in some cases, the gangrenous disposition is something *super*-added to the small-pox by the condition of the air which the patient breathes.

The main point, in the treatment of gangrene, is to support the general strength, until the diseased part has gone through the requisite process for throwing off the slough, and repairing the consequent loss of substance; at the same time, it is important to counteract the morbid tendency of the system, by improving the quality of the blood. Both of these indications are met by the use of tonics, stimulants, and a generous diet, with or without the aid of specific medicines. Chloride of Soda or Kreosote, internally or externally, are useful remedies, and may be aided by the inhalation of Chlorine-gas, as it issues from moistened chloride of lime. Arsenicum, Secale, Muriatic-acid, Bark and Wine, Carbonate of Ammonia, Opium, and Camphor have all been used, with more or less success.

Prognosis in Small-Pox.—1. If vomiting continues after the eruption is completed, the patient's life is in great danger, even although the small-pox be not confluent.

2. Excruciating pain in the loins is generally followed by a bad small-pox, and the more violent the pain the greater the danger.

3. Encephalic symptoms, such as severe headache, stupor, delirium, flushed face, strong beating of the carotid and temporal arteries, somnolency, or fits of convulsions in children may all pass away safely when they merely accompany the initiatory fever, for they subside spontaneously when the eruption comes out well.

4. Great shortness of breath, coming on about the fifth day of the eruption, scarcely leaves any hope that the patient will survive.

5. If the maturative process be accompanied by an exceedingly tender state of the surface, it is not a very favorable sign.

6. General tremors, low delirium, a quick and tremulous pulse, a dry tongue, collapse of the features, cold extremities, and subsultus-tendinum are generally the precursors of death.

7. The coming on of the menstrual flux, in cases attended with purpura, and hæmorrhages from other parts, is of a very serious character, and almost always fatal.

8. Pleurisy is a most frequent accompaniment of small-pox, and will most likely be followed by empyema. Blood-letting is said to be of no use, and death usually happens on the third or fourth day, from the invasion of the thoracic symptoms.

9. Extreme youth predisposes to an unfavorable termination, and few persons over forty years of age escape.

10. The average of deaths is one in six.

11. If there is no tumefaction of the face and eyelids, death takes place on the ninth or tenth day, if the disease is discrete; on the thirteenth or fourteenth, if it is confluent, according to Von Sweiten, Stoll, Sydenham, and Trousseau.

12. It is very seldom that a pregnant woman dies of small-pox without aborting or giving birth to the child. A consumptive female lives to give birth to her child, though she may sink exhausted a few hours afterward.

13. The danger, in small-pox, depends upon: 1. The quantity of the eruption; 2. On the condition of the mucous membranes; 3. On the state of the fluids; 4. On the state of the brain and nervous system; 5. On the age of the patient; 6. On his habit of body; 7. On the circumstances in which he is placed.

14. Confluence is always unfavorable, especially on the face, nor is the danger always apparent.

15. If the pustules on the extremities acuminate well, and exhibit a crimson areola, a good ground of hope exists. If they are flat, with a clarety areola, while the eruption on the face is white and pasty, no reasonable hope of recovery can be entertained.

16. Hoarseness, at an early period of the disease, is always to be looked upon with suspicion. A natural tone of voice is of good omen, even though the eruption be full and confluent, with a disposition to cellular complication.

17. Everything which indicates putrescency, and a dissolved state of the blood, is unfavorable. Petechiæ, mucous hæmorrhages, menorrhagia, and vesicles filled with blood preclude the hope of benefit, even from the most judicious treatment.

18. A tranquil state of the nervous system conduces to recovery. In severe confluent cases, this is the sole reliance. Quiet nights, composure of manner, a contented disposition, and confident hope of recovery are good signs.

19. Restlessness, a succession of sleepless nights, constant moaning, and despondency are very bad signs.

20. Children who grind their teeth seldom recover.

21. Persons above forty seldom recover, even from the semi-confluent small-pox.

22. Children are endangered by an amount of eruption that can scarcely be called semi-confluent.

23. The most favorable age is from seven to fourteen.

24. A state of plethora is unfavorable.

25. Constitutional debility is equally bad.

26. A strumous diathesis is very unfavorable.

27. In some cases, when petechiæ exist, or spots of purpura, even of considerable extent, if no hæmorrhage takes place from internal organs, the prognosis is very much less unfavorable.

Unfavorable signs, during the first stages, are not of such fatal import as when they appear during the secondary fever, especially when there is an absence of the usual redness in the intermediate spaces; distribution of petechiæ in the interstices; the development of a black spot, hardly so large as a pin's head, in the centre of each pustule; a lurid or purple color of the pustules, or imperfect development of them, or their sudden subsidence without a remission of the symptoms; sudden suppression of salivation or of urine; hæmaturia or hæmoptysis; absence of swelling of the hands and feet, when the eruption is copious, are all bad signs.

Mortality.—In the last century, prior to the discovery of vaccination, 199,665 persons died of small-pox in England; from 1775 to 1800, eight out of every hundred deaths, in England, were caused by this disease; and, as late as 1838, no less than 16,268 persons, in England and Wales, fell victims to it.

Of 637 *confluent* cases, under ordinary treatment, in the years 1837 to 1841, no less than 304 died; of 267 semi-confluent cases, only 20 died; of 143 examples of the confluent and semi-confluent *modified*, only 8 died; and of 373 discrete and varicelloid cases, only 3 died. Total, 1420 cases, with 385 deaths, of which the confluent cases supplied 304.

Under Fleischmann's treatment, in the Homœopathic Hospital of Vienna, there were 11 deaths in 136 cases, or 1 case in 12—about 8 per cent. It is not stated whether the cases were confluent or not. Now we have seen that the discrete form is scarcely ever dangerous, while the confluent is never free from peril; the distinction, therefore, is of the greatest importance. The secondary fever is but slightly marked in the discrete small-pox, while it is very intense and perilous in most instances of the confluent; and it is at this period that death, in the fatal cases, oftenest occurs. Again, it is not stated whether the patients had been vaccinated or not; yet this is also a very important point, in forming an estimate of the relative value of treatment in small-pox. In 1838, of 712 cases, of all kinds, admitted into the London Small-Pox Hospital, there were 187 deaths, or 27 per cent., or 1 case in every 4 under regular treatment; of these, 302 had been vaccinated, with 30 deaths, or 10 per cent., or 1 in every 10. Hence, even if we admit, for the sake of argument, that all the cases treated homœopathically by Dr. Fleischmann had been vaccinated, the results of his treatment were at least two per cent. better than the old-school treatment of vaccinated cases. But 392 of the 712 cases had not been vaccinated, with 157 deaths, or 40 per cent., or 1 in every 2½ under regular treatment—a tremendous loss. And what makes the matter worse, is that, in 1781, before vaccination was introduced, there were 646 cases admitted into the same hospital, of which 257 died, or 40 per cent., or 1 in every 2½. Hence the dominant-school treatment of small-pox did not seem to lead to better results in 1838 than it did in 1781, or fifty-seven years before.

PREVENTION OF SMALL-POX.

I. Inoculation.—Inoculation was the method first in vogue for the mitigation of small-pox. In Watson's cogent and forcible English, "All the world," he says, "knows that small-pox may be imparted to a healthy person by inserting beneath his cuticle a small portion of the matter taken from a variolous pustule: this, perhaps, is not very surprising; but it is surprising that the disease so received should be much milder than if contracted in the ordinary way." But such is the fact, be the explanation what it may; and for many years it was the only practice resorted to. The practice was first introduced into England by Lady Mary Wortley Montague, who had her own daughter inoculated; this was followed by the inoculation of a child of Dr. Keith, who had visited Miss Wortley, and this by the inoculation of several condemned felons. As these experiments all resulted successfully, some of the members of the royal family were next subjected to it. Lady Mary had first seen the practice followed while residing with her husband at the Ottoman Court; but, five years previously, Dr. Emanuel Timoni, a graduate of Oxford, settled at Constantinople, wrote to London to Dr. Woodward, giving him an account of the practice. This was communicated to the Royal Society, and, in 1715, Mr. Kennedy, an English surgeon, who had travelled in Turkey, gave similar information to the English public in an essay; and the following year M. Piglarini, Venetian Consul at Smyrna, gave publicity to it in the "Philosophical Transactions." The Chinese, however, claim to have been in the habit, for many centuries, of *sowing* the disease, by putting some of the crusts into the nostrils. This, however, differs from inoculation, as the mucous surfaces being entire, and the effluvium received directly into the lungs, it differs in no essential point from the natural way of taking the disorder. It is said, however, that a true engrafting of the disease has been in use by the Brahmins, time out of mind.

The practice was not thoroughly established, nor properly appreciated until the middle of the century (1750); but its efficacy, in mitigating the severity and danger of the disease, in saving life and preventing deformity, was signally great. The mortality, in the natural small-pox, was estimated at one in five. It is really higher. Mr.

Marson infers, from the records of the Small-Pox Hospital—where, however, the mortality is likely to be above the average—that the natural small-pox destroys about one-third of all whom it attacks. Baron Dimsdale, a great inoculator, declared that not one in fifteen died of the engrafted disease. Two brothers, named Sutton, who had introduced or rather revived a very improved method of treating the disorder, professed to have inoculated 20,000, without fairly losing one. But these, doubtless, were vastly exaggerated statements. Dr. Gregory says, that the average number of deaths at the Inoculation Hospital was only three in a thousand. The National Vaccine Board speak decidedly of one in three hundred, as the proportion of the inoculated that will surely die from the operation.

In the inoculated disease, the period of incubation is comparatively short; the pustules are seldom numerous, and still more seldom confluent, and the secondary fever generally slight or wanting. It may also be mentioned that the roseolous rash, which often precedes the confluent eruption, frequently also happens in the inoculated disease; Watson says, *more* frequently than in the casual disease. After inoculation, it is looked upon as a favorable sign, though, when preceding the confluent eruption, it is usually the harbinger of a severe disorder.

The great and fatal objection, however, to the practice of inoculation, was, that while it mitigated the disease, and protected for the future the individual who had been thus inoculated, it spread the disorder far and wide over the land, in localities where the unaided disease would never have found its way—since each and every person thus inoculated was as capable of sowing the disorder as if the disease had been taken in the ordinary way. In this manner, small-pox appeared, and raged as it had never done before, simply because, though the inoculated were many, and had the disorder lightly, so also, as they were many, was the disorder more wide-spread and destructive, as the vast majority of the people were still uninoculated.

So unpopular did the practice become at last, that an order was passed, prohibiting its practice, and making penal provisions for its enforcement. Different modes of introducing the virus have been proposed, some of them awkward and unnecessarily painful. The most convenient, and one as effectual as any other, is, by means of a puncture in the arm, to insert a small portion of pus from a variolous pock, exactly as is done in the operation of vaccination. As regards preparation for it, the best preparation is a condition of perfect health—either plethora or debility being unfavorable. All excess should be avoided beforehand.

A far superior expedient was soon discovered, however, in the practice of *vaccination*, which has rendered the inoculation of small-pox not merely unnecessary, but, in most cases, perfectly unjustifiable.

Yet circumstances do arise sometimes, even now, in which it may be allowable and right to engraft the matter of small-pox; as when an unprotected person has been unavoidably exposed and there is no vaccine matter at hand. The advantage of inoculating in such a case, is, that the inoculated disease gets the start of the natural form, and is sure to run its course more mildly; the fever commences sooner than it otherwise would do. To show the value of the practice in such cases, and the protection it affords to persons whom we cannot vaccinate, we may mention a fact which Professor Gregory, of Edinburgh, was in the habit of relating, and which he heard from a naval surgeon:

"Small-pox broke out among the crew of a man-of-war, in a tropical climate, where no vaccine matter was to be procured. The men were almost all unprotected. Sixteen of them took the disease in the natural way, and of these nine, or more than one-half died. Of 363 who were inoculated, under the disadvantages of a hot climate and no preparation, not one perished."

The following is the course of the inoculated small-pox, when artificially produced: On the third or fourth day after the operation, a slight pricking pain is experienced in the part, a hard elevation may be felt by the finger, and a minute vesicle upon an inflamed base may be seen upon a close examination. On the fifth day, the vesicle is well formed, and has an umbilicated appearance. This goes on increasing, and forms, at length, a small tumor, like a phlegmon. At the end of the seventh day, rigors are felt, followed by fever, and on the eighth or ninth day a variolous eruption makes its appearance on different parts of the body. This is almost always distinct, and generally moderate. One hundred pocks are a pretty full crop. A rose-colored efflorescence has already been mentioned as sometimes preceding the eruption. The pocks generally pass through the several stages, as in the discrete variety, though, in some instances, they are said to be abortive. In the meantime, the original pustule has been advancing, and, on the tenth or eleventh day, is surrounded by an irregular areola of inflammation, while the arm is often much swollen, and pus escapes from the tumor. No secondary fever occurs, and the pocks scab and desquamate kindly.

Some physicians inoculate patients in whom small-pox has already broken out; others give them variolous matter internally, in the following manner: A pustule is opened as soon as it has reached maturity, a few drops of the matter are collected in a tumbler of water, and of this solution the patient is given a small spoonful every two or three hours. In the majority of cases, the matter is taken from the patient himself, and is supposed to be as useful as syphilization, in the treatment of the great-pox. In other cases, the matter is taken from strange subjects. I have no experience on this point, and should be much more disposed to rely upon true inoculation, or vaccination, or the administration of vaccine matter internally, than upon the variolous.

II. Vaccination.—That a disorder communicated to the human being from one of the brute creation should protect the former against the contagion of small-pox, is one of the most interesting facts in the whole history of medicine. How glimpses of a truth so remarkable were first revealed to the casual observation of certain peasants, and how the results of this chance observation were gradually matured into a rational and scientific form, by a mind deeply imbued with the best principles of sound philosophy, are related in Dr. Baron's life of Jenner.

Dr. Jenner found, among the great dairy-farms in Gloucestershire, a popular belief that no person who had had the *cow-pox*, (an eruptive vesicular disease, communicated from the udder of the cow to the hands of the milkers,) could take the small-pox. Satisfied, by inoculating with small-pox matter several individuals who had had the cow-pox eruption, that this was not an unfounded notion, he at length conceived the great and happy idea of propagating the cow-pox from one human being to another, and so preventing, in all cases, the perilous and disfiguring distemper of small-pox, which he hoped might thus be finally exterminated.

By degrees, Dr. Jenner ascertained that some persons, who had had sore hands from milking, were not thereby rendered proof against the contagion of small-pox; but this difficulty was soon cleared up, by the discovery that the teats of cows were liable to different kinds of eruption, and he learned, by close observation, which of these it was that produced in the human frame the protecting disorder.

Dr. Jenner set himself to trace, if possible, the origin of the disease of the cow. First, he found that it was peculiar to certain dairies; then, that, in those dairies, men were employed as milkers. Following up this clue, he further made out that these men had also the charge of the farm-horses. Next he learned that the teats of the cows generally began to exhibit the specific eruption at that time of the year when a complaint called the "grease" chiefly prevailed among the horses. Hence, he concluded that the malady was conveyed to the cows by the hands of the men, who had been dressing the heels of horses affected with the grease. Subsequent inquiries, however, have shown that this conclusion was not strictly correct.

Another difficulty which lay in Dr. Jenner's way, and which his perseverance and sagacity surmounted, was this: He found that some, who were casually infected from the true complaint in the cow, were not protected. This depended, as he afterward ascertained, upon the period of the disease in the cow at which the virus was communicated to the milker. The thick matter proceeding from the vesicle, late in its progress, produced, indeed, a severer local sore than the thinner matter of its earlier state, but it did not confer the desired protection. The same thing is observed in regard to small-pox. If the matter used for inoculation be taken from a fully-matured pustule, it does not so surely excite the disease as when taken from a more crude one.

The next important step, in this most interesting investigation, was to determine whether the vaccine disease could be transmitted by engrafting from one human being to another, and whether, if so transmitted, it retained its protecting power. The fourteenth of May, 1796, was the birthday of vaccination. On that day, matter was taken from the hand of Sarah Nelmes, who had been infected by her master's cows, and inserted, by two superficial incisions, into the arms of James Phipps, a healthy boy, of about eight years old. He went through the vaccine disease, apparently, in a regular and satisfactory manner; but the most agitating part of the trial still remained to be performed. It was needful to ascertain whether he was secure from the contagion of small-pox. This point, so full of anxiety to Dr. Jenner, was fairly put to issue on the first of July following. Variolous matter, taken immediately from a pustule, was carefully inserted, by several punctures, but no disease followed.

It is scarcely necessary to notice the objections which were made at first to the practice of vaccination. Some of them were merely foolish—as, that it was unnatural and impious to engraft the diseases of a brute upon a Christian. Others were untrue—as, that it introduced into the system new, unheard of, and monstrous disorders, other than the cow-pox itself. It triumphed over all these cavils, and, in six years from its first promulgation, the discovery was known in every region of the world.

It was soon found, however, that some, who had apparently had the cow-pow by inoculation, were, nevertheless, not incapable of taking the small-pox; and that these failures were, many of them at least, attributable to the mistakes that were made in the time or manner of performing the operation. It became necessary, therefore, to ascertain precisely the conditions requisite for the production of the genuine disease; and these conditions have been successfully investigated by Dr. Jenner and subsequent observers.

To learn to recognize the true vaccine vesicle, it will be necessary to examine it repeatedly and critically, or its peculiar characteristics may not be fully impressed upon the mind.

On the second or third day after the insertion of the vaccine matter into the arm, the puncture looks red and inflamed; on the fourth or fifth day, the vesicle becomes perceptible—a pearl-colored elevation of the cuticle, enclosing a minute quantity of a thin, transparent liquid. It gradually increases in magnitude till the eighth day, when it should measure from a quarter to half an inch across. Like the pustule of small-pox, it is more prominent at its circumference than at its centre, and it consists of small cells, from ten to fourteen in number. By carefully puncturing one of these cells, a drop of the virus may be let out, the other cells remaining full. Up to the seventh, the eighth, or even to the beginning of the ninth day, the inflammation around the vesicle should extend to only a very small distance from it. After this, it spreads, and what is called the areola is formed: a circular red border, which continues to increase during the ninth and tenth days, and begins to fade on the eleventh, passing through shades of blue as it declines, and leaving a degree of hardness behind for two or three days more. By this time, a *dark* brown or *mahogany*-colored crust has formed over the vesicle, of a nearly circular shape; this becomes gradually harder and darker, and finally detaches itself about the twentieth day. The cicatrix which it leaves should be distinct, somewhat less than half an inch broad, circular, slightly depressed, marked (sometimes) by radiating lines, with a well-defined edge, and dotted with little pits, which seem to correspond to the cells of the vesicle. About the eighth day, there is usually some slight febrile excitement manifested, which soon subsides. This is analogous to the secondary fever of small-pox, and it appears to furnish the condition of the desired protection.

Of course it is of much moment to determine whether the cow-pox has run its course or not; and it is not always easy to say how far the progress of the vesicle may deviate from that which has just been described, without failing of its protective influence. A very ingenious *test* of this is to vaccinate the other arm, or some other part of the body, four or five days after the first vaccination. If the constitution has been properly affected by the first operation, the inflammation of the second vesicle will proceed so much more rapidly than usual that it will be at its height, and will decline and disappear as early as that of the first, only the vesicle and the areola will be smaller. In fact, from the time of the formation of the areola, the second vesicle is an exact miniature of the first. If the system has not been duly influenced by the first vesicle, the second will run its own course, increasing up to its eighth day, and so on. Should this be the case, this second vesicle may be tested by a third.

We find the germ of this criterion in the infancy of vaccination. Dr. Jenner vaccinated the children of his friend, Mr. Hicks, the first *gentleman* who consented to adopt the practice. This Mr. Hicks became afterwards an expert vaccinator himself, and it was his custom, in a doubtful case, to perform a second vaccination a few days after the first; and he remarked that "the second vesicle made immense strides to overtake the first."

After some time, it became apparent that Dr. Jenner's estimate of the protecting powers of the vaccine disease had been set too high. He had hoped and believed, as others also had, that the cow-pox would, in all cases, prove a perfect and permanent protection against the small-pox; but these hopes have been disappointed. Doubtless, complete protection is the rule; but, how thoroughly and regularly soever the vaccine malady may have proceeded, it is most certain that very many exceptions to this rule have taken place, and are constantly occurring about us.

But this, however, should not have depreciated the value of vaccination, as of late it has done, for it is a remarkable and most important truth, that the disease which may supervene after vaccination is much milder and shorter even than the inoculated, and, *à fortiori*, than the natural small-pox. This disorder has therefore been termed the *varioloid* disease, or, more properly, *modified* small-pox, or *post-vaccinal* small-pox.

In relation to this modified or post-vaccinal disease, several questions of the highest practical moment and interest have arisen, which, by slow degrees, and under careful and multiplied observation, may now be said to have found their solution.

The first is, Whether the protecting influence of cow-pox upon the human frame diminishes by lapse of time, and at length wears out?—There is ample evidence to show that sometimes, at least, it does. Certainly, in many, but not in all of those who have gone through the vaccine disease, vaccination, repeated at a distant period, reproduces in a greater or less degree its primary effects. A gentleman, who was vaccinated in 1799, has a son, nine or ten years old, who was vaccinated at the age of three weeks. Both of them have lately been revaccinated: the boy was somewhat affected by the renewal of the operation, *the father not at all.*

It may well be doubted whether *all* those who are susceptible of some impression from a second vaccination would become affected with small-pox under ordinary exposure to it. That *many* of them would thus contract the disease, and that all of them would be more or less endangered by the exposure, is too certain. And a second question immediately presents itself—namely, Whether this repetition of the operation of engrafting the cow-pox renews or adds to their security against small-pox?—Happily this question may also be answered in the affirmative, and answered by statistics of the amplest comparison. In his able and most conclusive digest of the whole subject, Mr. Simon shows, that, during the five years, 1833 to 1837, though small-pox infection had been imported sixteen times into different regiments of the army of Wurtemburg, there had ensued, among the 14,384 revaccinated soldiers, only one single instance of modified small-pox. Still more satisfactory experience is that of the Prussian army. In Prussia, as in Wurtemburg, the practice of revaccination grew out of the knowledge that the small-pox would attack a certain portion of those who had been vaccinated only in infancy. During the ten years preceding 1831, cases of post-vaccinal small-pox were increasing in number and fatality; and within the three years, 1831 to 1833, there had occurred no fewer than three hundred and twelve *deaths* by small-pox. For the last twenty years, the Prussian army has represented an almost entirely revaccinated population. And what has been the contrast?—One hundred and four annual deaths by small-pox was the last experience of the former system; *two* annual deaths by small-pox has been the average for the revaccinated army. Analyzing the forty fatal cases, for the last twenty years, we find that only four of the number were of persons, who, it is said, had been successfully revaccinated.

Similar facts, equally cogent with these, may be gathered from the experience of other countries. Mr. Marson, the resident surgeon to the Small-Pox and Vaccination Hospital, London, states that not one of the nurses or servants of the Hospital has had small-pox for the last twenty years. He holds that it is well, as a matter of safety, for all persons to be revaccinated at puberty, and especially those who have no cicatrix remaining. He recommends, also, as a matter of precaution, that all persons should be revaccinated on the appearance of small-pox in the house or neighborhood. But, thirdly, is there any ground for supposing that the wished-for protection ever fails to be conferred because the operation is performed too early?—None whatever, apparently. In fact, there is unquestionable evidence that, for the full attainment of its defensive purpose, gratuitous vaccination, at least, is performed too late in England. It appears, from official tables, that no less than one-fourth of the whole mortality from small-pox, in England and Wales, happens in infants less than one year old, and as much as eleven per cent. within the age of four months. Within the fifth year, the proportion reaches the enormous amount of from seventy-five to eighty per cent. These facts proclaim the necessity of *early* vaccination. It should be as early as is consistent with the safety of the child. Certainly, it should never be voluntarily delayed beyond the third or fourth month.

A fourth question is, How far the frequent failure, in late years, of complete protection can be ascribed to the circumstance that the vaccine virus has been repeatedly transmitted from one human being to another without any fresh recurrence to the cow, the original source of the disorder?—Dr. Jenner himself was not without apprehension that this might prove a cause of failure. For a year Dr. Watson had a seat at the National Vaccine Board, and he then had opportunities of satisfying himself that lymph, which had been transmitted without interruption from person to person ever since the time of Jenner, continued to generate what seemed a very perfect cow-pox vesicle. And it is the expressed opinion of the permanent members of that Board that the vaccine lymph does not lose any of its prophylactic power by a continued transit through successive subjects. M. Simon has, however, stated some strong grounds for suspecting that the occasional impermanence of protection may depend upon impairment in the specific power of vaccine contagion—an impairment arising in the transmission of that contagion through many generations of men. It was alleged by M. Brisset, in France, as early as 1818, that the past ten years had made a marked difference in the visible characters of the vaccine vesicle; that it has become necessary to establish, instead of Jenner's two vesicles, eight or ten points of infection. Dr. Meyer, of Kreutzberg, states, that on examining, in 1824 and 1825, nearly four thousand vaccinated persons, of all ages, he found the older scars much better marked than the recent ones; that, according to the testimony of many vaccinators, the proportion of cicatrices resulting from his own use of lymph recently obtained from the cow, were again after the old type. Dr. Gregory and Mr. Estlin, in England, have adduced similar facts, in evidence that the vaccine lymph, by passing through the bodies of many persons, loses, in process of time, some essential part of its activity.

This suspicion gathers force from a very curious result of the experience furnished by the Prussian army. It appears that where the vaccine supply has seldom or never been renewed from the cow, it has become easier to succeed in revaccinating a person, and very much in the same proportion that it has become easier for a patient to take post-vaccinal small-pox; and it is argued, How could the infantine generations of a country, year by year, successively derive less permanent constitutional impressions from vaccination, unless vaccine contagion had, year by year, undergone enfeeblement of its powers?

On this point, as on others, the statistical experience of the Prussian army is immense. The revaccination of recruits extends annually to some forty or forty-five thousand operations. It is reported upon annually. Its records run back twenty-four years. Its subjects are of like age, and under like circumstances. When this system of revaccination commenced, in 1833, the proportion of successful results (of those, that is, who again *took* the disorder) was thirty-three in every hundred. Now, the annual per centages of successful results, for the whole time during which revaccination has been practised in that army, run thus: 33, 39, 42, 46, 49, 50, 51, 54, 57, 58, 57, 57, 58, 60, 64, 64, 64, 61, 64, 69, 69,

69, 69, 70! *The last proportion of successful punctures more than double that with which the series commenced.* Supposing the first vaccination to have preceded the second by twenty years, *the vaccinations of* 1836—tested by the eventual resusceptibility to cow-pox—*were not half so stable as the vaccinations of* 1813.

In the fifth place, there are yet moot-points respecting the number of vesicles, and the degree of constitutional disturbance which are requisite to insure and prolong the protective power of vaccination. The constitutional effect will bear some proportion to the number of vesicles; and of these it would seem there should be several, and one or two of them, at least, should be suffered to pursue their course untouched. Mr. Marson believes that vaccination may be relied upon when four or more vesicles have formed, which have left good dotted cicatrices. During the five years of 1852 to 1856, of three hundred and fifty-three patients admitted, with small-pox after vaccination, into the Small-Pox and Vaccination Hospital, having each four or more vaccine cicatrices, only one died of small-pox.

I have seen a severe attack of varioloid, or rather a decided attack of discrete small-pox, in a young German woman, who had nine good vaccination-marks, each as large as a shilling, and distinctly pitted and seamed; five of these were on one arm, and four upon the other. They were arranged in rows, one row on each arm, extending from near the top of the shoulder, down below the insertion of the deltoid; so that nine vaccinations at the same time do not seem to be better than one. A second vaccination, some days or weeks after the first has run its course, is the most perfect safeguard against small-pox or varioloid.—It may be as well to add here, that I am a decided advocate for frequent revaccinations. I have been vaccinated at least a score of times, and am now not susceptible to its influence, as I have repeatedly vaccinated myself, even upon my hands and wrists. But vaccination has taken perfectly upon me three times: first, when an infant; second, when fourteen or sixteen years of age; third, when between twenty and thirty. I have been exposed to small-pox, of every grade of severity, every year, for upwards of twenty-five years, and, without the third successful vaccination, should probably have had at least an attack of varioloid.

The same gentleman who tells us that he has vaccinated between forty and fifty thousand patients, Mr. Marson asserts that one of the principal causes of failure in vaccinating, and of subsequent insecurity of the individual, even when the vaccination does take effect, is the want of care in the selection of the vaccine lymph. It is in its best state on the sixth or seventh day of the progress of the vesicle, say, the day week from the vaccination. It should be taken when the vesicle is plump, and just before the formation of the areola. Under no circumstances should it be taken for use later than twenty-four hours after the areola has began to form. If this rule were invariably observed, there would be fewer cases of severe small-pox after vaccination. There may be a worse arm, indeed, and a more apparently successful vaccination with lymph taken later, but the protection will be less perfect. He (Mr. Marson) contends—and there is every reason to believe him quite an expert vaccinator—that a serious error in vaccinating is the use of blunt lancets. It is impossible to have a lancet too sharp for vaccinating. The lymph should be introduced by a puncture of a valvular shape, from above downwards, so managed that the lymph, at each puncture, may gravitate into the wound. In this way, the lymph may be introduced in from one to five punctures, one-half to three-quarters of an inch apart.

In this country, where the scab or crust is so much more used than any other form of the virus, it is Dr. Wood's plan to reduce the virus to the consistence of pus, by the aid of water, upon a piece of glass, and then, holding the arm with the left hand, to ensure a slight degree of tension of the skin, he makes three punctures, each a line apart, disposed in the form of an equilateral triangle. This has the advantage, in the case of females, that while *one* of the punctures is almost certain to take, even if *all* should prove effective, but one pock results.

Another mode, is to make a number of parallel minute scarifications, these crossed by a similar number of transverse ones, and the virus is to be applied directly to the surface. Or the skin may be carefully scraped down with a sharp lancet, until minute points of blood or serum may be detected, and the virus is then applied directly to the surface, as in the preceding case. In any case, the only object is to secure an absorbing surface.

These, however, are minor points, in which each may consult his own experience, and, in a degree, his convenience. But I am myself inclined to think, from a careful comparison of the many different statements on the subject, that in this country, (America,) where the use of the scab or crust is so universal, and recourse to the fresh lymph so rare, we are fully as much and perhaps oftener visited with small-pox after vaccination than in England or on the Continent. It certainly has been so prevalent that many practitioners have felt it right to caution their well-vaccinated patients against exposure to any *chance* of contagion. It may be objected to this that the scab produces what *seems* a very perfect cow-pox vesicle, and that we are to abide by that. But the scar is not *always* to be taken as an index. It is a well-ascertained and parallel fact, that, though vaccination with *lymph* taken *after* the formation of the areola will produce a larger scar and a worse arm than the more benignant lymph of the earlier stage, the protection afforded is much less certain, and the danger to which the patient is subjected greater. Now, as the scab is the desiccated lymph and pus mingled—of all the stages indifferently—if its powers for ill have declined, and no malignant sore is produced, as in the case of tenth-day lymph, so also must its powers for good—i. e., its protective influence. I cannot but regard the use of the lymph, if carefully followed, as the more preferable practice.

The benefits which this safeguard of vaccination confers on the individual, are scarcely inferior to those which it is calculated to bestow on society. It unfortunately does not give complete protection against small-pox to all, but it gives complete protection to many. And we must recollect that small-pox itself is not a universal and absolute assurance against its own return. But the cow-pox relieves all from the necessity imposed by inoculation of coming within the sphere of variolous contagion. It renders many, I repeat, impregnable to that poison, if they do chance to be within its range; and its advantage to the comparative few, who suffer the double misfortune of being exposed to the contagion of small-pox, and of being affected by it, is this, that it gives safety, though not exemption—that it takes away the sting and peril of the variolous disease by curtailing it of the secondary fever. At the very worst, it leaves the individual liable, by a two-fold ill luck, to contract a form of small-pox not more dangerous than that which he would voluntarily accept by submitting to the operation of inoculation.

The protecting power of vaccination being definitely established, the question arises, Is it possible, after forty-five years experience, to determine the limits of that power?—The answer to this question is extremely difficult, but it may be approximated. It was found, on making the necessary observations, that somewhat more than one-third of the entire number of persons attacked with small-pox had been vaccinated; secondly, that the mortality among the vaccinated persons was very small. According to the author of one of the memoirs, more than one-third of those attacked, in the epidemics which occurred at Montbeillard, had been vaccinated, but there was no corresponding increase in the amount of mortality among the vaccinated patients; and the same result was observed in the epidemic of 1828, at Marseilles.

The fact, then, being established, that vaccinated persons can become affected with small-pox, and the proportion so attacked during the epidemics being nearly determined, a most important problem remains to be solved, viz.: What was the condition of the vaccinated persons affected, as regards the mere fact of their vaccination?—The authors of all the memoirs agree in stating that vaccinated persons were not affected indiscriminately, or by chance, as it were; on the contrary, the small-pox seems to make a kind of selection among them. With a few exceptions, it attacks those who have been vaccinated since a long time, and spares those who are recently so. It seems that children are seldom attacked until the ninth year after vaccination, and that it attacks by preference those who have been vaccinated fifteen, twenty, thirty, or thirty-five years previously. A general fact, which may be anticipated from the history of eruptive complaints, is that, after the age of thirty-five years, the aptitude of the vaccinated to contract small-pox becomes so slight that it may be considered as having vanished.

We may assume that the protective power of vaccination is absolute and general for the first five or six years, and even to the eleventh or twelfth year, to judge from the experiments on revaccination; and, after the foregoing period, a part, and a part only, of those vaccinated again become liable, especially under the influence of an epidemic, to contract small-pox. A large number of those vaccinated, probably remain completely protected during their entire life. Revaccination, at intervals of seven, eight, or ten years, will doubtless prevent both small-pox and varioloid. With a little care, varioloid could almost as certainly be eradicated as can small-pox.

Again, has the cow-pox, taken directly from the cow, a more certain and permanent protective power than vaccine matter that has been transmitted, more or less frequently, through the human constitution?—It would appear, from the very best authority, that the intensity of the new or fresh lymph, direct from the cow, is much greater; but, as regards the relation between the lesser or greater intensity of the local phenomena and the protective power of the *variolous* matter, experiments show that *the protective power of vaccine matter is not proportionate to the intensity of the local symptoms, but that vaccination with matter taken from the cow is more certain than vaccination with old vaccine matter.*

As to the means of renewal, the first mode resorted to was to transmit the vaccine matter back to the cow. Vaccine matter, thus regenerated, failed in less than one case in a hundred, while the failures of the old vaccine matter were nearly three per cent. But, by all means, the best mode is to obtain it direct from the cow.

The questions may be thus summed up:

First, The preservative power of vaccination is absolute for the majority, and temporary for a small number; and even in the latter it is absolute until adolescence.

Second, Small-pox rarely attacks those who have been vaccinated in infancy, before the age of ten or twelve years; from which time, however, until thirty or thirty-five, they are particularly liable to small-pox.

Third, Even in those cases in which it fails to protect the individual from an attack of small-pox, vaccination, nevertheless, so modifies the economy as to render the symptoms of small-pox milder, abridges its duration, and considerably diminishes its danger.

Fourth, Vaccine matter, taken directly from the cow, causes local symptoms of greater intensity; its effects are also more certain than those of old vaccine matter, but, after being transmitted for a few weeks through the human subject, its local intensity disappears.

Fifth, The preservative power of vaccine matter does not seem to be intimately connected with the intensity of the symptoms of vaccination; nevertheless, it is prudent to regenerate vaccine matter as frequently as possible, to preserve its protective power.

Sixth, The only mode of regenerating vaccine matter deserving of confidence is to procure it direct from the cow.

Seventh, Revaccination is the only method known of distinguishing those vaccinated persons that remain fully protected from those that do not.

Eighth, The success of revaccination is not a certain proof that the person in whom it succeeds was liable to contract small-pox; it merely establishes a tolerably strong presumption that they were more or less liable to the variolous infection.

Ninth, In ordinary periods, revaccination should be practiced at least after fourteen years; but sooner, as already remarked, especially during epidemics, which now occur every four years; in short every eight or ten years is safest.

Abortive Treatment of Small-Pox.—It has long been customary to vaccinate persons supposed to be attacked with varioloid or small-pox. It has also been proposed and tried with success to vaccinate the patient thoroughly and by many points, (thirty or forty,) so soon as it may be ascertained that the symptoms arise from small-pox contagion. It is asserted that the disease is greatly modified and ameliorated by it.

As a general rule, it may be stated that, where vaccination has been performed within less than four days after exposure to the small-pox infection, the disease has been uniformly prevented. Williamson, in the case of an infant, born prematurely at the eighth month, and whose mother had been sick with small-pox for six days, and who died of confluent disease on the eleventh day, vaccinated the child on the third day after its birth. The vaccine disease ran its course regularly and fully, and the babe escaped the variola, although it must have been exposed in utero for six days, and for three days after birth.

If vaccination be delayed more than four days after the small-pox incubation, there is reason to believe that a successful vaccination will modify the small-pox but not entirely prevent it. The premonitory symptoms of modified small-pox have been known to appear eight days after successful vaccination, the patient having been vaccinated on the fifth day after exposure.

Numerous cases have occurred where vaccination and varioloid have both run their course, in the same individual, at the same time, but each in a modified form: the vaccinia is prolonged, while the variola is shortened, the secondary fever prevented, and no cicatrices left behind

Vaccine Treatment.—The homœopathists have been in the habit of using vaccine matter internally for many years But lately a communication has been made to our Secretary of State, the Hon. Lewis Cass, and made public in the *American Journal of Medical Sciences*, for October, 1857. The vaccine virus is there recommended by a Dr. Landell, of Porte Alegre, Brazil, administered internally, for the cure of small-pox. It is not a new suggestion; but, apart from the unpleasant idea attaching to it, it would appear unobjectionable. The fact, however, that most animal poisons are changed, and rendered harmless and innocuous in their passage through the alimentary canal, would somewhat militate against its extensive trial.

Dr. Landell directs us to dissolve the virus contained on a pair of plates, or a capillary tube, which is about four or six drops of vaccine lymph, in four or six ounces of cold water, and give to the patient a tablespoonful every two or three hours. He says, that "It mitigates the symptoms, modifies the variety, and cures the disease. Under its use, the fever, the delirium, the hoarseness, diarrhœa, pneumonia, cerebral congestion, and finally the secondary fever disappear.

"Beginning the treatment on the second or third day of the eruption, the small-pox becomes more like varicella or varioloid than anything else, although the epidermis is thickened and congested, it will be dry in five days without any suppuration.

"Beginning the same treatment on the fourth or fifth day of the eruption, the small-pox becomes like the true vaccine, the pustules fill and dry in the space of ten days, *with* suppuration."

He always advocates opening the vesicles two or three times after the third day, when they contain any fluid, "to prevent the secondary fever," and recommends gargles of Nitrate of Silver, and Chloruret of Lime or Soda.

He casually speaks of having given vaccine inwardly, as a remedy in whooping cough, and with benefit. In some cases, the whooping or convulsive cough disappeared in two hours, only a simple cough remaining, which yielded in four to twelve days.

The homœopathists have been using Vaccinin internally for many years. According to Rückert, Schellhamer says that the sixth dilution of Vaccinin causes varioloid to dry up rapidly in children, but does not accomplish so much in adults; still he supposes that it shortens the course of the disease. I have used the first trituration in infants of only a few months old, without any bad effects; on the contrary, unvaccinated infants, exposed to confluent small-pox in the same house, have escaped the disease entirely, although the grandmother had the varioloid and the father the confluent small-pox, although repeated vaccinations by myself and other physicians have failed to produce any local effects. In one instance, many months afterwards, the vaccination took perfectly, although the infant had taken at least twenty doses of Vaccinin internally. Another unvaccinated infant, in a different house, whose vaccination also failed repeatedly, but who did not take any Vaccinin internally, took the discrete small-pox quite severely, from exposure to varioloid in the father. Rummel says, he has repeatedly seen a rapid interruption of the course of varioloid from the use of the third dilution of Vaccinin; the pustules dried up in five or seven days, without leaving any pits. In a case of small-pox, confluent on the face, hands, and feet, in which it was used, no scars were left; but we have no proof that this was not an example of the modified-confluent variety. Hencke, on the authority of Rückert, has experimented with Vaccinin since 1839; in that year, he treated one hundred and ten persons with it. In fifteen persons, of various ages, who had all been previously vaccinated, he succeeded in preventing the eruption, although they had already commenced to complain of lumbar pains, lassitude, alternate chills and heat, loss of appetite, nausea, and oppression of the stomach. They recovered in four to six days, some of them after critical attacks of vomiting, and did not again take the disease, although they were obliged to live with small-pox patients. Still, some of these cases may have been examples of variola without eruption. I had two cases of the kind, in a family where the father had varioloid, and an unvaccinated little girl had a severe attack of discrete small-pox; both the mother and the child's nurse had very severe attacks of *variola sine eruptione;* they were both sick in bed for several days, with high fever, severe backache, nausea, and vomiting, and then recovered rapidly without the occurrence of a single pimple; they took no Vaccinin internally, and their external vaccination failed.

In many other cases, Hencke did not succeed in preventing the eruption, although he gave several doses of Vaccinin very early in the disease; still, it ran its course like mild varioloid: the salivation and throat-affection were very slight, and the eruption, although very copious, only came out for twenty-four or forty-eight hours, and never progressed to the pustular stage, but formed pearl-colored, semi-globular vesicles, with a depression at the apex, and which dried up in from five to seven days, without secondary fever.

Hencke also thought Vaccinin useful when given late in the eruptive stage; for the salivation and throat-affection abated speedily, the secondary suppurative fever was scarcely perceptible, and the pustules began to dry up on the ninth or tenth day of the disease, and sixth or seventh of the eruption. They either turned brown, and began to dry up, so that they soon formed brown and empty shells or crusts, which was the case especially on the extremities; or else they broke, discharged their contents, and formed larger or smaller yellowish brown scabs, especially on the face, from whence they soon dried up and fell off; the urine was brownish red, and deposited a thick brick-red sediment. But few secondary affections, or ulcerations, or scars occurred. Hencke at first used fresh vaccine lymph, well shaken up in alcohol; afterwards the second dilution. Some years after, he treated six cases of natural small-pox, and four cases of modified, and supposed that he prevented or broke three cases in the first stage by the use of Vaccinin. Bentzendorff, Gross, and Bethman have also used the Vaccinin with more or less success, but their cases are not well detailed.

Case 1.—A girl, aged fifteen, previously vaccinated, was attacked. The pustules were large and umbilicated; the hands and feet were considerably swollen, and she had such oppression of the chest that she could scarcely speak; very dry, hot skin; small, quick pulse; much thirst; dry, coated, blackish tongue and teeth. One half grain of the third trituration of Vaccinin was given. The anxiety and oppression abated speedily, also the violent thirst, followed by perspiration and sleep, and all danger seemed over in four hours. The subsequent course of the disease was regular and favorable.

Case 2.—A vaccinated person had violent premonitory symptoms of small-pox. The eruption came out on the fifth day, was umbilicated on the sixth, and Vaccinin, third dilution, was given on the seventh; on the eighth day, some of the pustules were covered with brown crusts, and the vesicles were filled with yellow matter, somewhat resembling chicken-pox; on the ninth day, all were dried up. The pustules only lasted four days in all.

Case 3.—A woman, aged thirty-eight, who had never been vaccinated, and who had been much exposed to small-pox, received two doses of Vaccinin on the first and second days of sickness. She vomited several times, and red pimples appeared on the face and hands on the evening of the second day, and her throat pained her, but not much; she had a restless night and no sleep. On the third day, her face was abundantly covered with small, red pock-pimples, with many vesicles; she was more comfortable, and had but little fever at night, as is usual. On the fourth day, the eruption had spread over the whole body, and the pustules on the face were filled with turbid benign pus. On the sixth day, the pustules began to dry up, and the patient was very comfortable. She was well in fourteen days.

In another case, in a previously vaccinated woman, aged thirty-six, but in whom no vaccine mark was visible, the disease ran a more severe course, and the patient was not well until the twenty-seventh day. The case does not seem to have been a confluent one, and only of average severity for a discrete case. I have given the first trituration in a case of confluent small-pox, in a previously vaccinated person: the case ran a very favorable course, no severe secondary fever occurred, and the patient convalesced rapidly, as I suppose a case of modified-confluent small-pox would do. Numerous small pits, but no large scars were left; the patient was convalescent in two or three weeks, although the fever, vomiting, and backache had been intense, and the eruption very copious and decidedly confluent. The Vaccinine was not given until the fifth or sixth day.

Variolin has also been used by Syrbius, Tietze, Schnappauf, Trinks, Attomyr, Schmid, Gross, Dudgeon, Hencke, and Liedbeck. The success is apparently great, but not greater than with Vaccinin. I regard it as a dangerous remedy to be carried about indiscriminately, and that its use should be discouraged.

Medical Treatment of Small-Pox.—In few diseases has medical opinion undergone a greater or more beneficial change than in this. Under the impression that the eruption was an effort of nature to rid the system of noxious matter, which, if retained, must prove fatal, it was deemed important to favor, instead of repressing the process. It was known that heating and stimulating measures promoted the eruption. Hence arose the practice of sedulously excluding fresh air from the sick-room, heaping up bed-clothes upon the patient, giving him hot drinks, and not unfrequently administering stimulants. Now that the the greatest danger in small-pox is known to arise from the copiousness of the eruption, it will be readily understood how fatal must have been the disease under the old system of practice. To Sydenham belongs the credit of changing the current of medical sentiment in this respect. Having practically ascertained the effects of an opposite plan of treatment, he recommended it in his works, and refrigerant measures are now universally admitted to be the most efficient in the cure of the disease.

Gregory says, it is a melancholy reflection, but too true, that, for many hundred years the efforts of physicians were rather exerted to thwart nature, and to add to the malignancy of the disease, than to aid her in her efforts. Blisters, heating remedies, large bleedings, opiates, ointments, masks, and lotions, to prevent pitting, were the great measures formerly pursued, not one of which, he says, can be recommended.

Gregory does not believe that certain drugs possess the power of promoting the eruption of small-pox, or of producing a favorable kind of eruption. Nor that medical means possess the power of controlling the secondary fever of true unmodified-confluent small-pox, and its necessary consequence, pitting. He thinks that all that can be done is, 1. To moderate the violence of febrile excitement; 2. To check and relieve local determinations of blood; 3. To support the powers of the system when it flags; 4. To combat concomitant disease. It remains to be seen whether the homœopathic practice cannot advantageously supersede some of the ordinary expedients still in vogue with the majority of physicians.

The *ordinary homœopathic treatment* of small-pox, in the first stage, is to give *Aconite*, every hour or two during the primary fever, in alternation with *Bellad.*, if there be much headache or delirium. If severe backache is present, with pains in all the limbs and bones, *Bryonia* or *Rhus* are often given, either one alone or in alternation. If there is much vomiting, *Tartar-emetic*, *Ipecac.*, *Cuprum*, or *Zincum* are often used. If there be great drowsiness or stupor, *Opium* or *Stramonium;* while great restlessness or sleeplessness are often combatted with *Coffea* or *Bellad.* If the delirium persists, in the second stage, and the eruption does not come out fully, *Stramonium;* if the lungs suffer, and cough, with oppression of the chest occur, *Tartar-emetic*, *Phosphorus*, or *Ipecac.;* children often require *Bellad.* or *Stramonium* to allay nervous excitement. If the second stage progresses favorably, some physicians give *Thuja*, others *Tartar-emetic*, either alone or in alternation. In the suppurative stage, *Tartar-emetic* ought to be the favorite remedy, but *Mercurius-solubilis* is more frequently used, especially when there is much salivation. In the black small-pox, *Arsenicum* is regarded as the most frequently applicable remedy; when the debility is great, *Arsenicum*, *China*, and *Rhus*, also when typhoid symptoms occur, with dry, brown, and cracked tongue. If the eruption be suppressed, Cuprum and Sulphur are sometimes used. During the fourth stage, or that of desiccation, *Sulphur* is regarded as the best remedy; but, if diarrhœa occur, *Mercurius* is given in alternation with it; while, if the debility or itching are excessive, *Rhus* is often relied upon. The above is Pulte's plan.

Kretschmar gave Bryon., 30, one drop every twenty-four hours, to relieve the headache, nausea, vomiting, lumbar, dorsal, and muscular pains; as these disappear in a few days of themselves, he, of course, could not expect to effect much with one dose only per day. Against the throat-affection, with difficulty of swallowing, he used Arsenicum; also to remove hoarseness, and the diarrhœa in the suppurative stage; the latter often proved obstinate, still he thought the Arsen. held it in check till recovery took place. Mayrhofer used Acon., second dilution, in one-drop doses, every four hours, during the eruptive stage; Merc., 4, in the suppurative period; but, in severe cases of genuine small-pox, he administered tablespoonful doses of a solution of one-half drachm of Acid-muriat. dilut., in four ounces of water, every two or three hours. Dr. De Verneul gave Aconite during the first stage, with Bellad., if there was severe headache; in the second stage, he used Sulphur, if the eruption did not come out fully, either alone or in alternation with Merc.-sol.; in the third stage, if petechiæ, or a threatening putrid condition was present, he gave Carb.-veg. in alternation with China. He treated three hundred and ninety cases, with twenty-two deaths, and three hundred and sixty-eight recoveries; many of his patients had been vaccinated, and the older the vaccinated patient was the more severe was the disease Previous to his time, there had been one hundred and fifty-eight cases, under old-school treatment, with forty-two deaths, and one hundred and sixteen recoveries.—RÜCKERT.

Dr. Williams, of Kensington, has reported, in the *Philadelphia Journal of Homœopathy*, vol. 4, page 175, eight cases of small-pox treated with Causticum, third centesimal dilution, and Merc.-corrosiv., third dilution; the doses were repeated every hour, for the first four days, afterwards every two hours. The first case was convalescent on the tenth day—it is not stated whether the patient had been previously vaccinated; but five other cases are reported, all recovering within nine days, although none had been vaccinated. Dr. Williams supposes that when the thirtieth dilution is given, *just before* the eruption comes out, it relieves the pains in the head and nervous symptoms quite as promptly as the third; nature undoubtedly does more than either dilution. Dr. W. also treated sixteen cases of varioloid with the same remedies, but in the thirtieth dilution; none overran six days, and, in the majority, the eruptive stage only lasted four or five days.

A weak solution of Corrosive Sublimate, viz., one grain to eight ounces of distilled water, applied by means of compresses wet with it, is also said (not by Dr. Williams) to produce very marked effects, in causing the disappearance of the pustules, even after they have fully matured; but we have no security that the authors of this practice have not unwittingly based their favorable opinion upon its application in modified cases. And I have not the slightest hesitation in asserting that I have not a particle of belief in the efficacy of the thirtieth dilution, in any otherwise fatal and non-self-limited disease. Discrete and semi-confluent cases of small-pox are much more frequent, even in unvaccinated persons, than confluent, and these are comparatively not dangerous, and naturally leave but few scars. Of four hundred and thirty-eight cases of varioloid, under old-school treatment, only two died; while of fifty-eight unprotected cases, sixteen died, and some that recovered were disfigured for life.

Dr. J. Redman Cox, of Philadelphia, gives Acon., Bellad., or Bryonia in the first stage; after the pimples appear, he invariably gives a dose of Vaccinin every four hours, till the fifth or sixth day. For sore throat, he gives Merc.-viv., or Merc.-iodatus; in cases verging on typhoid, he found Arsen., Bry., and Rhus-tox., very efficient; in cases with bloody urine and purple-colored petechiæ, he says, Canth., Uva-ursi, and Arsen. had a most happy effect. In albuminuria, he gave Gallic-acid, probably in massive doses. He thus claims to have treated forty-seven cases of *confluent* small-pox, some of which *were quite mild*, a few very severe, and others malignant; without losing a case, and without leaving a pit, mark, or scar. As the remedies were used in the third, sixth, and ninth dilution, it is very probable that the Vaccinin was the most useful part of the treatment, although we are not told how many cases had been vaccinated, and hence cannot infer how much nature and partial vaccine protection did for them.

Where so many different remedies are said to be so very useful, we naturally become somewhat suspicious of all, unless they are given in doses sufficient to produce a decided effect, either for good or evil; or a thorough knowledge of the natural course of the disease convinces us that some agent must have modified its course. The striking peculiarities of the modified-confluent small-pox are familiar to few physicians only; vaccination, like good blood in a horse, will often tell at the end of the race with disease, and it often proves the best friend of those who condemn it most. In the *British Journal of Homœopathy*, vol. 9, page 480, we find a case in point. Kate Buckly, aged fifteen, vaccinated when young, had been sick six days; had a thick crop of pustules on her face, *becoming confluent* without much swelling; pulse 96, tongue very foul. Had taken Sulphur, 6, for several days, and now got Bellad., 3, and Merc., 3, every second hour, in alternation. On the next day, the eruption was fully developed, with an immense *confluent crop* on the face and arms, the features were swollen, eyelids closed, throat sore, headache severe, thirst troublesome, bowels costive, and pulse had run up to 120. The same remedies were continued for eight days in all, the case progressing favorably, when Sulphur, 6, was again given, to promote desquamation. It is self-evident that nature effected this cure.

The physician will probably be required first to prescribe for *fever*, *headache*, and *vomiting*. The latter is often very intense, continuing for two or more days, and frequently accompanied by tenderness of the epigastrium on pressure. It generally subsides of itself when the eruption appears; but, Heberden says, if the vomiting be continued after the eruption is completed, the patient's life is in great danger, even though the small-pox be not confluent.

In ordinary practice, if the stomach remains very irritable during the initiatory fever, saline effervescing draughts and Opium are generally used, aided by mustard-poultices to the epigastrium and feet.

In the homœopathic practice, *Tartar-emetic* is regarded as the most appropriate remedy, not only against the gastric derangement, but also to moderate the fever and control the eruptive disorder. Billing, a well-known allopathic medical writer, says, he knows full well that emetics will allay vomiting, and that Tartar-emetic will cure the vomiting of cholera quicker than any other remedy; and that it will, perhaps, astonish many to learn that Tartar-emetic relieves nausea and vomiting, in like manner as sedative remedies do, and that the nausea and vomiting in inflammation of the stomach can often be relieved by means of repeated small doses of Tartar-emetic. Eberlee (see "Materia Medica") says, that Schonheyder and Burdach have found Ipecac. very useful in habitual vomiting from morbid irritability of the stomach, but it must be given in very small doses.

Another large class of cases will commence with a chill, more or less severe, followed by fever, with severe pains in the head and *small of the back*, aching in the bones, and general soreness. The *lumbar* pain is one of the most common precursory symptoms of small-pox, is often of a great degree of severity, and is not met with in either scarlet fever or measles, at least to a degree at all marked. An excruciating pain in the loins is generally succeeded by a bad attack of small-pox, and the more violent has been the pain the greater the danger; still, a mild attack of varioloid sometimes follows severe pain in the back, and the reverse of this is also true. The backache is supposed to arise from congestion and irritation, and Bryonia and Rhus are regarded as the most useful remedies, although Aconite will also relieve the severe muscular pains, and lessen the attending fever.

As regards the treatment of the *initiatory fever* of small-pox, it very often happens that the disease is not suspected until the eruption appears, and the ordinary antiphlogistic or anti-febrile treatment is pursued in both schools. In the dominant school, the surface is kept moderately cool, a brisk cathartic is given, effervescing saline draughts are used, also James' powder, &c.; and, if there be severe pain in the head, back, or epigastrium, more urgent than these measures can control, a small quantity of blood is sometimes taken from the arm. Still, it is well ascertained that bleeding will neither eradicate the fever nor materially diminish the amount of the eruption. Gregory says, it has been supposed that blood-letting interrupts the process of nature, repels the eruption or retards it, and so weakens the constitution that the due concoction of the pustules is never effected; but, although many a small-pox patient has been bled unnecessarily, and too largely, yet he thinks that a moderate bleeding does no harm, and, if the fever runs high, often does great good. And he even goes so far as to assume that if the pulse be sharp or very full, the headache severe, with accompanying epistaxis, then blood-letting is not only very useful but absolutely indispensable; for the eruptive process is often impeded by the excess of blood in the body, and the violence of the arterial excitement. Huxham says, we should bleed in the onset of these fevers, for the same reason that we draw off part of a fermenting liquor to prevent the splitting of the vessel. By drawing off some blood he thought he prevented over-distending, inflaming, and rending the vessels of the human body. Gregory assumes that the object in bleeding is to unload and relieve the lungs, liver, or brain, and that whenever these organs are gorged, and their functions impeded by a load of stagnant or inflamed blood, when intense headache, extreme irritability of the stomach, oppressed breathing, with a full, laboring pulse, give evidence of such general or local congestion, then bleeding should be resorted to, although he admits that it has no effect on the quantity of eruption; for, he says, the most confluent eruption has succeeded to the most vigorous employment of the lancet. Still, he thinks that one must bleed in order to relieve internal congestion, but not so as to impair constitutional power; while to bleed simply because small-pox is expected, and to prevent confluence, is uselessly to expend that force which will soon be required to repair the injuries to the surface. Watson rather slights blood-letting, saying, that as the principal object in the treatment of small-pox is to prevent, if possible, a copious eruption, upon which the severity and peril of the disorder entirely depend, it has been thought that bleeding, by its antiphlogistic power, and perhaps by letting out with the blood some of the accumulating and fermenting virus, might lessen the number of the forthcoming pustules; but he says we cannot ensure this result by blood-letting, and, should the eruption prove confluent, suppuration to a large amount is inevitable, and all the resources of the constitution will be required.

As small-pox is always aggravated by its concurrence with a state of plethora, it may, perhaps, be necessary or allowable to bleed once, when a severe case of small-pox occurs in a too full-blooded subject, simply to reduce the whole mass of blood to the natural healthy standard. The patient should, if possible, have nothing else to contend with but his disease; on the same principle, if he have a foul stomach, loaded bowels, an excess of bile, &c., before he is attacked with the disorder, these morbid states should be rectified as early as possible, and by evacuant means if required. In the regular practice, laxatives and purgatives are often used more or less freely, to allay fever and diminish the amount of congestive irritation of the system, and also the virulence of the eruption. The compound cathartic dragees, Citrate of Magnesia, Seidlitz Powders, or Congress Water, are generally used when rather urgent symptoms are present, or at least troublesome constipation. Similar or more powerful laxatives are often given when the febrile symptoms do not abate as they ought in the regular course of the disease, or are attended with congestion of some important organ, and constipation.

In the homœopathic school, blood-letting is avoided, and *Aconite* and *Tartar-emetic* are relied upon to abate the primary fever. Aconite is regarded by some as an antiphlogistic sudorific remedy, which lessens the force and frequency of the pulse, and tends to produce copious perspiration, without heating the patient. It has also been supposed that it will remove the muscular and lumbar pains, in like manner as it does the syphilitic pains, although the remedy itself is apt to cause pains in the limbs, especially so-called bone-pains and pains in the joints; still the celebrated Storck thought that the acridities which attacked the nerves and bones were solved by the Aconite, brought into the circulation, and then cast out by the profuse sweats and urinations which the remedy is apt to cause. As a topical remedy for rheumatic and neuralgic pains, Aconite is invaluable, while its internal use is often equally beneficial, and, of course, can be brought to bear on parts which cannot be reached by an external application; and there is no reason why it should not relieve variolous pains as well as the syphilitic, neuralgic, and rheumatic.

Tartar-emetic is admitted, in all schools, to be a most powerful antiphlogistic and anti-febrile remedy; while the homœopathists suppose that it sustains a peculiar and specific relation to small-pox and other pustular diseases. The action of Tartar-emetic on the circulation and respiration is said to be that of a sedative; it has reduced the pulse from one hundred and twenty to thirty-four beats per minute, in nine days, and the respiration from fifty to eighteen. It causes sweating, without any very marked vascular excitement; promotes secretion and exhalation from the gastro-intestinal mucous membrane, and from the liver and pancreas, while it renders the mucous membranes, especially of the air-passages, moister.

All these effects of Tartar-emetic render it a proper remedy in many febrile diseases, in the opinion of physicians of almost all schools; but it is also a powerful local irritant, causing an eruption of painful pustules, resembling those of *variola* or ecthyma, and even Pereira regards these irritant properties as peculiar or specific. But it is not only emetic, but, of all emetic substances, creates the most nausea and depression; and we have seen that the outbreak of small-pox is often attended with an unusual amount of vomiting.

Besides all this, Tartarized Antimony produces a pustule hardly to be distinguished from the eruption of small-pox. According to Wood, of Philadelphia, when Tartar-emetic is kept for some time in contact with the skin, it produces inflammation, with a peculiar and quite characteristic eruption. It operates with much greater facility in some persons than in others, with so far as it appears the same delicacy of cuticle; so that its influence is probably dynamic. An increased heat is felt in the skin, with a prickling sensation; and, on examination, the surface is reddened with numerous red, papulous spots. The pimples become converted into vesicles or pustules, some of which are small and hemispherical (*variolæ discretæ?*); others are large, from half an inch to an inch in diameter, flat, with a dark crust in the centre (*variolæ confluentes?*). The smaller ones are semi-globular; the larger ones, when at their height, are flattened, are surrounded with an inflammatory border, contain a pseudo-membranous deposit (*variolous slough?*) and some purulent serum, and have a central dark point. When they have attained their greatest magnitude, the central brown spots become larger and darker, and, in a few days, desiccation takes place, and the crusts are thrown off. If the Antimonial be continued, the eruption takes on an ulcerative form, and scars are not unfrequently left behind, having all the appearance of small-pox scarring.

This pustular disease, caused by Tartar-emetic, does not always need an actual application to the skin to produce it. It has sometimes followed its internal administration. (See "New Materia Medica," pp. 400 to 410.)

According to Wood, it also produces a pustular eruption in the throat and fauces, and occasionally in the intestines (internal use); and white aphthous spots have been observed on the velum and tonsils. A severe inflammation of the throat (angina-antimonialis) has sometimes followed its employment.

It has also been proposed to make of it a substitute for vaccination. It has been stated that if the virus from a Tartar-emetic pustule be introduced into the arm of another person, vesicles are produced not to be distinguished from the cow-pox or vaccine vesicle; that they excite fresh pustules by inoculation, and that these confer the same immunity as regards the contagion of small-pox. How far this may be true, remains to be proved; but Dr. Lichtenstein claims to have inoculated thirty-one patients in this way with complete success, and that not one of them took the small-pox during an epidemic.

The antimonial treatment has been thoroughly tried by a number of physicians. It always allays the fever, and calms the arterial excitement. It may prove useful in the diarrhœas which often attend small-pox, for in cholera and choleraic diarrhœas, Dr. Billing and other physicians of the opposite school testify to having employed it effectively. It was observed that the mortality under the use of Tartar-emetic, in cholera, was only nineteen per cent., while under Mercury it was thirty-six per cent., and under stimulants fifty-eight per cent.

To Liedbeck, of Stockholm, belongs the credit of introducing the Tartar-emetic treatment of small-pox; he used from one-half to one grain of pure Tartar-emetic in sixteen ounces of water, and gave a tablespoonful every four hours. He says that the tongue becomes cleaner after the first dose, while the fever and skin-affections abate, and the whole disease assumes a milder character and course; even the difficulty of swallowing was relieved, if the remedy was given early enough. If there was an offensive smell from the mouth, and salivation, he rubbed a small quantity of mercurial ointment from ear to ear; in twelve to twenty-four hours after, the patient was able to swallow with more ease.

At a later period, Liedbeck gave two or three drops of Antimonial-wine per dose, every three or four hours; he thought that larger doses were apt to cause nausea and vomiting. He claims not to have lost a patient since 1839, and thought that it allayed the excessive itching and the fever better than any other remedy. Trinks did not find it so useful. I have repeatedly put one-fourth to one-half a grain of Tartar-emetic in a tumbler of water, giving one or two teaspoonfuls per dose, every one, two, or four hours, and seen nausea, vomiting, and diarrhœa subside under its use, both in varioloid, small-pox, and other diseases. I have seen smaller doses used in confluent small-pox, such as the first dilution, in solution, without beneficial effect. It should be avoided in the later stages of the disease, when the debility is great.

Mackenzie (see "Diseases of the Eye," p. 504) says he has seen Tartar-emetic productive of the best effects in abating the inflammation and promoting the absorption of any abscess which may have formed in the cornea, from secondary variolous ophthalmia; but he often gave it so as to vomit and purge freely.

In the sixth number of *Braithwaite's Retrospect*, p. 125, we learn that various eruptions of the skin yield favorably and rapidly to Antimony. In all forms of impetigo (a pustular disease) and encrusted sores, the rapidity with which the Antimonial treatment effects a cure is truly marvellous; exaggerated cases of herpes yield with extraordinary rapidity—ten or fourteen days being sometimes sufficient in cases where other treatment required three or four months.

Hence, in every view of the case, from old-school theory and new-school theory, and from the experience of both schools, Tartar-emetic is evidently a remedy which must prove very useful in some of the forms and complications of small-pox. But it should be used in reasonable or rational doses; neither in unreasonably large or irrationally small quantities.

In the *British Journal of Homœopathy*, vol. x., p. 262, the frank and honest Dr. Dudgeon reports a case of modified small-pox, treated with Tartar-emetic, fifth dilution, one-half drop every eight hours. I regard such doses as utterly inefficient, and Dr. D. says this was one of those cases of modified small-pox where, although the eruption was considerable, and the symptoms severe, the disease declined very suddenly; thereby showing that the influence of the vaccination, though not powerful enough to prevent the disease, is still felt by the system, and renders the variola perfectly innocuous. He does not suppose that the little medicine he gave had any influence in bringing about the speedy recovery; for he has observed, under allopathic treatment, and no treatment, equally rapid convalescence in cases of the modified disease, even when the invasion of the disease was much more severe, the eruption much more extensive, and *even when it has had a completely confluent character.* The disease, in such cases, seems to experience a sort of blight, when the pocks become filled, and the much dreaded suppurative fever is scarcely or not at all perceptible. The pocks do not seem, as in natural small-pox, to fill with pus, but wither away, with only a milky-looking fluid in them, and *produce no destruction of substance,* so as to cause no disfiguring pock-marks.

Asthenic and Typhoid Cases.—In another class of cases, in the first and second stages of the disease, the circulation is apt to be languid, the pulse small and feeble, the skin pale, and the extremities cold; the patient may lie on his back, sunk and exhausted, the eruptive nisus is prevented by depression, and nature appears obviously unequal to the task. In ordinary practice, warm brandy and water is given, the patient is covered with bed-clothes, mustard poultices are applied to the centre and extremities of the circulatory system, and from ten to thirty drops of Laudanum are given, to be repeated in four hours. Part of this treatment may not only be very useful, but is, perhaps, indispensable. But there is a question if Opium is not a dangerous remedy in this condition, however much its secondary depressing and venous effects may be obviated by the simultaneous use of warm brandy and mustard poultices. Its use is based upon the following effects of this drug: According to Wood, when a moderate dose is taken, it causes a slight feeling of warmth in the stomach; in ten or fifteen minutes, a sensation of fullness in the head is experienced, which is soon followed by a universal feeling of delicious ease and comfort, with an elevation and expansion of the whole moral and intellectual nature; in from one-half to two, three, or four hours, this exaltation fades into a corporeal and mental calmness, which, in a short time, ends in sleep, after which the patient experiences a state of greater or less depression, indicated by languor and restlessness, a relaxed surface, a rather feeble pulse, and not unfrequently loss of appetite, nausea, and even vomiting. The first operation of Opium is supposed to be that of a stimulant to the surface; for, within ten or fifteen minutes after its administration, the pulse is, in general, moderately increased in frequency, fullness, and force, and, at the same time, the surface of the body becomes warmer, and the face somewhat flushed; with the increased frequency of the pulse, the respiration is also somewhat quickened. Corresponding with the condition of the circulatory and respiratory movements, is that of the blood itself: it not only retains its florid color for a time, but may give a bright tint to the complexion during the stage of excitement; but, as the pulse and respiration become slower, the change from venous to arterial is less thoroughly effected, and the blood becomes darker hued, and the venous hue upon the surface, and particularly in the face, is often conspicuous. When the period of excitement is passed, and that of calmness or drowsiness supervenes, the pulse is apt to become somewhat slower, retaining, however, its fullness and force for a time; it then gradually relaxes, and finally participates in the general depression which follows the direct influence of the drug.

Watson says, about the eighth or ninth day wakefulness, restlessness, and sometimes tremors are apt to come on; and the proper remedies for this set of symptoms, in small-pox, as well as in continued fever, are opiates. He adds, in variola, when given in full doses at bed-time. their good effects are often very conspicuous the next day. When the pustules are livid and intermixed with petechiæ, and putrid symptoms occur, the disorder generally proves fatal; in such cases, in the regular ordinary practice, it is customary to prescribe Bark and acids, in addition to the wine and opiates. And we are told that the proper plan of managing the patient, during the continuance of the secondary suppurative fever, is to keep his bowels moderately open, by gentle laxatives or enemata, and to give opiates once or twice a day; the latter are thought the more necessary on account of the irritation of the skin. Still, Opium often causes the most excessive itching of the skin. Wood says, (see "Pharmacology," vol. i., p. 722,) "The itching sensation in the skin, which Opium is apt to produce, is sometimes attended with pricking, may occur in any part of the body, and is often very annoying to the patient, and may even prevent sleep; in some instances, it is attended with a *miliary*, *erythematous*, or *urticarious* eruption."

Frank reports several cases of *variolæ malignæ* treated with Opium. In one case, a little girl, aged eight years, after the small-pox spots had come out on the second day, they soon receded, and an array of the most dangerous symptoms occurred, such as twitchings and epileptic attacks, with high fever without thirst, involuntary stools, &c. On the evening of the third day, there was great restlessness, her respiration was at times heavy and sobbing, at others, short; her chin hung down, her face and limbs were cold, forehead and abdomen very hot, eyes dull, inability to swallow, pulselessness, and hippocratic countenance. Five drops of tinct. Opium were given internally, and she was rubbed with a weak solution externally; in half an hour the patient became more quiet, a profuse perspiration broke out, followed by an abundant small-pox eruption, from which she happily recovered. In another case, a boy, who had an unusually copious eruption of confluent small-pox, especially on the face, became suddenly exhausted on the ninth day of the attack, and the sixth day of the eruption. His pulse was small and quick, he had several thin stools, and the pustules, which had raised slowly, suddenly became collapsed, and a few of them became black, while the rest contained a thin, watery pus; at times, the skin was red and burning hot. He took tinct. Opium steadily for three days, first in one, then in three-drop doses, every two or three hours. He recovered perfectly.

From the above, it is evident that unless the quantity and repetitions of Opium be carefully managed, and well sustained by stimulants, it may, in its secondary effects, aggravate the nausea and vomiting which so frequently attend bad cases of small-pox, and increase the venous condition and vascular depression which mark unfavorable cases.

In the homœopathic school, *Rhus-toxicodendron* is much relied upon in the above described state of vascular paralysis or depression, when nature is obviously unequal to carry out the eruptive nisus. The exhalations from this plant, and much more the contact with it, as is well known, will cause violent itching, erysipelatous redness, considerable swelling, and finally a pemphigus, measly, scarlet fever like, or suppurative inflammation of the skin, which remains for several days, attended with fever, and then disappears, followed by desquamation of the skin. It will be seen that this is a most likely remedy to bring a suppressed eruption to the surface. It is also regarded as a stimulating and strengthening remedy, which has been found most useful in paralysis by Alderson, Horsfield, Dufresney, Elz, Van Mons, Ratier, Buchheim, Monte, Rossi, Brera, Blangy, Mangrat, Henning, Flemming, Ossaun, Heyfelder, Hildebrandt, and others. According to Sobernheim, it removes depressed and paralyzed conditions of the nervous system, is equally well adapted to remove depressed and paralytic conditions of the vascular system, and, at the same time, develop eruptions upon the skin. Tartar-emetic is generally regarded as most suitable when the febrile action runs high, and the eruption is copious and active; *Rhus*, when the nervous and vascular energies are depressed, the eruption flabby, discolored, livid, the pulse small and feeble, skin pale, and extremities cool. But there is another view which may be taken of the action of Rhus, and that is its alterative and curative action on eruptions, even when similar to those which it is apt to produce; for, on the authority of Sobernheim, an excellent writer on the materia medica of the dominant school, Dufresney, Lichtenfels, and Baudelocque have found it very serviceable against obstinate herpetic eruptions, and Delille-Flayac has even removed fungous growths by its internal use. In depressed states of the system, with suppressed or deficient eruption, it must be given in large doses, properly supported, perhaps, by warm brandy and other stimulants. In the acutely inflammatory eruptive stage, if used at all, it must be administered in quite small quantities. In depressed and paralytic affections, from one-fourth to two grains of the extract or powdered leaves are often given per dose, by allopathic physicians, and repeated every four, six, or eight hours, until ten grains are given per day. They also give teaspoonful or even tablespoonful doses, three or four times a day, of an infusion prepared with ten to twenty grains of the herb to six or eight ounces of hot water. The tincture is often given in five, ten, or fifteen drop doses, gradually increased to twenty-five. I have no experience with these large doses, but I have repeatedly given from ten to twenty times as much as the largest homœopathic doses, with none but good effects. Waring (see "Therapeutics," p. 442) corroborates its beneficial qualities in paralytic states, and says, in general it operates as a gentle laxative, notwithstanding the torpid state of the bowels of such patients. It proved successful in four cases of paralysis, in which it was employed by Dr. Alderson, of Hull, England, Dr. Duncan, and Dr. Fresnoir, in doses of one grain of the dried leaves, continued until four or five grains were given daily, or until a pricking sensation was experienced in the affected part.

According to Rückert, Dr. Horner's treatment of small-pox was limited to Aconite and Rhus-tox. mainly, both in hospital and private practice. If the inflammatory symptoms were predominant, he gave Aconite, and repeated it every two or three hours until they abated, which was generally in one or two days; then he gave Rhus, every two or three hours, and assures his readers that in very numerous cases no other remedy was required. Mayrhofer reports the case of a girl, aged eighteen years, who was seized with small-pox shortly after being worn out with nursing a sick friend. There was burning fever, excessive exhaustion, urgent thirst, noises in the ears, dry, cracked tongue, the lips and teeth were covered with a tough brown mucus, the abdomen was distended, and the small-pox eruption was flabby and depressed, while the areolæ of many of the pustules were lived, instead of being bright red. He gave one-eighth of a grain doses of extract of Rhus-tox. every three hours, and, on the following day, was astounded at the favorable change which had taken place. The typhoid symptoms had disappeared, and the eruption was in a state of active development and reaction; the disease now ran a regular course, and terminated in health.

Of course this remedy must be given in sufficient quantity and frequency. A case is reported in the *Philadelphia Journal of Homœopathy*, vol. ii., p. 377, in which a lady, pregnant eight months, took Rhus, 6, for three days, for the premonitory symptoms of small-pox; but, on the evening of the third day, the fever increased, and she became restless and frequently delirious, and remained so with little variation till the sixth day, when premature delivery suddenly took place, and the small-pox eruption appeared. She died on the tenth day of confluent disease. The doses of Rhus were probably altogether too small.

According to Pereira, this plant produces "in certain individuals, exposed to its influence, violent itching, redness, and erysipelatous swelling of the face, hands, or other parts which have been exposed to its influence. These effects are followed by vesications, and desquamation of the cuticle. In some cases, the swelling of the face has been so great as to have almost obliterated the features."

According to Merat and Deleus, the results of the inhalation of the atmosphere of Rhus-toxicodendron develop themselves in a few hours, and sometimes after some days; they consist of itching, swelling, redness, pain, and pustules, which are more or less vesicular, on the part which has been in contact with the plant, and even on those parts which have not been in contact, as the face, scrotum, eyelids, &c. They are generally accompanied with fever *malaise*, and oppression, lasting for several days, &c.

While the pustules are in process of maturation, the patient should be in a large cool room, covered lightly with bed-clothes; all flannel covering next the skin, if any be worn, should be removed. In all cases, even of moderate intensity, it is proper to cut the hair close, and to maintain it during the whole course of the disease; it is much better for the hair to do this, and also for the patient; for the head is kept cool, delirium is more easily relieved and prevented, cleanliness can more readily be enforced, and the risk of cellular inflammation of the scalp is diminished. I have seen much suffering and filth engendered by neglect of this simple precaution, in severe cases of small-pox. I have found the hair matted together with offensive pus, huge scabs, held down near the scalp by the hair, with much putrefying matter beneath them, so that it was impossible to cleanse the head without removing the hair, which it would have been infinitely wiser to have done at an earlier period.

The diet of the patient, in the earlier stages of maturation, should consist of tea, bread and milk, arrowroot, rice, milk, farina, hominy, &c.; roasted apples, grapes, oranges, and ripe sub-acid fruits are grateful to the patient, and useful adjuvants to the antiphlogistic remedies. Lemonade, apple water, tamarind water, toast water, flax-seed tea, barley water, or milk and water should be the ordinary beverages. At a later period of the disease, more decidedly nourishing means will probably have to be used. Thorough ventilation of the room and house should be constantly kept up. Wine-whey, and beef tea are often required later in the disease, and even more powerful stimulants, if the debility be great or progressive. In the advanced stages of the secondary fever, the system of the patient requires maintenance and support; for the abundant suppuration and extensive cutaneous irritation combine to exhaust its strength, as is often shown by the weakness of the pulse, dark and dry tongue, blueness, paleness, or coldness of the extremities; stimulants and nutritious diet may now be called for: milk and milk punch, raw eggs, with or without wine, or boiled, or egg nog, animal broths, malt liquors, light bitter ales, wine, or even brandy may be required, aided, or not, by Muriatic or some other acids, or by Quinine, Iron, &c., according to the preferences of the different schools.

As regards *petechial small-pox*, Gregory says, this variety admits of no essential relief from medicine; he can scarcely say that he could palliate even the most pressing symptoms. Bulkley says that mild cases of this form of disease occasionally recover under the free use of stimulants, when the hæmorrhage from internal organs is not very profuse, nor very protracted; while, in still milder cases, where petechiæ exist, or spots of purpura, even of considerable extent, and the prostration is not great, and no hæmorrhage takes place from internal organs, the prognosis is very much less unfavorable. He has seen varioloid, (not small-pox,) with this complication, pass favorably through its stages without interruption, the purpura disappearing in the course of a few days. Still, Bulkley admits that others sink at once, without hæmorrhage, and without reaction enough to develop the variolous eruption. When the hæmorrhagic diathesis is accompanied by a hot skin and excited circulation, Gregory thinks that the loss of a little blood from the arm has appeared to him more effectual than any other measure; but this must always be regarded as a very hazardous remedy. When the febrile symptoms are not prominent, the patient should not be allowed to make the slightest exertion, not even to rise up in bed. One of the most prominent philanthropists of this city, died almost instantaneously, while sick with black small-pox, and after making a comparatively slight exertion—he fell dead, and literally never spoke or moved. Gregory says he prescribes infusion of roses and acids in petechial cases, more in conformity with general usage than with expectation of real benefit; while port wine and brandy may be given when the powers of life appear to fail. The homœopathists rely upon Arsenicum, Rhus, Muriatic-acid, or Phosphorus.

Arsenicum.—Kreussler says that much may be expected from Arsenicum, in nervous and putrid small-pox, when the patient suffers constantly from a burning heat, with a very frequent, quick, small pulse. Hartmann recommends it when the pustules become flabby and surrounded with a livid areola, with dryness of the tongue, and blackness of the lips, gums, and mouth; also when the eruption recedes suddenly and disappears. It has often been used against the inflammation of the throat, hoarseness, and diarrhœa, and when maturation does not take place properly.

As Arsenic is generally regarded as a tonic remedy, it may at least prove useful in some asthenic, adynamic, or putrid cases of small-pox. As it is useful in many skin-diseases, it may also prove beneficial in some varieties of small-pox. Wood (see "Therapeutics and Pharmacology," vol. ii., page 318) says, cutaneous eruptions are the affections in which Arsenic exercises its most valuable powers; and, so far as his observation goes, there is no single remedy which equals it in efficiency, not even Mercury, if the syphilitic eruptions be excepted. As it is most useful in scaly eruptions, it may be beneficial in the desquamating stage of small-pox, and some of the accidents which attend that period; but, as it is next most useful in chronic eczema (vesicular) and impetigo (pustular), it may also prove salutary in the vesicular and pustular stages of small-pox. Waring (see "Therapeutics," page 77) says, for a long period, Arsenic has been known to exercise a beneficial influence in cutaneous affections. The celebrated Bateman employed it extensively and speaks highly of its efficacy, and, more lately, Dr. Hunt, of Margate, has strongly advocated its use in skin-affections. As it has been used in furunculus successfully, by Dr. Schweich, and in onychia-maligna, Mr. Luke regards it almost as specific; it may be given with benefit against the boils and abscesses which sometimes succeed small-pox, and against the malignant inflammations and gangrene, which may also be expected in some cases. As it has been used successfully in some intermittent and remittent fevers, it may also prove salutary against the variolous fever; as it has been found beneficial against neuralgia and rheumatic affections, it may relieve some of the nervous and muscular pains which attend small-pox. I believe that in all these cases it has been found useful by homœopathists.

Among the other remedies which have been found useful against small-pox, are:

Belladonna.—Mr. Erasmus Wilson, in his work on diseases of the skin, page 86, says that the Belladonna treatment recommended for scarlatina is also applicable to small-pox. "I have seen," he says, this remedy exhibited, with the greatest benefit, both as a prophylactic and as a curative measure." It is probably most homœopathic in those cases preceded by an erythematous or scarlatinous redness of the surface, particularly in the confluent form; and still more strongly is it homœopathic if there be cerebral complications, pain or heat of the head, delirium, or coma. If the delirium run high or be furious, it might be alternated with Veratrum-viride or Aconite-rad. As, according to Pereira, it "causes dryness of the mouth, throat, and fauces, difficulty of deglutition and articulation, a feeling of constriction about the throat, nausea, and sometimes actual vomiting, and now and then swelling and redness of the face," it would be highly homœopathic in those cases where anginose symptoms predominated, where the nausea was persistent, or where the tumefaction and swelling of the face was most distressing; also in those severe cases where the disease overwhelms the nervous system almost from the outset, and the patient lies in a lethargic and soporose condition. Pereira says that "convulsions from Belladonna are rare, but lethargy or sopor occurs subsequently to the delirium.

If the disease involve the eyes, threatening those destructive disorganizations which occasionally take place, this would still be a prominent remedy; although, according to Pereira, it produces injection of the conjunctiva with a bluish blood; protrusion of the eye, which in some appeared as if it were dull and in others ardent and furious.

Dr. Mandeville (see *Rankin's Abstract*, December, 1858, page 54) uses a Belladonna ointment, composed of half a drachm of extract of Belladonna, rubbed up with half a drachm of spermaceti ointment, and three and a half ounces of olive oil, with the addition of two and a half drachms of Chloroform, as a local application to the face or any other part of the body of which the small-pox patient complained of being itchy. He supposes that the Belladonna and Chloroform ointment allows the eruption to force its way more kindly through the cutis-vera, probably relaxing the skin in the same way that it relaxes the sphincters. The patients invariably expressed their sense of relief soon after its application—some saying that it made the skin pliable; others, that it made it feel cool; others, again, that it made it moist; but all felt it relieved the sensation of itching or tingling. Another remarkable fact, which he has observed since he commenced using this ointment, is, that none of the confluent cases were pitted, except in three instances, and those very slightly indeed; and he could perceive, after the scales became detached, the places where the original pustules were, had an elevated, instead of a depressed base, so that the subsequent absorption left the skin in its normal condition. He applied this soft liniment with a large camel's-hair brush, three or four times a day. In erysipelas, Waring (see "Therapeutics," p. 92,) says,

"The internal use of Belladonna, in repeated doses of one-sixteenth of a grain, is often very beneficial in reducing the excitement of the arterial system and in procuring rest;" he adds, "It is best given after the exhibition of Aconite." The celebrated English surgeon, Liston, says, after Aconite, in doses of one half-grain of the extract, every third or fourth hour, has performed its office, in abating vascular excitement, so that the necessity for the abstraction of blood is done away with, Belladonna, in doses of one-sixteenth of a grain, is productive of the greatest benefit. The equally celebrated dermatologist, Erasmus Wilson, confirms this view of the beneficial effects of Aconite, and observes that it proves especially useful in checking the heart's action, and in promoting cutaneous transpiration, and adds that, in small-pox, he has seen Belladonna exhibited with the greatest benefit, both as a prophylactic and as a curative measure.

The celebrated Fleischmann, of the Vienna Homœopathic Hospital, reports the case of a man, aged twenty-four, admitted with the first traces of small-pox eruption, which had rather a violet or livid hue. On the third night he became delirious, in an extreme degree. The next day he spoke confusedly, his head was hot, eyes glittering and congested, tongue dry, thirst excessive, and eruption coming out very slowly. Bellad., second decimal dilution, was given every four hours, but, on the fourth night, he was so delirious that he had to be confined, and his pulse rose to 124; the eruption was beginning to maturate. Bellad. was now given, in the first decimal dilution, every two hours, when he became quiet, recovered his senses, and had some sleep; the majority of the pustules were filled with matter. From the sixth day onward, convalescence progressed so rapidly that he could leave the hospital on the eleventh day.

Camphor.—Hartmann recommends this remedy when the eruption suddenly dries up, and the swelling of the face quickly subsides, which, he says, although generally fatal symptoms, the vital powers may sometimes be aroused by frequent doses of it internally, and by bathing the body externally with warm spirits of Camphor.—RÜCKERT.

According to Wood, when Camphor is applied locally, it causes heat, more or less redness, and pain; in large doses, it causes uneasiness or pain in the stomach, and even nausea and vomiting. A moderately large dose is followed by a slight increase in the frequency and, perhaps, fullness of the pulse, and of the warmth of the skin, and occasionally by some perspiration. In the course of twenty minutes, there may be a slight exhilaration of the spirits, or a feeling of comfort induced, which, however, is much more observable in depression or uneasiness, from nervous or other disorders, than in health. Thus far the medicine acts as a nervous stimulant. A larger dose will occasion decided narcotic symptoms. With or without previous excitement of the circulation, there will be a feeling of giddiness, perhaps, also, of languor or lassitude, with more or less mental confusion or unsteadiness, or, perhaps, some disorder of vision or hearing. These symptoms are soon followed by heaviness, mental hebetude, and a disposition to sleep, during which the general sensibility is impaired, the pulse—whether previously excited or not—usually becomes slower, though, perhaps, still full, and the temperature of the skin somewhat lowered. In great excess, Camphor sometimes causes nausea and vomiting; if not speedily thrown off the stomach, it causes anxiety, vertigo, disordered or obscured hearing and vision, delirium, insensibility, convulsions, and deep stupor, attended with diminution in the frequency and force of the pulse, paleness of the face, and coolness of the skin, which is sometimes bathed in a cold sweat, followed, in an hour or two, by unconsciousness. Wood says it is a singular fact that some of these cases of poisoning have commenced with symptoms of high circulatory excitement, with flushed face, and other symptoms of determination of blood to the head, and were followed by a state of depression; while, in other cases, the depressed condition occurred first, and the symptoms of excitement, succeeded by fever, have followed afterwards.

In small doses, of from one to three grains, Wood says, it often answers an admirable purpose as a nervous stimulant, relieving slight pains, vague uneasiness, nervous headaches, muscular twitchings, restlessness, and jactitation, and frequently enabling the patient to sleep. In full doses, it has been employed to stimulate the brain in depressed states of its functions, to relieve pain, allay spasms and some other nervous disorders; also in idiopathic fevers, when there is general uneasiness, restlessness, jactitation, tremors, twitchings, or startings of the muscles, slight delirium, wakefulness, &c.; again, in the low typhoid state of febrile diseases, when the pulse is frequent and feeble, the tongue and skin dry, and the patient has low, muttering delirium. It is supposed to act here as a stimulant to the brain and nervous system, and to cause perspiration, thus relieving the system from the sedative influence of depraved blood or some absorbed poison.—It has often been employed in the retrocession of cutaneous eruptions, in order to relieve internal irritation by its calming influence, and to favor the return of the eruption by its diaphoretic action. As it is very much used as an external application in various painful affections; such as rheumatic or neuralgic pains, sprains, bruises, &c., it may be useful in relieving the intense lumbar pains which precede bad or malignant cases of small-pox; and, as it has often been applied successfully as a stimulant to gangrenous, flabby, and indolent ulcers, it may occasionally come in play in the latter stages of confluent variola.

Dose.—Wood says, as a simple nervous stimulant, it may be given in doses of from one to three grains, repeated every hour or two. For its full effect, as a cerebral stimulant, the medium dose is from five to fifteen grains; for a very powerful effect, in painful neuralgic or spasmodic affections, from ten to twenty grains.

Iodine.—Schmid, of Vienna, reports the case of a lady, aged thirty, in the second half of pregnancy, and just recovering from a threatened miscarriage, when she was attacked with severe symptoms of small-pox and nervous disorder;—the eruption came out on the face and hands, with pain in the throat, and inflammatory redness, burning pain in the larynx, and along the trachea, frequent paroxysms of anxiety, oppression of the chest, and tendency to fainting, especially at night; sometimes she attempted to get out of bed, at others, she wished to be carried about, and behaved like a sick child. On the following night, she had turns of exhaustion, as if she would sink and die. The eruption did not come out fully, and paralysis of the heart or speedy death was expected. After various apparently appropriate remedies had been given, without benefit, on the seventh day of the disease, ten grains of *Iodine* were dissolved in half an ounce of Alcohol, and two drops given per dose, every half-hour during the day; in the evening, she was much better, and the doses were repeated only every hour; the next night was spent in quiet sleep, without anxiety, sinking turns, or oppression. On the eighth day, the small-pox eruption appeared fully, and ran a favorable course, although the Iodine was given until the twelfth day, in less frequent and smaller doses. The next month, she was safely delivered, and able to nurse her child.—RÜCKERT.

It is not difficult to divine the reasons which led Schmid to use Iodine in this case. Wood (see "Pharmacology," vol. ii., page 326) says that a very common result of the continued use of Iodine, even when no obvious irritation of the stomach is produced, is soreness of the throat, or some degree of inflammation of the air-passages. This catarrhal affection of the nose, throat, and air-tubes may, in fact, be considered as one of the most positive signs of its operation on the system, just as salivation is regarded as a sign of the action of Mercury, and, when present, should lead to a temporary suspension of the medicine, or a diminution of the dose. It often produces peculiar effects upon the skin, for it occasionally gives rise to eruptions on the surface, either *erythematous*, *papulous*, *eczematous*, or impetiginous (pustular); hence, it would be apt to reproduce a delayed or suppressed small-pox eruption.

Mercurius-Solubilis.—According to Rückert, Rummel says, that, in the last stages of small-pox, diarrhœa is apt to arise, which may be relieved by Mercurius; he also believes that it is generally indicated in the suppurative stage, on account of the salivation which attends it. Kreussler supposes that Merc.-sol., one dose daily, is a specific remedy against true, simple small-pox, which may also be called catarrhal, on account of the catarrhal symptoms which attend it. I should suppose that a purely catarrhal small-pox must be a very simple and innocent affection. He adds, that the irritative fever scarcely requires Aconite, and that only occasionally is a single dose of Bellad. required before the outbreak of the eruption, when Merc.-sol. may immediately be given. Such mild cases hardly require any treatment. He also supposes that it is the principal remedy against varioloid. Hartmann thinks that if the suppurative fever is excessive, on account of the great quantity of the pustules, while the attending affections of the nose, throat, and eyes are very troublesome, and attended with salivation, that we will rarely meet with a more specific remedy than Mercurius.

In regular practice, Mercury is not used in small-pox for its specific effects upon the disease; but is occasionally given in the beginning of the attack, in one or more full doses, to act freely upon the liver and bowels in bilious and plethoric subjects, and again when the maturation of a large crop of pustules excites much fever, in order to cause a drain from the blood-vessels, and diminish arterial action. In variolous ophthalmia, it has been pushed so as to touch the mouth; and in the bronchitis, when it does not yield to Tartar-emetic, several two-grain doses are sometimes given, but generally not more than three.

The skin-diseases (*eczema-mercurialis*) produced by Mercury, partake more of the scaly and eczematous character than of the pustular; yet, Wilson says, that in the more severe forms of it, the vesicles increase in size, and their transparent contents become opaque and purulent. In some instances, where febrile symptoms are present, the efflorescence occupies a large extent of surface, sometimes the entire body, and assumes the appearance of rubeola; in the more advanced degree—the *hydrargyria febrilis*—the invasion is marked by rigors, nausea, pains in the head, &c. The fauces are always more or less inflamed in these cases, and the inflammation of the mucous membrane often extends to the bronchial tubes. In the worst form, the face is enormously swollen, the eyelids closed, the throat tumefied and painful, and the color of the efflorescence a deep purple hue. The desquamation of the cuticle endures for quite a long period.

It will be most homœopathic in those cases where some morbillous complication exists, or the inflammation of the fauces is severe. In cases, too, where the desquamation of the skin is tardy, it will be highly appropriate. It would probably be particularly useful about the time of the secondary fever, to allay and mitigate the constitutional disturbance.

All this is just what we find to be the clinical experience with Mercury. The principal homœopathic indication for the use of Mercurius is supposed to be the presence of salivation: but there is nothing specific in this in small-pox, for it simply arises from the irritation of small-pox pimples in the mouth. It never fails to accompany the second stage of confluent small-pox, and the salivary discharge either begins with the eruption, or within a day or two after; it is then thin and copious, resembling the ptyalism of Mercury. About the eighth day, it becomes viscid, and is expectorated with difficulty; while, in bad cases, it ceases for a day or two, and then returns, or else disappears altogether. Children are not so liable to this salivation as adults; but in them a vicarious diarrhœa often appears, but not constantly, nor so early in the disease. It is frequently profuse, unless checked, and often persists until the disease terminates. Mercury is also regarded as indicated against this symptom.

Merc.-Corrosivus.—According to Frank, (see *Frank's Magazine*, vol. iv., page 224,) a solution of one grain of Merc.-corrosiv., in six ounces of water, applied to portions of the face and to the eyelids, in the suppurative stage of small-pox, produced such rapid improvement, that these places were quite smooth, while the uncovered parts were still going through the suppurative and desiccative process. In another case of confluent small-pox, in which the solution was applied to the entire face, the same happy results occurred to the whole of it, which had taken place in parts only in the other instance. Many other cases are given with like results. Sometimes one grain to three ounces of water, or one grain to six ounces, or from two to four grains in six ounces, or three grains to one pound of water were used. The same solutions were used with great effect as gargles, in severe affections of the throat, accompanying small-pox, aided occasionally by Bellad.

Phosphorus.—Fleischmann reports a case, with severe premonitory symptoms, in which the numerous pustules were filled with blood instead of pus, (*variola sanguinea,*) in the maturative stage; a violent cough set in, attended with copious and frequent expectoration of blood, without pneumonia being present, and, for ten nights in succession, a large spit-cup was filled with black, coagulated blood. The patient recovered under the use of Phosphorus.

I have seen cases of profuse hæmoptysis, during the course of confluent small-pox, which recovered perfectly. Fleischmann treats the majority of his cases of pneumonia with Phosphorus, which may also be used in the greater part of the chest-affections which attend bad cases of small-pox, with the exception of pleurisy. (For remarks on the use of Phosphorus, see page 213.)

Phosphoric-Acid.—Altschul reports a case, in a patient aged eighteen years, in which the pulse was excessively frequent, soft, empty, and compressible; the hot skin was not turgescent, but relaxed and flabby; the urine light colored and spastic, and there were frequent involuntary jerks of the muscles. The eruption appeared scantily, the vesicles were flat, and the heat of the skin continued after the imperfect appearance of the eruption; the tongue was dry, thirst excessive, nights restless and sleepless, and a frightful fear of death overpowered the patient. The vesicles did not fill with pus as usual, but huge watery blebs, like those caused by blisters, and as large as a walnut, appeared on the forehead and cheeks; they broke, and left raw, painful spots; the stools were loose. Phosphoric-acid was given every four hours, and, after the third dose, a very unexpected improvement occurred. The night was quiet, sleep refreshing and dreamless, and a more cheerful frame of mind ensued. Several new vesicles appeared, but filled with pus; the diarrhœa ceased, and the sore places healed. The patient was able to leave his bed in a few days.

Sulphur.—According to Rückert, Hartmann and Franz have advanced the idea that Sulphur might prove a prophylactic against small-pox. Rosenthal gave it in twenty-seven cases, with the premonitory symptoms of variola, varioloid, or varicella, and the eruption did not appear. Also in fourteen cases of true small-pox, in the second stage, and thought that the course of the disease was much shortened, especially if Aconite had been previously given; and in nine cases of varioloid, in the eruptive stage, and thought that no new pimples appeared after the Sulphur was given, and those already present dried up rapidly. He did not place very great stress upon his experiments, as he was aware that a *febris variolosa sine variolis* sometimes occurs.

Lobethal thinks that Sulphur moderates the severity of the symptoms at the outbreak of the eruption, and promotes the action of Mercurius, which he thinks so useful in the suppurative stage. Tietze regards Sulphur as very useful to prevent and cure scrofulous affections occurring after an attack of small-pox.

Sulphur is insoluble in water, but is soluble in alkaline solutions. When taken internally, it is dissolved by the alkaline matters contained in the alimentary canal, and when absorbed into the blood, which is always alkaline, it is still further acted upon; so that, when its use is long continued, a sulphurous odor generally exhales from the body, and can, at times, be detected in the sweat, urine, and milk. It generally causes a slight increase of secretion from the skin and bronchial mucous membrane, attended with some augmentation in the frequency of the pulse and temperature of the skin, showing a gentle excitement of the circulatory system. It is, perhaps, more useful in chronic rheumatism than in any other disease, except some skin affections; but has had a great reputation in bronchial disorders from the earliest times, especially chronic catarrh, when attended with dyspnœa. Among the cutaneous affections, in which, after scabies, it is most useful, are: porrigo, and chronic impetigo, both pustular diseases and chronic eczema.

It has also been proposed to apply Sulphur-ointment, by means of slight friction, to the entire surface of the skin. This ointment may be composed of Sulphur—two drachms to the ounce of lard—and used three times a day, at as early a stage of the disease as possible. The effects of the remedy, it is said, are contraction and hardening of the papulæ, diminution of the tumefaction of the skin, and subsidence of the gastro-intestinal irritation.

Thuja-Occidentalis, (*Arbor-vitæ*).—In 1849, the well-known Bönninghausen advised the use of this remedy as a specific against small-pox. In the first case in which he gave it, the pustules dried up on the fourth day, the scabs fell off on the eighth day, and no scars were left; but he does not say whether the person had been previously vaccinated or not. From that time on, he used it both as a remedy and a preventive, and always, he asserts, with success; he finally became so infatuated about it that he proposed it as a substitute for vaccination. Horner found it useful in the epidemic of 1854 and 1855. Trinks says that it produces no effect, either against the eruption or the attending fever. Croserio gave it in one case of benign small-pox, after he had, in imagination, allayed the primary fever and headache with Acon., 300, and Merc.-solub., 300, on the second day after the outbreak of the eruption, when these symptoms naturally subside of themselves. He then gave three globules of Thuja, 300, and noticed no perceptible effect for the next three days; but on the fourth day—i. e., the sixth day of the eruption—the pustules began to disappear promptly, and left no scars. This was probably a case of the five or seven-day pock.

The *British Journal of Homœopathy*, vol. xiii., p. 172, contains very just remarks about Bönninghausen's supposed discovery. We need only say he assumes that Thuja, in the two-hundredth dilution, is a remedy of sufficient power to cure true small-pox, without inconvenience and without the least danger, in less than eight days, without leaving the least disfigurement or mark upon the skin, and without introducing into the human body the seeds of another disease, often worse than the small-pox itself, as vaccination often does. It should be remembered how carefully vaccination and revaccination are insisted upon in Prussia, where Bönninghausen lives, and how few opportunities he must have of treating true unmodified small-pox.

Thuja resembles Sabina very much in its action; both are said to possess anthelmintic and emmenagogue powers. Boerhaave recommended a distilled water, prepared from the leaves, in dropsy; a decoction of the leaves has also been a popular remedy in intermittent and remittent fevers, rheumatism, cough, and scurvy. An ointment made from the fresh leaves, has been used successfully in rheumatic and neuralgic affections; a poultice of the cones, is said to remove the worst rheumatic pains; the oil has been used beneficially as a vermifuge. The plant has an agreeable balsamic odor, and a strong, balsamic, camphorous, and bitter taste, which has been compared to that of tansy. All authorities agree in giving Hahnemann the credit of introducing its use in condylomata and warts; latterly, it has been advanced as a specific in cancer, since the cure of the celebrated Field-Marshal Radetzky with it, of a cancerous fungus of the eye. It is now in common use, by physicians of all schools, in cancer. I have seen it used in ten-drop doses, three times a day, for months together, in a case of suspected cancer of the stomach, occurring after cancer of the breast of several years standing; it enabled the patient to retain her food, when almost all other remedies had failed, so that she got in the habit of taking a dose of Thuja before eating, in order to settle her stomach. Dr Bleifuss gave it successfully, in the same doses—ten drops, three times a day—against chronic styes upon the lids; and removed a chronic derangement of the stomach at the same time, marked by the sudden rising of offensive air (*anea fœtida*) several times a day, a constantly coated tongue, loss of appetite, and a musty sweetish taste in the mouth. The eruptions against which Thuja is regarded as specific, are: Red, smooth spots or maculæ; burning vesicles; moist, suppurating erosions; tubercles or nodes, with a reddish or brownish base, and passing over into suppuration on their summits, like boils, styes, &c.; warts and condylomata.*

External Treatment.—*Exclusion of Air and Light.*—As regards the exclusion of light, though there would appear to be some facts in favor of the supposition that it renders the course of the pustules more mild and less apt to scar; yet, the reasons for it appear so inadequate that it is more than probable that a coincidence has originated the idea. Touching the exclusion of air, however, there would appear to be more to recommend it. All lesions of surface, and many eruptions, are mitigated and assuaged in a remarkable degree by excluding the irritating contact of the air; and, no doubt, the inflammation excited in the skin by the presence of the morbid deposit in small-pox is heightened by exposure to the atmosphere. But, as air and light are generally both excluded when the experiment is tried, it is hard to separate their effects. M. Serres placed a glass capsule over a small-pox pustule, and observed the effects produced by excluding air and light. He found that in proportion to the exclusion of both was the development of the pustule checked, and that, when they were completely shut out, the pustule became shrivelled, and quickly dried up.

* See "Drug Provings," by the late lamented Dr. James W. Metcalfe. Published by Wm. Radde, No. 300 Broadway, New York.

M. Serres says that he never reaped such successful results in the cure of small-pox as he did at La Pitié, during one year that the patients were placed in a kind of cellar, which was very dark and ill ventilated. This, however, is so complete a return to the times of John of Gaddesden and of Mead, that it is more than probable that the patients recovered *in spite* of their surroundings, rather than in consequence of them. That an ill-ventilated apartment should conduce to safety or convalescence in an uncleanly disease is hardly to be admitted at the present day; but the coolness may have had some effect.

A great many masks and external applications have been used, from time immemorial, in order to prevent pitting and scarring of the face. Gregory says, all the attempts made with the use of masks to prevent pitting end in disappointment. But Bennett, of Edinburgh, has much confidence in external applications; he has tried Mercurial ointment, thickened with starch, in numerous cases, and is satisfied with the good effects of the practice. In one unvaccinated case, the most confluent he had ever seen, in which the entire face was so crowded with the papules and vesicles of the incipient stage that there was literally not room to place a pin's head anywhere on the sound skin, and it was evident that the whole surface of the face would, under ordinary circumstances, become one mass of suppuration, with horrible disfigurement, excessive agony, great swelling of the eyelids, dreadful suppuration and fetor of the discharge, violent secondary fever, and frightful cicatrices; yet, from the moment the plaster was applied, all smarting and pain in the face ceased, the eyelids did not swell, no suppuration occurred, there was no secondary fever, and, on the mask leaving the face, there was no pitting or suppuration. Bennett had no doubt that the external treatment really checked the progress of the suppuration and modified the disease. As he met with numerous instances in which slight salivation followed the use of the Mercurial plaster, he was led to substitute common Calamine, or impure Oxide of Zinc, saturated with olive oil; this forms a tough, coherent crust, which remains on the face, and answers well. I have been in the habit of using Magnesia ointment for the same purpose, made with one or two drachms of Henry's Magnesia to an ounce of simple cerate. This is a very cleanly, pleasant, and efficacious application; it forms a thick but flexible layer over the face, as dense and soft as a kid glove. The Magnesia prevents the ointment from becoming rancid from the heat of the skin, and prevents the putrefaction of the discharge; in short, it retains the whole surface of the face in a sweet and healthy condition.

Nitrate of Silver.—An apparently successful ectrotic method, (Εκτιτρωσκειν, to abort,) is that by the Nitrate of Silver. Of course, it has always been a great point to obtain some means of preventing the pitting of the face. This method is said to answer the purpose completely; but, to be effectual, it ought to be done as early as the first or second day of the eruption. Each individual pustule has had the apex removed, and the pointed extremity of a stick of Nitrate of Silver inserted into the opened vesicle. Its further progress, it is said, will be instantly arrested. The proceeding is necessarily attended with much pain, where the number of pustules is great, and requires a considerable time for its performance. Wilson also thinks that it augments the febrility and nervous irritability of the patient; but those drawbacks are declared to be trivial compared with the great advantage gained in the case of youths and females, where pitting is so much to be deprecated. To obviate these objections, however, it has been proposed to paint the entire face with a very strong solution of Nitrate of Silver, and this, certainly, so far from causing pain, is said to afford comfort to the patient, by allaying the itching; but it has been found that its advantages were deceptive, as the work of suppuration and destruction would go on unchecked beneath the mask formed by the blackened cuticle.

The Arabian physicians were in the habit of opening the pustules after suppuration had commenced, pressing out the liquid contents, and washing the surface with warm milk and water. Wilson recommends the same practice, substituting decoction of Poppies for the milk and water.

Mercurial Plaster.—The supposed power of Mercury to modify the influence of variola upon the system has been long believed in; but some recent experiments are said to prove that, applied externally, it also possesses the power of neutralizing the variolous poison. It has been applied in the form of a plaster, either Mercurial ointment, thickened with starch, or *emplastrum vigo cum Mercurio*, to the whole face, leaving merely a space for the mouth, nose, and eyes; a little Mercurial ointment is applied to the eyelids. The plaster is allowed to remain for three or four days, according to the amount of the disease. It should not be applied later than the second day, as after that period it is inoperative. Its effect, its advocates claim, is to arrest the eruption at the papular or vesicular stage; it never becomes purulent, and the skin between the pustules never becomes inflamed or swollen. But, however much it may fail as an ectrotic in the pustular stage, its efficiency is still said to be very marked in modifying the local inflammation. According to Briquet, "it exerts a specific action on the cause, whatever that may be, which produces the variolous pustule."

One of the preparations most commonly used is the *emplastrum de vigo cum Mercurio.* In the first experiment with it, a strip of the plaster was placed on the arm of the patient, while a similar strip of Diachylon plaster was placed upon the other arm. Under the Mercurial plaster, the development of the eruption was arrested; under the other plaster, no modification took place. In a second case, the face of the patient was covered with a plaster, a part of which he tore off during the night;—the denuded surface was the seat of suppurating pustules, while the rest of the visage escaped, the pustules being aborted. In a third case—a man, affected with violent confluent variola—the pimples were small, scarcely raised above the level of the epidermis, and surrounded by a brilliant red areola. The vigo plaster was applied, and allowed to remain on seven days; and, on its removal, it was found that no suppuration had been established, except four pustules near the mouth, where the plaster had not touched.

CHICKEN-POX.

Varicella.

Definition.—The disease consists of a specific vesicular eruption, somewhat resembling that of varioloid, attended with fever, and runs a definite course in eight or ten days.

Pathology.—This disease derives an importance, which it does not of itself possess, in consequence of its resemblance to small-pox, with which, in the modified form, it is considered by some to be identical. It is, for the most part, peculiar to childhood and early adult age, but its epidemic influence is very inconsiderable, and its extension easily under control. That it is contagious, has been proved by inoculation. The theory of the disease, therefore, is that a poison is absorbed and infects the blood, and, after a given period of latency, gives rise to primary fever, which lasts from twenty-four to seventy-two hours, when the eruption appears, and runs a course of eight or ten days. The fever is much mitigated on the appearance of the eruption, and entirely subsides with it.

There is a slight fever very generally observed at the outset, of short duration, preceding the eruption. It is of a mild character, and though, for a few hours, it may seem severe, it never passes into a brown tongue stage. The eruption has three stages—that of pimple, vesicle, and incrustation; and, after the fever has lasted from twenty-four to seventy-two hours, a number of scattered red papulæ appear, which become vesicular, and, perhaps, in a few points, pustular, on the first day. On the second day, the vesicles, which are almost always widely separated, are umbilicated, and filled with a whitish or straw-colored lymph. On the third and fourth days, they attain their greatest magnitude, when the central bridle ruptures, and they become acuminated; shortly afterwards, they burst and shrivel, except those few which contain purulent matter, and have much inflammation around their bases. The fifth day, they begin to crust, and, in four or five days more, the crust falls off, leaving, for a time, red spots on the skin, generally without, but sometimes with a pit or depression. The few pits are permanent, and the cicatrices generally whiter than the original texture, and the patient is consequently scarred or marked in a few places.

The eruption is not, at first, universal all over the body, but usually consists of a series of crops of scattered vesicles, which succeed each other at intervals of twenty-four hours, and die away in the order of their occurrence. It usually appears first on the breast and back, and afterwards on the face and extremities. The number of crops may be limited to one, or two, or three, while in others, again, a new succession will appear every twenty-four hours, for ten or twelve days.

Varieties.—Of the chicken-pox there are three kinds, the *varisella lenticularis*, the *varicella conoides*, and *varicella globata*. The symptoms of all these varieties are similar, their only difference being in the size and form of the vesicle, the varicella globata being the largest.

The fever which precedes this eruption is occasionally as severe as that preceding small-pox or measles; but it generally, though not constantly, remits on the appearance of the eruption, and does not return as it ripens.

The globate chicken-pox, known also as the swine-pox, is vulgarly called the "hives," in some districts of England. The eruption consists of large vesicles, not quite circular in form, but often a little larger than the pustules of small-pox, surrounded with a red margin, and containing a transparent fluid, which, on the second day of the eruption, resembles milk whey. On the third day, they subside, shrivel, and present a yellow tint. Before the conclusion of the fourth day, they are converted into thin, blackish scabs, which dry and fall off in four or five days more.

Differential Diagnosis.—1. Chicken-pox emits a peculiar odor, different from that of small-pox, and less decidedly partaking of the variolous fetor.

2. Chicken-pox appears indiscriminately, and almost equally all over the person, beginning first on the trunk in general, and then appearing on the face and scalp; while small-pox appears first on the face and neck, and the pustules are more numerous on the face than on any other part.

3. Chicken-pox eruption is generally complete in the space of twenty-four hours, or solitary vesicles come out irregularly afterwards, at different points; but, in small-pox, the eruption begins in the

evening of the third, or morning of the fourth day, and proceeds regularly for the ensuing three days, until it is complete.

4. While variolous pustules are, on the first and second day of the eruption, small, hard, globular, red, and painful, and communicate to the finger a sensation similar to that which would be excited by the presence of small round seeds under the cuticle, in chicken-pox, almost every vesicle has, on the first day, a hard, red margin, but communicates to the finger a sensation like that from a rounded seed, flattened by pressure.

5. On the second or third day of the eruption of chicken-pox, the individual bodies are vesicles containing serous fluid, and giving them a whitish aspect.

6. These vesicles are surrounded by little or no inflamed areola, and do not, naturally and independent of external violence, proceed to suppuration.

7. Chicken-pox may confidently be distinguished from small-pox, on the third and fourth days, by the state of the vesicles, some of which, being left entire, are shrivelled and wrinkled, while others, whose ruptured tops have been closed by incrustation of their fluid, are marked by radiating furrows. None present depressions on their apices; and, as they do not suppurate, they incrust and disappear sooner than variolous pustules.

8. The marks left by chicken-pox, when it does leave marks, are round and elliptical, and less frequently irregular than those of small-pox, and, in general, smooth and shining. Lastly, it is said by Luders that, while small-pox is formed in the cutis-vera or corion, the chicken-pox eruption is formed in the tissue situated between the corion and cuticle.

Treatment.—Rhus and Cantharides are the most homœopathic remedies, although the general treatment is simple, and may be conducted mainly with reference to the symptoms, as the disease itself is never severe, and generally proceeds to an entirely favorable termination. Among the symptoms, the most important are the fever and the itching of the pimples. Aconite and Antimony will abate the fever and inflammation about the vesicles more readily than most other remedies, and will also allay the itching, although an occasional mild laxative remedy may be required, if the patient is naturally plethoric, or has indulged in rich food, or an excessive quantity of his ordinary diet, or is naturally costive or bilious. Chicken-pox rarely or never le ves any bad consequences; it is hardly ever suppressed, and taking cold is not attended with the bad results which follow the like accident or carelessness in scarlet fever or measles. Some authors think that tenesmus and strangury are common attendants on chicken-pox, but we have never observed them; and that bilious-rheumatic and bilious-nervous symptoms are frequently met with, and recommend Bryonia and Rhus for the former, for which Colchicum and Mercurius are, however, better remedies, and Belladonna and Rhus for the latter.

MILIARIA.

Miliary Eruptive Disease.—Miliary Fever.—Sudatoria.—Millet-Seed Rash.—Hydroa.—Sudamina.

Definition.—An eruption of innumerable minute pimples, occurring in successive crops, with white summits, upon the skin of the trunk and extremities, preceded and accompanied by fever, anxiety, oppression of the chest and respiration, copious sweats, of a sour, rank, fetid odor, peculiar to itself. The base of the pimples, and the skin around, are red and irritable.

Pathology.—The specific nature of this disease, authors are not agreed upon at the present day. All physicians are not disposed to admit that, in miliaria, a peculiar disease exists, with a characteristic eruption and definite course, such as the variolous pustules and course of small-pox exhibit. Certain it is, however, that a peculiar epidemic disease has prevailed in different parts of Europe, at different periods in the world's history, the nature of which is described in the above definition; and although, in its pure form, it seems now to have disappeared from England and this country, yet there can be no doubt that a specific disease of this description prevails, epidemically, in many parts of continental Europe and Asia, and is sufficiently common as a symptomatic affection in this country. The disease of these epidemics has been described under the various names of "sweating sickness," "miliary fever," "sudatoria," "miliaria," and the like. Rayer has given an accurate account of the disease, and it has been studied by Dr. Aitkin, with peculiar advantage, in the military hospitals of Scutari, during the Crimean war; also by Dr. Foucart, in the south of France. The temperature and physical climate of that country, with the relaxed habits of the Turks, appear to favor greatly the production of the disorder.

Symptoms.—Nearly two-fifths of all the cases have no premonitory symptoms. The patient may go to bed well, when, suddenly in the night, a profuse perspiration occurs, followed by heat of the skin and some quickness of the pulse; there may be some headache and nausea, followed by some oppression of the chest, feeling of contraction in the region of the heart, and an annoying pressure in the epigastrium; and, at times, there may be fainting-fits, trembling, chilliness, formication, nausea, and vomiting. The symptoms are often like those of the extreme discomfort which attends waking at night, after overloading the stomach. Occasionally, many of these symptoms arise without any perspiration, especially the intense oppression of the chest, and feeling of suffocation, heat of the skin, restlessness, headache, pressure on the epigastrium, and the abdominal pulsation. Foucart terms these cases, "*suette sans suers.*"

The fever, which precedes the eruption, is ushered in by chills, intense and general, shivering anxiety, oppression of the chest, restlessness, a sense of great feebleness and imminent fainting, with pains in the head, loins, and limbs. In a few hours, nausea, flushing, and profuse sweat supervene, but without any diminution of the dyspnœa, the anxiety, or pectoral oppression; but rather with an aggravation, in the form of short, irregular, panting, and sighing breathing, as if proceeding from a sense of weight under the sternum, with a feeling of internal heat, wandering pains, and sometimes cramps of the hands and calves of the legs. The pulse is generally rapid, small, and feeble, in a few cases hard, often variable, irregular, or intermittent at every ninth, twelfth, or sixteenth beat. The tongue is coated with a white, foul, or yellow fur, indicative of a sluggish condition of the alimentary canal, and the bowels are constipated, from the first day of the disease throughout its whole course. The sweat which accompanies this febrile state is profuse, and emits a peculiar smell, of a rank, sour, fetid odor. The perspirations generally precede the eruption for two or three days. The patient is constantly covered with sweat, his skin is hot, but of a natural color, his pulse somewhat quick and full, and his urine decreases in bulk, so that, finally, only a small quantity is passed, once or twice in twenty-four hours, and it may be entirely suppressed. In the course of the second day, the tongue becomes more or less thickly coated; thirst may or may not be present. On the third or fourth day, the eruption is apt to appear; but, in dangerous and anomalous cases, it may not break out before the fourth or fifth week, attended with pricking pains in the skin and limbs, and increase of the dyspnœa and anxiety; the patient sometimes improves rapidly after the exanthem comes out, for the perspirations cease, and a more normal action of the skin ensues. Relapses are not uncommon, but are of no great importance; still, convalescence may be protracted and much disturbance of the stomach remain.

From the fifth or sixth day, up to the twenty-first, an itching sensation is felt in the mammary and epigastric regions, and the inner surface of the arms, and the skin of those parts is found to be diffusely rough and irregular, with numerous elevations not larger than pinheads. In a short time, the summits of these become pearly white, the cuticle being elevated by a slight opaque sero-albuminous fluid—crop

after crop breaks out, and continue from three to seven days, followed **by a** corresponding desquamation of the cuticle. The eruption is generally confined to the neck, breast, mammary and epigastric regions, and the inner surface of the loins and legs. In severe cases, miliary vesicles appear at the junctions of the skin and mucous membranes, and then they are apt to become aphthous.

A deranged state of the gastro-enteric mucous membrane, indicated by nausea and vomiting of bilious matter, and eructations, flatulence, and diarrhœa, frequently complicate the disease.

Varieties.—Six forms have been described, viz.: first, a mild; second, a malignant; third, the idiopathic; and fourth, the symptomatic; and two more, named, from the red or white color of the eruption, *miliaria rubra et alba.*

The *malignant* is rendered so chiefly by the occurrence of violent inflammation in some of the internal organs, especially of the stomach, lungs, kidneys, and brain; and the danger of the disease is chiefly due to these complications, and not merely to the retrocession of the eruption, which, however, is very apt to take place. Such malignant forms have been known to terminate fatally in two or three days, but more frequently in from seven to twenty-one. These cases are apt to be attended with raging delirium, death-like anxiety, insupportable palpitation of the heart, violent pains in the nape and back, cramps, and sopor; the voice fails, and, with or without the outbreak of the eruption and profuse sweats, the body gradually becomes cool or cold, and a collapse sets in, in which the patient may die in one or two days. These severe attacks and rapid deaths often arise from the intensity of the epidemic disorder; but are, at times, brought about by improper treatment, with heating drinks and superabundant clothes.

In the more malignant form, this disease is infectious and contagious, and occurs epidemically. It appears to correspond with the sweating sickness of the sixteenth century, a disease which is no longer met with in England and this country, but which still occurs in France and Italy, and occasionally in Germany.

The *sudamina*, however, or the *characteristic eruption of miliary fever, may accompany almost any febrile complaint*, and, in such cases, it appears to be due more to the great heat and perspiring state of the skin than anything else. It does not appear to affect either the grade or form of the fever, as it may accompany indifferently either the mild or malignant variety, the inflammatory or the typhous. Thus, we may see it in the typhus, typhoid, and enteric fevers, also accompanying scarlatina, as a precursor of the eruption of small-pox, in the milk-fever of puerperal women, in phthisis, rheumatism, &c. The best known condition that favors the symptomatic variety is copious and continued sweating; but we often meet with it in enteric and typhoid fever, where there has been no sensible perspiration.

There are seasons when the symptomatic variety is more prone to accompany diseases than at others, as if an epidemic influence might occasionally give a tendency to it, and on such occasions it is apt to appear in connection with diseases which, at other seasons, it does not affect. In this form, as an accompaniment of other diseases, it is not supposed to be contagious. As before said, it may attend any affection accompanied by excessive heat of the skin and profuse perspiration. Hence, it is occasionally met with in the eruptive fevers, viz., in measles, scarlet fever, and small-pox; also in simple, remittent, and typhoid fevers, and most inflammatory affections accompanied by profuse perspiration, such as acute rheumatism and puerperal fever. Occasionally, it has arisen among puerperal women, then spread to others, and become epidemic. It so rarely occurs as an idiopathic affection in temparate climates, and when a cooling regimen and treatment of fever is adopted, that most English, French, and American authors confound true miliaria with simple sudamina. The two affections resemble each other closely, and may seem identical; but a true and often dangerous variety of true idiopathic miliaria does sometimes occur, and requires great skill in the management of it.

At first, the vesicles are so small as scarcely to be visible, unless upon close inspection, and attention is often only called to them in consequence of a feeling of roughness which they impart to the fingers. If the surface be now viewed obliquely, it may be seen to be thickly studded with little glistening vesicles, almost as transparent as water, and looking very like minute, almost microscopic drops of clear sweat upon the skin. They gradually enlarge, become hemispherical, and assume a pearly aspect, in consequence of the liquid which they contain becoming opaque and somewhat milky. Sometimes they are formed on a red base, and consequently have a reddish tinge, *miliaria rubra;* sometimes they rest upon the skin, in a perfectly natural state as regards color, and are either transparent or whitish, *miliaria alba.* They are usually quite distinct, and irregularly scattered over the surface; though occasionally collected together in spots, so as to present a clustered appearance, and, in some instances, coälescing into the form of bullæ of considerable size. They may be dispersed over all parts of the body, but appear most abundantly upon the neck and trunk, and are rarely found on the face. In some instances, they are attended with itching or tingling, and in others it is absent. Each vesicle soon dries up, running a course of four or five days, but it may be followed by successive crops.

It may sometimes greatly obscure the diagnosis of scarlatina. I recollect being called to a case (a child) where, for some thirty-six hours, I was greatly perplexed as to what the disease might be; the symptoms of scarlatina being of the most indefinite sort, while the eruption of miliaria was strongly marked. The child had no sore throat, no coated tongue, but little fever, and did not appear much amiss. The eruption was not uniform, was strongest on the back of the arms and front of the thighs, was of a dusky instead of a bright red, and was everywhere visibly raised above the surface in minute granules, and great numbers of these raised points had increased to the size of large miliary vesicles, filled with a lactescent looking fluid, many of them half a line to a line across. Moreover, the child had not been out of the house, and no scarlatina prevailed in the vicinity.

I pronounced it unequivocally scarlet fever, and enjoined great care and watchfulness. My diagnosis was eventually fully sustained. The family doubted, the children were thoughtlessly exposed and carelessly looked after, and, by the time the first child was commencing upon the desquamative stage, two others broke out with the characteristic rash of scarlet fever, and one with well-marked anginose symptoms. This latter, from careless exposure, suffered a premature retrocession of the eruption; secondary fever came on, with a soporose state, hæmaturia, albuminuria, and, at length, almost total suppression of urine, and his life was only saved by the most vigilant care and watchfulness.—SNELLING.

I have repeatedly seen most abundant crops of miliaria in connection with ship fever; in some of the more marked cases, it seemed as if the whole chest, back, and abdomen were covered with an almost confluent, flattish, white vesicular eruption, intermingled with the maculæ of typhus. Typhoid fever is very commonly attended with sudamina about the clavicles; and rheumatism, on the Continent, is frequently accompanied by a true and copious miliary eruption.

Treatment.—The management of simple miliaria may be limited to cooling drinks, sponging the surface with tepid water, light clothing, not allowing the profuse sweats to stagnate and corrupt in the body- and bed-clothing, but preventing this by sufficiently frequent changes. The advantage of keeping the patient cool was exemplified in Foucart's treatment of the epidemic in 1849, in the south of France. Of 1549 patients, treated with the heating and sweating method, 84 died; while, of 1455, none died who, having their bed- and body-clothes changed frequently, were supplied with abundance of fresh air and cooling drinks.

The great oppressions of the chest, stomach, and heart are among the most troublesome of the symptoms. Ipecac., Camphor, Musk, and Arsenicum have been used with benefit. Foucart used emetic doses of Ipecac.,—i. e., from twenty-four to thirty-two grains; but these large quantities are generally unnecessary, although, he says, they are invariably beneficial, especially if followed, in one or two days, by a saline laxative. If the oppression of the chest is great, and the eruption does not come out properly, Mustard, and even blister-plasters have been used with supposed benefit. If the perspirations are excessive, bathings with Vinegar and water, or Camphor water, or simple dilute Alcohol, have found many advocates. But the really specific remedies are Arsenicum, Rhus, Cantharides, and Ranunculus-bulbosus, although Bryonia is thought to be the most useful remedy by many.

Arsenic.—Among the reasons why Arsenic may be selected as a remedy, we may instance: First, its beneficial effects in some zymotic and miasmatic fevers, like some of those which are apt to be attended with miliaria; Second, its curative powers against many eruptive diseases, especially of a vesicular or scaly character; Third, its successful use against angina-pectoris, asthma, and other pectoral affections, and the advanced stages of typhus fever and chronic rheumatism. We may expect, in virtue of its tonic powers, to ward off the tendency to collapse, and, with the aid of other remedies, to rescue the patient from that state if he should fall into it; to relieve the oppression of the chest and anxiety, which are such marked attendants of this disease; and to exert a beneficial and specific action upon the skin.

Musk is indicated when adynamic inflammation occurs in connection with miliaria, especially when attended with delirium, general failure of the vital forces, and dangerous prostration. It is all the more useful if the inflammation be an adynamic pneumonia, or an attendant of a pernicious fever, even in the stage of collapse of pernicious miasmatic or congestive fevers. Musk will also relieve painful spasms of the muscles, stomach, or bowels. There is no remedy or combination of remedies which is so efficacious against hiccough, while it will remove some of the various nervous affections which attend miliaria, such as subsultus, asthmatic oppression of the chest, palpitations, &c.

Cantharides may be used when there is partial or complete suppression of urine in malignant cases. Watson says that Dr. Elliotson refers to some examples of its success against ischuria-renalis in the hands of Sir Astley Cooper, and of another surgeon who took the hint from Sir Astley. If the oppression of the chest be very great, and is not relieved by Ipecac., Musk, or Arsenicum, it may be allowable, in very dangerous cases, to apply an irritant to the chest, in order to bring out the eruption if it be tardy in its development. The Cantharides eruption is somewhat similar to that of miliaria, and it may take on a vicarious action. If the urine be suppressed, in addition to great difficulty of breathing, a trituration of Cantharides should be given internally; and Sir Astley Cooper and other distinguished practitioners have successfully applied a large fly-blister upon the loins. Given in moderate doses, it produces a feeling of warmth in the throat and stomach, followed by a sense of heat or uneasiness in the urethra, with a disposition to micturate more frequently than in health, some increase in the quantity of urine, and a slight excitation of the genital organs. If too large doses be given, there will be a constant disposition to pass urine, which, instead of being increased in quantity, is often much diminished, coming away in a few drops at each effort, and often very high colored or bloody. With these local phenomena, the pulse may become more frequent and tense, the skin hot, the breathing hurried, with more or less nervous disturbance, and a general febrile condition. The homœopathists suppose Cantharides to be frequently useful in those cases which occur in connection with puerperal fever, although Aconite and Veratrum-viride are well-tried remedies in this affection.

Bryonia-Alba.—Some physicians assume that the appearance of sudamina, during the progress of any disease, will generally be an indication for the use of Bryonia. Hirschel says that it is indicated in rheumatic miliaria, from its special affinity to the rheumatic process, and to the serous and fibrous membranes, when it occurs as an accompaniment of acute gout, rheumatic fever, rheumatic pleurisy, or puerperal peritonitis. Bryonia is supposed to be somewhat similar in its action to Colocynth and Colchicum. The peasants of Lorraine and Franche Comté use it fresh, as a purgative; while the ancient German physicians improperly regarded it as a reliable emetic, and called it the European Ipecac. In large doses, it is a severe and drastic remedy. In the homœopathic school, it is regarded as a rheumatic remedy, *par excellence*, with some specific action on the liver. It is often found useful against rheumatic pleurisy, rheumatic miliaria, acute rheumatism, many painful affections of the fibrous and serous membranes, constipation, torpor of the liver, yellow-coated tongue &c. It may be used against miliaria, when there is much constipation. a coated tongue, severe rheumatic pains in the limbs, back, and chest, with tendency to pleurisy or pneumonia, with or without retrocession of the eruption.

Nitric Ether and Bitartrate of Potash.—Among the cooling drinks which have been most used in miliaria, in addition to simple cool water, lemonade, and tamarind water, many physicians have given Seltzer or Saratoga water, Cream of Tartar water, a dilution of Sweet Spirits of Nitre, or of Citrate of Magnesia. All these are more or less pleasant, simple, and useful drinks. When the urine is scanty, and the bowels very costive, Cream of Tartar is commonly given in ordinary practice. Wood even goes so far as to place it at the very head of the diuretic class of medicines, and thinks that no remedy or combination of medicines will be found to cure so large a proportion of dropsical cases as the Bitartrate of Potash. When given in small and frequently-repeated doses, so as not to purge, it operates as a diuretic, and often very powerfully so, at the same time producing a refrigerant effect on the system. As regards the *Nitric-ether*, it is regarded as a nervous stimulant, well adapted to the febrile diseases of children, and to those of a typhoid character in adults, when there is much functional disorder, as restlessness, wakefulness, twitchings of the tendons, starting in sleep, mental irritation, fretfulness, &c.; it will often very happily allay these symptoms, and even ward off delirium and convulsions. When given somewhat freely, diluted in a large proportion of cold water, the patient being at the same time kept cool, it often acts with considerable energy as a diuretic. In suppression of the urine, when not dependent on nephritis, it often answers an admirable purpose. This condition not unfrequently attends febrile diseases, and sometimes occurs in children without assignable cause, unless it may be some disturbance in the nervous functions; in such cases, Wood says, the Nitric-ether is habitually resorted to, and often with complete success. The solution of Bitartrate of Potash is used, in ordinary practice, when constipation is the more urgent symptom, whether the urine be scanty or not, while the dilute Nitric-ether is relied upon when scantiness or suppression of urine is the more prominent phenomenon.

If the eruption do not come out fully, a weak preparation of Croton-oil should not be forgotten in the treatment of miliaria. Theoretically, it would seem to be strongly indicated. Wood says of it, that "When rubbed on the skin, or simply kept in contact with it, after a considerable time—sometimes sooner, sometimes later, but generally in the course of a day or two—it produces a diffused redness of the surface, which is almost from the beginning, attended with a countless crop of minute eczematous vesicles. These increase, run together, and, at length, if the application be continued, form one complete pustulated surface."

MEASLES.

Morbilli.

Definition.—The eruption of a crimson rash, consisting of slightly elevated, minute dots, disposed in irregular circular forms or crescents, preceded by catarrhal symptoms about the eyes, nose, and bronchia, for about four days, and accompanied by inflammatory fever. It affects the system only once, as a rule, and often prevails as an epidemic.

Pathology.—That a poison is absorbed and infects the blood there can be no doubt, and, after a given period of latency, acts on the great nervous centres, producing a continued fever, which does not remit on the appearance of the eruption, but runs on throughout the whole disease. The fever thus established—at the end of three, more generally of four and in some few instances of five days—is followed by a peculiar secondary or specific inflammation of the skin, and of the mucous membranes of the eyes, nose, mouth, fauces, and bronchia, in addition to the fever. In a few cases, the poison has certain tertiary actions, and produces inflammation of the substance of the lungs or of the pleura. As the primary fever lasts from three to five days, and the eruption from six to seven days, the whole duration of the disease is from nine to twelve days. Whenever the tertiary actions occur, the disease is so much more prolonged. The law that fever precedes the specific action of the poison has scarcely a recorded exception, and, consequently, though the pyrexia may vary greatly in intensity, it is uniformly present. It does not always happen, however, that the functions of the mucous membrane are disordered as well as the cutaneous surface. There are cases where no catarrhal symptoms exist, and such cases are described as "*morbilli sine catarrho*." Such cases occur during epidemics of the disease, and are but few in number.

Since the affection of the skin is uniformly present, whilst that of the mucous membranes is sometimes absent, the cutaneous eruption is necessarily the great characteristic of the disease; but, the morbillous eruption being evanescent after death, we can only imperfectly trace its pathology. It first appears as a circular dot, similar to a flea-bite, slightly prominent, and sensible to the touch. Its color is of a deep raspberry hue, and, in rare instances, as in the morbilli-nigri, is livid or black. In severe cases, also, especially if the patient be of tender age, the eruption assumes a papular form, and, when at its height, occasionally a vesicular appearance; the latter being most common on the arms, the neck, or the breast. The color of the eruption is evanescent on pressure, but returns on the finger being removed.

The patches of the eruption are extremely numerous, so that they leave little of the healthy skin intervening between them, and they not unfrequently become coälescent, forming large maculæ, sometimes of a semi-lunar form. The principal seats of the eruption are the face and back, while the parts least affected are the popliteal and pudendal regions. The inflammation of the cutaneous texture extends, in some degree, to the subjacent cellular tissue, for the face is tumid and swollen, but not so as to close the eyelids.

The eruption does not at once cover the whole body, but consists of three crops, each of which follows the other at an interval of twenty-four hours, the duration of each crop being from three to four days. The course of the measles, then, in its most simple and uncomplicated form, is, that on the third or fourth day of the primary fever, the first crop appears on the face, neck, and upper extremities; on the following day, the second crop covers the trunk; and, on the third day, the third crop appears on the lower extremities, so that the whole body is covered with the eruption, which is then at its height. On the next day, (the fourth of the eruption,) it begins to decline from the face, neck, and upper extremities; on the following day, it fades from the trunk; and, on the sixth or seventh day, it is evanescent over the whole body. The eruption terminates by resolution, followed by a furfuraceous desquamation of the cuticle of the body generally.

The inflammation of the mucous membranes of the eyes and nasal fossæ generally commences either with or before the primary fever, and precedes the eruption by some days. This inflammation is, perhaps, for a few hours, confined to fixed spots, and is marked by itching at the mucous orifices; then it becomes diffuse, and quickly changes to the serous; for a profuse watery discharge from the eyes and nostrils shortly follows, technically termed "coryza." This affection usually continues until the decline of the eruption, and in some cases to a later period.

The mucous membrane of the mouth and fauces also inflames, but the irritation differs from that of the eyes and nose in not being accompanied by any discharge. In other respects it is exactly similar to the cutaneous eruption; for a number of maculæ, more or less confluent, are seen upon the palate, uvula, tonsils, and velum pendulum palati, and they equally terminate by resolution. They appear, also, at the same time with the eruption on the face, neck, and upper extremities, but do not decline till the eruption fades from the body generally.

The bronchial and tracheal mucous membranes are usually attacked either before or at the same time with the buccal membrane; but whether the inflammation of which they are the seat is marked by the same characteristic eruption is not determined, for few patients die at this early period of the disease. The cough and expectoration, however, which accompany it, are constant, and the latter shows that it partakes of the same serous character as that of the ocular and nasal membrane. Again, towards the close of the disease, or even as late as the third or fourth day after the eruption has disappeared, the poison not unfrequently affects the substance of the lungs or pleura, and this constitutes the most dangerous complication of measles. When the substance of the lungs is affected, a serous exudation pervades that tissue, and the quantity of fluid effused is frequently so considerable as often to stream from the lungs when divided. In severe forms of the disease, either the red or grey hepatization of the lungs may supervene, but these results are rare. The pleura does not at all times escape the morbid action; and the diffuse, the serous, the adhesive, and even the purulent inflammation may invade that tissue, and either destroy the patient or retard his recovery. Diarrhœa, also, is often an accompaniment, which renders it probable that the mucous membrane of the intestines may be a surface on which any exudation peculiar to the disease may take place.

Varieties.—The symptoms of measles result from the fever and the consecutive local lesions. The varieties of the disease, however, are extremely few, for no instance is known of a morbillous fever without the secondary or specific actions following; but the poison is supposed, sometimes, to limit its action to one membrane, as the cutis, and to exhaust itself on that tissue, and hence the "*morbilli sine catarrho.*" The varying intensity of the disease, also enables us to divide measles into two grades: 1. *Morbilli-mitiores*, and 2. *Morbilli-graviores.* The primary fever may make its attack suddenly, or be preceded for a few days by symptoms of a common cold, and, in general, the latter is the case; but in no instance is the primary fever, which may be prolonged, and accompanies the eruption, of any great intensity; for, although many succumb, from the severity of the local lesions, yet no instance is known of the patient being overwhelmed or destroyed by the general depressing power of the poison, as in typhus and scarlatina. The prostrating action of the poison, however, is considerable, and always sufficient to confine the patient to his bed for a few days, and to leave him, for a short time after the disease has subsided, weak and debilitated. The type of the fever of measles, consequently, differs greatly from that of typhus or of scarlatina, and the formidable brown tongue, so grave a symptom in the latter, is hardly known in the former, or only seen in a few fatal cases.

MORBILLI-MITIORES.

The essential characters of this affection are, that the poison produces a benign primary fever, and a specific inflammation of the skin and mucous membranes; the fever not subsiding till the eruption dies away.

The symptoms of measles may be divided into three stages: The first embraces the primary fever, or the period before the eruption, and may last from three to five days; while the second stage embraces the period of the eruption, and lasts from six to seven days. These two stages very commonly comprise the whole disease, whose usual course is from nine to twelve days. The third stage includes any inflammatory action which may be caused by the tertiary action of the poison, and therefore only occasionally exists.

The early symptoms of the primary fever are seldom severe, and greatly resemble those of an ordinary but severe catarrh. They are shivering, alternated with heat, frequent pulse, headache, derangement of the bowels, sometimes accompanied by nausea and vomiting, and these affections are so considerable that the patient takes to his bed. At the end of a few hours the fever becomes continued, and the specific action of the poison commences, by the mucous membranes of the eyes and nose inflaming, so that the light is painful; the senses of smell and taste are lost, followed by a copious discharge of serum from the nose and eyes.

The buccal and bronchial membranes may become affected at the same time, and the patient is then troubled with a frequent cough, which has this peculiarity, that it occurs in paroxysms. The cough does not remit until about the seventh day, and is often accompanied by hoarseness, by a sense of constriction across the chest, by diarrhœa, and sometimes by ischuria. The duration of the first stage is three, four, five, or even six days.

The second stage commences with the appearance of the eruption, the fever is often aggravated, but the occasional nausea and vomiting seldom last beyond the fourth day. The fever, therefore, together with the coryza, sneezing, coughing, hoarseness, and diarrhœa, continues with unabated severity till the eruption has reached its height, and is fully out over the whole body, which is on the third or fourth day after its first appearance. From this period, in favorable cases, all the symptoms begin to decline; and, on the eruption disappearing, the cuticle desquamates, and the disease terminates on the ninth, tenth, or eleventh day from its commencement.

In a few cases, however, on the subsiding of a benign eruption, or about the ninth, tenth, or eleventh day of the disease, and in some instances earlier, the pectoral symptoms do not decline as they ought to do; but the tertiary actions of the poisons are set up, and inflammation of the substance of the lungs or pleura takes place, prolonging the duration of the disorder, and endangering the life of the patient. The inflammation of the bronchial membrane is denoted by the expectoration of either a thick, viscid mucus or of pus, and which may or may not be streaked with blood, while the mucous or sonorous rattle will point out the peculiar seat and extent of the mischief. If the substance of the lungs be inflamed, the breathing is more difficult, the cough more troublesome, and the countenance livid; but the loud mucous rattle which accompanies it seldom allows us to hear crepitation, or to determine the absence of respiration in any given portion of the lung. If the pleura be inflamed, we have, in addition to the cough, severe pain in the side, and an impossibility of filling the chest with air, except in a very limited degree; but this is rarely accompanied by dullness on percussion, by bronchophony or ægophony, assuring us that fluid is effused into the cavity of the chest.

MORBILLI-GRAVIORES.

The characteristic of this severe form of measles is the eruption suddenly becoming black, or of a dark purple with a mixture of yellow The early writers on measles describe this form of the disease as being much more common in their time than we find it to be at the present day. Sydenham considered this appearance as extremely formidable, and that persons so seized were irrecoverably lost, unless they were immediately relieved by bleeding and a cooler regimen. Willan says that he has seen this discoloration, but thinks more lightly of it.

The eruption is sometimes greatly delayed, from causes not quite manifest. Excessive purging is sometimes thought to have this effect, or anything which greatly debilitates the system, hereditary or acquired unhealthiness of constitution or the peculiar malignity of the disease. The occurrence of the eruption is, therefore, to be looked for with anxious care, as the appearance of it, even though late, is in itself a favorable indication.

If the eruption also suddenly disappears, or "goes in," it is no less an unfavorable omen, and is apt to be followed by dangerous results diarrhœa, dyspnœa, coma, convulsions—all of which unfavorable signs may again disappear on the reappearance of the eruption.

Diagnosis.—The diseases with which measles may be confounded are scarlet fever, and some forms of syphilitic eruptions. The diagnostic symptoms between measles and scarlet fever are numerous; and there are many differences, both in their general laws and particular symptoms, by which they may be readily distinguished. Thus, the periods of latency of the poisons are different—that of scarlet fever being from two to ten days, while that of measles is from ten to sixteen days. The exanthema, in scarlet fever, seldom appears later than the second day of the primary fever; in the measles, it is delayed till the fourth day. In scarlatina, the patches of the eruption are large, and the surface they cover ample; but, in measles, they are not larger than flea-bites, and, when most coälescent, the clusters are small. The color is also different, being bright red in scarlet fever, while in measles it partakes more of a raspberry hue. The affections of the mucous membranes are also different in the two diseases. In scarlatina, the tonsils are almost constantly greatly enlarged and ulcerated, while in measles they are little or not at all affected. In scarlatina, the eyes are free from coryza, while in measles this is the most prominent symptom. The tertiary actions of the poison are also different, being, in scarlatina, inflammatory actions of the joints and dropsy, while in measles they are inflammations of the lungs or bronchiæ. And, lastly, in measles, the fever usually subsides on the disappearance of the eruption; but, in scarlatina, the fever often continues many days or weeks after the eruption has run its course, or till the sore throat has healed.

Prognosis.—The mortality from measles varies greatly in different years. During each of the four last years, the proportion of deaths from measles, in every 1000 deaths from other causes, has been, in

1851, 24; in 1852, 14½; in 1853, 11¾; in 1854, 21½. Percival says that out of 3807 cases of measles, 91 died, or 1 in 40. Watson says that, in one year, at the London Foundling Hospital, 1 in 10 died; and in another, 1 in 3. In the same establishment, also, in 1794, out of 28 cases, none died; in 1793, out of 69 cases, 6 died; in 1800, out of 66, 4 died; and the aggregate of these data will give us an average of 1 death in 15, so that the prognosis in every case of measles is favorable. The prognosis, however, is more favorable in the country than in large towns; for it appears by the Registrar-General's Reports that the proportion per cent. of the population that died of measles in London is much greater than in England and Wales.

The chief danger arises from bronchial and pulmonary inflammation, and the danger of this is greater after the disease has began to decline, than during its progress. Croup also sometimes supervenes, and cuts off young patients. Measles, in any of the malignant forms described, is highly dangerous; and the danger is greater in the old than in the young; in cold than in warm weather.

Causes.—The measles appeared at the same time and in the same country with scarlet fever, and has subsequently followed nearly the same course. They both now prevail all over the world, are little influenced by season, are constantly sporadic, and occasionally epidemic. Their poisons, it would appear, must consequently have a similar origin; but it can scarcely be doubted that there is more than one specific cause. (?)

Measles, though incidental to every period of life, is most frequently contracted in childhood, when it is difficult to trace the effects of accidental circumstances, so that our knowledge of the predisposing causes are most imperfect. Both sexes, however, appear to be equally liable to the infection. With respect to the influence of season, it is generally supposed that measles break out in the beginning of winter, increase till the vernal equinox, and then die away towards the summer solstice. The number of deaths from this disease, registered in England and Wales, shows that the influence of season is exceedingly trifling.

Propagation of the Disease by Contagion and Infection.—It is admitted by all authors that a patient laboring under measles generates a poison which is both infectious and contagious.

This disease, like scarlatina, is greatly infectious; and, in like manner, no susceptible person can remain in the same room, or even in the same house, without hazard of taking the disease. In the year 1824, it was imported into Malta by some children belonging to the Ninety-fifth Regiment, and spread extensively on that island, so that many died. This circumstance was the more remarkable as the measles had not been seen on that island for many years. The infecting distance of this poison, it will be plain from what has been stated, must be considerable; indeed, it is often impossible to isolate it in our public schools, or other large establishments, where it sometimes appears.

Complications and Sequelæ.—In a majority of cases, if an epidemic of measles be prevailing at the time, we may suspect the existence of the disease, at an early period, by the presence of irritation and redness of the conjunctiva, especially that of the eyelids, the lachrymation, suffusion, and watery condition of the eyes, sensibility to light, stuffing of the nose, coryza, sneezing, frequent, hoarse, and scraping cough, slight constriction of the chest and partial dyspnœa, fever, headache, and thirst. But occasionally the premonitory symptoms are so slight that the child is scarcely supposed to be sick before the eruption makes its appearance.

In quite a number of cases, considerable *drowsiness* is present during the first stage, and the child, if undisturbed, sleeps quietly for many hours, or the greatest part of one or two days, waking only from time to time, for a short while, and then sinking off to sleep again. This symptom is not alarming, unless there be other signs of local disease of the head, or unless it pass into coma, or alternate with marked delirium; in such cases, the state of the bowels and kidneys should be carefully inquired into. If there be scantiness of urine, with retention of urea in the system, Colchicum will prove one of the most useful remedies. If there be an overloaded state of the stomach and bowels, with or without torpor of the liver, Mercurius or some gentle laxative should be given. The systems, or stomach and bowels of many young children, are often much disordered previously to the contraction of measles; the physician has to deal, not with a pure and uncomplicated zymotic affection, but with errors of diet, or consequences of carelessness, or gluttony, in addition to the impending eruptive disorder. These, of course, should be first removed; for it will be the height of folly to administer the specific remedies against simple and uncomplicated measles, in a case complicated with other serious derangements.

In a few cases, *convulsions* may precede the outbreak of the eruption; these generally arise in nervous and sensitive children, and cease as soon as the eruption makes its appearance. I have seen but five or six cases in nearly twenty years practice; Meigs, but 5 cases in 314 cases of measles; Rilliet and Barthez, only 1 case in 167; none of them terminated fatally. If they occur in teething children, the gums should be lanced if they require it; if excited by the presence of indigestible food, and indurated and impacted fæces, that should be removed from the system as speedily as safe or convenient, by means of Castor oil, injections of Flax-seed tea mixed with sweet oil and molasses, or with Castor oil, &c. It is much more important to dislodge the fermented and fetid products of impaired digestion, and to evacuate the morbid and irritating accumulations arising from a torpid state of the intestinal canal, than it is to pay attention to the most trivial external symptoms. If spasms ensue, from scantiness or suppression of urine, Colchicum, Apocynum, Digitalis, or Cantharides may be required. If they arise from simple excitability of the nervous system, Agaricus will often prove a useful remedy, while Conium is a most efficient palliative. If they occur from the great violence of the fever, and are attended with restlessness, irritability, and delirium at night, Aconite or Veratrum-viride will afford the promptest relief.

The *cough* of measles sometimes reaches a troublesome degree; it usually appears on the first day, is infrequent and slight at first but is apt to become more annoying as the case progresses, until it assumes a peculiar character on the third or fourth day, which may often lead to a suspicion as to the true nature of the attack. Before the eruption makes its appearance, it is laryngeal, hard, dry, rather hoarse, and generally occurs in short and frequent paroxysms; at the same time the voice is often hoarse. In a few cases, it may increase to *true laryngitis*. Rilliet and Barthez met with this complication in 35 out of 167 cases, and Meigs with only 8 cases out of 314. I have met with it in only a few instances, although the amount of catarrhal hoarseness which often attends the disease might lead some physicians to enumerate many more cases. It is rarely fatal, unless it assumes the pseudo-membranous form, which seldom happens. For this troublesome cough and hoarseness, *Conium* and *Antimony* are not only palliative but curative, as far as it is possible to cure a self-limited disease.

Conium appears to act as a direct sedative to the sensibility of the part with which it is brought in contact; it is also sedative to the nervous centres, especially those of the spinal marrow, and indirectly depresses the circulation. In doses insufficient to produce any obvious pathogenetic effect, it appears, not unfrequently, to exert a soothing or composing influence over nervous disorder or irritation. In full doses, it may cause some giddiness, dull headache, dimness of vision, a feeling of weariness in the limbs, and general muscular weakness, with, perhaps, some faintness, without the slightest sign of previous exhilaration of any kind, while the pulse is somewhat depressed. In poisonous doses, it may cause complete paralysis of the upper and lower extremities, loss of vision and speech, and true palsy of the respiratory muscles, with asphyxia, the heart continuing to contract long after respiration has ceased. Judd found it, in full but not poisonous doses, to cause great languor and drowsiness, often profound sleep for two or three hours, the muscular excitability being lessened, and the circulation and general temperature being reduced. It may be used to relieve pain, relax spasm, and allay nervous irritation in general; it will lessen the irritation of the eyes, which is apt to arise in measles, and prevent the occurrence of scrofulous ophthalmia. It will appease the troublesome cough which attends the disease, and prevent the development of scrofulous or tuberculous disease about the throat, air-passages, or lungs; it has even been used successfully in whooping cough, and other spasmodic coughs, and in asthma. In virtue of its powerful influence over the nerves of motion and the muscles in general, it will allay twitchings and tendency to convulsions; it will remove scrofulous tumefactions of the glands, or ulcerations which may remain after an attack of measles, in scrofulous or otherwise unhealthy subjects. In short, it will palliate many of the annoying attendants of measles, and prevent various of the after-effects which are so much dreaded in this disorder. If the fever runs high, or the threatenings of croup or laryngitis are severe, it will have to be aided by Aconite, Antimony, or Veratrum-viride.

The cough of measles may increase to *true bronchitis or pneumonia.* Rilliet and Barthez, in 167 cases of measles, met with 24 cases of simple bronchitis, 58 of lobular broncho-pneumonia, and 8 of pneumonia without bronchitis. Meigs, in 314 cases, met with only 24 of bronchitis, and 6 of lobular pneumonia. The most common period for the occurrence of bronchitis and pneumonia, is during the primary stage of measles; this disease consists in a specific eruptive inflammatory irritation of the skin and mucous membranes, of which that on the skin ought to predominate; but, in some instances, from a peculiar idiosyncrasy, or from the influence of cold and accidental exposure, the eruptive disorder is checked upon the surface, and increased upon the mucous-membranes, and broncho-pneumonia or pharyngo-laryngitis may arise. When bronchitis or pneumonia arises in the first stage of measles, it almost always retards the outbreak of the eruption, or renders it irregular or imperfect. When it occurs in the second stage, it may cause a partial or complete retrocession of the eruption; but, in both instances, the internal more severe disorder prevents the development of the disease upon the skin, and it is not merely the retrocession of the eruption which causes the internal complication. Hence, the physician should not devote all his attention to the bringing out of the eruption upon the surface, but should properly heal the internal affection. When this is lessened, the eruption may come out itself; but it is quite possible for the disease to run its course upon the internal skin or mucous membrane, and the patient recover with little or no eruption upon the external surface at any time; but this is not desirable, if it can be arranged otherwise. When the rash does appear, in such cases, it is often pale and scanty, or somewhat abundant on one part of the body and scanty on another, or it appears and disappears alternately. At length, it may come out fully, and the threatening symptoms pass away; or the eruption may persist in its pale and imperfect condition, and the little patient recover slowly but perfectly from the whole disease, and the complication which has become the most important part of the sickness; or, in bad cases, the symptoms grow worse and worse, and the child succumbs. I have never had a fatal case of measles, either during the disease proper, or in consequence of any of the complications or sequelæ, although I have witnessed them in the practice of others.

If the eruption is delayed until the fifth, sixth, or ninth day, or comes out scantily or irregularly, and if there is more drowsiness or irritability than usual, or the pulse is more frequent and stronger, and the breathing accelerated or oppressed, the chest should be carefully examined, in order that some pulmonic complication may not be allowed to steal on unawares upon the patient. In bad cases, the dyspnœa may become excessive, the respirations increasing to forty, fifty, or even sixty or eighty per minute; the pulse becomes rapid and small, the face pale and anxious, the child restless and irritable, with broken and irregular sleep, or dull and soporose. In the beginning of pneumonia, the cough may seem to be slighter than the ordinary measles cough; in bronchitis, it is apt to be still more severe and troublesome.

According to Gregory, rubeolous pneumonia, from its frequency and danger, requires close attention; it may occur either in the progress of the eruption or during its decline, and is often a slow, creeping, insidious form of inflammation, which too frequently throws the practitioner off his guard; for no positive complaint may be made, the child may only droop, and appear weak and exhausted, and the common practitioner may simply direct some mild tonic, supposing that the disorder has unduly weakened his patient. In the meanwhile, pneumonic engorgement creeps on, the lungs become more and more congested, and, at last, solidified; then a convulsion may occur, the dyspnœa increases, the child becomes drowsy, the feet cold, the pulse sinks, œdema of the lungs occurs, with fluid effusion from the bronchial mucous membrane, another and another convulsion may occur, rattles are heard in the throat, and the child dies. There is reason to suppose, if the alarm be taken soon enough, that the mischief is not irreparable in the first stages; although Gregory thinks that he speaks within bounds when he assumes that nine-tenths of the deaths by measles occur in consequence of the sub-acute form of pneumonia above described. He does not recollect ever having seen a case of rubeolous pleurisy.

Gregory supposes that, in perfectly regular measles, the cough, hoarseness, and other mucous symptoms should begin to abate on the first appearance of the eruption, and says he has seen the cough cease instantly, as if by magic. I am sure that this is not commonly the case, but, more frequently, the cough continues troublesome until the decline of the eruption and whole disorder, and that it is not always a bad sign when the catarrhal symptoms do not subside on the outbreak of the eruption, and the cough continues, the child becoming restless; but it is not favorable if dyspnœa comes on after the sixth day of the eruption, the child continuing to droop, its hands remaining hot, its nights unquiet, with thirst and scanty urine, and true secondary fever sets in, which may run on to the rapid development of tubercles in the lungs and the formation of small abscesses;—in the course of four or six weeks more, the child may emaciate, become consumptive, and die, more rarely from the development of tubercles in the lungs alone than from general tuberculosis in many organs.

The *ophthalmia* which succeeds measles is of the kind usually called scrofulous; there is often scrofulous photophobia to such an extent, and the irritability of the retina so intense, that it is impossible to open the eyelids, even by force. There is some redness of the conjunctiva, but not proportioned to the intolerance of light. This state of the eyes may continue for weeks, or even months.

Conium, internally and externally, is one of the best remedies for this disorder; a weak ointment of Conium or Stramonium may be smeared over the outside of the lids several times a day, for the relief of the excessive photophobia, with rapid relief, as I have repeatedly witnessed. It is far superior to lotions of simple warm water, or warm milk and water, or sassafras-pith mucilage, alone or mixed with rose water, which are more frequently recommended as external applications.

Pain and inflammation of the ears are very apt to come on during the course or decline of measles. They may come on slowly, marked by more or less uneasiness in the ear; or set in suddenly at night, with a severe paroxysm of earache, which may be more or less obstinate, and followed or not by a discharge from the ear, which may subside rapidly, or persist for a long time.

The local treatment of this affection is much more rapid and efficacious than internal remedies, and, of all applications, I prefer Majendie's solution of Morphine. The whole meatus may be filled up with the solution, then a bit of cotton, moistened with it, be lightly applied to the external meatus, in order to retain a portion of it. This process may be repeated every hour or two; but, in a large proportion of cases, one application is sufficient to afford speedy and permanent relief. This method is far superior to the application of poultices to the ear, although I also often direct the use of a many-folded napkin, wrung out in warm water, to the painful ear, to be renewed as often as it gets cold. Sweet oil and Laudanum. roasted onions and all similar disgusting and irritating applications should be discouraged, although, too frequently, they have been used before the physician is called.

A slight *diarrhœa*, or even a rather smart one, often precedes or attends the progress or decline of measles, and requires little or no interference in the majority of cases, except when it tends to excess, as it does in a few instances. It doubtless arises from eruptive irritation of the intestinal mucous membrane, and may be regarded as part of the disease, almost as much so as the irritation of the nasal, ocular, and pulmonary mucous membranes. Meigs says that the bowels may remain in their natural condition in measles, or there may be slight constipation or diarrhœa; but that constipation is most frequent, according to his experience. Mine is just the contrary; but this probably varies in different epidemics and seasons, although Meigs subsequently admits that a slight diarrhœa is a common event in measles, and occurs in a considerable number of cases, although it was severe in only seven out of three hundred and fourteen. Rilliet and Barthez regard the intestinal complications as the next most frequent after the pulmonary affections, in hospital practice. They think that about one-third of all the cases present the appearances of eruptive irritation, or erythematous inflammation of the intestinal membrane; that one-fifth offer the signs of follicular enteritis; one-seventh of ulcerative inflammation. In a few cases dysentery may arise, probably from the same causes which would excite the disease in non-rubeolous subjects. The symptoms of intestinal irritation are more or less abundant diarrhœa, which, singularly enough, does not exert much influence upon the external appearance of the measles, which usually pursue their regular course. Sometimes, however, it is attended with an increase of fever and, in the worst cases, interferes more or less with the regular progress of the eruption. It rarely or never is the chief cause of a fatal termination, but it increases very much the danger of the pulmonic attacks, which are less serious when they exist alone, but become exceedingly dangerous when complicated with intestinal inflammation. Gregory says that a sub-acute form of muco-enteritis is apt to arise when secondary fever occurs; the child then cries exceedingly, which it does not do in pulmonary inflammation, and draws up its legs to the belly; the stools are frequent, unhealthy, green, very offensive, and often ejected with force; the tongue is red, at first, and may become aphthous, ulcers may form at the angles of the mouth, the countenance is anxious, while emaciation and marasmus occur rapidly.

Other *eruptive* and *scrofulous* troubles are apt to arise after measles; eczematous runnings behind the ears are frequent, and the glands of the neck may harden, or advance to indolent abscesses. In these cases, Iodide of Mercury, Conium, and Baryta-muriatica are among the most useful remedies.

Treatment.—As measles is a self-limited, and generally not a dangerous disease, a large portion of the treatment may be expectant and palliative. Fever may be moderated, itching of the skin allayed, cough lessened, restlessness appeased, wakefulness and fretfulness removed, costiveness obviated, and diarrhœa checked, when any of these symptoms or others become annoying. Some suppose that one remedy can be found to accomplish all these desirable ends, and that such specific medicines have been discovered, viz.: *Aconite*, *Pulsatilla*, *Euphrasia*, and *Sulphur*, all of which have been assumed to possess specific powers against the whole complex of phenomena which attend measles. In the simple form of the affection, or the so-called catarrhal eruptive variety, Aconite and Pulsatilla are supposed to be all-sufficient. In the inflammatory variety, Aconite and Antimony, or Veratrum-viride are decreed to be the most useful remedies; in the gastric variety, Pulsatilla and Ipecac. are most frequently relied upon; in the malignant form, with petechiæ and hæmorrhages, Hammamelis, Phosphoric-acid, and Arsenicum are often used, with more or less effect; in the typhoid or nervous form, Rhus, Arsenicum, China, and Phosphoric-acid are thought useful. If the cough is very hoarse, resembling croup, Aconite and Antimony will often prevent danger, or Hepar-sulph., or Phosphor., or Bromide of Potash, or Mercury and Antimony may be given. If inflammation of the lungs arises, Aconite and Antimony will often remove it, although an occasional dose of Mercury, or a course of Veratrum-viride, followed by Phosphorus or Sulphur, may be required. If the eruption become suddenly suppressed, some will rely upon Bryonia, Sulphur, or Pulsatilla; while others suppose that Opium acts more specifically upon the skin than any of these remedies, and will reproduce the suppressed eruption more certainly and promptly. For excessive diarrhœa, China, Pulsatilla, Sulphur, Phosphoric-acid, or Arsenicum are used by some, while others maintain that a few small doses of Opium will remove the disease, and prevent the tedious and uncertain hunting after a supposed specific remedy.

The celebrated Kopp, from his experience in several epidemics, places great reliance upon the use of *Aconite*, assisted, or not, by Pulsatilla or Bryonia. He says he never treated the disease more satisfactorily; he thought the fever abated decidedly, the eruption became less burning, hot, and swollen, and the cough moderated. Watzke had thirteen cases recover, in five days from the commencement of the attack; fifty cases in seven days; eighteen in nine days; and only five cases dragged on to the tenth, eleventh, or twelfth day. Kirsch lost only one case out of seventy-eight; but he found *Pulsatilla* the most generally useful remedy, although he occasionally used Aconite, Bellad., and Bryonia, for fever and disorders of the head or lungs. When the cough was croupy, he gave Aconite and Hepar sulph. He never witnessed any serious after-diseases. Ozanne lost two cases out of seventy-three; one died of laryngitis, and the other of pneumonia. In one instance, the whole force of the disease fell upon the lungs, and there was little or no eruption. In the majority of cases, he relied upon Aconite and Pulsatilla alone, although, when delirium was present, he used Bellad.; when there were signs of irritation or inflammation of the small bowels he gave Veratrum, and Ipecac. when there was troublesome vomiting. He thought that Aconite lessened the frequency of the pulse, and Pulsatilla rather quickened it. In a large majority of cases, he relied upon *Aconite* alone, and found it to lessen the irritation of the eyes, fauces, trachea, and larynx. Heichelheim treated fifty-three cases without losing any, although some of them were left with a chronic cough, attended with pains in the chest, emaciation, night-sweats, and febris-lenta; while others had discharges from the ears, abscesses in the skin, affections of the bones, and chronic eruptions, in the shape of small boils. The principal complications bore an active inflammatory character, and occurred in the third stage, or that of desquamation. Schroen treated his cases symptomatically; he thought that Aconite hastened and aided the favorable outbreak of the eruption, that Belladonna removed the inflammation of the eyes and photophobia, that Hepar-sulph. was efficient and even absolutely specific against the peculiar measly cough, even when croupy, and Bryonia generally removed pains in the chest. In three cases, in which the eruption receded, the membranes of the brain were attacked;—one recovered under the use of Arsenicum, 2, and two died. Mayrhofer thought that children with light hair and skins were more violently attacked than those with dark. The most frequent consecutive affections, in his experience, were ophthalmia, with excessive photophobia, and occasional ulcerations of the cornea, for which he used Bellad., followed by Mercurius-solubilis and Hepar-sulphur; persistent diarrhœa and tedious cough, against which Nux-vomica and Pulsatilla were useful; and pleurisy and pericarditis, the former of which he cured with Bryonia, the latter with Tartar-emetic. Weber treated eighty-seven cases without losing one. Tietze, fifty-four cases, and lost three; he used the thirtieth dilution exclusively, and hence, perhaps, his comparative ill success. He gave Aconite in the first stage; Aconite and Bryonia if the fever ran high, the cough and eye-affections being severe, with constipation; Aconite and Pulsatilla if diarrhœa was present, and, if these remedies did not avail, he used Mercurius and Chamomilla; but, if the diarrhœa was very profuse and exhausting, he gave Phosphorus and Arsenicum. Croupy cough was speedily relieved by Aconite, Spongia, and Hepar-sulph. If the eruption came out tardily, Bryonia proved useful, if the lungs were principally affected; Pulsatilla and Mercury if the bowels were most in fault; and Belladonna if the head was affected. But, if these remedies failed to hasten out the eruption, Sulphur almost always had the desired effect; still there were some disappointments. Occasionally, the fever, cough, and diarrhœa commenced anew in the desquamative stage, and he used the ordinary remedies. Thus, we have given an outline of the practice of some of the most prominent European homœopathists.

In the regular practice, I have seen some very severe cases treated throughout with *Paregoric:* convulsions were removed, cough and diarrhœa allayed, wakefulness, restlessness, and excessive itching moderated, and a degree of general comfort produced which was very pleasant to witness, and must have been still more so to have experienced. I have treated many cases with Ipecac. and Opium, Aconite and Opium, or Pulsatilla and Opium, in alternation, with vastly more success and comfort to my patients than when I timidly and bigotedly avoided Opium under all circumstances.

In the mildest form of the disease, nothing more is requisite than to keep the patient on low diet, allay cough and irritation, attend to the state of the bowels, and prevent exposure to cold and wet; for the tendency to bronchial and pulmonary inflammation renders caution in this latter respect peculiarly necessary, especially as this disorder does not bear exposure of the surface to cold as well as either small-pox or scarlet fever. Demulcent drinks may be used with benefit against the cough and diarrhœa, or even the constipation, when it is present; flax-seed tea, infusion of slippery elm, or decoctions of the saccharine fruits may be used when constipation prevails, and solution of gum Arabic when diarrhœa is troublesome. If the bowels are not moved naturally for several days, and these demulcent and laxative drinks do not open them, injections of flax-seed tea may be given, to which Castor-oil may be added, if necessary. More severe purgatives may produce overpurging, and thus, perhaps, disturb the regular progress of the eruption, and it should always be held in mind that diarrhœa is very apt to occur spontaneously, and a little overactive treatment may precipitate it too profusely. If the fever runs high, a little sweetened Spirits of Nitric-ether is often used in ordinary practice, aided or not by small doses of Antimony. Bleeding is seldom or never resorted to, Meigs having used it twice only in two hundred and fifty-seven cases, although Wood supposes that the disease bears the loss of blood well, except that excessive bleeding interferes with the outbreak of the eruption, and favors its retrocession when it is already out; still, he only uses it when signs of decided bronchitis or pneumonia present themselves, or the laryngeal inflammation be threatening, or convulsions with tendency to stupor occur.

The convulsions which occur in children, in the early stage, sometimes require nothing more than a warm foot-bath, and cold to the head, as they frequently subside spontaneously without injury; they only require close attention when they are persistent, or often repeated, and followed by stupor, or when they occur in the later stages of the disease, especially when consecutive to severe bronchitis or pneumonia.

Aconite.—Hahnemann was the first to recommend the use of Aconite in measles. Bethman treated thirty-six cases with it, with marked success; he says, if given before the eruption was fully developed, it seemed to stay the whole disorder, and that no consecutive diseases followed. Stapf once regarded it as the principal remedy in measles: he sometimes used the tincture, and thought that the fever was moderated by it in an extraordinarily rapid manner, that local inflammations were prevented, or were lessened when present, especially those of the chest and eyes; the children recovered more rapidly than usual, scarcely ever had consecutive diseases, and could be allowed to run about much sooner than under other treatment. Kammerer thought that, when given in the incubative period, it often broke up the whole disease, and that no eruption appeared. When used during the eruptive stage, it ran a mild course, and the eruption commenced to abate in twenty-four hours. He regarded the appearance of a moderate bilious diarrhœa as a beneficial and critical occurrence, which might be imitated by artificial means when it did not occur naturally; but, if the diarrhœa and cough persisted too long, and secondary fever arose, he again resorted to Aconite with success. Weber thought Aconite more of a specific than Pulsatilla. Hartung, physician to Field-Marshal Radetzky, generally gave Aconite three times for three days; if a troublesome dry cough remained, Chamomilla generally removed it. Hartmann found Aconite to lessen the active fever, hard, quick pulse, dry heat of the skin, hot, red face, red and painful eyes, and photophobia, the painful hoarseness, with short, dry, and frequent, or hollow cough, the pains in the sides and chest, to procure sleep when disturbed by dreams and sudden startings; it also removed the bleeding of the nose, frequent vomiting, diarrhœa, and pains in the bowels. Schwarze thought it produced much alleviation in robust and plethoric children, when there was distress in the head, burning in the eyes, great intolerance of light, and much thirst. Some cases were relieved by one dose, others only by frequent repetitions of the remedy.—Heichelheim says that his treatment of measles was generally very simple; he gave Aconite in the first stage, when the fever ran high, with a full, hard pulse, excessive thirst, dry and troublesome cough, pains in the chest, and delirium at night. If there was threatening of pneumonia, he gave Bryonia in addition. He soon began to regard it as a specific, even when chronic cough set in, with hectic or febris-lenta, with inflammatory irritation of the lungs; he gave several doses of Aconite, followed by Sulphur and Sepia, although he occasionally found Dulcamara very useful. Muller relied almost exclusively on Aconite; also Mayrhofer, who thought it shortened the course of the disease, always kept the skin moist, and prevented secondary troubles. If the head and eyes were much affected, he gave Bellad. in addition. Tüllf thought that Aconite was the main remedy, that it allayed the fever, removed the symptoms of croup, and prevented pneumonic troubles, even when the capillary bronchi were affected.

The action of Aconite is now well understood: it is an arterial sedative, promptly and efficiently reducing the action of the heart and arteries, moderating fever, cooling the skin, and more apt to produce perspiration than to increase any of the other secretions or excretions. Hence, it is well adapted for the relief of febrile skin-diseases, and measles among the rest; it tends to develop the eruption, at the same time that it lessens the heat and irritation of the system; it relieves pain and restlessness, allays cough, prevents a tendency to bronchitis, pneumonia, and croup, and thus materially aids in conducting the disease pleasantly and safely to its natural termination. It is suitable even when the eruption is copious, and the fever intense, with an almost equal amount of irritation upon the mucous membranes as there is upon the skin, with quick respiration, stitches in the chest, troublesome cough, congestion of the air-tubes and lungs, and more or less stupor; also when the eruption recedes, the skin being cool and covered with perspiration, the face and whole body pale, the pulse thread-like and uncountable, the respiration short, quick, and panting, with groaning; also when there is congestive irritation of the brain, marked by constant automatic motions of one or the other hand, or spasms of the arms and legs, gritting of the teeth, and loss of consciousness. It may require from twelve to twenty-four hours to remove some of the danger in cases similar to the above.

Arsenicum has been used successfully when typhoid symptoms were present; when there was great anxiety, restlessness, and palpitation; when the eruption was faint or receded, and the face was dingy, with bluish or sallow streaks; when there were sordes about the mouth, or puffiness and paleness of the face, vomiting or diarrhœa, great debility and exhaustion. The action of Arsenicum is manifold: in small quantities, it is regarded as an irritant or stimulant, and sometimes as a tonic; it has a special tendency to the mucous membranes, especially of the eyes and nose, and is regarded as a useful remedy when the severest effects of measles fall on these parts, although it is equally specific in its effects upon the bronchial and intestinal mucous membranes. It is also one of the most remarkable of those mineral substances that are used to counteract blood-disorders. Headland says that it is capable of exciting no less than three kinds of action in the blood, which operations result in the counteraction of periodic disorders, convulsive diseases, especially choreas and certain cutaneous eruptions; and supposes that it must, of necessity, be a various and obscure agency which is gifted with the power of arresting and controlling so great a variety of morbid actions. Others infer that it is simply so powerful a remedy that it implants its own action upon the organism, and thus excludes all minor influences. It has been assumed that its principal action upon the blood is to enter into such union with the blood-globules as excludes the iron which should normally combine with them. Hence, it is thought to be the natural enemy or antagonist of Iron, and that this is its natural antidote; thus the great tendency of Arsenic is to produce dropsy and chlorosis, while Iron antidotes these affections; again, Iron not only removes the vomiting and diarrhœa caused by Arsenic, but will cure many affections of the stomach and bowels, even true Asiatic cholera, when the symptoms are similar to those caused by Arsenic. Iron will also remove many rheumatic and neuralgic pains similar to those caused by Arsenic; thus Hutchinson cured over two hundred cases of prosopalgia with Iron. Neumann says it will almost instantly remove very violent nervous pains, which are entirely rebellious to the most powerful narcotics. Iron, it is also assumed, will cure ulcers similar to those caused by Arsenic; while Neumann says it exerts remarkable curative powers against chronic suppurations and ichorations, and will cleanse foul ulcers better than any other remedy.

To return to the action of Arsenic. When given in slight excess, it is apt to bring on œdema of the face and redness of the conjunctiva, and its continued use may bring on a cutaneous eruption—described by Mr. Hunt as a kind of ptyriasis—together with failure of the appetite, general depression, a quick, small pulse, hurried respiration, and sometimes dropsical swelling of the feet. These actions prove its homœopathicity to some forms of febrile eruptions; but the majority of physicians only use it in chronic skin-diseases. The celebrated Gibert, of Paris, cured four cases of ptyriasis with it, to which Arsenicum is certainly homœopathic; also acne and impetigo quite rapidly; lichen in twenty-five days; chronic erythema in one month; frambœsia in three and a half months; lupus in five weeks, of which Hunt cured seventeen cases; prurigo was improved. Of 98 cases of psoriasis, 40 were cured, 38 improved, and 20 not benefitted; while of 119 cases, treated without Arsenic, 59 recovered. This prominent action in skin-diseases would lead us to infer that it might exert a beneficial action in some of the severer and more malignant forms of measles, if experience had not already proven the fact. It may prove as homœopathic to some skin-affections as it is to some intermittent and remittent disorders.

Dr. A. T. Thomson, on the authority of Headland, states that the action of Arsenic is liable to exacerbations and remissions, and sometimes even intermissions, and Headland adds: "Thus we may suppose that there is a certain degree of analogy between its operation and that of the malarious poison, by virtue of which it may exert a corrective power over the working of the latter in the blood." It is also useful in other intermittent disorders, besides ague, as in various kinds of intermittent neuralgia; it has been given successfully in some varieties of intermittent pulse, which are not due to organic disease of the heart, for the celebrated Darwin cured a case in which the beats of the heart intermitted regularly once in every three or four beats, by the administration of four drops of a saturated solution of Arsenious-acid, three times a day.

Belladonna.—Heichelheim and many others recommend this remedy when there is congestive or inflammatory irritation of the brain or its membranes, marked by either coma or delirium. Hartmann advises it when there is excessive thirst, which the patient cannot allay, on account of painful irritation of the throat, which is rather rare in measles; when there is a troublesome dry, spasmodic cough; when the eyes are congested, glistening, and watery, and there is anxious restlessness of mind, excessive irritation of the nervous system, and sleeplessness. Belladonna is supposed to act primarily upon the blood, next upon the brain, then upon the ciliary nerves and vagus. Others suppose that it acts as a paralyzer upon the sympathetic nerves, and that the redness of the skin and apparent congestions produced by it are owing, not to active turgor of the blood, but to paralysis of the sympathetic nerve, as first explained by Claude Bernard. According to his well-known experiments, when the cervical branch of the sympathetic nerve which unites the cervical ganglions was cut through, there followed immediately an increase of *heat* on the corresponding side of the face, which could be very easily appreciated by the hand, and which was found to be from four to six degrees, centigrade, higher by the thermometer. When the superior cervical ganglion of the great sympathetic nerve was entirely extirpated, Bernard found the same effect produced, in even greater intensity, and, at the same time that the heat was increased, the circulation of the blood became more active. This new phenomenon of increased calorification continued for a long time, for Bernard found it to last, at times, for several successive months. With the aid of these facts, we can reconcile the apparently opposing actions of Belladonna, in producing paralysis of some of the motor nerves and muscles, and apparent excitement in parts of the vascular system. One of the first manifestations of its action is paralysis of the ciliary nerves, marked by dilatation of the pupils; next, paralysis of the glossopharyngeus, characterized by difficulty of swallowing and dryness of the throat, with more or less sym pathetic nervo-paralytic congestion and redness of the throat; next, by a sub-paralytic affection of the vagus, some of the fibres of which, especially those of the acessorius, bring about the connection between the musculo-motor and regulatory system of the cardiac nerves, and account for the varying and often contradictory action of Belladonna upon the circulation and respiration. In the higher degrees of its action it causes paralysis of common sensation and of the sphincters and extremities.

As Belladonna produces an eruption somewhat similar to that of scarlet fever and erysipelas, it cannot well be strictly homœopathic to the essential substratum of measles; it can, at most, be more or less analogous, in some of its actions, to more or fewer of the phenomena of measles, and probably is, if not antagonistic, at least very different in its essence and most prominent manifestations from this disease. However this may be, it has been used most successfully in whooping cough by many eminent practitioners, and may, and often will relieve the troublesome cough of measles quite materially; it also exerts a specific action upon the eyes, and has been used successfully, in both schools, in some ophthalmic affections. Wood says it is often employed to diminish the sensibility of the retina or optic nervous centre, especially in that not uncommon condition of the eye in which, altogether independently of inflammation, light is extremely painful to it. It has also been used beneficially against spasms of the eyelids, spasmodic contractions of the iris, and photophobia; hence, there is nothing to prevent its proving useful against some of the eye-affections which attend measles. As it produces great redness of the skin, it may be used, in exceptional cases, to throw out the eruption of measles when it is suppressed or scanty.

According to Wood, among the chief indications which Belladonna is calculated to fulfil, are, first, to relax muscular spasm and rigidity, and second, to subdue pain. He says, in painless spasms it is often highly beneficial, and not only affords relief, but makes a permanent impression on the nervous centres, which sometimes proves curative. He says it will seldom cure epilepsy, but will often ameliorate the symptoms; while, in the non-epileptic convulsions of children and puerperal women, it has been highly recommended. In infantile cases, he thinks its use should be confined to the convulsions which depend on some extra-cranial irritation, such as teething, or spasm of the bowels. In both instances it is said to be best adapted to those attacks in which there is a frequent recurrence of the paroxysms. In another spasmodic affection, viz., asthma, it has been strongly recommended. In muscular rigidity, its local application has been found very useful in a number of different affections—viz., in constriction of the sphincters of the anus and neck of the bladder, and in spasms of the urethra; while rigidity of the os-uteri, it is well known, will sometimes yield to it, and also dysmenorrhœa, which is a spasmodic affection of the body of the uterus. All this experience would render it a suitable remedy in some of the attacks of convulsions which attend measles.

Stramonium is very similar to Belladonna in its action, both upon the brain, nervous system, and skin. Müller used it, at times, in preference to Aconite, when there was a decided irritative or erethistic fever, the face being red and bloated, with great heat of the body and profuse sweats, attended with a peculiar kind of anxious delirium, in which the children thought they saw frightful figures, rats and mice, from which they sought to escape or hide, especially if there was some spasmodic trouble about the throat, which rendered swallowing difficult. It moderated the fever, removed the delirium, after it had caused quiet sleep, and favored the outbreak of the eruption; the attack then ran a regular course, except the troublesome cough, to allay which other remedies were required. He used the twelfth dilution, and it is more than probable that the delirium, &c., were removed by the spontaneous appearance of the eruption, while larger doses would, perhaps, have proved as useful against the cough as the same quantities of Belladonna have so frequently been found efficacious against whooping- and other severe coughs.

Bryonia.—According to Kreussler, as quoted by Rückert, Bryonia is often useful when a troublesome cough remains after measles, especially if it is dry, but sounds hollow, and is attended with pain in the larynx. Hartmann recommends Bryonia when the organs of the chest are predominantly affected, especially when the cough is short and dry, sometimes actually spasmodic and gagging, causing vomiting of food and mucus; also when there is a profuse flowing catarrh, often attended with bleeding from the nose; difficult, short, and anxious respiration, aggravated by violent stitches in the chest, which are excited anew by the incessant cough and the deep inspirations which it causes; rheumatic pains in the limbs, red inflamed eyelids, constipation. It is claimed that Bryonia removes or moderates all the above symptoms, and thus allows the eruption to appear more abundantly upon the surface. It is thought still more useful when the eruption suddenly fades from the skin, and when the persistance of the chest-symptoms enables us to infer that it is this which prevents the eruption from reäppearing. Hartmann assumes that Bryonia is more reliable under these circumstances than any other remedy. Heichelheim often found Bryonia beneficial when the normal catarrhal affection was increased to such an extent as to amount to inflammation of the lungs; he says one or two doses were generally sufficient. Tülff thinks that his experience enables him to say positively that Bryonia possesses the power of throwing out a delaying eruption, and thus of allaying the violent commotions in the nervous and vascular systems consequent upon this retention; but then its beneficial effects cease, and it is subsquently only useful against the dry, gagging cough, which often excites vomiting, and leads one to fear the occurrence of bronchitis.

Bryonia is a rheumatic remedy, more nearly approaching Colchicum in its general action than any other medicine; hence, it is suited against many of those catarrhal and rheumatic affections which so frequently complicate measles. The tendency to take cold in this disease is well known, and the proclivity towards internal, inflammatory, rheumatic, and catarrhal affections, especially of the pulmonary organs, forms the great danger of the disorder. Bryonia has no special specific relation to the miasm of measles, or to the essential principle of this disease, and hence is not strictly homœopathic to the purely morbillous chest-affections; but if, from accidental or other exposure to cold, a rheumatic affection of the chest is superadded, Bryonia will come in play. The purely morbillous chest-affections are best met by Pulsatilla and Sulphur, while Aconite and Tartar-emetic may often be required to aid the Bryonia.

Ipecac. is often given in alternation with Bryonia. Hartmann thinks it most indicated when the eruption is delayed or appears imperfectly, attended with anxious oppression of the chest and excessive irritability, both of which are increased at night, and do not allow the patient to sleep; a very troublesome tickling cough is often connected with this state. In such cases, if Ipecac. and Bryonia do not afford prompt relief, Ipecac. and Opium will generally quickly render the patient very comfortable. Wood regards Ipecac. as an irritant of considerable power. Applied to the skin, it is capable of producing inflammation and a vesicular eruption; the dust, in contact with the eyes, occasions redness and high irritation; particles of the powder, inhaled by certain individuals, cause severe irritation of the air-passages, exciting, in some, violent sneezing, and in others a complete paroxysm of spasmodic asthmatic dyspnœa, followed by copious expectoration. In very minute doses, it increases the appetite and facilitates digestion, probably owing to a very gentle exercise of its irritant property; in somewhat larger doses, it acts as a diaphoretic and expectorant, appearing to have a special tendency to the broncho-pulmonary apparatus. In still larger doses, it nauseates, causing coolness of the surface, paleness of the face, softness of the pulse, and moisture of the skin, whence it is frequently used, in regular practice, as an antiphlogistic remedy, in some fevers and inflammatory irritations. It is possible that Euphrasia and Pulsatilla may combine irritant with antiphlogistic properties, somewhat like Ipecac. and Tartar-emetic.

Drosera has been used by Stapf and Tietze, to relieve the troublesome cough and hoarseness which oftentimes attend measles, especially if the cough is so severe as to resemble whooping cough, and attended with vomiting and lividity of the lips and face. It may be used alone or in alternation with Ipecac. or Bryonia, or even Opium if absolutely necessary. The Drosera-rotundifolia was used as early as the sixteenth century, by herbalist-physicians, under the supposition that the permanent moisture of the sun-dew would render it an excellent remedy to restore vital moisture in persons laboring under consumption; but Gerard states that those who took it died sooner than those who were treated by other means. Still very able physicians, such as Forest, Schenk, Holland, Valentin, and Chomel, have used it, with more or less success, in different kinds of cough, arising from bronchial attacks and phthisis, and Ossiander in chronic asthma and palpitation of the heart.

Hepar-sulph.-calcarea is regarded by Heichelheim as almost specific against the ordinary measles-cough, and many croupy coughs. He says, if croup symptoms develop themselves, even if the fever is excessive, while the dry cough has a bellowing sound, and vexes the patient night and day, a few doses of Hepar-sulph. will soon loosen the cough, promote expectoration, and abate the threatening symptoms; but he does not regard the measles-croup as dangerous as the sporadic croup, however threatening the symptoms may seem. In ordinary parlance, the liver of Sulphur is regarded as a diaphoretic remedy, which increases the secretions from the skin and lungs. In olden times it was supposed to act inimically upon the red globules of the blood, and to exert a liquefacient action upon the fibrin and other plastic portions of this fluid; from these notions, it was used by ancient physicians, with more or less success, in croup, dropsy of the brain, tubercular phthisis, and various forms of ophthalmia. It was rescued from oblivion by Hahnemann.

Phosphorus is recommended strongly by Tülff when pneumonia develops itself in the course of measles. He says it is indispensable, and the presence of the highest fever does not contra-indicate its use, although it is most serviceable in the second stage, or that of *ramollisement rouge*; he thinks it injurious in the first stadium, and useless in the third stage, or that of grey hepatization, unless aided by Sulphur, Carb.-veg., or Arsenicum. He also advises it in catarrhus-suffocativus, when the bronchiæ are filled with mucus and a loud rattling is heard while coughing or breathing. I think it much more safe to rely upon Aconite, Tartar-emetic, or Veratrum-viride in the first stage of pneumonia, upon Mercurius and Tartar-emetic in the second period, and Phosphorus in the third stage of inflammation of the lungs. In small doses, Phosphorus excites the nervous, vascular, and secreting organs;

it causes an agreeable feeling of warmth at the epigastrium, increases the frequency and fullness of the pulse, augments the heat of the skin, heightens the mental activity and the muscular powers, and operates as a powerful sudorific and diuretic. Pereira says, in some of the exanthemata, such as measles, it has been administered to promote the reäppearance of the eruption, when this has receded from the skin. Beck says, of all the stimulants, Phosphorus is one of the most prompt and energetic; taken in moderate doses, it produces a sense of warmth in the stomach, together with a very powerful general excitement, quickens the circulation, augments the animal heat, promoting, at the same time, all the secretions, especially those of the skin and kidneys, and exciting the venereal appetite. If used at all in the primary stages of pneumonia, it should be given in very small doses; in the later periods of the disease, when better nourishment and Camphor or Ammonia are thought indicated, Phosphorus may be used in larger quantities. The mistake that Heichelheim probably made, was in giving as small doses in the third stage as he did in the first and second.

Schwarze gave it to a delicate little girl, who already had had a few measly spots for three days, still the eruption remained pale and inclined to recede; she had but little fever, and was very languid. In four hours after taking Phosphor., the fever arose, and more eruption appeared, and, under a repetition of the remedy, the whole body was fully covered with measles in thirty-six hours. Troublesome cough and photophobia were relieved by Bellad. Phosphor. has also afforded speedy relief in several cases of measles, when the dry cough was attended with inclination to vomit or actual vomiting.

Camphor is recommended by Hartmann when the eruption is delayed, and there is the greatest debility of the body, with difficulty or inability of moving any of the limbs, and great paleness of the face, with coldness and blueness of the skin, frequent chills and rigors, chattering of the teeth, spasmodic rigidity of the body, and cold sweats. Hartmann says these few symptoms are so characteristic for Camphor that its place cannot be supplied by any other remedy, and thinks no other drug arouses the reäctive powers of the skin so rapidly as it, by which the outbreak of the eruption is favored, and all other anxiety removed. He recommends the first to the third dilution of Camphor to be given every half-hour, and the limbs to be rubbed with several drops of spirits of Camphor on flannel. I regard it as perfectly useless to give a high dilution of Camphor internally while the strong odorous tincture is used externally. I am also inclined to deny the homœopathicity of minute doses of Camphor to the above-described conditions of exhaustion, depression, coldness, and almost of collapse; it requires overwhelming doses of Camphor to produce these effects, while moderate doses are antagonistic to them, and cause an increase in the frequency and fullness of the pulse, and warmth of the skin, some perspiration, exhilaration of spirits, and feeling of comfort. In short, in moderate quantities, it acts as a nervous stimulant; high dilutions will not produce the above effects, even when the skin is naturally warm and the pulse active, as in health, much less rescue a prostrate and almost collapsed patient from his exhaustion and depression. It requires quite large doses to do this; for, even in health, moderately large doses are requisite to induce some warmth of the skin, greater frequency of the pulse, and decided increase of perspiration, which, under favorable circumstances, may pass over into a profuse warm sweat. These must be regarded as the primary effects of Camphor, and, if the dose be considerably increased, burning pain in the stomach will arise, with congestion to the head, great redness of the face, sparkling of the eyes, great anxiety in the præcordia, and, perhaps, nausea and vomiting, from irritation of the stomach. This state of over-excitation will be followed by signs of depression, such as coolness of the skin, paleness of the face, drowsiness, &c.; but very large doses may overwhelm the powers of the system, and produce depressing effects from the commencement. Wharton and Stille report a case, in which a man took, for the relief of priapism, an enema containing *ten drachms* of Camphor. Immediately afterward, he had sensations of *cold*, alternating with heat in the lower bowels, and these feelings extended along the spine to the neck, and spread over the whole body; he was then seized with vertigo, had grotesque hallucinations, an excessive frequency of the pulse, embarrassed respiration, vomiting, strangury, and was greatly prostrated within two minutes after taking the injection; the delirium increased, the features were *pale* and composed, the eyes fixed, and the pupils dilated, the skin became covered with clammy perspiration and was *ice-cold*, the pulse frequent and thready, and the impulse of the heart very feeble. When violently aroused, he regained his consciousness for a moment, complained of distressing nausea, extreme *chilliness*, and great desire to sleep; vomiting of a yellow watery fluid was succeeded by great prostration. By the assiduous employment of stimulants, both internally and externally, he was rescued from this very precarious condition, and recovered entirely; the only durable result of the Camphor was complete *aphrodysia*, which lasted several weeks. From such effects as these the early Arabian physicians, who introduced Camphor into the practice of medicine, regarded and employed it as a *refrigerant*. Like views induced Hahnemann to recommend it as homœopathic to the cold stage of cholera, and Hartmann and others as homœopathic to the collapse-stage of many diseases and eruptions. A leaning towards its refrigerant action leads Wood and others to say that the *ardor urinæ* of gonorrhœa may be alleviated by injecting an oleaginous solution of Camphor into the urethra, and the tenesmus from ascarides and dysentery by administering the same solution in an enema; and twenty or thirty grains of Camphor, added to a poultice and applied to the perinæum, is said to allay the chordee, which is a painful attendant on gonorrhœa, and the vapor of Camphor has been inhaled into the lungs, with benefit, in asthma and spasmodic cough. The *depressing* and *cooling* effects of Camphor on the genital organs is almost undoubted, and has led to its use in a great number of spasmodic and nervous disorders, when connected with urinary or genital diseases; the cases of this nature to which ordinary experience has proved it best adapted, are dysmenorrhœa, puerperal convulsions, and other nervous affections of the puerperal state, also certain forms of mania, especially puerperal mania and that arising from the abuse of spirituous liquors. Gooch thought it especially useful in controlling uterine irritation, dysmenorrhœa, irritable uterus, &c.; it is also much employed in certain forms of melancholy, to relieve despondency, cause mental quiet, and produce sleep. "Especially is this true," says Beck, "when the mental disease has any connection with the sexual organs, such as puerperal mania and nymphomania." Dierbach recommends it in wasting disorders excited by excessive loss of semen and frequent pollutions; against *satyriasis*, *furor uterinus*, and *hysteria libidinosa;* against mania, when connected with an excited state of the genital organs, chordee, painful erections, &c. In many of these cases, in addition to its internal use, Dierbach says it may be sewed up in little linen bags, or in belts, and worn around the body.

Camphor is also recommended, in the regular practice, in small-pox, measles, scarlatina, and miliary fever; but Pereira says it is only admissible when the circulation flags, and the temperature of the body falls below the natural standard; in such cases it is sometimes employed to determine to the skin, as Pereira regards its leading effects —when given in what he regards as small or medium doses, of five or ten grains—as that of a vascular excitant; for he has seen it increase the fullness of the pulse, raise the temperature of the surface, and operate as a sudorific.

Euphrasia.—Hartmann says this remedy is often indicated in the first stage of measles, against the irritative or so-called catarrhal symptoms, such as great inflammatory irritation of the eyes, intolerance of light, profuse secretion of mucus on and from the lids, violent flowing catarrh, with aching pain in the forehead, and troublesome dry cough. Tülff says it is often used, with great success, against the morbillous inflammation of the eyes, but thinks the internal use of the remedy should be aided by the external application of compresses, and bathings with a solution of twenty drops of the tincture in two ounces of water. Drysdale corroborates the above testimony by an experience of several years with the use of Euphrasia, aided or not by Aconite, against the morbillous irritation, or catarrhal inflammation of the eyes and nose, which attend the first stage of measles. Boyce thinks that, in several instances, it aided the outbreak of the eruption, even when this had been delayed several days or even two weeks, and when typhoid or cerebral symptoms occurred in consequence, or the eruption was dark like petechiæ.

Euphrasia, or Eye-bright, has been used in eye-affections from time immemorial—long before the homœopathists began to use it; but Hahnemann rescued it from oblivion. Its name, in all languages, seems to point to some specific action on the eyes or brain. Its Greek name (Εὐφρᾶσια) means delight, joy, happiness; the Romans called it *ophthalmica* or *ocularia;* the Swedes, Dutch, Danes, and Germans, *ogentrost*, or eye-comfort; the French, *cassé-lunettes*, or herb which renders spectacles unnecessary. It has also been called brain-herb and milk-thief.—Frank says there seems to be little doubt that it acts specifically upon the mucous membranes of the eyes and nose, also somewhat upon the brain, while it has a domestic reputation for drying up the milk. It has a pleasant, meadow-like smell, and a mild taste, which is neither bitter nor astringent. The tincture should have a light or dark green color; when it has changed to a violet-brown shade it is old and worthless. Shenstone and Milton have sung the praises of Euphrasia in affections of the eyes; the former says it enables dim eyes to see far around, the latter that the visual nerve may be purged with Euphrasia and films removed. Kranichfeld thought that three-drop doses of the tincture, once a day, caused an aggravation of a catarrhal ophthalmia and nasal catarrh, followed by commotion in the bowels, as if diarrhœa would occur, and sleeplessness in the morning. He also reports a cure of blepharo-ophthalmia glandulosa catarrhosa chronica, marked by itching, redness, and profuse secretion of mucus from the eyes, of two years standing, in eight days, with one-drop doses of the tincture every twenty-four hours, aided by bathing the eyes, three or four times a day, with Aqua-euphras.-officinal. A man, aged sixty-two, was cured, in ten days, of a chronic catarrhal inflammation of the eye; and a woman, aged twenty-one, of an acute attack, of fourteen days standing, in six days: one drop of the tincture was taken every evening, and the eye washed with Euphrasia water, four or five times a day. Euphrasia, perhaps, approaches Pulsatilla more nearly in its action on the mucous membranes than most other remedies. Hamilton says that Bauhin, in 1580, asserted that the earliest notice of Euphrasia as a medicine is in the works of Tragus. It was employed as a remedy in diseases of the eyes by Frischius, Haller, and others, and has been a domestic remedy in these diseases from time immemorial, throughout the whole of Europe.

Frischius recommended it in suffusions and cataracts. Hildanus, Villanova, and Veleot in weakness of the eyes. Arnaldus Villanova, who died in 1313, was the author of "*vini Euphrasiati tantopere celebrati.*" How long before him Euphrasia was in repute for eye-diseases it is impossible to say; but, in a book of Gordon's, published in 1305, among the medicines for the eyes, Euphrasia is one. The Highlanders of Scotland make an infusion of it in milk, and anoint the patient's eye with a feather dipped in it. In 1836, Kranichfeld, of Berlin—doubtless getting his information from homœopathic sources—employed it with success in rheumatic and catarrhal inflammations of the eyes and lids, in coughs, hoarseness, earache, and headaches, which have supervened on catarrhal affections, and in glandulous, catarrhal, and scrofulous blepharophthalmia. It is a pleasant plant to the eye; Hamilton says that no gem can equal this brilliant and lasting ornament of the turf in the fall of the year, after the harvest: then the grassy downs are still glowing with the tufted Euphrasia, its beautiful whiteness tastefully variegated with purple and pale yellow. Geoffrey and others mention that a Swiss lost his sight, instead of improving it, by the immoderate use of Wine of Euphrasia. Lobel states that it produces inflammation of the eyes, and that a friend of his nearly lost his eyesight by the use of it. Some assume that Euphrasia is an acrid remedy, and cures ophthalmia in the same or a similar way that Nitrate of Silver and Corrosive Sublimate do; others that it is a homœopathic antiphlogistic remedy, like Aconite or Veratrum-viride, but exerting a specific influence upon the eyes and mucous membranes; it is probable that it has a mixed irritant and antiphlogistic power, somewhat like that of Ipecac. or Tartar-emetic.

Chamomilla.—Among the remedies which are given for some of the accidents that attend measles, Chamomilla has frequently been used when diarrhœa occurred, with or without retrocession of the eruption; in some cases, the diarrhœa subsides rapidly under its use, and the eruption comes out again fully. The German Chamomilla, or Matricaria-chamomilla, differs very widely from the Roman Chamomile, or Anthemis-nobilis; the former is often called the Catnip of the homœopathists, as it is so frequently used by them to allay the colic and crying of infants, to soothe pain from teething and flatulence, to quiet the nervous system, and promote perspiration. It is often given, in alternation with Coffea, when there is great nervous excitement, excessive irritability of the patient, much sensitiveness of the skin and all the senses to external irritations, even when there are slight convulsions, some gritting of the teeth, and entire sleeplessness, on account of the great hyperæsthesia of body and mind, and the incessant short, dry cough. If these remedies fail, Opium may be given in alternation. Chamomilla is also supposed to act specifically on the liver, and, when that organ is disturbed in measles, it may be given, either alone or in alternation with Mercurius.

Pulsatilla is, doubtless, the most frequently used remedy in measles, both as a palliative, preservative, and curative means. Schwarze is, perhaps, the most earnest advocate of the protective powers of Pulsatilla against measles; he says he has often employed it in families in which several members were already attacked with the disease, which did not then spread to the others; he only gave the ninth, twelfth, or fifteenth dilution, in one-drop doses, every fourth evening, for fourteen days, then omitted it for eight days, and resumed it again. He has grace enough to add that, if the measly spots have already appeared on the face, the remedy will not prevent the complete outbreak of the disorder, but will render it much milder. He repeats that several observations have convinced him that it is a preservative remedy. He gives a case, in which a boy, aged four years, began to complain during the prevalence of an epidemic of measles; he was hot and cold by turns, coughed and sneezed much, was hoarse, and had red, sensitive, and watery eyes; it is not positively stated whether he had actually been exposed to measles, or merely had a catarrhal fever. He took Pulsat., 15, and was much sicker for twelve hours, when he steadily recovered, without the outbreak of any eruption. Schwarze says he has noticed the same thing in several other, already apparently contaminated children, and feels convinced that Pulsat. possesses the power of counteracting the miasm of measles when already operative in the human body. His cases would have been much more satisfactory if he had stated positively that the children had been fully and fairly exposed to measles, and were not merely the subjects of some catarrhal affection. Hartmann also claims to have observed the preventive powers of Pulsatilla; he says, if given early enough, it will completely prevent the disorder. Genzke gives his experience very frankly: he gave Pulsat., 3, to seventeen children, one dose every third day; the result was that nine of them took the measles and eight escaped; to four of the subjects the antidote was only given after the measles had already broken out in the house. All his cases ran a mild course, apparently made so by the previous administration of the remedy; yet he honestly states that the whole epidemic was a very mild one. Tülff says he never could convince himself satisfactorily of the specific powers of Pulsatilla against measles, and has never witnessed anything like prophylactic properties.

On the other hand, Hartmann declares it is wonderful how Pulsatilla will favor the outbreak of the eruption; others say, when the measles recede, Pulsat. will bring them out again, especially if there is much hoarseness and affection of the larynx; another authority asserts it may be well known that Pulsat. will drive out the eruption of measles in two, four, or six hours; still he has noticed it in a special manner in four cases, both in adults and children. The remedy certainly seems to blow both hot and cold: to antidote the miasm, and develop it; to destroy it, and throw it out.

Pulsatilla is also recommended when the brunt of the disease falls on the bowels, causes acute intestinal catarrh, and disturbs the regular course of the disease; also when the ears are severely inflamed, and when tubercular consumption threatens to develop itself. Watzke reports a case, in which a scrofulous girl, aged twelve years, who had had shortness of breath and an eruption about the knees for a year, was attacked with measles. The desquamation took place with difficulty, the shortness of breath increased, attended with constant oppression and acute stitches in the chest; the cough was very troublesome and dry, with a scanty, white, mucous expectoration; she became very weak, much emaciated, lost her appetite, slept little, was very restless, and perspired profusely towards morning; she had frequent alternations of chills and heat, with hectic spots on the cheek, and small, quick pulse. She recovered perfectly in ten days, under the use of Pulsat., 3, a dose night and morning. Bethmann reports a case of inflammation of the ear, occurring fourteen days after the retrocession of measles, from taking cold. There was hardness of hearing, increasing rending pains in the head, especially behind the right ear, from which a yellowish watery fluid ran; the region behind the ear was inflamed and swollen, the mouth was dry, face swollen and red, pulse hard, small, and 110, with sleeplessness. Pulsat., 12, was given, and a recovery occurred by the third day.

Although Pulsatilla is mentioned by Dioscorides and Pliny, still we are most indebted to Storck and Hahnemann for our knowledge of this remedy. As early as 1771, Storck recommended it as an effectual remedy for many chronic diseases of the eyes, particularly amaurosis, cataract, and opacity of the cornea; he also thought it useful in nodes. nocturnal pains, ulcers, caries, indurated glands, scrpiginous eruptions, melancholy, and palsy. Two cases of amaurosis, three of cataract, and seven of affections of the cornea were either entirely cured or greatly benefitted by it. In almost all cases it excited quite severe pains in the diseased eyes; frequent and profuse urination was caused in eight cases; increase of menstruation was induced in three cases, and return of menses, which had been suppressed for a year, in one case; dysmenorrhœa was removed in one case; diarrhœa was excited in five cases, in some of which the passages were very offensive, but not debilitating, and ceased under the continued use of the Pulsatilla. From these experiments and cures by Storck, Hahnemann became acquainted with the virtues of Pulsatilla in affections of the eyes, stomach, and bowels, and the urinary and genital organs. We are more particularly interested at present with Storck's ophthalmic cases, as measles, it is well known, is often attended and followed by severe affections of the eyes. Storck used from seven to fourteen grains of extract of Pulsatilla, rubbed up into a very fine powder in a marble mortar, with one drachm of white sugar; of this preparation he gave from twenty to thirty grains, three times a day.

Case 1.—A man, aged twenty-one, after having had venereal ulcers of the throat, was attacked with syphilitic ophthalmia of both eyes. He could see a little, indistinctly, with the right eye, but the left was entirely blinded by an albugo; the right parotid gland was also enlarged and hard. Mercurials and antimonials were given without benefit. The weaker powder of Pulsatilla was given by Storck, in scruple doses, every night and morning. The remedy caused increased pain in the eyes and lachrymation, followed by salivation and improvement of sight; when the salivation ceased, an offensive diarrhœa occurred. After this treatment was followed up for five weeks the patient could see quite well with the right eye, and better with the left, as the albugo had commenced to disappear. Then the same doses were given three times a day, followed by a renewal of the pains in the eyes, increased lachrymation, and more profuse and frequent discharges of urine; but, in a few days, the pains in the eyes lessened, and the parotid began to soften, and, at the end of two months, there was a still greater improvement of the sight. The stronger powder was now given, in thirty-grain doses, three times a day, and in four months the patient was quite cured, both of his eye- and parotid-affection.

Case 2.—A woman, aged twenty-eight, had been blind for several years, with a thick *pannus* over both, but more particularly over the whole left cornea. The weaker powder was given, in twenty-grain doses, three times a day, and, in fourteen days, the opacity began to grow thinner, and the patient could easily distinguish light from darkness. The stronger powder was now given, in fifteen-grain doses, three times a day, and, in six weeks more, the right eye was quite restored, and there was every prospect that the left would be so also. The remedy caused violent pains about the eyes and slight diarrhœa.

Case 3.—Scar and opacity of the whole left cornea, remaining after the bursting of an abscess, in a girl aged twenty. Many remedies had been used, without benefit, when the weaker powder was given as above; she was cured in two months. Soon after the commencement of the treatment, her menses, which had been suppressed for a year returned, and continued to do so regularly.

Case 4.—Complete amaurosis of the right eye for twelve years, and of the left eye for a year and a half, in a woman aged thirty-nine; many remedies had, of course, been used in vain. The weaker powder was given as above, followed by the occurrence of very violent, rending, dilacerating, boring, and lancinating pains in the eyes, and profuse lachrymation. In the course of three weeks, her menses, which had been suppressed for several years, returned again freely; at the end of six weeks she could plainly distinguish light, and her pupils had become moveable; at the end of five months, she could see objects with her left eye, could distinguish colors, and was able to walk alone, she also began to see a little with her left eye. Her menses continued to return every three weeks.

CASE 5.—Cataract for seven years, in the left eye of a man, aged sixty-two; his right eye was also very weak, and had gradually become so dim, that he not only could not attend to his work, but could not walk alone in the street. The stronger powder was given, in thirty-grain doses, three times a day, and, in twelve days, he could work a little with the right eye, and also distinguish candlelight with the left.

The equally celebrated Kopp cured a case of erethismus-oculorum, or morbid sensibility of the retina, with ten-drop doses of the strong tincture, three times a day; no aggravation or other unpleasant effects were noticed. Also severe pains in the eye, in another case, with the same doses. This experience would encourage us to use the remedy in some severe eye-affections, and it is a question whether smaller doses would effect equally good cures.

Dierbach asserts that Pulsatilla will throw out offensive sweats and pustular eruptions, and that it often acts as a powerful diuretic; that suppressed hæmorrhoids and menses will reappear under its use, and that it will excite cough, frequent sneezing, headache, dimness of sight, vertigo, and trembling of the limbs. He thinks it is an exceedingly active and useful plant, and when it fails the apothecary or herbalist is in fault, by delivering a poor article. On the same authority, it was used as early as the sixteenth century, by Zorn, to throw out the eruption of measles and small-pox, as he was well acquainted with its diaphoretic powers. Clarus says, in ordinary practice, it is now only used in those cataracts and amauroses which arise from some suppressed eruption; he says it actually seems to possess the power of retarding the development of cataract. Sobernheim believes that it is a still more powerful remedy than Aconite; it belongs to the acrid family of the ranunculaceæ, in company with Ranunculus-bulbosus, Sceleratus, &c., of which the common name is "crow-foot," or "butter-cup." The same author says it acts most specifically upon the eyes, next upon the skin, mucous membranes, and genital organs; it may cause a vesicular eruption, irritation to sneeze and cough, an itching feeling in the urethra, attended with increased inclination to pass water. The active principle of the drug—the anemonin—acts quite as specifically upon the eyes, but in a different way, as does Belladonna. Sobernheim states most positively that it worthily retains the reputation given to it by Storck, in diseases of the eyes. It is not as useful in purely dynamic affections of the eye, as in those which follow of measles, or from the suppression of some eruptive affection, or connected with some rheumatic derangement, or from a metastasis or suppression of some disorder of the mucous membranes, especially those of the nose, ears, stomach, bowels, bladder, or uterus.

Sulphur is thought to be almost as specific against measles, by some physicians, as Pulsatilla. It is used when the eruption does not come out fully; when obstinate eruptions remain after measles; when a scrofulous or tuberculous affection threatens to arise; when a troublesome cough and tendency to hectic fever develop themselves; and when an annoying diarrhœa occurs.

Some allusion has been made to the action of Sulphur on page 317. It has been supposed to exert a specific action in measles from its well-known influence upon the *skin;* for, when large doses have been taken internally, the skin exhales a sulphurous smell, and silver articles allowed to remain in contact with it are blackened. Vogt says, when taken for a long time, it gives a peculiar tint to the skin, and Hahnemann noticed brownish spots and other ephemeral cutaneous eruptions from its use. Rayer says, after using warm Sulphur baths for several days, they often produce an eruption of small, red, accuminated, pruriginous elevations, and of red spots, which appear first upon the limbs, but soon spread to nearly the whole surface of the body; a febrile movement, with thirst and loss of appetite, is developed; the sleep is restless, and the urine cloudy and muddy;—but, in from one to two weeks, these symptoms disappear in the order of their coming, the epidermis separating in branny scales, but the skin continues to itch for some time longer. Sulphur is regarded as homœopathic to the diarrhœa which often attends or follows measles; for, in large doses, it is apt to cause thirst and diarrhœa, to augment the secretion of intestinal mucus, and procure abundant and semi-fluid dejections. In doses of from a scruple to a drachm it creates some movement in the abdomen, and a loose discharge from the bowels, without colic; but whatever flatus escapes has the odor of sulphuretted hydrogen, and a sense of anxiety and extreme depression ceases upon the free discharge of this gas. In chronic cough, with profuse expectoration, its virtues are sometimes conspicuous, even in allopathic practice, and it is very useful in the cough which often remains after measles.

Sulphuric-acid was used by Hartmann with success in a case of black measles, attended with ecchymoses and hæmorrhages. When Sulphuric-acid is sufficiently diluted for internal use its action is supposed, in the dominant school, to be tonic, astringent, and inspissating, both locally and generally, as it is absorbed by the blood-vessels; it is said to strengthen the appetite, quench thirst, acidify the milk and urine, lessen the frequency of the pulse, and render the blood darker and more coagulable. In accordance with these views it has been used in those cases of hæmorrhage which are supposed to arise from "a dissolution of the blood," particularly in *scurvy* and *purpura*, in which affections it is pronounced superior to all other mineral acids; it is particularly efficient, also, in hæmorrhages from mucous membranes, and Chapman thought it sometimes effectual in restraining moderate uterine losses. In typhoid fever, and measles of a typhoid type, when there are flushed cheeks, burning skin, dry tongue, thirst, hæmorrhage, or profuse sweats, J. P. Frank thought it useful; while others rely upon it in a later stage, when the complexion is husky, skin harsh and dry, tongue black, with hæmorrhage from various organs; and Neumann even prefers it in acute stages of typhus fever, when there is active delirium, full pulse, and other signs of an inflammatory character. In diarrhœa, even of a severe character, so as to amount to cholera-morbus, it is a most useful remedy; and its action on the skin is also manifested by its curing itch and prurigo as rapidly as Sulphur.

Veratrum-album has been used by Kreussler when the diarrhœa was profuse and the exhaustion of the patient great, the eruption being very pale. There is no doubt of the homœopathicity of Veratrum-album to diarrhœa; in very large doses it causes, in all cases, a burning heat in the stomach, and vomiting, with anxiety, tremor, vertigo, weakness of the limbs, faintness, syncope, aphonia, interrupted respiration, feeble pulse, slight convulsions, distortion of the eyes, dilated pupils, dimness of sight, wandering of the mind from debility, sometimes prolonged insensibility and cold sweats over the whole body. After a severe dose there often remained, for several days, debility, tremulousness, muscular twitching, and a sense of constriction and distress in the præcordial region.

General Treatment.—When called to a case of measles I have the patient well rubbed over, from neck to feet, with *sweet oil*, several times a day; I am confident this allays the excessive itching, moderates the fever, prevents taking cold, renders the skin less sensitive, while it keeps up its secreting functions more freely, prevents the retrocession of the eruption, and lessens the danger of internal disease of the bronchiæ, lungs, and bowels. In mild cases I should give Sulphur or Pulsatilla, either singly or in alternation. If the feverish, inflammatory, or chest-symptoms are severe, I rely on Aconite and Antimony, or Aconite and Veratrum-viride. If the cough, vomiting, or diarrhœa prove troublesome, I often use Pulsatilla and Ipecac., or Chamomilla and Pulsatilla, or, in very severe and obstinate cases, Pulsatilla and Opium, or Ipecac. and Opium.

In malignant measles, *Arsenicum*, *Sulphuric- or Muriatic-acid*, often prove useful. In this form the eruption is apt to appear unusually early, as early as the second day of the disease; and, besides cough and dyspnœa, the complaint is marked by extreme debility, and attended with dysenteric diarrhœa. More may die of the intestinal affections than of the pectoral; Watson lost nineteen out of one hundred and eighty-three patients. The same remedies may prove useful when the malignant character of the disorder is manifested by the occurrence of gangrene, either internally or externally; and when, in this low form of measles, the rash is irregularly and imperfectly developed and of a livid color.

In regular practice, tonics, such as Bark, Wine, and Camphor, are only given when the pulse is small and feeble, skin cold, and eruption full and livid; they are never given when the skin is dry and burning, notwithstanding the appearance of adynamic symptoms; but the cooling tonics are used, such as the mineral acids.

As before said, as a general rule, a most important part of the treatment of measles relates to the remedies employed for the pulmonary symptoms, which, in the outset, almost always depend upon bronchitis; but the inflammation, in severe cases, is apt to spread insidiously from the mucous to the other tissues—the bronchitis may become pneumonia, and we find, after death, some portions of the lungs hepatized, usually small portions, while more frequently it is extensive inflammation of the bronchial mucous membrane we have to dread. In these cases Phosphor., Sulphur, and Ant.-tart. are reliable remedies, which may be aided by Aconite and Veratrum-viride, according to circumstances.

The *diarrhœa* which succeeds measles on the ninth or tenth day requires no special treatment, unless it is excessive; for, when the rash is about to decline, a spontaneous diarrhœa often sets in, and appears to have a beneficial effect in abating the febrile symptoms; if this natural curative process should fail to occur, it may even be imitated by the exhibition of a very gentle aperient, and, when the dysenteric symptoms are severe, it is well to unload the bowels. Rademacher says he has often noticed tenesmus with retention of fæces in the latter stages of measles. He convinced himself that the fæces were retained by an examination of the rectum with the finger; a gentle laxative remedy not only acted as an evacuant remedy, but allayed the tenesmus, while it produced a gentle and almost natural diarrhœa. He is confident that he has saved some lives in this way; although, as a general rule, the German writers are opposed to the use of laxatives in measles, finding that a thoughtlessly-given purgative may produce a long-continued and troublesome disorder of the bowels.

In ordinary practice, simple diaphoretic drinks, as the Acetate of Ammonia, or spirits of Nitric Ether, or Camphor-water, are relied upon in mild cases; in severer attacks, especially when the inflammatory or pectoral symptoms are severe, Nitre and Tartar-emetic are often used.

In the hæmorrhagic, or black measles, Sulphuric-acid is frequently given, aided or not by Camphor. When the eruption suddenly disappears, some think opiates by far the best remedies to act upon the skin, provided the lungs or brain are not too much affected. Folt, and others, have found this remedy exceedingly useful in allaying the irritation of measles; he says, many times it will remove the most troublesome cough, and it is his principal reliance when the bowels are much affected with diarrhœa or pain.

It is generally said that measles occur but once: I have witnessed at least a dozen instances in which they occurred twice, and once where the same subject was attacked three times.

The contagion of the disease was well marked as it occurred at Malta and the Feroe Islands. In the latter place measles had been unknown for sixty-five years; it was then imported by a man from Copenhagen, and, in the six subsequent months, of seven thousand seven hundred and eighty-two inhabitants of the Feroe Islands, no less than six thousand underwent the disease. The immediate and rapid diffusion of the contagion was extraordinary.

During the last winter (1859–60), roseola, or rose-rash, has been unusually prevalent in New-York, and, by many physicians, was very generally mistaken for measles; in fact, in most instances, the resemblance was so strong to "rubeola sine catarrho" that many, relying upon the epidemic prevalence of roseola, decreed almost all eruptive affections to be cases of this disease; numerous others mistook the affection for a hybrid of measles and scarlatina. In many cases, although the eruption was abundant, the patients were able to be up, and the whole affection disappeared in two or three days; in other instances it lasted for a week or ten days. Any one who has seen much of roseola will agree with Wilson that it is distinguished from other exanthemata by *negative*, rather than positive characters; and that the diseases with which it is most likely to be confounded are rubeola, erythema, urticaria, purpura, and scarlatina. Although non-contagious and non-infectious, still the epidemic influence may be so great that many are attacked in the same house; and I have seen a new-born babe take it a week after its mother had recovered from it. In general appearance the rash resembles rubeola, but, on closer examination, is found to consist of patches of larger size and more irregular form; and, at a later period, the difference is still more striking, in consequence of the change of tint to a dark roseate hue, which may be followed by petechial or ecchymosed spots and a discoloration like that which follows a bruise. Although there is generally little or no cough, still occasionally there is some, and more or less redness of the fauces.

SCARLATINA.

Scarlet Fever.

Definition.—An infectious and contagious febrile disease, usually commencing with vomiting, on the first or second day of which, or sometimes a little later, a *scarlet* efflorescence generally appears, first on the fauces and pharynx, and then on the face and neck, from whence it spreads over the whole body, and commonly commences to terminate in desquamation from the fifth to the seventh day. The fever is often accompanied with an affection of the kidneys, more frequently with severe disease of the throat and neck, or of some internal organ, sometimes followed by dropsy. The whole disease generally occurs only once during life.

History.—By whom the term *scarlatina* was first used is not well known, but the *mild variety* of the disease undoubtedly existed in the East in very remote times. It probably invaded the world soon after small-pox and measles; and it was doubtless looked upon as a sort of spurious measles, for the Arabian physicians described a species of measles which, from the extent of the desquamation recorded as having succeeded it, we may be assured was scarlatina. It continued for many centuries to be confounded with rubeola, and, when this error was corrected, they still continued to believe in the distinct nature of the two different forms—viz., scarlatina-simplex and scarlatina-anginosa. In the year 1610 an *epidemic angina*, accompanied with a scarlet eruption, invaded Spain, passing over in 1618 to Naples, then under the rule of Spain. Of the early Spanish writers (Ludovic Mercatus and Michel Heredia), the latter is peculiarly full and clear in his description of it. According to Gregory, the first Italian authors are Sgambatus, "*De pestilente faucium affectu Neapoli sæviente*" (1620), and Œtius Clerus, "*De morbo strangulatorio*" (1636). Sennertus noticed the same disease in Germany about 1625. Diemerbrœck, of Utrecht, in 1640, described, under the title of *purpura*, a disease which he believed to be a variety of measles, but which was evidently scarlatina. But Diemerbrœck was as ignorant of any connection between his so-called "*purpura*" and the "epidemic angina" of Ludovic Mercatus, as was Sydenham, after him, of the connection between his scarlatina and the putrid sore throat of the Continent. The milder type (scarlatina-simplex) was seen by Sydenham, in London, between the years 1670 and 1675. He describes it as a disease more in name than in essence, and fatal only through the officiousness of the physician. He was ignorant of any connection existing between it and the *angina-putrida-maligna* of the continental authors of that day.

Scarlet fever in its mild form (*scarlatina-simplex*), first reached Edinburgh in the year 1680. Sir Robert Sibbald, physician to King Charles II., of Scotland, says: "It is so recently introduced, and so little understood, that I cannot venture any observations on its theory or treatment." It appeared in London again in 1689 and the three following years, and was a *severer epidemic* than that witnessed by Sydenham. In 1747–8 a severe epidemic of the *anginose variety* appeared in London, and its historian was Dr. Fothergill, then a young man, just entering on his professional career. His work was entitled, "An Account of the Sore Throat attended with Ulcers: a disease which hath of late years appeared in this city and various parts of the nation." He distinctly traced the disease "to a reception into the habit of a fermentative or putrid virus or miasm, *sui generis*, by contagion, and principally by means of the breath;" but he confessed his inability to explain the cause of its peculiarly malignant or putrid tendency, nor did he suspect its connection with Sydenham's scarlatina. This tract placed its author at the head of the profession in London, and, in compliment to him, it was long called the Fothergillian sore throat.

From London, where it appeared and was described as above by Fothergill in 1748, it spread to Plymouth, in the years 1751–53, and was described by Huxham. In 1778, an epidemic devasted Birmingham, and was described by Withering; and here we find, in the first edition of his work, a formal diagnosis drawn between the *scarlatina-anginosa* of the old authors and the *angina-maligna* or ulcerous sore throat of Fothergill—making the *third* distinct disease which was supposed to exist; but, in 1793, a second edition appeared, wherein he candidly acknowledged his error, and taught the identity of the two last-named varieties, a doctrine which has never been questioned since that period. Sauvages and Cullen (1767 and 1792), as we have seen, had previously separated them in their nosologies, and Dr. Withering writes in his work (1793), "From the most assiduous attention to this disease, during fifteen years, I am now persuaded that the *scarlatina-anginosa* and the *angina-gangrenosa* are one and the same disease; that they owe their existence to the same specific contagion; that the varieties in their appearance depend upon contingent circumstances, and that their greatest differences are not greater than those of distinct and confluent small-pox;" and to this he should also have added the identity of origin of the *scarlatina-simplex*.

It prevailed in Dublin from 1834 to 1842, and an account of this epidemic has recently been published by Dr. Kennedy. His work was the latest, and, at the same time, one of the most valued monographs which had been published up to that time. It is said to be peculiarly rich in details of post-mortem appearances. This brings us down to our own day.

By this we see that nosologists were at first led to divide one and the same complaint into two (perhaps three) independent maladies, to which Cullen and others assigned the respective names of *cynanche-*

maligna and *scarlatina*. Cullen and Fothergill's definition of them both is very much the same. They both specify inflammation of the fauces, a cutaneous rash, and fever. But, in the definition of scarlatina, the rash is dwelt upon and described, and the fever is called synocha; while in that of cynanche-maligna the ulceration of the throat is more insisted on, and the fever is said to resemble typhus. The truth is, that these two kinds of disorder are both caused by the same contagious poison; for the malignant sore throat may be caught from a patient who has mild scarlet fever, and the mild scarlet fever may, in like manner, be contracted from one who is suffering under the malignant sore throat. The two forms graduate insensibly in different cases towards each other, and it would be impossible, even if it were desirable, to draw any strict line of separation between them. Many would say, and probably with truth, that their difference is this: in the one form the poison of the disorder is seeking its vent principally by the throat, in the other by the skin.

For convenience of description, and for the better direction of the treatment, authors have generally abided by these distinctions forced upon them by the history of the disease, and speak of three *varieties* of scarlet fever: 1. *Scarlatina-simplex*, in which there is a florid rash, and little or no affection of the throat; 2. *Scarlatina-anginosa*, in which both the skin and the throat are decidedly implicated; and 3. *Scarlatina-maligna*, in which the stress of the disease falls upon the blood and the throat. The epithet *maligna* marks truly the fearful character of this latter form of the malady. To these three varieties Dr. Copland has added a fourth, which he names *Scarlatina-latens*. This addition is warranted by the fact (certified now by the testimony of several observers) of the manifestation of certain well-known and remarkable sequelæ of scarlet fever in persons who had been living with others sick of that disease, but in whom its primary and diagnostic symptoms had not occurred, or had occurred in so slight a degree as to escape notice. I have seen severe cases of hæmaturia and dropsy in persons much exposed to the miasm of scarlet fever, with some fever, but without any sore throat or eruption

Pathology.—After a definite period of latency the peculiar poison of scarlet fever induces a disorder of the blood, which is, in the first place, made manifest by a febrile state, and a disturbed condition of the great nervous centres. This fever—termed the primary fever—having lasted for one, two, or three days, does not subside, but the secondary actions of the poisons are set up as a peculiar eruption, preceded, followed, or accompanied, in a majority of instances, by a sore throat. The eruption runs a given course of six to eight days, but the duration of the affection of the throat is more indefinite, and varies from eight to twenty or more days. The fever continues during the eruption, and as long as the sore throat exists; but, this being terminated, it subsides, and the original disease is at an end. In a few instances, however, tertiary actions succeed, as dropsy or inflammations of the bowels, kidneys, or joints, diseases quite as formidable as any which had preceded them. As in or during contagious fevers, the poison of scarlet fever acts on the blood and nerves, and thence on the brain and its membranes, often causing the usual forms of irritation of those parts, modified in their course and effects by the nature of the specific febrile disease.

That fever precedes the specific actions of the poison upon the skin is so general a rule that it has few exceptions, and the pyrexia has, at times, been so severe as occasionally to destroy the patient before the more peculiar actions of the poison could be set up. Again, the law that the great specific action of the poison is on the skin, causing the eruption or exanthem, has likewise only a few exceptions. Of this eruption there are several forms, such as smooth, papulose, phlyctænoid, or vesicular. These are all evanescent after death.

In the *smooth* eruption the surface of the inflamed skin presents no inequality to the sight or touch: this is the true scarlet fever of Sydenham and Hahnemann. The scarlatina *papulosa* is when the papillæ of the skin are enlarged, and the appearance is that of roughness or "*goose-flesh*," or as if Cayenne pepper were sprinkled over the skin: this is now the most common variety. The third form is when the eruption is accompanied by a number of *vesicles*, filled with serum, which ultimately shrivel up and desquamate: this is sometimes called the *miliary* species. Whatever the ultimate form of the eruption may be, its first appearance is that of innumerable small bright-red puncta, separated by interstices of healthy skin, as if brick-dust or Cayenne pepper had been sprinkled over the surface. These puncta quickly become confluent, so that in a few hours the redness becomes general over the parts attacked. The color, in ordinary cases, is in the first instance a yellowish-red, like that of Cayenne pepper, or a bright red, like that of a boiled lobster; but, on the decline of the disease, it becomes deeper, and more resembles that of red sand or the beet-root, while, in some peculiar and severe cases, it is livid and intermixed with petechiæ. But, whatever tint the eruption may assume, it has this peculiarity: that it disappears on pressure, and again returns from the periphery to the centre on the pressure being removed. The color is also brighter and more vivid in the flexures of the joints, and about the hips and loins, than over the rest of the body. The termination of this inflammation is generally by desquamation, and the scaling off generally begins with the decline of the eruption, and is followed by a succession of exfoliations. A few days after the commencement of the desquamation *albumen may be detected in the urine in small quantity*, and continues to be given off for several days, along with a considerable amount of epithelium from the uriniferous tubules. Occasionally the squamæ from the skin are so large as to preserve entire the whole epidermis of the palms of the hands or soles of the feet; and there are preparations in some cabinets of cuticular moulds of the entire hand, like a glove. In a few instances, however, the termination is by ulceration and sloughing of large portions of the integument.

Whatever be the color or description of the eruption, it does not attack all parts of the body simultaneously, but appears partially, or in a succession of crops, in an order which may be thus stated: On the first day it spreads universally over the face, neck, and upper extremities; on the following day over the trunk, but less general on the back than on the abdomen; and, lastly, on the third day, it has extended itself over the lower extremities. The duration of each crop is about three days, when it disappears; and, in the order of attack, it fades from the head and upper extremities on the fourth day, from the trunk on the fifth day, and from the lower extremities from the sixth to the eighth day. The order of attack, however, which has been mentioned is not constant; for, in many instances, the eruption appears first on the trunk, and in some few cases on the lower extremities, and only on the second day very faintly on the face and upper extremities. The disease attains its height usually from the fifth to the ninth day, when, in favorable cases, all the symptoms begin to decline. The primary fever does not subside on the appearance of the rash, as is the case with small-pox, and sometimes in measles, but continues, with various degrees of violence, throughout its progress. The pulse is often 120 to 130 in a minute, and sometimes beats with considerable force. The temperature of the skin is frequently 105° to 106°, or even 112° Fahrenheit, and is dry, with a sensation of burning heat.

The virus frequently falls on the mucous membranes of the eyes and nasal fossæ in a more moderate degree than upon the throat and skin; but excites a somewhat similar eruption on those parts, at first consisting of a similar distinct punctated or dotted appearance, which changes in a few hours to one of diffuse redness. The inflammation of the ocular membrane has also this peculiarity, that it does not distress the sight; for the eye bears light without inconvenience, and in no case is it combined with ordinary coryza, as in measles. Neither is sneezing a consequence of the affection of the nasal membrane; and only in severe and malignant cases is there much discharge from the nostrils. As the eruption attacking these parts generally appears with the first crop of the exanthem, so does it generally die away with it. The nasal inflammation usually terminates by resolution; but, in a few instances, the alæ of the nose ulcerate, and very rarely mortify.

The lingual and buccal mucous membranes are also often the seat of a similar exanthem, presenting nearly the same appearance as in other parts, and sometimes preceding all of them. The *papillæ* of the tongue are generally singularly elongated and enlarged, and stand up salient and erect, and of a deep scarlet color, above the thick white mucus which coats the lingual membrane, whence the term "strawberry tongue" has often been applied to it. This affection lasts longer than the former, and usually terminates by resolution; although, in a few instances, the buccal membrane ulcerates and very rarely mortifies.

The *sore throat*, or inflammation of the faucial membrane—though not quite so constant an affection as that of the skin, yet almost always does exist—is often of much longer duration, and a much more grave disease: it may either precede all the symptoms, or else occur at any period of the fever. The redness of the throat is generally present before that of the skin; and, if it occur in connection with some soreness of throat, with great quickness of the pulse, the presence of the strawberry tongue, and be preceded by sudden and rather severe vomiting, we may often predict the presence of scarlet fever before the eruption shows itself. This inflammation, at first punctated, then diffuse, usually runs into the exudation of coagulable lymph, or even into ulceration. The character of the ulcer, when it does exist, is so completely in unison with the state of the constitution as to enable us sometimes, according as it is slight or severe, to divide scarlatina into two great varieties, or into *scarlatina-simplex* or *mitior*, and *scarlatina-maligna* or *gravior*. The first or sthenic form is marked by a greatly enlarged or swollen state of the tonsils, which are of a vivid or bright-red color; are covered with coagulable lymph in patches, and, when ulceration takes place, the ulcers are seldom deep, or the sloughs slow to come away, but the patches of coagulable lymph and sloughs usually separate about the fifth or sixth day; so that, in mild cases, the sore throat is healed about the eighth or tenth day, or, in more severe ones, about the fifteenth or twentieth. In malignant cases, or in scarlatina-gravior, the tonsils are much less tumefied and enlarged, but much more loaded with blood, and of a deeper and sometimes of a livid color. The patches of coagulable lymph are larger and more diffluent; the ulcers, also, are deep and formidable, and the sloughs are thrown off later in the disease. They are likewise slow to heal not till the end of three weeks, or, in severe cases, not till four or even six weeks have elapsed, during which period the fever continues, and the patient remains in considerable danger.

The inflammation of the throat may extend to all the neighboring parts, and an abscess may form in the cellular tissue of the neck, or in the glands, or in the pharynx, or pus issue from the ears; for the tympanum has often been eroded, and, in a few instances, the inflammation has extended to the larynx, and the patient has died of croup.

Besides these disorders, the glands of the neck often enlarge, and occasionally suppurate, and, singular to say, sometimes not till after the sore throat has healed, and at other times when there has been no very apparent previous affection of the throat at all—as if these parts were the seat of a specific action of the poison.

The inflammation of the skin, like that of the buccal mucous membrane, is often accompanied by some inflammation or inflammatory œdema of the sub-cellular tissue. This affection takes place as soon as the rash appears, and often causes the hands to swell so that the patient is unable to bend his fingers, and his face also frequently becomes tumefied and painful. The serum effused is, however, in mild cases, soon absorbed, and this phase of the disease terminates without any unpleasant consequences. In severe attacks, however, it has a tendency to terminate in ulceration or in mortification. In children the toes of one foot have been known to slough off, and in some the integuments of the leg have mortified, from the knee to the foot; while in others mortification commenced in the upper lip, and spread till one-half the cheek was eaten away. Some have been known to die of mortification of the rectum, and others of a similar affection of the pudenda.

Such are the primary and secondary affections of scarlatina; but the poison has also occasionally some tertiary actions, as on the cellular tissue, causing dropsy; and on the synovial membranes of the joints, or upon the heart, glands, ears, bowels, liver, or kidneys.

The *dropsy* which sometimes occurs after scarlet fever must be considered as a tertiary action of the poison. It usually commences between the fifteenth and twenty-third day of the disease, and almost uniformly not till after all the other symptoms have subsided. The patient is liable to it during the period of desquamation, and for a considerable time afterwards, although the foundation of it is often laid very early in the disease. It begins with puffiness of the face, and afterwards shows itself in the hands and feet. In some few instances the anasarca is rapid and general, the whole cellular tissue filling so quickly as sometimes to destroy the patient in a few hours, the cavities of the chest and abdomen frequently filling at the same time. According to the observation of Dr. Wood, and many others, it has occurred more frequently after *mild* than severe cases. Its forms are, therefore, anasarca, ascites, hydrothorax, hydropericardium, and even hydrocephalus; and, in whatever part it appears, heaviness, approaching to stupor, is a common attendant; and, during its progress, *œdema of the glottis* must often be watched for and relieved. The dropsy is generally accompanied with *scanty and albuminous urine;* and, although the presence of albumen without diminished secretion is almost a regular phenomenon in the course of the disease, yet, if the urine become highly albuminous, and diminished in quantity, the dropsical complications may be apprehended. The urine should be watched and examined during the whole course of the attack.

Intercurrent inflammations of the synovial membranes have been described by Withering, Sennertus, Heberden, and others; but they are rare in modern times. This disease may attack the wrist, ankle, or knee-joints, and usually terminates by effusion of serum; but, in some cases, the cavities of the joints contain pus. This inflammation seldom occurs till after the eruption has subsided, and is generally a tertiary phenomenon in the course of this specific disease.

Such are the morbid phenomena which have been observed in the ordinary course of scarlatina, and with sufficient constancy to be attributed to the specific action of a poison; but these appearances are only to be found when the disease is of moderate intensity, and the patient survives some days. In the most severe and rapid cases the patient dies, not from any organic lesion, but from the intensity of the shock, in the first instance, on the blood and nervous system; for Britonneau, Tweedie, and Sims all speak of having examined the bodies of those who had died early in the disease, in which there was scarcely any appreciable local lesion: coma, convulsions, or other violent cerebral affection carrying off the patient.

Diagnosis.—Scarlet fever is still more frequently mistaken for measles, diphtherite, and roseola than any other diseases. Although scarlet fever and measles were so long confounded together, the differences between them are well pronounced, and, when once understood, are easily recognized. Measles is distinguishable, then, from scarlatina:

First.—By the presence, at the outset, of catarrhal symptoms; by the sneezing, the cough, the defluxion from the eyes and nose which precede the rash. There is, doubtless, in many cases of scarlatina, a running from the nose and eyes, but not till late in the disease; at any rate, not prior to the eruption. And scarlatina generally commences with *vomiting*, which rarely precedes measles.

Second.—By the absence of severe inflammation and ulceration of the throat: symptoms which always accompany severe cases, at least of scarlet fever.

Third.—By the character of the eruption itself. The rash in measles is more elevated above the surface than in scarlatina, and of a darker color. In measles it is said to present somewhat the appearance of a raspberry, and, in scarlet fever, to have that of Cayenne pepper, or brick-dust, or of a boiled lobster. In measles the papulæ are collected into semi-lunar groups, leaving interstices of healthy skin; while the redness of scarlatina commences in minute points, which speedily become so numerous and crowded that the surface appears to be universally red. They begin on the face, neck, and breast, and extend to the extremities, pervading, at last, every part of the skin. The scarlet color is deeper in general about the groins and in the flexures of the joints than elsewhere.

Fourth, and lastly.—The rash of measles, in its most regular form, appears on the *fourth* day of the disease; that of scarlatina on the *second*.

Differential Diagnosis of Scarlatina and Measles.

a. SCARLATINA.	MEASLES.
1. Period of invasion short, and generally marked by sudden and severe vomiting.	1. Period of invasion rather long.
2. Anginose symptoms predominate.	2. Coryza and bronchitis predominate.
3. Redness of skin uniform or regularly punctate.	3. Redness of the skin is in irregular blotches.
4. Cerebral symptoms inclined to be frequent and violent.	4. Cerebral complications unfrequent and but little violent.
5. Swelling of the hands and feet.	5. No swelling of the hands or feet.
6. No nummular sputa.	6. Nummular expectoration.

Differential Diagnosis of Scarlatinous-angina and Diphtheria.

b. SCARLATINOUS ANGINA.	DIPHTHERIA (*angine-couenneuse*).
1. Appears during the course of a scarlatinal epidemic.	1. Appears without any epidemic of scarlatina being present.
2. Invasion is sudden and violent.	2. Invasion insidious.
3. Tonsils more bathed in exudation than covered with false membrane.	3. Tonsils covered with unmistakable false membranes.
4. The exudation is produced upon a surface of *a scarlet redness.*	4. The diphtheritic false membrane is produced upon a surface which presents *an inflammatory redness.*
5. Exudation white, opaque, caseiform, easily detached by the finger-nail.	5. Exudation grayish, tenacious, receiving with difficulty the impression of an instrument.
6. Exudation invades simultaneously the whole extent of the fauces, and sometimes the posterior nares.	6. The false membrane commences by patches upon the tonsils, and is propagated thence towards the larynx.
7. Slight tendency to invade the respiratory passages.	8. Great tendency to invade the respiratory passages.

Differential Diagnosis of Scarlatina and Roseola.

c. SCARLATINA.	ROSEOLA.
1. Contagious.	1. Not contagious.
2. Occurs but once.	2. May recur a number of times.
3. Often followed by severe sequelæ.	3. Not followed by sequelæ.
4. Pursues a definite course.	4. Pursues no definite course, but may come and go.

The eruption of roseola is also said to be more generally confined to the chest or trunk, and to commence upon the extremities; while, in scarlatina, it has a tendency to appear first upon the face, and afterwards to invade successively the whole body. As roseola may be accompanied with fever and severe sore throat, or with catarrh, it is sometimes impossible to distinguish between it and mild cases of scarlatina or measles. It is only after the doubtful complaint is over that a correct inference may be drawn from a general survey of its cause, course, and effects.

Symptoms of the Disease in its Various Stages and Modifications.—Although, as we have seen, several varieties of scarlatina are described by authors, it is not to be supposed that they are equally distinctly defined in nature. The different forms often run into each other. Yet it not unfrequently happens that the characters of each variety are tolerably well marked, and, as is usual, we may, for convenience sake, divide it into scarlatina-*simplex*, scarlatina-*anginosa*, scarlatina-*maligna*, and scarlatina-*latens*.

Scarlet fever, of whatever description, essentially consists of fever, a blood-affection, and certain local inflammations; but among the more striking *occasional* phenomena of this disease is the sudden and remarkable depression of the mental and physical powers of the body which the poison often produces: a depression so great as sometimes to cause the death of the patient in a few hours, without any febrile reaction or any very sensible local lesion of the throat or other parts being discoverable after death. On the other hand, a few instances have occurred in which the febrile reaction is so great as to destroy the patient in an equally short time, and with a similar absence of all pathological phenomena: the affection of the skin being suppressed, the sore throat wanting, and the patient dying as from an overwhelming inflammatory poison. But first we will turn our attention to the different stages of the disease; for the symptoms of scarlet fever, under ordinary circumstances, may be divided into three groups.

The *first stage* occupies the period from the commencement of the disease till the appearance of the eruption, and is technically termed the "*primary fever*." The *second stage* is that from the appearance of the eruption till its entire subsidence—of course termed the *eruptive* period; while the *third stage* is reckoned from the disappearance of the eruption till the termination of the disease, and is often called the *desquamative* period. The duration of the first stage is one, two, or three days; that of the second from two to eight days; while the third stage may either not exist at all, or vary from a few hours to two or three weeks—making the whole duration of the fever from eight to thirty days or more. These stages are not, as in typhus, usually marked by fixed and peculiar changes in the appearance of the tongue; for, except in the more severe forms of the disease, it continues coated with a white mucus, or red, moist, and raw throughout the whole course of the disease. In *scarlatina-anginosa* or *maligna*, however, it becomes brown or black in the second, or at the commencement of the third stage.

First Stage.—The primary fever may be, and often is very sudden in its attack; or the patient may complain for some days of slight indisposition, languor, and lassitude. But the disease may, and, perhaps, generally does want these prodromata, and it usually sets in at once, with nausea, vomiting, shivering, lassitude, and rapidly-augmenting debility, followed almost immediately by a frequent pulse, hot dry skin, flushed face, furred tongue, anorexia, thirst, and great muscular weakness. Generally our attention is first called to nausea and vomiting; sometimes more or less headache, or other symptoms of nervous disorder occur, such as restlessness, morbid vigilance, delirium, stupor, coma, or convulsions. All these are very much like the symptoms of typhus; but still there are signs which serve to distinguish it; for the pulse of typhus, instead of being full and strong, is small, weak, and rapid, and the heat of the skin more ardent, and these phenomena continue throughout the whole course of the disease. The fever of scarlatina varies, however, from a mere febricula to the severest forms of the typhoid type; while the initial vomiting may be as severe as that which precedes small-pox.

The onset of many cases is generally sudden. A child is well, or so slightly ailing on one day that the change from its usual condition is not noticed at the time, though it may be recollected afterwards; but, on the following day, or often within twelve hours, or even less, the symptoms of the disease become marked and characteristic. In a large majority of cases the eruption is already visible at the first visit. Frequently the patient has been put to bed well in the evening, and, becoming restless and feverish in the night, is found in the morning with fever, sore throat, and very considerable eruption; or, as happened in one of Dr. Meigs' cases, a child gets up in the morning apparently well, breakfasts as usual, goes to church, and, falling sick while there, comes home, and, a few hours later, shows the eruption over the neck and upper part of the trunk, and has fever and sore throat.

Watson thinks that the first thing of which a feverish patient usually complains is sore throat, with some stiffness of the neck, and, on examining the fauces, there will be found—without, indeed, so much swelling of the tonsils as occurs in quinsy or common sore throat—a diffused redness, sometimes of a dark claret color, including a large part of the palate. In a short time it may be perceived that the tonsils and velum are covered irregularly with whitish exudations, or gray aphthous crusts; or, perhaps, a sloughy kind of ulceration is left by the separation of these crusts.

As Gregory vividly says, everything about scarlatina is rapid; the incubation is short, the invasion violent and unforeseen, the eruption quickly evanescent, and desquamation has begun almost before the fever has completely left the patient. It is the quickness and rapidity which constitutes one of its most marked and striking characteristics. A child may go to bed well in the evening, and wake in the middle of the night with scarlet fever, and the fever may be all the more hard and violent from its very quickness, though the *subsequent disease* is not necessarily severe in proportion to the violence of the primary symptoms: a mild disease has often followed a severe primary fever. Meigs relates a case where a child was playing in the garden, and its mother, a remarkably intelligent woman, remarked upon his appearance of robust and hearty health. A quarter of an hour after this he felt sick at the stomach; he came into the house, and went up to the nursery, looking pale and pinched, with a cold skin, and nearly fainted in the nurse's arms. He had then, in the course of an hour, three copious and watery stools, each one accompanied with vomiting. Dr. Meigs saw him one hour after this—dozing, very pale, with pinched features, sunken and half-closed eyes, cool surface, and with the pulse at 128, and rather feeble. There was no eruption. At six, P. M., he had a hot dry skin, with the tongue heavily coated, the fauces swollen, and showing flecks of exudation upon the tonsils, the pulse at 128, and a well-marked scarlatinous eruption coming out abundantly. The case pursued a very regular course, without dangerous or malignant symptoms of any kind.—I have seen many very sudden cases, where the disease was already in the house; some of the children would go to bed well, after being bright and merry during the evening, and then be suddenly attacked at midnight with sudden vomiting.

But the invasion, though sudden in nearly all cases, is not always so precipitate as this. When we come to analyze the early symptoms we find that the first one observed in many cases is fever, with considerable acceleration of the pulse, heat of skin, and muscular debility, attended or not with vomiting. Simultaneously with the fever there is, in a large number of cases, more or less soreness of the throat, and generally, even when no pain is complained of, there is redness, or redness with swelling of the fauces; and, to repeat, in a majority of the cases, *vomiting* occurs, or, at least, some degree of nausea, and, of course, complete anorexia, more or less acute thirst, loose or but slightly constipated bowels; the child may be quiet and dull, or else restless and irritable; but sometimes delirium occurs, with flushed face, and the eyes are often slightly injected. Meigs thinks that these symptoms precede the eruption but a very short time—not more than twelve hours or less, and rarely over a day.

The *tongue* is a very important diagnostic mark. In the *scarlatina-simplex* and *anginosa* it is often covered at the outset with a white cream-like fur, through which are seen projecting the red and exaggerated papillæ, the edges of the tongue being likewise of a bright-red color. The red points gradually multiply, and the white fur clears away, and, at length, the whole surface of the tongue becomes preternaturally red, clean, and raw looking. After becoming thus clean, as well as red and rough (the "*strawberry tongue*"), it will sometimes, when the disease goes on unpromisingly, get hard, dry, and brown, as in continued fever. But more commonly the tongue is moist throughout the attack; but it may also become pinched or diminished in size, from contraction of its tissues.

The *pulse* is another most important point to be noticed in making an early diagnosis. In this disease, above all others, does it show a tendency (especially in children) to run up to an extraordinary degree of rapidity, and the threatening symptoms may often be decided to be coming scarlatina from this circumstance alone, even though the tongue may be natural, and the faucial inflammation slight or wanting. Meigs thinks that frequency of the pulse is, perhaps, the most marked early symptom of the disease. He has rarely, even in very mild cases, found it less than 140, and in not a few it has been, he says, in the first few days, and in children of four or six years old, even as high as 168 or 170. Occasionally, and as an exceptional case, it may be much lower. Meigs saw one case in a boy five years old; it was 96 on the second day, and only 88 on the third, though there was still a good deal of rash upon the skin. It is also generally proportionally weak to the amount of debility and general muscular weakness existing.

It should be borne in mind that often the very first intimation of the real nature of the disease is given by a feeling of roughness of the throat, and some pain in deglutition, and these symptoms will materially aid in the diagnosis.

Second Stage.—The second stage commences with the eruption, and lasts until its entire subsidence. The rash generally appears from twelve to thirty-six hours after the first invasion of the fever, and shows itself first upon the face and neck, whence it extends rapidly over the whole surface. It continues to increase in extent and intensity, so as to reach its maximum about the third or fourth day. It breaks out first in minute red points, dotted upon a rose-colored surface, forming patches of irregular shape, of considerable size, level with the skin, *disappearing under pressure*, divided at first by portions of healthy skin, but running rapidly together, and giving to large portions of the surface a uniform Cayenne pepper or scarlet color. The eruption is not generally equally diffused over the whole body, but is more marked upon one portion than upon another. It is often most intense upon the back, and is then of a deeper color than elsewhere, not unfrequently assuming a purple hue. It is generally very well marked on the abdomen and thighs and about the articulations, and assumes in those regions a particularly bright tint.

It does not ultimately always cover the whole surface, but, in some very mild cases, and, as we shall find when treating of the grave cases, in the latter also it may occur only in patches of moderate extent upon different portions of the body, leaving us, at times, in some doubt as to the real nature of the rash. A certain degree of roughness is sometimes occasioned by enlargement of the papillæ of the skin in various parts of the body, particularly on the extensor surface of the limbs, but these are evidently independent of the characteristic eruption. The skin upon some parts of the body, especially the face, hands, and feet, often present a swollen appearance, rendering the movements somewhat stiff. There is, in most cases, a feeling of burning, irritation, and itching in the skin, the latter of which symptoms increases as the malady progresses. On the arms and legs the eruption occasionally differs somewhat from that which is visible on the trunk; is more spotty, more papular, and the papulæ are somewhat prominent, while over the body there is a general punctuated blush. In some cases of scarlatina parts of the red surface are closely studded with little transparent vesicles, containing a thin colorless liquid, and resembling what has already been described as the eruption of miliary fever or *sudamina*: they show a tendency to appear more especially on the thorax and on the front and sides of the neck. The liquid is soon reabsorbed, and the cuticle under which it has been enclosed shrivels up, turns white, and comes off in a thick white scurf, so that the part from which it has been separated looks as though it had been powdered, at first sight. I have seen them occupy more especially the front of the thigh, the back of the arms, and outside of the fore-arm, and occasionally they are interspersed with minute pimples and pustules.

As regards the time of coming out of the eruption, the older authors differ from the modern writers. Cullen stated the time, from the first invasion of the symptoms to the appearance of the eruption, to be four days; in this he is undoubtedly wrong. Watson states it at two days, or, "upon the second day of the disease," to use his own words, and Meigs, in his work on "Diseases of Children," sets it at twelve hours in most cases, and rarely more than twenty-four. Dr. Wood, of Philadelphia, says that the rash makes its appearance, in most cases, upon the second day of the fever, often, however, earlier or later, and sometimes at the very commencement of the disease, if the statements of the friends or attendants can be relied upon. It is this last clause which probably gives the clue to the discrepancy. The primary symptoms differ so much in severity that, in many instances, they may challenge the attention for a few days previous to the eruption, while at others they have been so absolutely inappreciable as to lead to the impression that, *in some instances*, the rash may be the first symptom of the disease.

The period of incubation, like all the rest of the phenomena, is generally short; for *rapidity* is the great characteristic of the disease. Gregory, in speaking of it, says that it invaded his own family in April, 1839. Rigors occurred in one member of it on the last Saturday in April. On Sunday, languor and lassitude, with dryness of the skin, were the chief symptoms. At six o'clock on Monday morning the eruption appeared. On the following Saturday, at two, P. M., his eldest daughter sickened; so that the incubative period could not have exceeded seven days, and was probably only six. Withering says that he has known patients begin to complain as early as the third day from exposure to the contagion, and he (Gregory) says that he cannot contradict the assertion, though he has never seen a case of incubation so short as this.

The eruption generally reaches its height about the fourth day, and then remains stationary for one, or, less frequently, two days, after which it begins to decline. Its decline is marked by a diminution in the intensity of the color, which, from scarlet, becomes red, then rose-colored, and, growing paler and paler, finally disappears entirely about the sixth, seventh, or eighth day. In some very mild cases, however, the whole duration of the eruption is not over two or three days, and in such the color it imparts to the skin is never very bright or deep, nor is it accompanied by intense heat, or by much irritation or itching.

The color has been compared to that of brick-dust, Cayenne pepper, or a boiled lobster, but it is often darker, though not so dusky as that of measles. It disappears under pressure, and returns when the pressure is removed. Whatever increases the general excitement has a tendency to deepen it. Hence the color is more intense during the exacerbations of the fever, and is increased when the patient cries, or is otherwise agitated.

The symptoms which preceded the eruption do not subside on its appearance, but persist, or are even augmented. The febrile movement continues unabated; the pulse is full, strong, and frequent, running up very soon after the onset to 120, 140, 150, and often to 160. As before mentioned, this *frequency of the pulse* is, in fact, one of the most marked phenomena of the disease, and even in mild cases it is seldom found less than 140, and it *may* be as high as 168 or 170. The skin is burning hot and dry, as a general rule, and loses its usual softness and suppleness. The expression of the face is usually natural. The eye is often animated, and slightly injected. The respiration is generally easy and natural, though sometimes, when the fever is violent, it becomes quickened. The auscultation and percussion signs are natural, unless some complication exists. There is often rather a frequent cough, which is dry, and evidently depends on the guttural inflammation, and not on any bronchial or pulmonary irritation. It exists during the early period of the eruption, and declines with the inflammation of the fauces. It will rarely be mistaken for the peculiar measles-cough.

The voice is seldom altered, beyond having a nasal sound, so long as the disease is simple and regular. If the voice becomes hoarse or whispering it indicates a dangerous extension of the inflammation from the pharynx to the larynx. The anorexia continues until the eruption begins to decline, and the thirst is craving up to the same period, when it moderates. At first the dorsum of the tongue is covered with a whitish or yellowish-white fur, of variable thickness, while its tip and edges are of a deep red color. After two or three days, and during the course of the eruption, the coating just described disappears from its tongue, and its whole surface assumes a deep red tint and a shining appearance, which makes it look like raw flesh. At the same time it is often much diminished in size, while its papillæ become enlarged and projecting. This condition generally lasts from six to ten days, after which it returns to its natural state. It is commonly moist throughout the attack. Vomiting is rarely troublesome in mild cases, though it often occurs severely in the beginning of the attack. The bowels continue nearly in their natural condition; in some few cases slight diarrhœa occurs, but, more frequently, there is moderate constipation. The abdomen is natural in most of the cases; sometimes, however, there is slight pain and tension for a few days, which coincide generally with some enlargement of the liver, or more rarely of the spleen. The urinary secretion is usually more or less reddened, as in other febrile diseases.

The temperature of the skin, as indicated by the thermometer, is not unfrequently 105° or 106° of Fahrenheit, and is asserted to have reached 112°. The highest, however, observed by Andral and Roger was 106° Fahrenheit. The fever often exhibits exacerbations towards evening, and is occasionally attended with restlessness or delirium, and sometimes with comatose symptoms. Occasionally there is continued irritability of the stomach, but this is not very frequent.

Of late years, however, and in this country, the prevailing type of scarlatina has been rather typhoid than otherwise, and it is comparatively rare to find the great heat of skin described above. The temperature in this (the typhoid) form is not unfrequently about natural, and sometimes even below this standard, and with this variety an anginose affection of the worst character is often associated.

The affection of the *throat*, in some cases, never exceeds that already noticed as occurring, even before the appearance of the eruption. But generally it very soon becomes the most prominent and distressing symptom, being attended with swelling within and without, painful deglutition, and sometimes impeded respiration. Generally speaking, when it has not formed one of the initiatory symptoms of the disorder, the *faucial inflammation* comes on early in the second stage; the pharynx is reddened, and in some instances swelled; the tonsils enlarge and become red; the submaxillary and lymphatic glands of the neck are somewhat tumefied and tender to the touch, and in some bad cases become exceedingly large and hard. When the case is at all severe, deglutition is generally painful, and in some instances extremely so. Still the absence of complaint of sore throat in a child, or the fact of its swallowing without hesitation or apparent difficulty, is no proof that angina does not exist; since, generally, in a good light, much greater redness than natural, and, in many instances, redness and swelling combined, may be found. As the eruption progresses, and the tongue loses its coat and becomes red, the inflammation of the pharynx usually *augments*, the redness becoming deeper, and the tonsils are more swelled and painful, and in a good many, but not in all the cases, dotted over with small white spots, or with whitish and soft false membranes. The throat affection is rarely severe enough, however, to constitute a serious danger in mild scarlatina, while, in many of the malignant cases, it is a frequent cause of a fatal termination. During the eruption the nostrils are either dry and encrusted or there is some coryza. In bad cases the affection of the nostrils is often exceedingly severe: the nose is blocked up with false membranes and thick secretions; still the discharge is profuse and the nose often excoriated. It is said to be an absolutely fatal sign when this nasal affection occurs in connection with much, and hard swelling of the parotid and submaxillary glands. The strength of the child is reduced for the time, but there are no signs of excessive prostration, and the decubitus is indifferent. There is almost always more or less disorder of the nervous system, sometimes amounting only to headache and restlessness, while, in other instances, there is great irritability, wakefulness, and occasional delirium, especially at night.

According to Gregory, along with redness and swelling, if the fever be active, portions of coagulated lymph will be seen upon the tonsils and fauces. These are often mistaken for ulcers, but in many, most severe cases of anginose scarlatina there is no actual breach of surface, only excessive engorgement with effusion of lymph.

Deglutition often becomes so painful that the patient would rather suffer thirst than attempt to quench it with the certainty of experiencing excessive pain. We should always be on our guard whenever intense pain occurs, whether it be in pleurisy, jaundice, enteritis, rheumatism, or scarlatina. It should be remembered that *death* may be caused by excessive pain, as in crucifixion; at all events, serious mischief. In the case of angina, excess of pain is frequently followed by extension of inflammation to the cellular membrane subjacent to the ear and to the brain.

It is often difficult to examine the state of the throat, from the extent of the cellular inflammation of the neck and throat, but we may often form a good judgment of what is going forward there by taking as our guides the pulse and the degree of pain in deglutition. That actual ulceration does take place in a certain proportion of cases is undeniable, but the exudation of coagulable lymph is the more frequent pathological condition.

Third Stage.—The third stage is that of *desquamation* and decline. The eruption reaches its height, as already stated, about the third or fourth day; then remains stationary for one or two days, and afterwards declines gradually, so that no traces are visible on the sixth day; yet, in some rare cases, it may linger until the ninth or tenth. In other very mild attacks the whole duration of the eruption is not over two or three days. By the third day it has disappeared entirely. This is not, however, very common, except in those cases which are followed by dropsy. The other symptoms, both general and local, decline with the eruption: the pulse loses its frequency, and falls to its natural standard; the heat of the surface first subsides, and then disappears, but the skin remains somewhat harsh; the redness and swelling of the tonsils and pharynx diminish; the spots of the false membrane, if these be present, are absorbed and thrown off; the deglutition becomes easy, if it had been difficult, and soon all signs of throat affection vanish; the tongue cleans off, becomes reddish and glossy, and after a time returns to its natural state.

At the time that the subsidence of all the symptoms take place, desquamation begins. It dates, therefore, from about the sixth day, though it may be either earlier or later. It commences in most of the cases on the face and neck, though, in a few instances, it appears first on the abdomen. It then extends gradually over the body, and becomes general. About the thorax and abdomen it occurs in the form of minute points, like those which result from the desiccation of sudamina; on the face it is in the form of thin light scales or squamæ; while on the extremities large flakes of the epidermis become separated from the derm, and are pulled off by the child, or rubbed off by his movements in bed. These flakes are sometimes so large on the hands and feet as to form complete moulds of the fingers and toes, or even of the feet and hands. The whole process usually occupies some ten or twelve days, but may be prolonged even into the third week. It is generally accompanied by roughness and dryness, and some itching and irritation of the skin. Not unfrequently the surface beneath the exfoliation is left tender and irritable for some time afterwards.

It is during the desquamate-period that ulceration of the ears and nostrils, the swelling of the parotid and submaxillary glands, and the throat affection are apt to assume a serious form.

Alleix says, after mentioning that the desquamation is heralded by an alteration in color, from scarlet to dusky red, and *this* gradually fading out, "that, nevertheless, in some cases, it commences while the color is still persistent;" and sometimes even, as is corroborated by Vieusseux and M. Mondière, *it is not until one, two, and even three weeks after the eruption that desquamation appears;* and Jahn has *seen it recur from time* in the same patient.

Before quitting the general description of the disease, it should be remarked that, though the above is a correct description of the usual symptoms of the milder and some of the severer cases of scarlatina, the reader would be greatly deceived were he to expect to find always and invariably this exact train of morbid phenomena. On the contrary, both the mild and the grave cases vary so much that it would be impossible to describe them accurately by one or two portraits. Taking the above sketch as a standard, then, of numerous cases, the observer will find that many will fall short of it in all their features, while others deepen gradually in their shades, so to speak, until they pass into the truly grave type. Those that are milder in their type than the above sketch, may be so in such a degree as to make it very difficult, and in many cases impossible, to determine positively whether the child has had the disease or not. Indeed there is but little doubt that children may sometimes have the disease so slightly that it is not discovered by either the physician or parents, and, being protected by this attack, are in after life classed among those insusceptible to the disease. Meigs says that some of the cases he has seen have been so very mild that but for the existence of the disease amongst other members of the family, they might have passed unobserved; and that, in one case, he was sent for to see a patient who had had the eruption for three days, and yet who was so slightly sick that he was sent for from school, to which he had gone. It was a well-marked case, and the child had no troublesome symptoms afterwards, notwithstanding the exposure he had undergone.

SCARLATINA-SIMPLEX.

This form is known also by the names of *scarlatina-mitis* and *scarlatina sine angina.* It is the simplest form of scarlet fever, and is limited to the fever and eruption, without any very severe affection of the throat.

The symptoms of this variety are often extremely mild, so that the patient is frequently not confined to his bed. The primary fever, except that the pulse is rapid, is little more than a mere febricula, and is not aggravated on the appearance of the eruption. The rash appears at the end of twenty-four or forty-eight hours, and the crops follow each other according to the usual order of succession, appearing first on the face and neck, and upper extremities; on the following day on the trunk; and on the third day on the lower extremities, when the disease has reached its acme. On the fourth day the rash begins to decline, and fades from the face, neck, and upper extremities; on the fifth day it disappears from the trunk, and on the sixth or seventh day it is evanescent over the whole body. The color of the rash is always more florid during the night than during the day, and, on its declining, desquamation takes place. With the disappearance of the eruption the fever of this variety ceases, and the disease terminates; but it often leaves the patient in a state of considerable debility for several days, and may be followed by albuminuria and dropsy, and, in some rare cases, by fatal convulsions, arising from almost complete suppression of urine and retention of urea.

This is the variety seen and described by Sydenham, and for which Belladonna may prove a prophylactic, even in small doses, and is the only remedy required in the majority of cases. Still it is better not to prevent this form, as it is far preferable for as many children as possible to have it, as it prevents the subsequent occurrence of malignant attacks.

It is very important, even in these mild attacks, to watch for the appearance of any signs of derangement of the kidneys, such as dark, smoky, or scanty urine. This condition precedes the occurrence of dropsy for some time, and also the severe attacks of headache and vomiting which precede fatal convulsions. The physician should hold himself to blame for negligence who allows either dropsy or convulsions to occur before his attention has been directed to the state of the kidneys and urine. Apocynum, Digitalis, Mercurius, Arsenicum, Hellebore, Kali-hydriod., and Apis have all proved useful in the premonitory stages of these affections, and have prevented attacks of dropsy and convulsions. Some assume that Belladonna is not at all suited to these states of the kidney and the consequent dropsy, and that it is a fair question whether some kidney-remedy would not prove a better or more specific prophylactic against the whole disease; still Belladonna sometimes exerts a tremendous diuretic power, but not when given in small doses.

The post-scarlatinal convulsions deserve more attention than they have received. We, of course, do not refer so much to those which sometimes accompany the development of the fever, but those which occur at a later period, when a careless observer might consider convalescence as confirmed. The majority of cases which I have witnessed occurred after the mild forms of scarlatina. The period of accession may vary from the third to the fortieth day from the invasion of the fever; it always betokens great danger, as Gregory, of seven cases, lost five. The pathology is well understood; for the disease almost always arises from derangement of the action of the kidneys, accompanied with a depraved condition of the blood, and some consequent irritation of the brain or nervous system.

If Belladonna be given, it should be used in quantities sufficient to act upon the kidneys; but it generally will have to be aided by Apocynum, Digitalis, Kali-hydriodicum, &c. Many persons are not aware that Bellad. exerts any diuretic effect; but Dr. H. M. Gray, who was accidentally poisoned with it, says: "One other fact, with reference to the effects of Belladonna, is worthy of note—viz., *its tremendous diuretic power*." He has observed that it does not seem to reach the kidneys until it has been some time in the system, and has exerted its specific influence upon the brain; but its power over the secretion of urine then appears to be very great. He is confident that he passed water at the rate of three pints an hour. I have witnessed similar effects, in the person of a friend who took a very large dose of Belladonna as an experiment: he was delirious for several hours, and then passed urine very frequently and copiously.

SCARLATINA-ANGINOSA.

1. In one form of this disease the specific action of the poison may be limited to one tissue—that of the throat; the eruption on the skin being altogether wanting, or appearing at a later period than usual, generally by one day, and then is less copious and less diffused than in the other forms.

There is seldom a season in which scarlatina has been in any degree epidemic that cases have not occurred in which patients, not having previously had scarlatina, are seized with severe fever and sore throat, unaccompanied by any eruption, and who, on subsequent exposure to the contagion of scarlatina, have been found insusceptible to the action of the poison; and hence it is inferred that the disease they have passed through must have been a variety of scarlet fever, or *scarlatina sine eruptione*, making itself manifest by a peculiar sore throat.

This form, therefore, essentially consists of (or, in other words, the symptoms that are never wanting are) the fever and sore throat. It has been stated that the state of the throat was constantly in unison with the state of the constitution, and consequently this variety of the disease, according to its severity, assumes all the symptoms which accompany scarlatina-simplex or the more severe forms, with the exception of the comparative absence of the eruption.

2. In another form, the essential character is that the secondary or specific actions of this poison fall quite severely on two tissues—on the skin and on the mucous membrane of the mouth and fauces, also somewhat upon the nose and eyes. This variety is liable also to be followed by the tertiary actions of the virus—such as dropsy, &c.—but in what proportions have not as yet been determined.

The fever which precedes the eruption in this variety of scarlatina lasts from twenty-four to seventy-two hours. The symptoms, however, are more violent than in the preceding species; for nausea or vomiting, great restlessness, headache, and some delirium frequently occur as early as the second day. The heat of the skin, also, is more considerable, and often is as high as 105°, while the pulse is quick, feeble, and fluttering, and shows the extreme debility the virus has occasioned. The primary fever having lasted its period, the specific actions of the poison are set up, and the eruption runs the course, which has been described in scarlatina-simplex; but its color is more intense, its duration more variable, and its attack more partial.

The *angina*, so marked a symptom in this affection, may precede the primary fever, may commence with the eruption, or may occur at some later day of the disease. It has many grades, and, in this form of scarlatina, they are generally sthenic. Thus, in slight cases, the throat has merely the sensation of roughness, with some pain in deglutition; at a higher degree the tonsils are enlarged, and covered with false membranes, and, in a few instances, ulcerated; while, in cases of still greater severity, they are swollen to a degree almost to occlude the fauces. In this latter case the act of deglutition is not merely painful, but, in many instances, impossible, and is impeded by a thick viscid mucus, which frequently requires the effort of vomiting to remove. The irritation of the fauces is sometimes propagated to the larynx, and the patient's voice is hoarse and inaudible, and perhaps he may ultimately die from this new affection. The parotid and submaxillary glands also often enlarge, sometimes previously to the sore throat, more commonly about the fifth day, and again after the throat affection has abated.

The degree of fever is usually proportioned to the severity of the angina, and is accompanied by headache, and sometimes by delirium. It does not abate on the appearance of the eruption, but continues until the throat has healed. If the false membranes come away early, or on the fourth or fifth day, the throat heals, and the fever perhaps subsides within a day or two of the eruption. It sometimes happens, however, that the false membranes do not separate till the fourteenth or fifteenth day; and, in this case, the fever runs on with equal violence after the disappearance of the rash, and the whole disease is sometimes prolonged for three weeks or a month. In this case the tongue may become dry or brown, but it seldom continues so more than a few hours. In the best marked and most exquisite cases of this form the affection of the throat and skin are, perhaps, equally intense, and equally a source of danger; in fact, it may be regarded as the standard or primitive type of the disease, or that from which all other varieties diverge. In the majority of cases the inflammatory type of fever prevails: the heat and redness of the skin being more remarkable than in any other known malady, the body seems like a living furnace of its own making. Heat of 105°, 108°, or 110° no system can long withstand. It burns and dries up everything: it kills the cuticle and hair, injures the structure of many internal organ, and deranges the liver, lungs, kidneys, bowels, and brain. Gregory attributes a large share of the evils of scarlatina-anginosa to the intensity of the animal heat. In these cases Aconite and Veratrum-viride are most useful and important remedies.

The rash, as before said, is abundant and vivid in color; it seems that a poison of a sthenic type was so abundant as to overwhelm the whole skin, and many of the mucous membranes with its affluence. There is nothing more desirable than that the eruption should be accompanied by a *moist* state of the skin; there is then much less risk of visceral obstruction or dangerous disorder of the brain and nervous system; the lungs less frequently become the seat of inflammatory engorgement; the endocarditis and pericarditis, which so frequently attend the renal affection, are less commonly observed; the renal affection, instead of being frequent, is rare. But blood of a depraved and vitiated quality often collects and stagnates in many of the mucous membranes, both thoracic and abdominal—causing either diarrhœa scarcely to be restrained, or ischuria-renalis, or some chest or brain affection.

3. In the *severe* forms of scarlatina-anginosa (described by some authors as "*scarlatina-gravior*") the specific actions of the poison are the same as in scarlatina-mitior; but the symptoms, both local and general, are more severe, and the tertiary affections more frequent—consequently the disease is more grave, and the danger more formidable.

The more remarkable symptom which distinguishes this form of the disease is the state of the tonsils. In the milder form of scarlatina-anginosa, previously noticed, it has been stated that they are either slightly affected or greatly enlarged, of a bright red; the false membranes are not very copious, and the ulcers comparatively superficial; but, in this severer form, the tonsils, though less swollen, are more gorged with blood, more livid in color, while the ulcers are foul, deep, and burrowing; the secretions of the mouth are also more copious, and generally impregnated with the offensive sordes of the sloughs; while deglutition, if less difficult, is, perhaps, infinitely more painful, and the mouth is often so tender that the slightest touch excoriates it. The ulcers, likewise, are slow to granulate, and only heal after a fearful struggle; and, in the worst cases, they spread in every direction, and the parts vesicate and mortify previous to the death of the patient.

The eruption also offers some peculiarities: being often later by some hours in coming out, its color darker and more livid, its duration more uncertain, and its distribution more irregular and capricious than in the milder form. The primary fever, likewise, is usually longer, the delirium earlier, and the depression more complete than in the milder variety; and, towards the close of the disease, the tongue becomes brown, and the symptoms closely resemble those of the last stage of typhus fever.

Such are its more marked characteristics; but it often happens that its progress is slow, silent, insidious, scarcely marked by any prominent symptom till the degree in which the constitution is subdued by this formidable poison is shown by the inflamed nasal membrane discharging its fetid ichor, causing mortification of the alæ of the nose, or mortification of the cheek or lip; or it seizes on some remote part, as the toe, the leg, or the whole of the lower extremity. But such cases ought, perhaps, more properly to be classed among the malignant cases.

As regards the *treatment* of scarlatina-anginosa, it is a disease which will often call in play all our pathological knowledge, and all our therapeutical skill; and as often, from the rapidity of its progress, it will give us but little time for reflection, it must be well studied beforehand, while we must well know how to act promptly and decidedly in cases of emergency. In a large number of cases the excessive rapidity of the pulse and great heat and redness of the skin will demand our first attention, and Aconite, Veratrum-viride, &c., will come in play; next the inflammation of the throat may require Aconite, Mercurius, and Belladonna. As soon as false membranes show themselves, Bichromate of Potash and Bromide of Potash will have to be given, either alone or in alternation with Mercurius and Belladonna. If some ulceration of the throat arise, Arsenicum, or Muriatic- or Nitric-acid may be relied upon; if profuse discharge from the nostrils and great swelling of neck ensue, Baryta-muriatica, Kali-hydriodicum, and Bromide of Potash may be required; if much delirium, with great scantiness of urine appear, Belladonna and Apocynum, or Digitalis may be given, or, if needs be, Opium; if much diarrhœa make its appearance, Arsenicum, Phosphor., Nitric-acid, or Opium may be given.

It is, of course, very important to keep the skin moist with frequent applications of sweet oil, sweet lard, or even mutton tallow when the skin remains obstinately harsh and dry.

It is a disease in the management of which intelligent medical men of all schools are more apt to differ than, perhaps, any other. In the dominant school, when the symptoms indicate high arterial action, some physicians check the first advances of the disease with antiphlogistic treatment, and take the chance of succeeding debility. But the scarlatinal miasm is very depressing, and the powers of life often sink rapidly, even without artificial reduction of strength ; some physicians, therefore, let the primary arterial action have its full play, from fear of subsequent exhaustion, and others even give tonics and stimulants from the commencement. Others limit the use of stimulants to the latter stages of the disease, and to those cases of angina-maligna, with undeveloped eruption, which, from the very onset, are characterized by depression or collapse of the vascular and nervous systems. Gregory says : "Common sense here dictates an early recourse to stimulants—to wine, brandy, cordial draughts, containing Ether, Camphor-julep, tincture of Bark, in such quantities as the stomach will bear, and the age of the patient justify." He adds, "On this point there is no room for doubt or cavil."

Some few in the dominant school use specific remedies, among which Ammonia and Belladonna are the most relied upon.

SCARLATINA-MALIGNA.

This form was formerly known as the malignant sore throat, or putrid sore throat of the earlier authors ; but the name is now generally applied to certain cases of extreme severity, into which some of the forms already described may pass, as if by insensible gradations. In others the violence of the attack is so sudden that the patient is at once struck down by the force or virulence of the poison, the type of the attack being at once adynamic, typhoid, and malignant. The extreme severity of the constitutional symptoms is marked by the smallness, feebleness, and irregularity of the pulse; the oppressed, short and quick respiration; the appearance of early raving, stupor, and sometimes coma, alternating with fretfulness and violence, dullness and suffusion of the eyes, flushing of the cheeks, and dark-brown furred tongue. The rash appears late, is of uncertain duration, and soon assumes a dark or livid color, or disappears in a few hours, and reappears again after several days if life is so far prolonged. Aphthous elevations in the throat, surrounded by a livid base, also become dark, and, bursting, they expose a surface of a dark gangrenous appearance. The passages of the fauces are always clogged up with much viscid mucus or phlegm, which produces a rattling noise in breathing, and increases the pain and difficulty of swallowing. The discharges are remarkably acrid which issue from the nostrils and posterior nasal passages, causing soreness, excoriations, and even blisters on the surfaces over which they flow. To this source the diarrhœa may be ascribed which is sometimes severe at this period, and generally adds greatly to the sufferings of the patient.

The severity of the symptoms may produce a fatal result on the second, third, or fourth day of the disease. Death frequently follows from gangrene occurring in the course of the œsophagus and alimentary canal. In other instances, in which the earlier symptoms were not very severe, the aphthous state of the throat may all at once assume a sloughing aspect, and carry off the patient at the close of the first week.

As these two last named varieties run so insensibly into one another a detailed description of the one could not be given without touching upon the description of the other; we have, therefore, preferred to pursue their description conjointly.

The symptoms which mark the invasion of grave cases of scarlet fever, though sufficiently alike in all to show the unity of the disease, differ very materially as to their degree of severity in different cases. Meigs says that, in one-third of his severe cases (16 out of 57), they were truly appalling in their character—marked by symptoms of the utmost violence and danger: the imminent danger was apparent from the outset. In the other two-thirds (41 in 57) they were either evidently severe and dangerous, though not appalling as the first, or they were much milder—more like those which mark the invasion of mild cases; but even under these circumstances they soon put on their grave and dangerous character.

According to Meigs, the first set of cases, or those in which the symptoms are most severe of all, usually begin with nervous symptoms. The onset is in some cases instantaneous. In one, the patient, a little girl two years old, whose brother and sister had been sick for some days with scarlatina, was put to bed in the evening in her usual health, which was strong and vigorous; she slept quietly through the night, but was found by the mother the next morning in a state of drowsiness, violent fever, and covered with a deep red scarlatinous rash;—she soon became comatose, and died on the third day. In another case, a boy, eleven months old, was a little fretful in the afternoon, but was put to bed in the evening as usual, and went to sleep. About ten o'clock the nurse heard a rustling in the bed, and, on going to it, found him in a violent general convulsion. The next morning he was covered with a scarlet rash, which became deeper and deeper as the disease went on On the second day he was nearly insensible, and had frequent attacks of convulsions; on the third day he had retraction of the neck, with spasmodic twitchings, and at the end of the day died comatose. In a third case, a boy, six years old, whose sister had been sick for a week with a mild attack, went to bed well. At three o'clock in the morning he was seized with vomiting and purging, paleness and coolness of the skin, and great exhaustion. At nine o'clock he was drowsy and dull; the skin was pale and cool, and the pulse extremely rapid; the vomiting and purging had ceased. At twelve, M., he was comatose, and had a convulsion. From this time he was comatose until he died, at six, P. M., of the same day, after an illness of fifteen hours. In a fourth instance the invasion was that of croup; after a few hours coma and convulsions came on; patches of eruption then appeared on the trunk, and death occurred in twenty-four hours from the commencement. The subject of this case, a boy, five years old, was thought to be so well in the afternoon of the day he was taken sick that he had been sent out to see a relation, and was seized while there. In the fifth case the onset was sudden, with violent fever, drowsiness, deep suffusion of the skin, and in a few hours insensibility, general convulsions, and death in thirty-six hours. In a sixth, a boy, four years old, the attack came on with vomiting, paleness, drowsiness, and then a scarlet rash; after a few days coryza and otorrhœa occurred; the tongue and lips became cracked and dry; and, in the second week, the child was comatose, with occasional attacks of extreme jactitation and the most violent hydrocephalic cries, which condition lasted two days. After this there was diarrhœa, extreme emaciation, loss of speech, and entire deafness. Gradually, however, the fever disappeared, the tongue cleaned off, and intelligence very slowly returned. In the sixth week convalescence was firmly established, and the child recovered perfectly, with the exception of his hearing, which remained very dull, in consequence of the perforation of both membranæ tympanorum. In a seventh, a girl, eight years old, whose brother was then sick in the house with the disease, was, in the morning, well. At breakfast she said she felt sick, and soon went to bed. At five, P. M., of that day she was attacked with a general convulsion, which lasted about fifteen minutes. The pulse immediately after the convulsion was 150. At eleven, P. M., she had another convulsion. Through the night she was very restless and wandering. On the morning of the second day there was a third convulsion, which, however, was very short. The pulse was now 160, small, and very feeble. The patient was very heavy and dull, answering questions slowly and with great difficulty; and during a part of the day she was comatose. On the third day she was better, the pulse having fallen to 152, and she was less dull, though she still continued very heavy and inattentive, unless aroused by persevering efforts. The limbs were cool, while the head and trunk were hot. The eruption was thick on the trunk and upper part of the extremities; elsewhere it was scanty. Wherever it existed it was of a deep red or purplish color, and the capillary circulation was sluggish and imperfect. On the fourth day her intellectual condition continued better; but the extremities were still cold, and the lymphatic glands and subcutaneous tissues about the lower jaw had begun to swell. On the fifth day the swelling had become very great, the stupor had returned, a profuse and disgusting coryza and otorrhœa had set in, and the edges of the eye-lids were inflamed and sore. On the sixth day the discharge from the mucous membranes of the head were very copious, and consisted of a thick, offensive, purulent fluid, intermixed with dull, whitish, grumous particles. The patient was now comatose or very restless; she swallowed with great difficulty; the swelling about the lower jaw and under the throat was enormous; the pulse was rapid and small; the eruption was very dark in hue; the cutaneous circulation was slow; the extremities were cold, and death occurred about the middle of this day.

In another case, the subject of which was a girl between three and four years old, the attack began with severe inflammation of the throat, causing great difficulty in swallowing; the rash on the first day was very extensive, and of a deep red color; the child was drowsy and heavy, or else delirious. On the second day she was comatose, and had strabismus and automatic movements of the limbs. On the third day the coma continued, and there were automatic movements of the extensor muscles, with retraction of the head. The eruption continued vivid, but was of a dark red color. Death occurred in the middle of the fourth day, in a state of coma, without convulsions. In still another case, a boy, between eight and nine years old, was suddenly attacked, while in good health, with vomiting, sore throat, and high fever. Twelve hours after the onset he had a severe convulsion, which lasted fifteen minutes. He soon recovered from this, however, and remained perfectly intelligent. On the second day the rash was moderate; there was violent fever, and the child was heavy, but when roused still intelligent. Early in this day a severe fit occurred. This was most violent, as severe as the worst epileptic convulsion; it lasted one hour and three-quarters. The pulse after this was 145. On the third and fourth days the symptoms improved very much, the pulse having fallen to 125 and 132, but he continued drowsy and heavy. The eruption came out most abundantly. The fauces were very much inflamed and somewhat ulcerated, and the external lymphatic glands were enlarged; but still the swallowing was not difficult. On the fifth day he was not so well, being more restless and heavy alternately. There had now come on much difficulty in breathing, and some croupal sound. The latter symptom increased through the day, until the dyspnœa became very great. Deglutition now became very difficult; the external swelling increased; attacks of suffocation, attended with the most painful and distressing jactitation, came on, and were renewed more and more frequently, and death occurred by asphyxia about the middle of the sixth day. In a tenth case, in a girl, five months old, convulsions occurred on the second day. These were followed by coma, lasting several days, and by enormous swelling of the lymphatic glands and subcutaneous tissues on the left side of the neck, and by a less degree of swelling over the right side of the neck. The glands of both sides suppurated, and were opened, and the child finally recovered perfectly. In an eleventh case, in a boy seven years old, an attack of general convulsions took place on the third day, after which there was delirium and coma alternately for several days, with coryza, angina, and offensive otorrhœa, lasting in all six weeks. The child recovered, but remained deaf.

In the malignant form of the disease, therefore, the symptoms are of a most virulent character. The onset is sudden: the child passes within a few hours from a state of apparent health into one of the extremest danger. Most of the cases begin with violent fever and great depression of the strength. The pulse soon becomes very rapid (140, 150, and 180), or so quick that it cannot be counted, and it is, at the same time, small and often irregular. The skin is dry and burning hot in some parts, in others cool, or even cold. There is generally nausea, or even vomiting, and these may be violent and constant. These are accompanied (but generally only in the severer cases) by colliquative diarrhœa and meteorism. Delirium often exists from the first, or else there is drowsiness and dullness of intelligence, verging gradually into coma. In the most violent cases the stupor or coma alternates with convulsions, which may cause a fatal termination in eighteen, twenty-four, or thirty-six hours.

When a case of this kind lasts over three, or even two days, the violence of the nervous symptoms almost always subsides; the convulsions cease to recur; the delirium is less violent; the coma gives way to drowsiness, or the patient becomes quite intelligent and observant; the pulse often falls in frequency, and the heat of the skin may diminish, and the eruption assume a more favorable appearance. All the symptoms seem, indeed, to be more promising, and very often the physician and friends may both be greatly elated by the improvement in the patient's condition. Nor are these hopes always illusory, since children do recover occasionally, even in cases that have exhibited the most threatening and malignant appearance at the moment of invasion. It happens unfortunately, however, in a majority of such cases, that the improvement which takes place on the third or fourth day is only momentary. The nervous symptoms subside, but new phenomena make their appearance, in the shape of severe inflammation, membranous deposit upon, or ulceration of the fauces, extensive swelling and induration of the lymphatic glands and subcutaneous tissues about the angle of the lower jaw and under the chin and throat.

In connection with the throat affection, which develops itself in this way, it is very common to have abundant purulent coryza, and often, also, otorrhœa. The symptoms assume, in fact, the features of the cases usually described under the title of scarlatina-anginosa, as we shall describe them in the second set of grave cases. It may be said here, however, that the anginose and general symptoms, which occur in cases beginning with violent nervous phenomona, are nearly always of the most dangerous and malignant character, and usually end fatally in two, three, or four days after their appearance.

The eruption in this class of cases varies according to the violence of the attack. In one of the severest, which proved fatal in fifteen hours, no eruption whatever appeared, and it was only known to be scarlatina by the character of the other symptoms, and by the fact that the sister of the boy had been sick, in the same house, with the disease for a week. In a case which terminated fatally in twenty-four hours the eruption showed itself in the form of scarlet patches about the face and upper parts of the body, twelve hours after the onset. In another case the eruption was moderate, but perfectly well marked and general. In thirteen other cases, which lasted, with one exception, not less than three days, the eruption was perfectly well marked. It covered the whole surface; was at first scarlet in color, soon ran into a deep red, and then became violet or purplish. The exceptional case was one which lasted thirty-six hours, and proved fatal in that time. In this case the eruption was well marked and extensive. M. Gueretin, in his account of the acute malignant form which he witnessed, states that the eruption was nearly constant. It generally occurs within twenty-four hours, though it may be delayed until the fourth or fifth day.

If no favorable change takes place in these severe cases, and when they do not prove fatal at once, the patient grows weaker and weaker; the delirium continues, or is replaced by coma; subsultus-tendinum, rigidity of the limbs, spasmodic twitchings, or general convulsions make their appearance; the eruption becomes more and more livid; the pulse grows smaller, more frequent, and irregular; the respiration is excessively embarrassed; deglutition becomes impossible, and the patient dies in from three to seven or nine days. In some few instances the child struggles on for several weeks, and dies in a state of utter exhaustion; or, having a constitution of great powers of endurance, at last surmounts the disease and recovers.

The invasion of grave cases is not always, as has been stated above, so violent as those which have just been described. In rather more than two-thirds of fifty-seven grave cases the onset was less threatening than in the other third; though the symptoms were severe and dangerous in most of these also, and, when not so at the start, very soon assumed the serious characters which make it necessary to class the cases in which they occurred as grave. The chief difference between the symptoms that mark the onset of grave cases of this kind and of those in which the symptoms are still more violent—which latter we have thus far been describing—lies in the character of the nervous phenomena: in the latter they are most severe, threatening, and dangerous, consisting of stupor, coma, and convulsions; in the former merely excessive agitation, restlessness, heaviness, or stupor. In one well marked case of the kind now under consideration, the patient, a boy between seven and eight years old, was attacked in the evening with headache, fever, and vomiting. On the following morning a faint rash was perceptible, which, by the afternoon of that day, was distinct, though not very full. The case now rapidly assumed unpleasant features: the pulse rose to 150; there was much drowsiness and delirium; and, on the fourth day, constant picking of the bed-clothes and at the fingers. In another case, in a boy between four and five years of age, the first sign of sickness was slight languor after dinner, which was followed by fever in the evening, and the development in the night of a scarlatinous rash. On the following day there was some pain in the throat, with redness; the pulse was 140, and the skin hot and dry; there were no nervous symptoms, except slight drowsiness. On the third day the pulse was 136, the rash was well out, and there were no unpleasant symptoms whatever. From this time, however, the symptoms gradually grew worse: the throat affection increasing, the cervical lymphatic glands becoming very much swollen, and the child growing more uneasy and restless, though retaining perfectly its intelligence. By the sixth day the grave character of the case was fully developed: the eruption being intense, and of a deep brick-red color, verging towards a purple. There was, at the same time, very great drowsiness, abundant discharges from the nasal passages of thick sero-mucous and purulent fluids membranous exudation in the fauces, with gurgling and great difficulty in swallowing, and an utter loss of appetite.

The mode of invasion is different, therefore, in different cases of the same degree of severity. In some, indeed, it may be mild; and it is not until the third, fourth, or fifth day, or later, that the severity of the attack shows itself unmistakably.

In this class of cases (the milder of the grave cases) the false membrane which is thrown out is rarely present on the first day. Rilliet and Barthez say that they have known it absent until the tenth or eleventh day. It appears first in small, thin, whitish, yellowish, or ash-colored points or patches, on one or both tonsils, or on the soft palate only, where it remains limited, or from whence it extends to the pharynx. The patches vary in extent, thickness, and adherence. They may remain from one to four or five days (more frequently the latter), and are then thrown off; but, in some few cases, they are thrown off after a day or so, and then reproduced. The mucous membrane beneath may be ulcerated, or it may be only in a high state of congestion and inflammation. There may be great fetor of the breath, sometimes almost intolerable, after the appearance of the false membrane.

The exudation of plastic lymph is not constant. There may be some cases in which the throat affection is very severe indeed, but in which there is no deposit of false membrane whatever; and in others the mucous membrane is of a deep red or even purplish hue, its consistence softened, and it is swollen, and covered with a layer of grayish or sanious pus. The tonsils are enlarged, infiltrated with pus, softened, and break down easily under the finger. In other cases there are ulcerations; which may be superficial, amounting only to superficial erosion, or they may extend through the mucous and submucous tissue, even to the muscles beneath. In still more rare cases we have gangrene; and it is important to be able to distinguish between a real slough and that state of the false membrane in which it assumes the appearance of a slough. By far the greater number of so-called cases of gangrene are nothing more than this appearance assumed by the false membrane.

An almost constant accompaniment is *swelling and inflammation of the submaxillary lymphatic glands* and surrounding cellular tissue. The tumefaction is generally confined at first to the glands beneath the jaw, and extends to the parts behind the angle of it, until the sides of the neck and throat become largely distended, so as to interfere with and prevent, in a great measure, the opening of the mouth. Swelling of the parotid glands is a rare occurrence. Barthez states that the tumefaction of the cellular tissue is often of the nature of active œdema. This tumefaction of the parts about the neck seldom takes place the third or fourth day. During the first two or three days the chief symptoms are the fever, the eruption, and the nervous phenomena, viz., restlessness and agitation, or drowsiness and stupor.

A delusive appearance of improvement may take place on the third or fourth day. It is just at this time, however, that the throat affection is apt to set in severely; and it rarely fails to appear in children who have presented violent symptoms during the first two or three days. The enlargement *may* terminate by suppuration, but generally ends by resolution.

Violent *coryza* is commonly observed in this form of disease: it may appear at once, or not for several days. The discharge is yellowish, granular, thin, very offensive, and highly acrid, so as to excoriate very much the upper lip. It often flows in surprising quantities, and generally continues up to the moment of death. As before mentioned, the occurrence of this coryza in connection with great external swelling of the glands of the neck is regarded as an absolutely fatal complication.

Otorrhœa is another symptom of this form, and similarly unfavorable. It generally occurs simultaneously with coryza. The discharge is at first thin and watery, and sanious, but becomes gradually thicker as the disease progresses. The quantity is extremely variable: it will sometimes fill the meatus and conchæ of both ears, and then flow out and make large stains upon the pillow. It is an unfavorable symptom, apt, if the child recovers, to result in deafness, which is too often permanent. When the coryza and catarrh exist in mild cases they do not assume the pecular character of violence which they bear in grave cases.

In most cases a loud gurgling, which is very characteristic, is heard in the throat, particularly when the child is asleep or dozing. It depends in part upon the collection of viscid and tenacious secretions in the throat, which embarrass respiration, and in part upon the existence of the coryza. The coryza is a symptom of very serious consequence at all ages, but especially in young children. There is generally some cough, which may be frequent and troublesome, though not usually so, unless there be a disposition to laryngeal complications. The voice is hoarse, gutteral, and sometimes whispering.

When the cough is very frequent, and still more when it becomes hoarse and croupal, in connection with hoarse and whispering voice, or aphonia, there is great reason to fear the extension of the disease into the larynx, which constitutes an almost necessarily fatal accident.

The occurrence of laryngitis is a disputed point: some say that it never occurs, while others again distinctly state having found the false membrane existing after death. Meigs is certain that it occurred in one of his cases.

Sequelæ of Scarlatina.—Gregory divides the sequelæ into: 1. Inflammation of the cellular tissue of the neck; 2. Desquamation of the cuticle; 3. A low degree of mucous enteritis; occasionally, 4. True debility; 5. Dropsy.

Desquamation of the cuticle is quite pathognomonic of scarlatina. It is hardly ever absent. In all bad cases, too, the hair comes off, as, indeed, it does after all long fevers accompanied with dryness and great heat of skin. The nails are sometimes thrown off, and some cabinets contain gloves of cuticle with the nails on.

When scarlet fever attacks a child between the ages of three and seven, while the second set of teeth is in process of formation, it very frequently happens that their structure is materially weakened and injured. These teeth in after life appear dark and imperfect, and are lost at a very early age. This is true also of the other exanthemata.

The whole process of desquamation requires careful watching. The period is one of low fever, often tending to inflammation. The urine is scanty and high colored during its progress. The tongue is white, the pulse quick, and the rest disturbed. The desquamation begins about the fourth or fifth day, and may continue three weeks; and many physicians (the Germans especially) often confine their patients to bed during desquamation, so conscious are they of the danger.

In the progress of this secondary or desquamative fever, inflammation may invade any of the great viscera, especially if the constitution be weak, and the contractile power or tone of the vessels small. Acute pneumonia or peritonitis may thus supervene, and prove the immediate cause of death. More frequently than is generally supposed some affection of the heart also arises. I have seen several cases of endocarditis, which, although not immediately fatal, were the cause of trouble for years afterwards.

The great safeguard against unpleasant occurrences during the period of desquamation is proper attention to the condition of the skin. If this be anointed with sweet oil, or lard from which the salt has been worked out in water, or with simple cerate, several times a day, during the whole course of the attack of scarlet fever, a good convalescence will almost always reward the physician.

In some cases a low degree of *mucous enteritis* accompanies the decline of the disease. The patient complains of exceeding languor and lassitude and total loss of appetite; diarrhœa is present, and the body emaciates; the tongue is red, and superficially ulcerated; the angles of the lip excoriated; the verge of the anus beset with eczematous vesicles; the mucous membrane of the bowels is tender, and is thrown into spasms and disturbance by the simplest food. Griping, therefore, is complained of, and a general soreness of the belly. All this may, and frequently does depend simply on congestion. In bad cases the membrane ulcerates, and much blood appears in the motions. Death may then ensue. In these cases Phosphoric and Nitric-acids, Arsenicum, and Opium are the most important remedies.

The *true debility* which succeeds scarlatina deserves mention. The muscular power is everywhere enfeebled; the slightest exertion fatigues; the heart participates in this general debility, and frequent syncope occurs; the clean tongue distinguishes this condition of the frame from secondary fever. In this state Arsenicum and Phosphorus are among the most useful remedies.

But, of all the sequelæ of scarlatina, *dropsy* is by far the most frequent and important. It seems to bear, also, a direct relation to the intensity of the disease; that is to say, the milder the disease, and the more the ordinary symptoms of scarlet fever may have been wanting, the more apt is the dropsy to ensue. In fact, so marked is this peculiarity that it alone has led to the discovery of a form of the disease called *scarlatina-latens*, in which the child, without having had any of the visible signs of scarlatina, at a certain time after having been exposed to its contagion is attacked with anasarca or some other form of dropsical effusion.

Dropsy occurs, perhaps, in about ten to twenty per cent. of all the cases of scarlet fever. It occurred in one-fifth of the cases of MM. Barthez and Rilliet, and in about one-ninth of those observed by Meigs. It occurs generally in the course of the second or third week of the disease—during desquamation; but there is no doubt that its access may be deferred to a later period.

It selects by preference those cases, as remarked above, whose course has been mild and symptoms slight or wanting; and, indeed, Dr. Tweedie states that it has never been known to follow a malignant case. This does not accord with Meigs' experience, however, as he states that he has seen it follow in six out of twenty-nine grave cases. The most frequent form is anasarca, then œdema of the lungs, hydrothorax, ascites, hydropericardium, and hydrocephalus, and in the order mentioned.

Gregory says he does not pretend always to anticipate when dropsy *will* supervene, but he does know when it *will not* occur; and that is when the pulse falls to the natural standard on the tenth day, and becomes soft, with a clean state of tongue, an abundant clear urine, and a natural aspect of countenance. But, on the other hand, he says it is very likely to happen to him whose pulse, after the twelfth day of fever, remains sharp and quick, and whose tongue continues obstinately white; whose sleep is disturbed, whose skin is dry, and who has a scanty urine, which becomes turbid on cooling. Such persons remain languid and weak after scarlet fever, and their appetite does not return. If tonics are given, to improve the appetite and recruit the strength, secretion is still further checked, and the probability of supervening dropsy greatly increased. In a large proportion of such cases the urine is loaded with albumen and is of low specific gravity.

The exciting cause, however, in those cases which otherwise look favorable, is generally believed to be cold. Meigs says that he has rarely known it to occur where the patient has been confined to the house until after the twenty-first day; while, on the other hand, he has seen it follow immediately upon a ride, in cool weather, on the fourteenth day.

The symptoms, as before remarked, generally supervene during the period of desquamation. The attack is sometimes very sudden, but, in most instances, it is slow and gradual. Effusion, however, is not the first evidence of trouble. There is, for a day or two, more or less constitutional disturbance; the child becomes languid, drooping, and irritable, and very soon after fever sets in, with dry and heated skin, frequent and hard pulse, anorexia, and thirst; there is constipation, scanty urine, and not unfrequently nausea and vomiting or headache. In some cases, however, these precursory symptoms may be much less marked, and indeed, so slight as to escape notice.

The effusion generally commences in the eye-lids, and there it should be looked for first, it then invades the lower extremities, and finally the internal organs. It has the peculiarity of not pitting upon pressure, at least in the first stage. In very mild cases the cause of the fever is only to be determined by a careful examination of the face, and, perhaps, a *cushiony* appearance of the backs of the hands and feet; and in these cases the symptoms soon subside, and the patient recovers with the restoration of the urinary secretion. In more violent cases all the symptoms are increased; the anasarca is general and great, and death may occur in the worst cases by asphyxia, occasioned by œdema of the lung, hydrothorax, or hydropericardium.

It sometimes happens that death occurs very rapidly after the invasion of the symptoms. It has been known to end fatally in thirty-six, fourteen, and even in twelve hours.

In some instances *no evidence of subcutaneous effusion* may be found; yet the symptoms may be proved to be due to the scarlatinal poison by the presence of albumen in the urine. The patient may be seized with severe headache and vomiting; for instance, after two days of slight ailment (marked by diminution of urine, feverishness, &c.) this is followed by *convulsive* movements, and this again in twelve hours by coma and death. The symptoms which mark the occurrence of internal effusion will depend, of course, upon the part attacked.

The particular condition of the urinary function should be attended to. It has already been stated that the amount of urine secreted is less than natural during the early period of the dropsical attack; but, while this is true, it ought to be observed that the patient also makes water more frequently than usual. There is, in fact, frequent micturition—a symptom occasioned, no doubt, by the acrid and irritating character of the urine. The diminution in the amount is usually a very marked symptom. It is sometimes almost, or even entirely suppressed for a considerable period, and during this time there is no distention of the bladder, as may be ascertained by percussion; there is, in fact, not retention, but suppression. In these cases what little urine is passed is dark, bloody, thick, and of a highly offensive smell.

In very mild cases of dropsy the urine is usually of a deeper color than natural, but still retains its transparency when first voided. It is apt, however, to become turbid on cooling, and to deposit a more or less abundant sediment. It has, in these cases, an acid reaction; its specific gravity is somewhat increased; when heated it becomes cloudy, and a small amount of a flocculent precipitate falls to the bottom. In severer cases the urine is very much diminished in quantity; it may be merely of a dark red color, but more commonly it is blackish or brownish in tint, or it is of the color of smoke or soot, or as if ink had been poured into the vessel; it throws down a deposit, which is generally of a reddish-brown color; when heated it yields a very large amount of coagulated albumen. If the spontaneous deposit be examined with the microscope in these cases it is found to consist of crystals of lithate of ammonia, of blood-globules, scarcely altered, and of mucous corpuscles and epithelial scales. The black or brown discoloration depends, of course, upon the presence of blood.

The danger to be apprehended depends entirely upon the form which the dropsy takes. So long as it is confined to the subcutaneous cellular tissue there is no danger whatever; when, however, it attacks the brain or lungs it is exceedingly dangerous. In these cases the condition of the patient is a faithful index of the extent of danger—the gravity of the symptom admitting of no doubt or hesitancy.

I have cured many cases of dropsy after scarlet fever with simple Cream of Tartar, faithfully followed up for seven or ten days, in doses of from one-quarter to a whole teaspoonful every four hours at first; then every six, eight, or twelve hours. It acts first upon the bowels, and subsequently upon the kidneys. In other cases Apocynum, Apis, Kali-hydriodicum, and Digitalis have been used with equal success.

The cases of *convulsions* after scarlet fever which I have seen have generally been preceded by severe headache and vomiting, just as in Bright's disease of the kidneys, the urine being invariably scanty. The treatment is similar to that which obtains in manifest dropsy, and relief ensues as soon as the secretion from the kidneys is reëstablished.

The above is a fair statement of the ordinary views of dropsy after scarlet fever; but more minute and satisfactory knowledge has been obtained. Thus Golding Bird recognizes two varieties or classes of cases of scarlatinal dropsy: the one arising from *simple debility*, which is usually speedily removed; the other caused by the fever and which is *highly dangerous*, inasmuch as the blood is poisoned by containing the uneliminated elements of the urine. The *dangerous variety* may also occur under one of three forms. In *one* the disease is very acute, and, if seen early, the urine is not only albuminous, but contains the coloring matter of the blood also. In a *second* class the urine is always albuminous, but contains no blood;

in these cases Digitalis and Apocynum-cannabinum are the most reliable remedies, but may have to be aided by Colchicum to eliminate the urea, and Tartrate or Iodide of Potash to increase the action of the kidneys. When the albumen has disappeared from the urine many allopathic physicians give Iron and Quinine. In the *third* class of dangerous cases, which are chronic, tonic medicines and nourishing support are said to be necessary from the first. Dr. Wilshire thinks that the *asthenic* cases are the most frequent, and has found that, in the greater number of cases, the Iodide of Potassium, in some bitter infusion, was of great utility, or that Quinine was frequently necessary in the later periods of the disease, and in those cases characterized by anæmic urine.

Some physicians do not believe the urea is retained in the blood in these affections; but Golding Bird has devised a simple method of detecting it. The suspected blood having been allowed to coagulate, the serum is to be decanted, and shaken up with an equal quantity of rectified spirits, which causes precipitation of the albumen. The mixture is then to be filtered, and the purified liquid, after having been evaporated to two drachms, is to be treated with an equal bulk of nitric acid and again filtered. This last strained fluid, being slowly evaporated on a watch-glass, will exhibit the feathery crystals of nitrate of urea.

Dr. Charlton describes the dropsy after scarlet fever as coming on in two different ways; in one its invasion is intense and sudden, the body being distended with fluid in twenty-four hours, with high fever, full pulse, and almost entire suppression of urine, and much oppression of breathing, in which he thinks one good general bleeding is followed by the most beneficial effects; in the other form the dropsical swelling comes on gradually, with little fever; but in both instances dangerous head and thoracic symptoms may occur, and fluid may accumulate in the pericardium, pleura, peritonæum, or general cellular tissue. He says Elaterium, in one-twelfth or one-sixth grain doses, every three or four hours, produces most rapid amendment. In some cases much benefit is derived from Iodide of Potash during convalescence. In patients left anæmic and debilitated, with tendency to scrofulous deposits, the Citrate and Iodide of Iron are most useful.

Todd thinks, in order to induce the dropsy, there must be: *First*, A particular state of the skin; *Second*, A peculiar state of the kidney; and, *Third*, A special state of the blood; and he thinks we will not find the disease fully developed without the concurrence of all three of these conditions, and if any of them are absent we will only have a threatening of dropsy, but the full-blown disease will not follow. Thus, if we find only the peculiar state of the blood, and the specific state of the kidneys, while the *skin* is normal, the dropsy will be slight, or altogether absent. Again, when the requisite conditions of the blood and skin are present, but the kidneys are healthy, dropsy will not occur; and, even if the predisposing state of the kidneys and skin both exist (and under such circumstances we could scarcely have a healthy state of the blood), yet if the condition of that fluid does not correspond with that which is favorable to dropsy, we may have other disorders, such as severe head affections, but there will be no dropsy.

In these cases the skin has a peculiar white, semi-transparent, waxy appearance, very characteristic of the disease; it is, also, dry, rough, and harsh, and, probably, in an irritated state, and its secretions are locked up, or prevented from being excreted, and retained in the system. The amount and importance of these excretions may be inferred from the following data: The perspiratory glands are scattered everywhere throughout the integument, being most abundant on the anterior portions of the body; thus, on the posterior portion of the trunk, the cheeks, and skin of the thighs and legs, there are about five hundred to the square inch, while on the anterior portion of the trunk, the forehead, neck, fore-arms, and back of the hands and feet, there are no less than one thousand to the square inch; and on the soles of the feet and palms of the hands as many as two thousand seven hundred in the same space. The whole number of perspiratory glands is not less than two million three hundred thousand; and the entire length of the glandular tubing is not less than one hundred and fifty-three thousand inches, or about two and a half miles. It is easy to understand, therefore, that a very large amount of fluid may be supplied from so extensive a glandular apparatus—viz.: no less than two pounds, avoirdupois, in twenty-four hours; while, under extraordinary circumstances, as much as three and one-half pounds have been lost in a single hour: the complete retention of so much fluid would almost produce a dropsy unaided. Of the solid constituents of perspiration, chloride of sodium is the most abundant; the salts of ammonia are evidently present in it, while the earthy phosphates and a little peroxide of iron also found. It also contains acetic, formic, and lactic acids and a sulphurous matter; *urea*, too, is a normal constituent. It has been fully demonstrated that carbonic acid and nitrogen are also given off in the liquid secretion of the sudariparous glands: four hundred and twelve cubic inches of carbonic acid gas are excreted from the skin of a full-grown man in twenty-four hours, and a little less than half as much nitrogen. Thirty-eight grains of mineral substances are cast out, and a quarter of an ounce of organic and volatile matters—more than the equivalent of many homœopathic doses. As additional proofs of the importance of the functions of the skin, we may add that the normal quantity of free *lactic* acid is always increased in the perspiration of rheumatic individuals. Sometimes *acetic* acid is found combined with the lactic, but acetic acid is more common in the sweat of consumptive patients; ammonia is present in gout, typhus and typhoid fevers, and some nervous affections; *uric acid* has been found in the sweat of rheumatic patients, and urate of soda in gouty individuals. Hence it is evident, if the perspiration be completely locked up, blood-poisoning must ensue, from the retention of injurious and poisonous substances. In scarlet fever, from some cause not easy of detection—but, in some instances, undoubtedly from exposure to cold—there is an arrest of the proper elimination of the scarlet-fever poison through the skin, its usual emunctory, and the ordinary excretion of waters and salts through that organ is checked; not obtaining complete egress there, the virus finds for itself another channel, and is thrown upon the kidneys. Its passage through these organs produces great irritation in them, the effect of which is, that water and salts are imperfectly eliminated, and thus the escape of water from the blood is prevented through its two ordinary channels—the kidneys and skin. (On page 224 the functions of the kidneys have been elaborately considered.)

The kidneys in scarlet fever are in a very analogous condition to that of the skin; there is a desquamative state in one, as well as the other. When we examine a scarlet-fever kidney we find it filled with epithelium, and the whole organ is enlarged and in a state of hyperæmia, as far as this great filling of the uriniferous tubes with epithelium will permit it to be so; this accumulation of epithelium creates an unnatural distention of the tubes, and the small vessels which ramify upon their walls become compressed, and thus the blood is thrown back upon the malphigian bodies. Hence but a small quantity of urine is secreted, and that containing serum or blood in large quantity; and this scanty secretion of urine is negatively a further cause for the accumulation of epithelium in the uriniferous tubes, as there is less fluid to wash or flood them out. The congestion of the malphigian bodies, when it exists to a certain extent, produces an effusion of liquor-sanguinis, or the serum of the blood, into the tubes, and the urine is merely albuminous and presents a peculiar smoky appearance; but, when it exists to a greater extent, it leads to a rupture of some of the malphigian vessels and the escape of all the constituents of the blood, and we find, by microscopic examination of the urine, an abundance of blood-corpuscules and fibrinous casts of the tubes, from the fibrine having moulded itself to their walls in the process of coagulation.

As a direct consequence of this obstruction to the escape of water from the skin and kidneys, a watery condition of the blood is induced; for two pints of water should be excreted daily by the skin and three pints by the kidneys. Now this water must be got rid of in some way or other, and when its usual channels of escape are cut off it is very apt to permeate the parieties of the blood-vessels. But why, asks Todd, do we find it in the cellular tissue; and why in that of the skin more than any other part? It finds its way into the areolar tissue of the skin, in consequence of the determination of blood to the skin due to its state of irritation; for, in order to reach the skin, the blood must pass through the subcutaneous cellular tissue. It would be wrong, however, to suppose that the effusion of serum is always confined to the neighborhood of the skin, for we often find it in the areolar tissue of the lungs, and in the serous cavities; in the former aided by the necessarily large flow of blood to the lungs, and in the latter favored by the comparative tenuity of the texture of the serous membrane, which offers a proportionately small obstacle to the escape of the serous parts of the blood. If it were not for this ready and copious escape of dropsical fluid into the cellular tissue, the internal organs, especially the brain, would be quickly involved, and dropsy of the brain or chest, with rapidly fatal results, would quickly ensue.

All this is favored by an impoverished, watery, and poisonous state of the blood. If the scarlet-fever poison is not properly and promptly eliminated, it interferes with the normal nutrient changes which should take place in the blood, and it is not improbable that some special chemical change in this fluid occurs; for Magendie found that the introduction of alkalies into the circulation caused great retardation of the current through the capillaries, and consequent dropsical effusion. We know that urea is retained, and carbonate of ammonia formed. Schoenlein was the first to suggest that the scarlatinous alkali is similar to, and as virulent as the narcotic alkaloids, such as exist in Stramonium, Belladonna, Rhus-toxicodendron, &c.

Tripe admits three varieties of scarlatinal dropsy: *First*, That in which the urine is not albuminous, but contains an unusual quantity of lithates; *Second*, That in which it is albuminous, with *sub-acute* nephritis; *Third*, That in which the urine is albuminous, with *acute* nephritis. Or, as he otherwise assumes: *First*, Dropsy from *debility; Second*, Dropsy with and from congestion, irritation, or sub-acute inflammation of the kidneys; and, *Third*, Dropsy with acute inflammation of the renal glands. In the *first* variety recovery speedily occurs from the use of mild purgatives, warm baths, and Muriate tincture of Iron. In the *second* variety, from derangement of the circulation of the kidneys, or congestion, or acute irritation, the symptoms may be at first slight, such as trifling fever, loss of appetite, lassitude, and slight aching of the loins; but after a few days the eye-lids puff up, the face becomes œdematous, and next the extremities and skin. If the urine has not previously been albuminous it now becomes so, and scanty, and of higher specific gravity; the microscope detects blood-corpuscules and broken-up epithelial cells; the salts of the urine are increased, especially the lithates, while the urea is diminished. The treatment consists in the use of the antiphlogistic diuretics, such as Digitalis,

Cream of Tartar, Spirits of Nitre, Apocynum-cannabinum, &c. In the *third*, and most important, but fortunately the most rare form of acute albuminous dropsy, the symptoms are more severe—viz.: increased heat of skin, thirst, furred tongue, quick pulse, great diminution or almost entire suppression of urine, and great lessening of urea; the dropsy sets in rapidly. The treatment is the same as in the second variety, but more active in proportion to the severity of the disease.

In Tripe's cases nine per cent. of the dropsies occurred in the first week of the disease; thirty-eight per cent. in the second; thirty-four per cent. in the third; forty-one per cent. in the fourth; and four per cent in the fifth week.

To give some idea of ordinary regular treatment we subjoin the following: In one case Todd ordered a daily warm bath, and a daily dose of pulv. Jalap compos.—*i. e.*, Jalap one part, to Cream of Tartar two parts; dose, one-half to one drachm—which carried off an abundance of watery stools. The next day the patient passed one and a half pints of urine, which had been deficient in quantity, smoky in color, with great abundance of albumen; and the dropsy had greatly diminished. In the following twenty-four hours he voided two quarts of urine; and from this time it is wonderful with what degree of rapidity the kidneys continued to secrete. On the third day he was relieved of two and a half quarts, and the dropsy had almost entirely passed away, although he had been suffering with almost universal dropsy, even of his peritonæum, and there had doubtless been some effusion into the ventricles of the brain, for he had been very drowsy and lethargic. There still remained a little smokiness of the urine, indicating the escape of blood; and, with a view of checking this and removing his anæmia, he got Citrate of Iron, under which he improved rapidly, and entirely recovered.

Brain Affections subsequent to Scarlet Fever.—If the dropsy be, as it were, suppressed, or rather do not manifest itself externally, a serious affection of some internal organ will arise; among these, disorders of the brain and spinal marrow are not uncommon. In 128 fatal cases, recorded by Tripe, no less than 51 were referable to this category. Thus, meningitis occurred in 6 cases; passive effusion in the cranial cavity in 7; with convulsions alone, or coma and convulsions combined, in 29; and coma alone in 5; total 51. All these cases may safely be regarded as arising from those derangements of the kidneys that cause the dropsies before described, and require similar treatment.

Heart Diseases occurring during or after Scarlet Fever.—It has long been known that scarlet fever is apt to be complicated with brain and spinal disease; but the possibility of the supervention of pericarditis and endocarditis is not so generally recognized. Even Watson, in his most brilliant and practical work on the "Practice of Medicine," erroneously says that the affections of the joints similative of rheumatism, occurring in the course of scarlet fever, may be distinguished from true rheumatism by the absence of cardiac complication. Heart-disease in scarlet fever may appear at the height of the disease or as a complication of the dropsical affections which arise afterwards. The attack may be insidious, or there may be severe pain, with rapid and tumultuous action of the heart, orthorpnœa, and great restlessness. I have seen endocarditis quite as frequently as pericarditis. That heart-disease should occur in the course of or subsequent to scarlet fever should not be surprising; for nothing is so well ascertained as that pericarditis and endocarditis very frequently follow obstructive and Bright's disease of the kidneys, and nothing is more familiar to the profession than that obstructive disease of the kidneys is not uncommon during convalescence from scarlet fever. It may owe its origin to two different sources—viz., the presence of the specific scarlet-fever poison in the blood acting as an irritant to the heart, or the existence of crystallizable compounds in the circulation which should have been eliminated from the system by the kidneys. These are much more important parts in the treatment than the consideration of trivial modifications of the symptoms. In Tripe's 128 cases, 12 were fatal from diseases of the heart and pericardium—viz., 4 of pericarditis, 3 of endocarditis, and 5 of effusion into the pericardium without dropsy of the other cavities. In these cases Aconite and Digitalis are the most important remedies, but may have to be aided by Veratrum-viride, Veratrum-album, Spigelia, Gelseminum, or Apocynum-cannabinum.

The *chest affections* arise from a mingling of uræmia with more or less decided congestive or inflammatory disorders. In Tripe's 128 fatal cases, no less than 40 were complicated with lung affections—viz., 3 with bronchitis, 16 with pneumonia, 4 with pleuro-pneumonia, 7 with pleurisy, 2 with peritonitis combined with pleuro-pneumonia, 1 with œdema of the lungs, and 7 with non-inflammatory effusion into the thoracic cavities. The most important remedies in these cases are Aconite and Antimony, Veratrum-viride and Digitalis, and Phosphorus and Apocynum-cannabinum.

Closely allied with these are the so-called *rheumatic affections* which follow scarlet fever; the poison retained in the system simply falls more decidedly upon the muscles and joints than upon the cellular and serous tissues. The treatment is very similar—Aconite and Bryonia, or Digitalis and Colchicum, or Veratrum-viride and Nitrate of Potash are frequently useful.

When an apparently rheumatic affection seems to invade *the neck* we must be more careful in our diagnosis; for the inflammation of the fauces and back of the pharynx may be propagated to the external fibrous coverings of the spine, and from thence to the meninges of the spinal marrow, and paralysis may ensue, or the disease may advance from the inter-vertebral substance to destruction of the ligamentous or cartilaginous structures, and even to caries of the bones of the base of the skull, or of one or more of the cervical vertebræ.

Neck Glands.—Corrigan describes a peculiar and very fatal form of scarlatina-anginosa, consisting in a rapid tumefaction of the parts beneath the angle of the jaw, *without* any corresponding inflammation of the throat internally. This swelling occasionally reaches an enormous size, and the child usually sinks under the sloughing of the cellular tissue, or from the effects of the pressure on the blood-vessels. It should not be opened, for it is not a case of diffused cellular suppuration, but the cellular tissue is merely infiltrated with a dirty-looking serous fluid. Iodide of Potash or Apocynum, in alternation with Arsenicum or Cantharides, will promote the absorption of the fluid and counteract the malignant poison in the tissues.

Prognosis.—1. The chance of recovery is much greater in scarlatina-anginosa when the eruption is florid and stands well out; although, in some cases, the more profuse and abundant the eruption the more dangerous the attack, simply because there is a greater amount of the disease, although it is well out upon the surface. But, even in this form of the disorder, there are many sources of danger, and various ways in which it may prove fatal. In the first place, many of the patients apparently die from inflammation or effusion within the head; they are attacked with violent headache, with furious delirium, which is followed by coma and death.

2. And, secondly, the state of the throat may be full of peril. As the disease proceeds—although the rash may be steadily persistent—the throat may become foul and sloughy; an acrid discharge from the nostrils—which are so stuffed and swollen internally that the patient can scarcely breathe through them—runs over and frets the upper lip; the parotid and submaxillary glands swell.

3. If the voice become hoarse or whispering it indicates a very dangerous extension of the disease from the pharynx to the larynx.

4. The symptoms which indicate a disposition to implication of the larynx are frequent hoarse and croupal cough, hoarse and whispering voice or cry, aphonia, and dyspnœa with stridulous respiration.

5. The anginose and general symptoms which occur in cases beginning with violent nervous phenomena, and especially with convulsions, are nearly always of the most dangerous and malignant character, and usually end fatally in two, three, or four days after their appearance.

6. In the second week of scarlatina-maligna, if death occurs, it is foretold by the quick, small, and weak pulse, by the rapid, languid, and oppressed respiration, frequent fluid acrid discharges from the bowels;

blood may be discharged from the nostrils, mouth, throat, bowels, or even from the kidneys; petechial spots appear on the skin, and the patient is at last destroyed with local manifestations of the morbid state in different parts and organs.

7. Violent nervous symptoms, occurring early in scarlet fever, augur great danger to the patient.

8. The *character* of the nervous symptoms is all-important, as the probable termination of the disease can be foretold more surely by a just appreciation of these phenomena than by any other means. Excessive jactitation or irritability, delirium, coma, and the hydrocephalic crisis, are all unfavorable symptoms, but not in the same degree as are those connected with the locomotive apparatus. MM. Rilliet and Barthez state that they have seen recoveries take place in cases in which the intelligence of the patient had been very much disordered, while of those who, *during the first fifteen days of scarlatina*, were taken with convulsions, convulsive movements, contractions—in a word, any symptoms affecting the locomotive apparatus—all, without exception, died. Exceptions to this rule have occurred in my own practice.

9. An extremely frequent or very violent pulse is an unfavorable sign; so, also, intense heat or unnatural coolness of the skin; deficiency or sudden disappearance of the eruption, or a livid or purple hue of it; slow and imperfect capillary circulation, as ascertained by pressure; the appearance of petechiæ, ecchymosis, or hæmorrhages; violent vomiting and colliquative diarrhœa; great violence of the throat-affection, whether from tumefaction, great abundance of pseudo-membranous exudation, or disposition to ulceration and sloughing, or severe coryza and otorrhœa.

10. A disposition to a typhoid state, indicated by dullness of the intelligence, dusky hue of the skin, frequent and feeble pulse, dry brown tongue, sordes on the teeth, meteorism, and diarrhœa, presents a grave cause for alarm.

Mortality.—In homœopathic practice, of 75 cases, 4 ended fatally; in Trinks' 92 cases, 5 died; in a mild epidemic observed by Knorre, of 153, only 3 died; in Urdemann's 40 cases, none died; in a more severe epidemic observed by Lorbach, no less than 20 cases died out of 96; Moschick lost 7 cases out of 60; in Lorbach's 12 cases of subsequent dropsy, 3 died. In all, 43 cases out of 528.

In allopathic practice, of 16 very grave cases, 11 died; of 41 of the less violent of the grave cases, 14 died; in 206 mild cases, the mortality was slight; of 263 cases of all kinds, 29, or about one-ninth terminated in dropsy. In all 28 cases out of 263.

Preventive Treatment.—Before passing to the consideration of the treatment of the developed disease in all its varieties and complications, it is proper to inquire how far it is possible to prevent the occurrence of the affection altogether, or, at least, lessen the susceptibility to the severest consequences of it. We have to intercept a disease which is neither a simple sthenic inflammation, nor yet one of simple debility or putrescency; a disorder in which strict antiphlogistic treatment is generally dangerous, and one which, on the other hand, is frequently aggravated by decided tonics or stimulants. Hence it must be a remedy which neither depresses excessively, nor excites or irritates too powerfully; yet it must be a medicine which will control an excessively rapid pulse without producing unusual debility; it should also restore the functions of the skin and kidneys without irritating either unusually; it must be capable of allaying a peculiar neuro-phlogistic state of the throat, skin, or many other organs, without disordering the stomach excessively; it must be competent to counteract a contagious disorder and its morbid influence upon the blood and nervous system; it should also be capable of eliminating urea and obviating uræmic blood-poisoning; it should also be an antihydropic remedy.

To Hahnemann belongs the great credit of first suggesting this important desideratum, and of pointing out a remedy to meet some of the above indications, but certainly not all of them. As is well known, Belladonna is the preservative means suggested by Hahnemann, and there is abundant but conflicting proof, for and against its use, both from allopathic and homœopathic physicians. We propose here to give the homœopathic experience against it, and the allopathic in favor of it; as these facts are less known than the contrary opinions, and have, doubtless, been less influenced by prejudice. Kreussler, a homœopathic author, says that he no longer readily advises the use of Belladonna as a preservative against scarlet fever, as he is convinced that it is not suitable in all cases. Kopp says abundant experience has convinced him that it is an uncertain prophylactic. Schroen, a most deservedly distinguished homœopathic author and practitioner, says that, in his experience, it could not be relied upon, as almost as many children who did not take it were not attacked by the disease, while others who did use it were not prevented from taking it. Lorbach had the same experience. Elb speaks still more decidedly, and says that many of his little patients who had taken it for several weeks were not only not preserved from the disease, but the severity of it, where it did occur, was not even mitigated. I have met with one case in which a little boy had taken it for three weeks; he was separated, although in the same house, from his two brothers and one sister, who were successively attacked with scarlet fever; his was the most severe case, and the only fatal one of the four. I have, however, met with numerous instances in which the attacks after taking Belladonna were decidedly milder than the preceding ones in the same house and family.

Aconite has been decreed to be as preservative against the scarlet rash as Belladonna is against the true smooth scarlatina. A number of other suggestions have been made for the same purpose. Dr. Sims reports that spiced syrup of Rhubarb, taken in such doses as will produce one loose stool per diem, was found by him to be the best preventive; he did not see one case, in which this was used, confined to bed, although several commenced the practice after they had been infected. Dr. Lee supposes that the liberal use of *Spirits of Nitre* will prove successful in anticipating a severe attack, and, in some instances, in arresting it altogether. It is useful by keeping the kidneys active.

Many physicians object to the use of *Belladonna* because they think it useless in very small doses, while larger ones produce symptoms, especially in the throat and brain, which are so similar to those caused by the disease that they are plunged into doubts as to which are effects of scarlet fever, and which of the remedy. Some practitioners use a combination of Aconite and Digitalis, to act both on the skin and kidneys. Others prefer a cold infusion of *Wild Cherry bark*, which, they think, possesses exactly the properties which are required —viz., tonic with directly sedative properties. It quiets excessive action of the heart, allays irritability of the nervous system, yet improves the appetite and digestion. Others use it when the first force of the disease has been broken, in the commencement of convalescence, when exhausting discharges still remain, and nervous irritability is yet manifested by lingering daily exacerbations of fever. It has the advantage of being a pleasant and harmless remedy, and often enables the system to pass with ease and speed through the milder forms of the attack. *Dulcamara* has been suggested, from its efficacy in skin diseases, and its tendency to promote the secretions from the skin, kidneys, and mucous membranes; *Sambucus* from its efficacy in burns, scalds, and excoriated surfaces, from its marked diuretic action and unquestioned powers in dropsy. Finally, *Angelica-archangelica* has been suggested as an agreeable and slightly stimulant tonic, from its efficacy in typhoid affections. Most of these remedies have the advantage of being pleasant to take, and harmless in ordinary doses, while their powers against disease are greater than is usually supposed.

In accordance with a previous promise we proceed to give some new allopathic authority in favor of Belladonna as a preventive of scarlet fever. Stille (see "Therapeutics and Materia Medica," vol. ii., p. 48) says: "This alleged power of Belladonna has done more, perhaps, than anything else to sustain homœopathy; and for that reason many regular practitioners have refrained from testing its truth. To do so however, is both impolitic and unjust; for the allegation is not in itself repugnant to belief, and, if really true, is too important to be slighted." And, on page 17, he adds: "On reviewing the whole subject, we [Stille] feel bound to express the conviction that the virtues of Belladonna as a protective against scarlet fever are so far proven that it becomes the duty of practitioners to invoke its aid whenever the disease breaks out in a locality where there are many persons liable to the contagion, particularly in boarding schools, orphan asylums, and similar institutions—whenever, in a word, it is difficult to place the healthy at a distance from the sick." Caspar Morris says that "It is quite possible that the influence of a slight narcotic on the nerves of organic life may so preoccupy them that they shall not yield to the impression of the epidemic or contagious principle." Wilson (see "Diseases of the Skin") gives no testimony adverse, while he volunteers much that is in favor of it; and also says it may be used with advantage after the attack and during the progress of the fever, and conjectures that Belladonna acts therapeutically, by virtue of its sedative effects on the nervous system; but assumes that any sedative means from which the stimulant property is as much as possible excluded would ensure the same desirable end. Meigs (see "Diseases of Children," third edition, p. 561) says he has used it a great deal during the last four years; and the impression he has received is decidedly favorable, so much so that he always makes use of it now when the cases are severe, and especially when the type of the epidemic is dangerous. In one family he gave it to nine children exposed directly to the disease, either from their being in the house in which it was prevailing or in the very room of the patient. Eight escaped the disease entirely, and the one who took it had it very mildly and safely. And, on the next page, he continues: "By far the most thorough and careful examination of this interesting and important matter that I am acquainted with has been made by Dr. Porcher, who states that his paper contains the results of an examination of about four hundred volumes, and gives his conclusions in the following words: 'In reviewing the testimony afforded by the preceding facts, our opinions are decidedly in favor of the prophylactic powers of Belladonna. However some may consider the evidence of a negative character, and therefore unworthy of confidence, yet, from its cumulation, from the careful way in which some observers conducted their inquiries, and from the possibility of some failures owing to the use of an inferior or badly prepared drug, I [Porcher] cannot but conceive that to discard it as utterly indecisive would be indulging a spirit of irrational incredulity leading to the rejection of any amount of merely presumptive proof. But, assuredly, under circumstances like these, granting that the efficacy of the means is only problematical, none should hesitate to employ measures so simple in their application and so safe in their consequences. The failure to avail ourselves of the prophylactic influence of Belladonna we cannot now but regard as a violation of those sacred obligations which force us to leave nothing untried which may contribute so largely to the mitigation or eradication of one of the severest inflictions of the hand of God!'"

Mild and regular cases rarely prove fatal. Of Meigs' two hundred and six mild cases, only three proved fatal.

Treatment.—In allopathic practice, Meigs says, the mild cases need but very simple treatment. Some mild laxative may be taken to commence with; then two to four drops of Antimonial wine, and eight to ten drops of Spirits Nit.-dulc. may be given every few hours, aided by inunction with—

℞.—Glycerine, ... ʒj.
Ung. Aq. Rosæ, . . . ℥j.—M.

Meigs adds that there can be no doubt that the employment of inunction in scarlet fever has proved a most useful addition to our former means of treatment. It has had the effect of allaying, in almost all cases, the violent irritation caused by the intense heat and inflammation of the skin; in nearly all cases it sensibly diminishes the frequency of the pulse, and in many this effect is very strongly marked; it removes, of course, the dryness and harshness of the skin, keeping it instead soft and moist; it lessens, or even removes the burning irritation and itching caused by the eruption. By these effects—to wit, lowering of the pulse and alleviation of the external heat, dryness, itching, and irritation—it cannot but, and evidently does, modify and diminish most happily the injurious effects of the disease upon the constitution at large. When the eruption is very intense, the skin very hot, and the febrile symptoms marked, the inunctions should be repeated every two or four hours, or oftener; in milder cases they need be used only three or four times in the twenty-four hours. I can corroborate this testimony from abundant experience; it interferes with no other more specific treatment, and, in fact, if I were obliged to rely upon any one mode of management, I should select that by inunction.

In many of the rather more severe cases dilute Phosphoric-acid may be relied upon; in still severer cases, Muriatic-acid. In many cases Aconite and Belladonna are useful, but in others Carbonate of Ammonia and Capsicum will come in play. But we propose here to treat of the remedies for scarlet fever somewhat in alphabetical order, but with due regard to the proper grouping of allied remedies.

Acetic-acid has been suggested in scarlet fever because it is regarded as a means of destroying contagion; because it has been regarded as antagonistic to almost every variety of narcotic poisoning—including Stramonium and Belladonna, which produce effects somewhat similar to those of scarlet fever—as an antidote to that alkaline state of the system which is present in typhus and scarlet fevers; while it has been used from time immemorial in fevers of a typhoid type, with languid capillary circulation, a doughy feel of the skin, and profuse sweats. Stille says, when much diluted, and applied to the hot, dry, and injected skin of patients laboring under typhus or scarlet fever, it appears to be more efficient than aqueous lotions in lowering the temperature of the body and quieting restlessness. Huss, of Stockholm, is the great advocate for the use of acids in typhus and scarlet fevers; he says the primitive change in these fevers, as far as is accessible to our understanding, seems to be a peculiar alteration in the blood; the chemical characters of this change are diminished proportion of fibrin and increased proportion of several inorganic salts, especially those of ammonia and carbonate of soda. This alteration in the blood is caused by the introduction into the system of some foreign matter or virus. Huss says numerous experiments have shown that, in animals which have for a long time been submitted to the use of alkalies, the blood has become destitute of fibrin and rich in carbonated alkalies. On the other hand, it has also been proven that the blood of animals to which acids have been given during a sufficient period has become rich in fibrin and almost destitute of carbonated alkalies. These two classes of remedies have, consequently, a contrary effect on the chemical composition of the blood, and acids must be considered as rationally indicated in typhus and scarlet fevers. But, even several centuries before these experiments were made, experience had confirmed the benefit from the use of acids in these fevers; therefore experience and theory agree perfectly on this point. Of late years, Dr. Isaac Brown has introduced the treatment with one-drachm doses of distilled Vinegar, as curative against scarlet fever and preventive against the subsequent dropsy; he says he has never seen a case of sequela where this treatment has been used, and similar testimony is afforded by Dr. Hunter, of Margate. I should prefer Phosphoric to Acetic-acid, but neither have as yet been much used in homœopathic practice, while the Muriatic and Nitric have.

Phosphoric-acid.—Huss says Phosphoric is not only the mildest of all the mineral acids, but is a natural constituent of the human body, and congenial to it. Its use may be continued longer than that of other acids without acting injuriously on the digestive organs; received into the blood it must, according to the laws of chemical affinity, form salts with ammonia, soda, and potash, and very extensive experience induces him to believe that the Phosphoric-acid, besides the ordinary effects of acids in general, possesses a more strengthening and regulating influence upon the central parts of the nervous system. This power it receives from its base, Phosphorus, in the same way that Muriatic retains the special power of Chlorine; hence, in these fevers it acts partly as an acid, and partly from its containing Phosphorus. However this may be, his experience places it in the first and most eminent rank of all the remedies he has tried in treating these fevers, especially from the safety and general benefit which follows its use. Huss generally gives from ten to fifteen drops of dilute Phosphoric-acid every other hour; but twenty, thirty, and more drops are safe—in fact, no quantity is dangerous.

Muriatic-acid.—The homœopathic experience with this remedy is as follows: Lorbach says it and Sulphuric-acid afforded him excellent results in malignant and sloughing anginas, and in bad cases of scarlet fever, when the internal parts were more affected than the external; when the bluish-red and blackish appearance of the same, the aphthous ulcers, the exfoliation of the surface of the tongue in large brown pieces, and the peculiar offensive smell from the mouth betrayed the septic and malignant character of the affection. Lobethal used it when the inflammation of the throat persisted longer and with greater intensity than usual, and when the patient was almost comatose from the commencement; when the eruption was profuse, rapid in its outbreak, and very red, the throat being very sore. He found it more useful than Bellad., though he sometimes gave them in alternation. Hartmann gave it under different circumstances—when the patient was so weak as to slide down to the foot of the bed, with burning heat of the whole body, excessive restlessness, feeble pulse, dark redness of the cheeks, red and dull eyes, bluish color of the skin, with irregular and scanty eruption, of scarlet color, but intermixed with many petechiæ, with oppressed breathing and offensive breath, acrid discharges from the nose, &c.

Aconite.—Before proceeding to the uses of Aconite in scarlet fever I propose to make a few remarks about the general action of this remedy. As early as 1843,* from a collection of over twenty cases of poisoning with this remedy, from the appearances in four post-mortem examinations, and from experiments upon myself, I arrived at the same conclusions which Fleming subsequently promulgated in 1844—viz., that, in its action upon the vascular system, it is similar to Digitalis. Veratrum-viride and Gelseminum have lately been found to be allied remedies. Thus, in half an hour after taking five drops of tincture of the root of Aconite, the pulse is found to be diminished in strength; in another hour both the pulse and respiration will be found less frequent. Thus a pulse which, in a normal state, beats 72 in a minute, will by that

* See *Homœopathic Examiner*, first series, vol. iii., p. 265.

time have fallen to 64, and the respirations from 18 to 15 or 60 per minute. Ten-drop doses will reduce the pulse to 56, and it will become smaller and weaker, although still regular, while the respirations will have diminished to about 13, presenting, at the same time, a slow, laboring character; great muscular debility will be experienced, and much chilliness felt, especially about the extremities, which are cold to the touch. The pulse has been reduced by Aconite to 40 and even 36. Next to depression of the vascular system it exerts a benumbing effect upon the *nerves of sensation*, causing numbness and tingling even of the tips of the fingers and toes and roots of the teeth, while the sensibility of the surface is much impaired. It also acts powerfully upon the skin, causing profuse perspiration. Hence Aconite is antipathic and antagonistic to many feverish, inflammatory, and excessively painful affections, and to some which may be relieved by free sweating. Digitalis acts as powerfully upon the vascular system, but not upon the nerves of sensation; still it exerts as peculiar and powerful an action upon the kidneys as Aconite does upon the skin. Hence, in feverish and inflammatory affections, if it be requisite to act both upon the skin and kidneys, these two remedies may be given in combination or alternation. They may be made very useful in scarlet fever; for, as Wilson says, the principle of treatment in this disease is to endeavor to purify the blood of the morbid poison it contains, and which is the cause of the disease, by calling into action the various emunctories of the system—viz., the skin, kidneys, and, in a lesser degree, the bowels; the former are more decided depuratives of the vascular system than the bowels. Veratrum-viride is also allied in its action to Aconite and Digitalis; its most remarkable quality is its sedative action on the pulse. Osgood was the first to state that, by the exhibition of full doses, the pulse, when ranging from 75 to 80 in a minute, may be reduced to 35 or 40 in the course of a few hours, and become small and creeping, with great coolness of the surface and often icy coldness; although it is apt to cause vomiting, yet the above effects upon the pulse and skin may be induced without either nausea or vomiting. Dr. Norwood and many others declare that, by its careful administration, nausea and vomiting may be avoided altogether, and the pulse reduced as low as 35 beats in a minute without the occurrence of either of these symptoms. But it is a dangerous remedy in unskilful hands; for the nausea and vomiting may become persistent and violent, in fact almost continuous, with great prostration. Yet, Stille says, alarming and apparently dangerous as these symptoms are, it does not appear that they have ever terminated in death; on the contrary, they have generally been dispelled with facility by suspending the use of the medicine and administering diffusible stimulants; still, in feeble subjects, a fatal result may occasionally ensue. Gelseminum is another very powerful and, it is said, unrivalled febrifuge, which has lately been introduced into practice. By enthusiastic partizans it is claimed to be the only remedy ever yet discovered capable of subduing, in from two to twenty hours, the most formidable and the most complicated as well as the most simple fevers incident to our country and climate—quieting all nervous irritability and excitement, equalizing the circulation, promoting perspiration, and rectifying the various secretions, without causing nausea, vomiting, or purging. If given in excessive doses it may cause a transient loss of muscular power, so that the patient is unable to move a limb or even raise his eye-lids; yet he can hear, and is conscious of all that is going on around him. In full, but not excessive doses, it causes double and clouded vision, and it is thought that, as soon as the heaviness or partial paralysis of the lids is induced, no more of the remedy should be given, even if these effects follow the first small dose; if carried to such an extent that the patient cannot open his eyes the relaxation produced by the drug may be too great for the system to recover from. It is also said to exert a powerful control over the nervous system, removing nervous irritability as well or more completely than any other known agent. Dr. Holcombe regards Gelseminum as holding an intermediate place between Aconite and Belladonna, and oftentimes promptly antiphlogistic when both of these invaluable remedies have seemed inefficient; he regards it as indicated when there are violent pains, referable to the cerebro-spinal rather than to the ganglionic system, and corresponding amount of intense burning fever, great nervous restlessness, sensitiveness to light and sound, mental agitation or anxiety, delirium, sleeplessness, curious sensation of falling, swimming, from giddiness, partial blindness or deafness. He regards it as especially applicable to nervous excitable subjects.

Homœopathic Experience with Aconite.—Knorre treated two epidemics of the milder form of scarlet fever with Aconite, thirtieth dilution, one or two doses daily; of one hundred and fifty-three cases he lost only six cases in all, or about one in twenty-five and a half. In some epidemics, under allopathic treatment, the loss has only been one in forty. Widemann used from the fifteenth to the twenty-fourth dilution of Aconite as long as the febrile condition lasted, and says he was generally successful. He only used Bellad., 30, when there was congestion to the head and sore throat; hence these must have been mild regular cases. Teller says when, in not absolutely malignant cases, there was an indescribable restlessness, constant tossing about in bed, sleeplessness, with alternating violent delirium, however much Belladonna might seem indicated, it would *not* afford relief, but Aconite was very useful, especially if aided by an occasional dose of Opium; he does not mention the size of the doses either of Aconite or Opium.

Trinks found Aconite very useful in several epidemics, in which he depended upon it almost exclusively; the size of the dose is not given. Hartmann and Gross also found it useful; while Kreussler, who seems as much opposed to Aconite as Dr. Hempel is in favor of it—says it is often given without any effect in scarlatina, even when violent pain is present, and sometimes seems to produce the most violent aggravations; but, as Kreussler advises us never to go below the twelfth dilution, and that an interval of six hours should always elapse before a second dose is given, it is easy to understand why he does not have faith in Aconite, and why the natural turbulent course of the disease should be mistaken by him for a succession of severe aggravations. Hahnemann, it is well known, had so much confidence in Aconite that he pronounced it a specific against scarlatina-miliaris, as distinguished from scarlatina-lævigata.

Dose of Aconite.—For young children I would unhesitatingly use from one to three drops of the tincture of the root, in a tumbler half full of water, giving from one to two teaspoonfuls per dose, every half, one, or two hours, in very severe cases; every two, three, or four hours in less urgent attacks. For older children from three to five drops are put in a tumbler half full of water, and given as above; while for adults, from five to ten or fifteen drops are put in a tumbler quite full of water, and one, or sometimes two tablepoonfuls given per dose. In allopathic practice, Dr. Wood, of Philadelphia, recommends *five drops* of the tincture of the root for adults, three times a day, and says it may be increased gradually after the first dose, until some sign of its action is afforded, such as tingling or numbness in the fingers or lips, or diminished frequency of the pulse. Dr. Stille only recommended three-drop doses, three times a day, and this smaller quantity is undoubtedly the safest to begin with.

Antiphlogistic Treatment.—All the above remedies are regarded as sedatives to the vascular system, and as more or less adapted to depress the pulse and remove febrile and inflammatory irritations. But this class of medicines must be used with caution in some cases of scarlet fever, and avoided altogether in others. As regards *bleeding*, Dr. Caspar Morris says it is unnecessary in the milder cases, and in those which assume a greater degree of severity his personal experience is very decidedly unfavorable to its employment. Dr. Graves, of Dublin, expresses himself strongly to the same effect; he describes the cases in which depletion was resorted to, and records the fatal results. Singularly enough, the cases which are attended by convulsions and high cerebral excitement, with a very rapid pulse, do not bear depletion; for the nervous system only appeared to be aggravated, although the heat of the skin suggested its employment. The derangement of the brain and nerves in this form depends on something more than the violence of the circulation, and originates in something altogether different from mere cerebral inflammation or congestion—that something is the result of an intense poisoning of the blood and system generally by the animal poisoning of the scarlet-fever miasm. Graves says he has never seen any good effects from blood-letting, even in those cases in which the nervous symptoms were most severe and the vascular excitement the most intense; and he has, alas, too frequently had occasion to mourn over its fatal influence! It is needless to multiply testimony to this effect. It is rendered evident that, to treat scarlet fever correctly, either some direct antidote must be found—like Mercury for syphilis, Quinine for fever and ague, Sulphur for itch, or Belladonna for scarlet fever, as is claimed by the homœopathists—or, if the virus cannot be neutralized, it must be eliminated from the system; and, with this view, *Aconite* often comes into play, as somewhat antidotal to the poison of scarlet fever, as antagonistic to some forms of fever and inflammation, and powerfully promoting the action of the skin. Digitalis will aid the sedative action of Aconite and act specifically upon the kidneys, while Veratrum-viride will sustain the action of both these remedies, and Gelseminum, with similar powers, will allay the threatening nervous symptoms. Infinitesimal doses will exhibit a false appearance of usefulness in the milder cases, of which Meigs only lost three cases out of two-hundred and six, under allopathic treatment; moderate doses—viz.: from one-eighth to one-fourth, or rarely one-half the quantities ordinarily used in allopathic practice of Aconite, Digitalis, Veratrum-viride, or Gelseminum, will suffice to place many of the severer cases in a comparatively safe condition; while, in the malignant and septic cases, probably all these remedies must be avoided.

Ammonium-carbonicum.—In 1800 an allopathic physician, Dr. Peart, of London, described his use of this remedy in a *very malignant* form of scarlet fever, as being singularly successful. He directed two drachms of the salt to be dissolved in five ounces or forty drachms of water, and two teaspoonfuls or two drachms of the solution to be given every two, three, or four hours—equivalent to from three to six grains per dose. Mr. Wilkinson, in 1822, extolled it extravagantly, declaring that he not only never lost a patient in this disease, but never had a case of the malignant kind that even appeared dangerous or gave him a moment's anxiety. Much more recently—viz., in 1851—he confirmed his original statement, and extended its applications to measles and other exanthemata. In 1833 it was proposed as a specific in every form and stage of the disease by Stille, and subsequently Bourdelocque and Bohel found it singularly efficacious when the disease was marked by ataxic symptoms, delirium, subsultus-tendinum, encrusted teeth, vomiting, a small irregular pulse, and involuntary discharge of fæces and urine, with a scanty or irregular eruption. Even in malignant cases, with production of *false* membranes on the buccal mucous membrane and its continuations, with *hæmorrhage* from the same parts, ecchymoses, delirium, adynamia, a small and frequent pulse, and anxious respiration, it *sometimes* availed to save life. In these accounts, Stille adds, some exaggeration must be suspected, were it only because the disease continues to be, in its severer forms, one of the most fatal of its class; besides, some cautious and experienced observers make a different report. Nevertheless, Stille adds, the value of the remedy is great, particularly when scarlet fever assumes the low type which it is apt to wear in the crowded families of the poor. Under these circumstances the celebrated Dr. Charles West has found it desirable to give Ammonia almost from the onset of the disease, and whenever the pulse presents the character of frequency and softness combined. Dr. Caspar Morris says that, in the severer malignant form, Carbonate of Ammonia has been highly recommended by some physicians; but one almost insuperable obstacle to its use is found in the difficulty of deglutition; for, even in those low forms of fever which are free from angina, the pungent character of the remedy makes it difficult of administration, and where there is much swelling or ulceration, it would be impossible that it could be swallowed, especially by a child. But he recommends, apparently, quite as objectionable a remedy; for he says *Capsicum* produces all the benefit which could be hoped from the Ammonia, and with less effort in swallowing. He says the treatment of those cases in which the eruption appears imperfectly developed from the first, or in which, after having been well marked, it recedes, or where the force of the attack falls upon the throat from the beginning, causing great tumefaction and difficulty of deglutition, must be very energetic. In all these cases this condition evidently results from the overwhelming influence of the poison on the blood and nervous system. Whether convulsions, or restlessness, or stupor complicate the case, or mere languor and exhaustion, all are but varying phases of one condition, and that a condition which is to be removed by appropriate stimulation; and it is in these cases that the *Capsicum* is productive of the happiest results. He confesses that it was with great reluctance that he was first prevailed upon to resort to a remedy apparently so little appropriate, and, he might have added, homœopathic, to the treatment of a disease in which the rapid circulation and heated surface seemed rather to call for remedies which should produce a refrigerant impression; and, to force a harsh irritating liquid into a throat already inflamed, was, he thought, little short of a refinement of cruelty. But the entire failure of the cooling treatment in such cases led him to test the opposite and more homœopathic course, and he can recommend it with entire confidence. Weak animal broths freely charged with Capsicum, he says, may be given with great safety, even to the youngest infant in this condition, and although it may not, and indeed rarely does so rouse the energies of the system as to cause the full development of the eruption, it will so excite the vital forces as to carry the patient safely through the regular period. Should there be much local disease of the throat it will receive great benefit from the passage of the *Capsicum* over it. Dr. Caspar Morris has often administered the simple infusion when the stomach rejected the broths, or when he desired to maintain a more constant local impression; a teaspoonful of Cayenne pepper in half a pint of boiling water, and of this a teaspoonful given every one or two hours to a child five years old and upwards, followed by a small portion of broth or wine whey, forms the ordinary dose. But, to return to the *Carbonate of Ammonia*, Dr. Schroen, one of the most distinguished, honest, and liberal of the homœopathists, adopted the Ammonia-treatment in 1842, after he had often been disappointed with Belladonna, Aconite, Bryonia, Mercurius, Rhus, Sulphur, &c. He claims that it is a homœopathic remedy, causing a red eruption on the chest, and redness of the whole upper part of the body, as if covered with scarlet rash. Schroen says, as soon as he commenced to use moderately strong doses, the results were gratifying and surprising: all the symptoms were moderated, the eruption did not develop itself so extensively and intensely, the redness was not so dark and general, the fearful head-symptoms either did not occur at all, or were amenable to Merc., Aconite, Belladonna, or Hellebore, which previously had been useless; he put from ten to twenty grains in two ounces of strongly sweetened water, and gave one-half or a whole tablespoonful every two hours; as a large quantity of sugar or syrup is necessary to render it tolerable to young children. Trinks denies its homœopathicity and specificity to scarlet fever, but admits that it is a valuable remedy when the eruption does not appear freely on account of the debility of the patient, and when great anxiety, oppressed, short, and very contracted breathing are present, with very quick pulse and threatening of paralysis of the heart or lungs, or when the skin has a livid appearance, and other signs of putrescency are present. The good effects of this medicine in the above state are supposed to be explained by the experiments of Wibmer on himself, in which from ten to twenty-five drops of liquor Ammonia caused a feeling of extreme tension in the temples, which, however, only lasted several minutes; the pulse was somewhat more frequent and harder in some experiments, while in others it remained unchanged, but in none was the circulation quickened beyond a few pulsations: to these phenomena were added a general enlivening of the feelings, a sense of increased strength, augmented warmth of the skin, a more abundant and easy flow of perspiration and urine, and, in bronchial affections, a greater quantity of sputa and ease of expectoration. The tendency to diaphoresis was greatly increased by warm drinks and external warmth.

As a matter of course, some other homœopathic physicians have not found Ammonia particularly useful in scarlet fever, and, among others, Dr. Elb, of Dresden. When experience at the bed-side is so conflicting we must endeavor to decide the question by a comparison between the known effects of the drug and those of the disease in question.

1. In the first place, Carbonate of Ammonia is an alkali, or antacid, and must partake in some measure of the properties of these remedies; now the blood is always alkaline, and a certain excess of alkali in this fluid is essential to the continued solubility of the albumen and fibrin, and possibly for other purposes. But, beyond the normal amount, it produces depressing effects, for the coagulability of the fibrin is probably impaired; and when in great excess the blood corpuscules are to a certain extent broken up and dissolved. In short, the alkalies, when given continuously and copiously, cause a scorbutic and dissolved state of the blood and all their consequences.

2. Although ammonia is a normal constituent of some of the excretions of the body, yet the blood naturally contains exceedingly small quantities of it; but in the sweat, especially that of the axillæ, the occurrence of ammonia is incontestible; in the pulmonary exhalation small quantities of this salt may always be recognized with great certainty; in the urine the normal quantity of it is exceedingly small. But, according to Lehman, in certain diseased conditions of the system very considerable quantities of ammonia are often found in the blood, as well as in the urine: thus Winter thought that the presence of an excess of ammonia and other alkaline salts in the blood—especially of carbonate of soda—explained some of the phenomena of typhus and other allied diseases, such as variola and scarlatina. It is by no means strange that, in the state of the system which prevails in many blood poisonings and in typhoid and septic fevers, the blood and urine should contain ammonia; for carbonate of ammonia is easily formed during the decomposition, putrefaction, or destructive metamorphoses of those organic substances which contain nitrogen. Hence Ammonia would seem to be more or less homœopathic to many typhoid and septic affections, malignant scarlet fever among the rest; but, although the result of decomposition and putrefaction, it may prevent these, just as alcohol, which is the result of fermentation and distillation, may prevent fermentation in other substances. Some form of acid, probably the Phosphoric, may prove the natural antipathic or antagonistic remedy for some of these affections.

3. Ammonia is also an irritant or general stimulant remedy. According to Billing, it is merely a local stimulant, exerting a temporary exciting action on the stomach, and from thence through the solar-

plexus on the heart and arteries; but in the stomach it quickly unites with the digestive acids, and then circulates through the system and blood, not as a diffusible stimulant, but as a *saline sedative;* for it is converted into muriate and lactate of ammonia by the muriatic and lactic acids which normally exist in the gastric fluids and juices. Hence its further action is somewhat like that of the Acetate of Ammonia, or Spiritus-mindereri; and Billing concludes that it may act as a sedative to inflamed capillaries, while its remote action may be somewhat similar to that of Aconite, Digitalis, Veratrum-viride, &c.

4. It may prove useful in some of the brain affections which attend the blood-poisoning with the miasm of scarlet fever, as it is a prompt and effectual antidote to *alcoholic* intoxication. Stille has seen a man who was taken up in a state of complete and helpless drunkenness speedily restored to his senses and the use of his limbs by a few drops of Ammonia in water, poured down his throat; and a very similar instance occurred in the wards of Dupuytren, while others are related by Prazza. If Ammonia will remove the coma of drunkenness, it has been conjectured that it may remove that of scarlet fever.

5. Poisoning by Prussic-acid and the virus of venomous reptiles and insects somewhat resembles the severe blood-poisoning of scarlet, typhoid, and other malignant fevers, while the efficacy of Ammonia in these seems to be well established; for Christison and Pereira regard Ammonia as the best antidote for poisoning with Prussic-acid; and Murray, of Edinburgh, was so convinced of its efficacy, by experiments which he made on animals and himself, that he did not hesitate to declare his willingness to take a poisonous dose of Prussic-acid, provided he could be certain that what he regarded as a sufficient amount of Ammonia would be at once administered to him. Its efficacy in the bites of the rattle and moccasin snakes seems to be well established; for Dr. Moore, of Mississippi, has published valuable testimony on this point; in some of his cases the symptoms were alarming, but were mitigated directly the Ammonia was made use of.

6. According to Wood, Carbonate of Ammonia is primarily irritant in its local action, and an energetic stimulant to the system. Taken internally it causes heat in the stomach, increases the frequency and force of the pulse, and produces a general glow through the system; but as a diffusible stimulant it is remarkably characterized by the brevity of its action, owing to its being rapidly converted into the muriate, lactate, or acetate of ammonia in the system. With its decided stimulant influence on the circulation and general organic nervous system it has a tendency to increase the secretions; for it often produces more or less diaphoresis, and sometimes operates as a diuretic; it also appears to act on the pulmonary organs, if not as a specific expectorant, certainly as a special stimulant of the respiratory

function; for we have seen that, even in the normal state, a small quantity of ammonia is exhaled from the lungs. Hence it may favor the depurating powers of the system in getting rid of the scarlet-fever miasm, by exciting the actions of the skin, kidneys, and pulmonary mucous membrane.

7. Huxham relates a case in which its long continued use was followed by a cachectic state of the system and depraved state of the blood, as indicated by hæmorrhage from the nose, gums, and intestines, pustular eruptions on the surface, dropping out of the teeth, and a general wasting of the body, with hectic symptoms. These effects depended mainly upon a constantly sustained excess of alkalinity of the blood, similar to that which occurs in erysipelas, small-pox, typhus, and malignant scarlet fever, to which diseases it must be more or less homœopathic in large and frequently repeated doses. Acute rheumatism is attended with an excessively acid state of many of the secretions and excretions, and probably of the blood; hence an opposite condition of the fluids of the body obtains in rheumatism to what is present in erysipelas, typhus, and scarlet fevers, and an opposite mode of treatment may be required in these diseases. Hence, if alkalies are exceedingly serviceable in rheumatism, it is probable that acids will prove the natural antagonists of typhus and scarlet fevers. This has been partially proven to be true.

In the milder forms of scarlet fever large and strong doses of Ammonia are unnecessary; if any are used they should consist of small quantities of the Carbonate, or somewhat larger of the Acetate. It is probable that the enthusiastic advocates of the ammoniacal treatment of scarlet fever use large doses in all the forms of the disease. Morris truly says that no habit can be more pernicious to the physician and less beneficial to the patient than that so often adopted by enthusiastic and superficial thinkers and practitioners, of omitting the consideration of the causes which modify and influence the progress of any form of disease, and merely filling the memory with modes of treatment and specific remedies, which may be employed empirically, without endeavoring to understand the principles which should determine their adoption, and regulate their application. There is no disease which more fully illustrates this common truth than that now under consideration. It is only from a careful study of its general history, as well as minute observation of the course of its symptoms in individual cases, that any suitable idea of treatment can be deduced. While the liability which the history of the disease has exhibited to frequent change in type, from simple and sthenic to irregular and malignant, demands a corresponding change in remedies and in the mode of treatment, renders the success of the practitioner equally dependent upon his freedom from routine treatment with any one remedy, be it Belladonna, Ammonia, &c., &c., and upon the soundness of his general principles, and the accuracy of his particular observation. Large doses of Ammonia are thought by some to be too homœopathic to the malignant and septic varieties of scarlet fever to be used thoughtlessly; but excessive anxiety on this point is not necessary, for Periera has given from fifteen to twenty grains three times a day for two or three weeks, without producing the scorbutic effects noticed by Huxham; and Pringle somewhat justly affirmed that we should no more refrain from giving Ammonia in low fevers because it induces dissolution of the blood when used long and immoderately, than we should reject table-salt as a condiment because an exclusive use of salted meat causes scurvy.

It is a question whether Ammonia can be used against the convulsions which sometimes precede and follow scarlet fever. Siebold has highly recommended it in cases of *puerperal convulsions* independent of an organic cause, but arising from irritability of the nervous system, and excited by debilitating influences. It is also one of the numerous remedies proposed for epilepsy, and the celebrated Pereira employed it extensively, and, in many cases, with obvious benefit; yet all the ammoniacal remedies cause convulsions.

It may prove homœopathic to the membranous croup and membranous pharyngitis which sometimes attend scarlet fever; for, Stille says, from excessive quantities of Ammonia, violent inflammation, (sometimes of the *pseudo*-membranous form) in the fauces and œsophagus has been observed.

Capsicum.—This remedy is used largely in the Thompsonian and in the Philadelphia allopathic schools of medicine; less so in the homœopathic. We have already quoted the experience of Dr. Caspar Morris, of Philadelphia; Dr. George B. Wood, also of Philadelphia, says it has been employed as a safe stimulant in the cold stage of pernicious fevers, and occasionally in low typhoid fevers; while in the low and malignant forms of scarlet fever it has been much and advantageously employed, and may be considered as among the best stimulants in this affection. He has himself given it frequently, and been satisfied of its beneficial effects. It is used both internally and as a gargle; in the latter mode of application Wood knows of nothing better adapted to that condition of the fauces in which the mucous membrane has assumed a dark red color, and has begun to slough, or appears to be on the point of doing so. But it has also seemed useful to him in almost all varieties of the sore throat of scarlatina, in which, *so far from irritating, it often soothes;* at least patients have frequently assured him that, though it burned their healthy mouth in its passage, it *had quite a contrary* effect on the sore and inflamed fauces, which it greatly relieved. Wood also says that, in the early stage of scarlet fever, there is sometimes great backwardness in the appearance of the eruption—a few purplish points only serving to indicate the nature of the case, and the vain struggle of the system to throw out the virus upon the surface; along with this condition there may be coma, or a disposition to it, with an appearance of general prostration. In such cases Capsicum may be freely used, both internally, in connection with other stimulants, and outwardly as a rubefacient. Dr. Stille, also of Philadelphia, says the most useful application of Capsicum is in the treatment of *tonsillitis*, and particularly of that form which arises in some cases of scarlet fever, and known as cynanche-maligna. The practice of employing it in the ulcerated sore throat of scarlet fever originated with the West Indian physicians, who used it very successfully for a kind of angina-maligna prevailing among the children of St. Vincent, which began with blackness, sloughiness, and ulceration of the fauces and tonsils: Dr. Stephens gave it to four hundred patients laboring under this disease, and it seemed to save some whose state had been thought desperate. Kreysig, Headley, Currie, Collins, and others, employed it in the malignant sore throat of scarlet fever.

Capsicum has at least a superficial homœopathicity to scarlet fever: it is a rubefacient, and the eruption of scarlet fever resembles the effect of a rubefacient applied all over the surface. All rubefacients cause fever and inflammation, and scarlet fever is often a decidedly inflammatory affection. Still Capsicum produces a true, frank, and open inflammation, while that of scarlet fever is perhaps never so; but generally assumes a peculiar, specific, so-called neuro-phlogistic, or dyscratic, and even septic, putrid, typhoid, or malignant form of phlogosis, attended with and arising from a profound poisoning of the blood.

Apis-mellifica.—This remedy is allied in its action to Cantharides, Arsenicum, Capsicum, Rhus, and other acrid agents. The virus of the honey-bee is secreted by a poison apparatus, which is found in female and neuter bees only; it is a transparent fluid, with a sweetish and afterwards acrid taste, and strongly *acid* reaction; it is so active that a single sting instantly kills another bee. The ordinary consequences in man produced by the sting of a bee are *pain*, *redness*, *swelling*, *and hardness of the part;* Pereira assumes that fatal effects might be produced if a swarm were to attack an individual. Alkalies and especially Ammonia are supposed to be antidotes. The poison apparatus of bees consists of two thin convoluted secreting organs, opening into a pyriform receptacle, from which a small duct passes to the sting. The sting is in itself a very irritating organ, apart from any poison which accompanies its use, for it consists of two separable portions placed side by side, the surfaces of which are barbed to the point; when forced into the flesh the two blades of the sting separate like the opened blades of a scissors, and the barbed sides act like small saws on the withdrawal of the instrument. No experiments on the healthy have been made with the pure virus, but it is probable that its action will prove very similar to that of Cantharides. The first uses of the Honey-bee as a medicine took place among the aborigines of this country; for the Indians were in the habit of making an infusion of this insect, and of giving a gill of it every half-hour in strangury, suppression of urine, &c.; they also supposed that this decoction possessed the power of destroying the sexual inclinations. A tincture of Honey-bees has also long been in use among the botanic physicians of this country, and, when given in doses of five, ten, or fifteen drops, three or four times a day, they recommend it highly in many diseases of the bladder and kidneys, as well as some uterine affections. Some Thompsonian practitioners assert that it will produce abortion in the pregnant female if its use be too long continued, or the doses be too strong.

It has been used by homœopathists in all the stages of scarlet fever, but more particularly against the dropsy which often follows it. Dr. Munger, of Waterville, New-York, was the first to report a well-attested case of scarlatinal dropsy cured by it; twenty-four days after a mild attack of scarlet fever the patient's face began to bloat, and the bowels to be unusually full and hard; two or three days subsequently her face was still more bloated, especially about the eyes; there was an anxious expression of countenance, the abdomen was very much distended, with a general anasarcous condition of the body; violent beating of the heart, pulse 160; respiration excessively labored, panting, and hurried, with inability to lie down; urine very scanty and high colored; skin hot and dry, with thirst, but no pain. Acon. and Ars., and Bellad. and Ars. were given without benefit; on the contrary the breathing became more labored, the pulse feeble, rapid, and intermittent, the extremities cool, and urine not increased. Acon., Helleb., and Digit. were given without effect, probably because the doses were too small. On the next day the symptoms were still more alarming: the face and lips livid, the respiration gasping and excessively rapid, pulse almost indistinct, with cold perspiration and coldness of the face and extremities. With little hope of benefit Apis, 3, was given every two hours; but, in the course of the same day, the lividity passed away, the perspiration became warm, the extremities ceased to be cold, the breathing easier than at any time, though still very laborious and hurried; the pulse more full and regular, and the urine began to be passed in considerable quantities. The Apis was now repeated only every four hours, and the next day the patient was better in every respect: was able to lie down for the first time, had passed three pints of dark urine; and from thence she continued rapidly to recover, passing large quantities of urine, with corresponding decrease of the dropsy, and was regarded as well on the eighth day of the treatment with Apis. Dr. Munger treated several other cases successfully with Apis, using the third dilution only—being perfectly satisfied with its operation. Lately, Dr. Joslin, Jr., has had considerable experience with it in the Protestant Half-Orphan Asylum, of New-York. He says a large proportion of the dropsical patients had the first stage of the disease in an exceedingly mild form, so much so that, in one or two of the fatal cases, they had scarcely been supposed to have had scarlet fever at all. One case had sore throat only, without scarlet eruption; another had merely a slight eruption, and neither had been obliged to go to bed. From the absence of more minute data we are obliged to separate Dr. Joslin's cases into two classes: *first*, the sub-acute; and *second*, the acute, or the moderately slow and rapid cases. Before going further we must express our gratitude to Dr. Joslin, Jr., for the manliness and honesty with which he has published his experience.

CASE 1—Had scarlatina slightly, and, forty-four days subsequently, was found with slight œdema of eye-lids, swelling of abdomen, frequent pulse, and swelling of glands of neck; gave Apis, 1. Next day was better, and improvement continued, interrupted but little by cough, diarrhœa, and frequent pulse, until convalescence ensued seven or eight days afterwards. This may be regarded as sub-acute.

CASE 2.—Twenty-four days after a slight attack of scarlet fever, treated with Acon., Bell., and Puls., 30, which did not prevent the occurrence of dropsy, the face, eyes, and feet were found swollen. Arsen., 30, was continued for four days without good effect; for very great dyspnœa occurred, so that the patient could not lie down, and passed only one gill of very dark urine in twenty-four hours; pulse frequent and feeble. Apis, 30 and 0, were given; but it was too late, as the patient died the same night. This case proves that Acon. and Bell., 30, did not eradicate the scarlet-fever miasm, and that Arsen., 30, will not always arrest the dropsy when it sets in rapidly.

CASE 3.—Sixteen days after a mild attack of scarlet fever, treated with Acon. and Puls., 30, inflammation and abscess of the glands of the neck occurred, followed by dropsy in ten days more, which was not prevented by Bellad., Merc., and Sulph., 30. The face became swollen, pulse 100 and intermittent. Apis, 1, was given, and a steady and gradual improvement followed for twenty days, when the patient was well. This may be regarded as sub-acute.

CASE 4.—Nineteen days after a very slight attack of scarlet fever, treated with Verat. and Puls., 30, dropsy of the face, eyes, and feet occurred, and proceeded unchecked by Sulph. and Ars., 30, until oppressed breathing, sleeplessness, obstinate vomiting, and suppression of urine occurred, which increased under Merc.-corr., Arsen., and Carb.-veg., 30, until death ensued on the fourth day after the dropsy sat in. This case proves that the high dilutions of well-selected remedies will not always prevent or cure the secondary effects of scarlet fever.

CASE 5.—Twenty-five days after such a slight attack of scarlet fever that the patient was never confined to bed, and treated with Bellad., 30, dropsy occurred, which increased rapidly, and ended in death on the third day, in spite of the use of Apis., 1, and Helleb. tincture. This case proves that Bellad., 30, will not prevent, and Apis and Hellebore, in moderately strong doses, will not always cure rapid and dangerous sequelæ of scarlet fever.

CASE 6.—About one month after a very slight attack of scarlet fever, treated with Acon., Bell., and Puls., 30, dropsy occurred, which was not checked by Apis, 30; but, after Apis, 1, was given, improvement went on steadily for fifteen days, when the patient was comparatively convalescent.

CASE 7.—Twenty-two days after a not very severe attack of scarlet fever, treated with Puls. and Bellad., 30, dropsy sat in, which was quickly relieved by Apis, 1.

CASE 8.—Twenty-five days after a moderate attack of scarlet fever, treated with Bell., Puls., and Bryon., 30, dropsy occurred, which was quickly relieved by Apis, 1.

CASE 9.—Similar to the above, was quickly cured by Apis, 1. Cases 10 and 11 were also cured by Apis, 1. Case 12 was treated with Bellad., Apis, Acon., and Lach., 30, and proved fatal in eight days. This case proves that high dilutions of well-selected remedies—Apis among the rest—will not always prevent or cure the secondary effects of scarlet fever. Case 13 was apparently saved by Apis, 1, although Bell., Acon., Op., and Hepar., 30, were given subsequently. In case 14 dropsy was not prevented by Bellad., 30, but was cured by Apis, 1. In case 15, dropsy was not prevented by Verat., Bellad., Hepar, Merc., and Carb.-veg., 30, but was rapidly relieved by Apis, 1. Case 16, was somewhat relieved by Apis, 1; but relapsed under Helleb., 3, and Apis, 30; was not benefitted by Bellad., 30, Lach., 30, and Camph., 200; then again improved under Apis, 1; then relapsed under Lach., 700, and Apis, 1; but improved a third time under a persistent use of the remedy, and recovered on the nineteenth day of the sickness.

Dr. Joslin adds that Apis was the only remedy he found to reduce the dropsy. The general action of Apis makes it evident that it is antipathic to dropsy from debility, and more or less homœopathic to the same disease when arising from active congestion, acute irritation, or actual inflammation of the kidneys.

Cantharides is very similar in its action to Apis, Rhus, and Arsenicum, and is equally, if not more homœopathic to scarlet fever and some of its consequences than Capsicum or Apis. From over-doses of Cantharides there is apt to arise an incessant desire to urinate, but a small quantity only of high-colored and scalding urine is voided with extreme suffering; the water is sometimes bloody, and a burning pain is experienced in the region of the bladder and kidneys; the urine under these circumstances is highly albuminous. This is an almost exact counter-part of the action of the scarlet-fever-miasm on the kidneys, at times, and the remedy should be used more frequently by the homœopathists than it as yet has been. It has been given in dropsy in the dominant school; but Wood says that the only circumstances under which it would be appropriate are when there is *great torpor* of the kidneys, without the least evidence of excitement in these organs; but Ferriar refers to several cases of general dropsy, occurring for the most part after scarlet fever, in which it effected a cure. In *albuminuria* it has been successfully employed by Monneret, who commenced with small doses, gradually increased to sixty drops of the tincture. Rayer also speaks of it favorably in doses of from four to twelve drops, but considers it dangerous in inexperienced hands. Of five cases treated with it by Dr. Wells, there was marked improvement in three, but it failed in two; and he observed that it sometimes increased the coagulability of the urine. In *passive* dropsy, Waring says, it is occasionally administered with the view of stimulating the action of the kidneys; given with equal parts of spirits Ether-nitrici, he has seen benefit derived from it, but regards it as inadmissible in sthenic and acute cases. In absolute *torpor* of the kidneys, with complete suppression of urine, the powdered Cantharides, in grain-doses, has been used successfully by Dr. Elliotson and Sir Astley Cooper; in these cases there is no pain, no sense of weight in the loins, the patient may be able to sit up and converse as usual, and seem but little sick. If any urine, however small the quantity, be secreted, there is hope of recovery, but if not, in a few days he will die comatose. In another set of cases some blood will appear in the urine for a day or two before the secretion is totally suppressed, and after death the kidneys will be found gorged with blood, and in these Cantharides is dangerous. Still, Watson says, the endeavor to force the secretion of urine by strong stimulating diuretics, would strike one, *à priori*, as hazardous; yet this practice has its allopathic advocates, and, Watson adds, if experience should declare in its favor, theoretic objections ought to be disregarded. Stille says many of the older writers furnish numerous examples of the usefulness of Cantharides in *chronic* affections of the urinary passages, in which the secretion or discharge of the urine is impeded; the work of Greenfield contains many of these, which would probably now be described as instances of *chronic* pyelitis and vesical catarrh. Stille approaches very near to a homœopathic explanation when he adds: "Doubtless, by thus substituting an artificial and temporary stimulation for a morbid and permanent one, the latter may be dissipated." The difference between the practice of some homœopathic and allopathic practitioners would merely seem to be that the former use very small doses in some *acute* affections, while the latter give larger doses of the same remedy in *chronic* varieties of similar diseases. On the same principle, in the dominant school, this remedy is used in a few chronic skin affections; thus the celebrated Cazenave says that the success of tincture of Cantharides in the treatment of *chronic eczema*, particularly in females, is surprising. Hence it may also be used in some of the low, torpid, or malignant forms of the scarlet-fever eruption; also in the ulcerations of the throat, external neck, and other parts which attend or follow severe cases of scarlatina; for Mr. Tait speaks highly of the efficacy of the tincture of Cantharides, both internally and externally, against the most obstinate ulcerations. It has been found particularly useful: 1. Where the granulations are exuberant, but pale, weak, and flabby; 2. Where there is a deficiency or total absence of granulations, the ulcers being deep and scooped out, with raised and indurated edges; 3. Where the granulations are not defective, but cicatrize irregularly, sometimes in the centre, and at other times on one side—the lymph which is thrown out and organized one day being absorbed the next.

But many physicians, and myself among the rest, prefer the previous use of another class of remedies in the early stages of dropsy after scarlet fever; among these may be mentioned *Nitric-ether*, of which Stille says, in that form of general dropsy which follows scarlet fever, it is eminently serviceable, as well as in extensive anasarca produced by suppression of perspiration. Wood says it frequently acts with considerable energy as a diuretic, and in *suppression of urine* not dependent on nephritis it often answers an admirable purpose; for this condition not unfrequently attends febrile diseases, and occurs in children without assignable cause, unless it may be some disturbance in the nervous functions; in these cases it is resorted to, often with complete success. Its effects are those of a nervous stimulant, with the property of increasing the secretion of the urine or perspiration according as it may be directed to the skin or kidneys. In the febrile diseases of children, and those of a typhoid character in adults, when there is much restlessness, wakefulness, twitching of the tendons, starting in sleep, mental irritation, and fretfulness, it usually acts very happily; it often seems to ward off convulsions, and, even when they do occur, it may be given in the intervals with excellent effects.

Phosphoric-ether may be used in cases of torpid dropsy requiring a more powerful remedy than the Nitric. In *Frank's Magazine* we find the following experience:

"Case 1.—After an attack of typhus fever a man was left with swelling of the legs and thighs; the dropsy extended to the scrotum and penis, and the urine was found scanty; soon the abdomen became distended, and its walls thick and hard; the pulse was weak and slow; skin pale. *Phosphoric-ether*, in five-drop doses, was given, and the urine quickly became abundant, and increased still more when eight drops were given at a time; the swelling of the abdomen, scrotum, and penis lessened as the profuse flow of urine sat in. The patient was comparatively well in six days; on the eighth day of treatment his appetite and strength had returned, and the medicine was omitted. He used in all one hundred and seventeen drops of Phosphoric-ether, containing about one and one-fifth grains of Phosphor.

"Case 2.—A woman, aged fifty-five, after typhus fever, was left with swelling of the thighs and legs, and almost entire helplessness; a general coldness extended from the navel to the feet. In four days after commencing the Phosphoric-ether profuse urination sat in, with general improvement; still the legs were very cold, but frictions with Phosphoric-ether were used, followed by profuse discharges from the bowels and kidneys and return of warmth and mobility of the legs. At first six-drop doses, three times a day, were used; then ten drops. After taking one hundred and twenty-eight drops she was entirely cured.

"Case 3.—A woman, aged fifty-eight, who had been abandoned by her two physicians, was found almost pulseless, her face and hands covered with a cold sweat, and deathly pale. Her eyes were dimmed and covered with a thick white film; respiration almost imperceptible; her whole body icy cold; abdomen much bloated, but not very hard; genitals, thighs, legs, and feet considerably swollen; the uterus was much prolapsed, and the os thick, but not hard or painful; the rectum was filled with hard fæcal masses; the sphincter-ani quite relaxed. At first three-, and finally five-drop doses were used for nine days: on the very first day the urine became more abundant, and two clysters, with six drops each of Phos.-ether, were followed by stools. On the ninth day the abdomen was almost natural; the uterus had ascended, the *os* was much smaller, but the rectum still remained loaded. Injections with ten drops of Phos.-ether were followed by profuse fæcal discharges, succeeded by excessive debility and profuse perspiration; but ten drops by the mouth soon revived her; regular stools now occurred, but the abdomen became painful; still in four or five weeks the patient was able to walk out, but became chilled and fell into convulsions; she was very pale, in a profuse cold sweat, pulse almost imperceptible, abdomen tense and painful. Six drops of Phos.-ether restored her; stools and urine were free, and, finally, the medicine purged her. She was entirely cured in two months."

The *Bi-tartrate of Potash* is another more safe and pleasant remedy. Wood says, judging from his own experience, he should be disposed to place it at the very head of the diuretics. Though there may be cases of *dropsy* which *Digitalis* will cure, and this medicine will not, and others of which the same observation may be made of *Scilla*, yet, on the whole, no one medicine, and, he thinks, no combination of medicines will be found to cure so large a proportion of dropsical cases as the one under consideration. When administered in small and frequently repeated doses it operates as a diuretic, and may be given in all varieties of dropsy when not forbidden by the presence of an exhausting diarrhœa. Though theoretically applicable more especially to the febrile and inflammatory forms of the disease, Wood has found it not less effectual in those of a contrary nature, as, for example, that which so frequently follows miasmatic fever after the disappearance of the febrile disease. Wood says it might be supposed to be contra-indicated by debility; but he has used it as often in the feeble as in the strong, and with not less success. I have used it repeatedly in dropsy after scarlet fever, and cured the disease without the aid of any other remedy.

Arsenicum is very similar in its action to Cantharides and Rhus; all of them produce serous inflammations, and Arsenicum is the most homœopathic of all remedies to dropsy, especially when connected with disease of the skin or kidneys. If its use is followed up for some time the urine is occasionally increased in quantity, more rarely perspiration occurs; but, if too long continued, the urine is sometimes completely suppressed, or mixed with blood; the conjunctiva becomes more or less injected, and, in a few instances, an eruption of urticaria, pityriasis, or psoriasis appears on the skin; the pityriasis chiefly affects the parts covered by the clothing, and has a dirty, brown, dingy, unwashed appearance, somewhat similar to that which occurs in Addison's disease of the supra-renal capules. Stille says urticaria has sometimes followed a single dose of the medicine; and that need not surprise us, for nettle-rash consists of circumscribed effusions of serum into the subcutaneous cellular tissue. Soon a characteristic *puffiness* of the face arises, with *œdema* of the eye-lids, which is at first visible in the morning, but is afterwards more permanent and extensive, occupying the ankles, limbs, and abdomen with a *dropsical* effusion. This is exactly what occurs in the dropsy after scarlet fever, and we may draw the inference that the scarlet-fever virus and the arsenical poison have many points of similarity in their action upon the system, the blood, and the kidneys. The production of *serous effusions*, as an ordinary effect, and of chronic anæmia as a consequence of prolonged exposure to arsenical influences, appear to Stille to furnish grounds for believing that it tends to disintegrate the blood-corpuscules, to diminish the proportion of fibrin, and possibly, also, to attack still more directly the vital principle upon which the normal qualities of the blood depend. Stille thinks this theory is not inconsistent with the results obtained by the administration of Arsenic in minute doses, and which have led to a *tonic* virtue being attributed to it; for under their influence the skin becomes warmer, the pulse fuller and more frequent, the muscular system more active, the whole organism invigorated, and freer, and lighter in its movements, while even the mind improves in activity and power; a fresh and healthy appearance is gained, with a certain degree of *embonpoint*, so that the subjects of it are distinguished by the freshness of their complexions, and by an aspect of flourishing health;—the respiration also becomes more free, so that they ascend without difficulty heights which would have been almost insurmountable without its aid, and even asthma has been removed by it. *Arsenicum* is so homœopathic to dropsy that a very large number of cases ought to be cured by it if the homœopathic law be a true one; even allopathic physicians may be prepared to admit that it may cure some cases of *passive* dropsy, occurring in debilitated and atonic states of the system. My own experience with it has not been favorable, although there is a great deal of homœopathic testimony both for and against it. Clotar Müller says that, after the unavailing use of Hellebore, he has relieved dropsy with Arsenicum when the accumulation of water has reached an extreme degree, attended with considerable dyspnœa, spasmodic cough, and constant vomiting, even after taking only a teaspoonful of water or tea. Lobethal says he prefers Arsenicum when the dropsical effusion is advancing in the chest and pericardium, and persisted reliantly in the use of the remedy, although it seemed useless at first, and claims to have obtained cures with the thirtieth dilution. Bosch says, in the asthenic form of scarlatina-narcosis, with coma and decomposition of the blood, he lost his patients when he relied on Acon., Bell., Rhus, or Zinc.; but when he gave Arsenicum and Phosphor. in alternation he saved quite a number. Teller lost patients treated with Arsenicum and Hellebore under similar circumstances; but when he gave Digitalis, in rather large doses of the tincture, he became more successful; he never saw any good effects from the dilutions. Gross reports the following case: A child, fifteen days after an attack of scarlet fever, was seized with dropsy of the face, abdomen, and legs, with oppression of the chest and short breathing; the urine was scanty, but the bowels were loose, and that probably saved the child, although it lay in somewhat of a stupor. He gave Arsenicum, 30, one dose daily; and on the third day profuse urination occurred, followed by a rapid recovery. Arsenicum is also much used during the course of scarlet fever, especially in the low and malignant types of the disease, in which Stille would say it acts as a tonic.

Helleborus-niger has been frequently used in the homœopathic school in dropsical affections after scarlet fever, and in dropsy of the brain. Thus Clotar Müller, in three cases, quickly removed considerable œdematous swellings which involved almost the whole body. Tietze claims to have cured four cases with the eighteenth dilution, and among others the following: A girl, aged eight, three weeks after scarlet rash, complained of piercing pains over the whole head, and dizziness; she had a pale, very much bloated face, so that she could scarcely be recognized; had a bitter taste in the mouth, and no appetite, with nausea, retching, and vomiting after drinking; constipation for three days; scanty discharge of very brown urine; no perspiration, skin hot and dry; abdomen swollen, but soft. The child was greatly dejected, was afraid of dying, and sat quietly and disconsolately all day. Hellebore, 18, was given, and three days subsequently the urine was still quite scanty and dark brown, shewing that the remedy does not act very promptly in these small doses, and must prove inefficient in some dangerous, rapid, and acute cases. At the end of eight days the bloating of the face had diminished, the urine was copious and yellow, the abdomen had lessened in size, and she perspired frequently and profusely; in thirteen days the dropsical swelling was entirely removed. Urdemann reports a case treated with Hellebore, 12. A delicate boy became dropsical after scarlet rash; his face was bloated, and respiration difficult; but on the seventh day of treatment the previously blood-red urine had become clear, and convalescence gradually supervened. Teller generally used Hellebore, 2, as soon as the first signs of dropsical swelling, associated with scanty urine, showed themselves; but if, as frequently happened, improvement did not occur in the course of a few days—but, on the contrary, the urine became still scantier, and the dropsical effusions in the chest and abdomen increased —he used full doses of the tincture of Digitalis; from the dilutions of which he never derived good effects. Buchner says the sphere of Hellebore ceases as soon as fibrinous casts of the uriniferous tubes are observed in the urine, as occurs in the severest cases. Robinson reports a case cured by Apis, in which Hellebore had failed. Joslin gave it repeatedly without success. Rückert cured two mild cases with Hellebore, 9, aided by Lycopod. and Sepia. Kapper treated a case with Arsen., 3, and Hellebore, 3, but was obliged to resort to other remedies. Knorre, an able homœopathist, recommends it in *large* and frequent doses in chronic dropsy. Hartlaub, in a case of hydrocephalus-acutus, in the second stage, with screaming, throwing the head backwards, with convulsive movements of the limbs, especially the right arm and left foot,—used Aconite, Bellad., Rhus, Arnica, and Hellebore in the high potencies, but failed to give relief; he then gave ten-drop doses of tincture of Hellebore, at first every fifteen minutes, then every half-hour, and finally only every forty-eight hours; and cured the child. Dr. Ozanne prefers the second dilution; but, in some of his cases, after the Hellebore had been taken two days, the urine still continued very scanty, and the breathing oppressed; but he adds that it *often* happens that the second dilution is not sufficient, and then advises the first. He thinks, in the treatment of scarlatinal dropsy, Hellebore is generally sufficient; but the patient must be carefully watched, for, although mere anasarca is not a serious symptom, nor the accumulation of water in the abdomen, yet acceleration or oppression of respiration is dangerous. When the Hellebore fails in the first dilution, he uses Arsenicum, instead of giving more massive doses. Dr. Dubs, of Philadelphia, has cured one case of anasarca with the first decimal dilution, three or four times daily, in six weeks, after the sixth had failed to afford any relief. Dr. Dorwell, an allopathic physician, (see "Cyc. Prac. Med.") has given it in anasarca and dropsy after fevers; under its use he has seen the dropsy gradually disappear without any extraordinary increase of the secretions; still he says it should be discontinued if severe effects follow large doses, but it may generally be resumed in a few days. Its use in dropsy dates from the time of Avicenna.

I have failed to find any proof that Hellebore really produces any dropsical swelling, or that it is decidedly homœopathic to dropsy. Hahnemann, in his treatise on the "Helleborism of the Ancients," alludes to their use of it in dropsy, and probably adopted the practice from them; hence the dose ought to be larger than that usually adopted by homœopathists. In accordance with our usual custom, we will endeavor to give some idea of the real *modus operandi* of the remedy.

We have made some allusion to the ancient use of Hellebore on page 11. Dierbach places it among the *purgantia amara hydragoga*, or powerful purgatives characterized by their bitterness and the production of serous or watery diarrhœa; and in company with Gratiola, Colocynth, Elaterium, Bryonia, and Gamboge. In small doses it stimulates the abdominal organs, increasing the secretions of the liver and pancreas, quickening the peristaltic movements of the bowels, and augmenting the catamenial and hæmorrhoidal discharges. In large doses it operates as an acrid irritant, causing vomiting, colic, profuse purging, thirst, &c.; in fatal cases the gall-bladder and ducts have been found distended with bile, of which a large quantity was found in the small bowels, whence is derived its reputation among the ancients as an evacuator of black bile; the liver is often congested, and the stomach and bowels irritated. It has also been supposed to act specifically on the brain, and Orfila says that it causes a remarkable stupefaction, which may have to be combatted by Coffee or Camphor. Wood says that the Hellebore of the ancients had a great reputation in the treatment of insanity and melancholy, and it was believed to operate usefully in these complaints through its purgative properties, though he admits that it is not impossible that its supposed narcotic influence may have had some instrumentality in the favorable results. The ancients also gave it in amenorrhœa, *dropsy*, worms, and skin diseases, pretty much as more modern physicians use Aloes and Cream of Tartar. Wood says that allopathic physicians employ it but little now, except in amenorrhœa, in which it is supposed to be useful by a specific action on the uterus, independently of purgation. Mead has recommended it most highly in amenorrhœa, saying that he found in it so singular a virtue that it hardly ever failed in answering his expectations, and, in proof of its efficacy, alleges that, when it failed to restore the catamenia, it produced some other discharge of blood. Stille has found it useful in suppression of the menses from cold. It was once famous for its use in the treatment of insanity, both of the maniacal and melancholic forms; and the species which grew in the island of Anticyra was so renowned for its efficacy in mental disorders that the ancient phrase "*navigare Anticyras*" was equivalent to saying one had become deranged. It was also used by the ancients in dropsy, but in full doses. Stille says it has been much recommended as a purgative in dropsy, and adds that, doubtless, like other drastic cathartics, it is capable of causing the evacuation of serous effusions; but he assumes that it exerts no specific control over even this common symptom of various pathological conditions, and, on account of its harsh operation when given in allopathic doses, is often less eligible than other medicines of the same class, and particularly Jalap. It is the basis of Bacchus' celebrated "hydragogue pills," composed of extract of Black Hellebore, Myrrh, and powdered Carduus-benedictus, in the proportion of half a drachm of the first two ingredients and five grains of the last, beat into a mass, and made into one-grain pills. These pills, which formerly had a place in the pharmacopœias of the seventeenth and eighteenth centuries, in doses of from one to six, three or four times a day, were strongly recommended on the Continent in *dropsical* cases, and were conjectured to unite an evacuant and tonic power; hence they were supposed particularly adapted to those cases of *dropsy* in which general debility and relaxation of the system occurs. Stephenson and Churchill, in their "Medical Botany," say that, under the hands of their inventor, they acquired so great a reputation that, after a trial in the military hospitals in Paris, the receipt was purchased by the French king, and published by authority; but, like many other nostrums, since their composition became known, Bacchus' pills have by no means supported the reputation which they had when kept a secret.—I have so long been familiar with the true *modus operandi* of Hellebore that I have felt no inclination to give it in infinitesimal doses in affections to which it is not homœopathic, and hence have not often used it in dropsy, preferring Apocynum, Digitalis, Hydriodate of Potash, Benzoate of Ammonia, and other prompt and reliable remedies.

Bryonia is somewhat similar in its action to Hellebore and Colchicum. It has been used more particularly when the eruption fails to appear on the surface, and the disease falls upon the internal organs, especially those of the chest. But Bryonia has a far more specific relation to rheumatic disorders than to the erysipelatous and scarlatinous, which are in some measure the antagonists in essence of the former. It can hardly be as homœopathic to a chest affection arising from the scarlet-fever miasm as it is to one originating in a rheumatic disorder. It may be specific against those complications of scarlet fever which distinctly arise from exposure to cold or wet. Goullon has cured several cases of post-scarlatinal dropsy in from two to five days with Bryonia. Käsemann treated a case successfully in which the face was swollen, abdomen distended, urine as dark as beer, the chest oppressed, and the skin dry; it seemed to induce perspiration, increased discharge of clearer and lighter urine, to relieve the breathing, and loosen the cough: in eight days the patient was comparatively well. The action of Bryonia has already been touched upon on pages 351 and 373. Dierbach says the remedy was well known to the ancient Grecian and Roman physicians; it was given in dropsy by Engerasius, Asclepiades, Scribonius Largus, and others; the latter also used it in asthmatic affections. It was regarded as a drastic purgative remedy, like Hellebore and Colchicum. In the Sydenham edition of "Paulus Egineta" we find that Męsne regarded it as a phlemagogue, deobstruent, and *diuretic* medicine, and relied upon it against many coughs, asthmas, and *pleurisy*. Old Culpepper, in his "Complete Herbal and English Physician," says "It does mightily cleanse the chest of rotten phlegm, and wonderfully help the dry, old, and long coughs of those that are troubled with a shortness of breath." Serapion ascribes to it, among other secretory virtues, that of producing a great flow of milk. Galen used it in rheumatism and gout; Trautmann in arthritic hemicrania; Alexander Trallian in dropsy, pleurisy, stitches in the side, sciatica, white swelling; Loniger in asthma and spitting of blood. Dioscorides gave it in coughs. Hahnemann, whose extensive erudition made him acquainted with the works of these authors, revived the ancient uses of this efficacious and powerful remedy.

Colchicum-autumnale, as already said, resembles Bryonia and Hellebore in its action. Clotar Muller, who is one of the most learned and practical homœopathists, has given it with success in two cases of post-scarlatinal dropsy with scanty discharge of almost ink-like and decidedly albuminous urine. Colchicum was originally proposed by the celebrated Stoerck, as a remedy in dropsy, and he claims to have used it very successfully. Others have since been equally fortunate, and among them the equally distinguished Mason Good, who was a very emphatic eulogist, for he ranked it next to Scilla in power. Clark, of Philadelphia, and Aran, have reported instances of its success. In *scarlatinous dropsy*, Dr. Maclagan frequently found it of much service, particularly when the urine became very scanty, and indications were seen of approaching coma; he thinks that the *urea* retained in the blood is the cause of the symptoms, and that Colchicum causes its discharge. The same writer proposes it in the advanced stages of Bright's disease, as a means of depurating the blood. Dr. Tait thought that he was very successful in treating *scarlet fever* of an inflammatory type with it, and subsequently the celebrated Bennett, of Edinburgh, gave it in a case marked by alternate delirium and coma, and scanty urine without sediment; the cerebral symptoms disappeared, and a large quantity of urine, rendered turbid by urate of ammonia, was voided. The distinguished Chelius, of Heidelberg, was the first to notice that Colchicum increases the quantity of uric acid which is thrown out of the system through the kidneys; Kuhn noticed the same effect. Dr. Shervins maintains that it promotes the evacuation of urea, as well as of uric acid. Hence, as many of the dangerous symptoms in Bright's disease and post-scarlatinal dropsy arise from the retention of urea in the system, it is easy to understand the benefit which must sometimes ensue from the use of this remedy in these diseases. I have repeatedly given it, with marked good effects, and often substitute it for Bryonia and Hellebore when they seem indicated but do not act as promptly as is desirable.

Belladonna.—The similarity of the action of this remedy to scarlet fever is striking in some particulars, especially *on the skin;* thus Stille (see "Therapeutics") reports a case of poisoning with it, in which the face, upper extremities, and trunk of the body exhibited a diffuse scarlet efflorescence *studded with innumerable papillæ*, very closely resembling the rash of scarlatina. In another case, published in Hamilton's "Flora Homœopathica," the whole body, except the face, became red, and was *covered with miliary vesicles.* These cases prove that Belladonna is homœopathic to scarlatina-miliaris and- vesicularis, as well as to the smooth variety. Pereira and many other authorities simply say that an exanthematous eruption, like that of scarlet fever, has been noticed after large doses of Belladonna, without any more accurate description of the exanthem.

The *throat affection* produced by Belladonna is described as if the tongue, mouth, and fauces were as devoid of moisture as if they had been composed of burned shoe-leather; the secretions of the glands of the mouth and the saliva were entirely suspended; about the pharynx the sensations were most distressing, inducing constant attempts at deglutition, and finally exciting suffocation, with spasms of the fauces and glottis renewed at every effort to swallow; a little saliva, white and round, like a ball of cotton, was occasionally spat up. In the few cases in which the throat was examined, it was simply red and dry; there was no pseudo-membranous exudation.

It undoubtedly operates on the system through absorption into the blood, for its active principle has been detected in the urine, and the urine of a rabbit which had been fed upon it produced dilatation of the pupil of a cat to the eye of which it had been applied. Hence it is capable of meeting a blood-poisoning like that produced by the scarlet-fever miasm on its own ground.

It may also be capable of eliminating this and other blood-poisons from the system *through the kidneys and urine;* for Dr. H. M. Gray, who experimented on his own person, says the power of Belladonna over the secretion of urine seems very great; he is confident that he passed, in the course of an hour, three pints of urine, accompanied with slight strangury at the neck of the bladder. I have also witnessed this effect in another case of accidental poisoning. In the case of a child, towards the end of the attack, the diuretic effects of the plant began to be experienced, the patient evacuating an *enormous* quantity of limpid urine. Dr. Gray speaks of its diuretic power as *tremendous*, but has observed that it does not seem to reach the kidneys until it has been some time in the system, and has exerted its specific influence on the brain. In fact, in the majority of cases, it lessens the quantity of urine first, and increases it afterwards; thus, in one case it caused inability to pass water, or only in drops and with great difficulty, so that the catheter had to be used. In another case but little urine was passed for twenty-four hours, but then it came away copiously. Hence it may relieve the dropsy after scarlet fever as other diuretics do.

The action of Belladonna and other narcotics *upon the blood*, as compared with that of scarlet and other malignant fevers, requires a somewhat minute examination on our part. Although we do not expect to arrive at the exact truth, we hope to make very close approximations to it, in some directions at least.

Normal blood is a thick opaque fluid, varying in color, in different parts of the body, from a brilliant *scarlet* to a dark *purple;* it is scarlet in the arteries, and more or less purple in the veins. This difference in color is owing somewhat to the different proportions of *carbonic acid* and oxygen in the two kinds of blood; for in arterial blood the proportion of oxygen to carbonic acid, by volume, is as ten to twenty-five, while in the venous blood it is only ten to forty: *i. e.*, there is nearly twice as much carbonic acid in venous blood as in arterial. The blood alters its hue from purple to scarlet by giving up carbonic acid and absorbing a fresh quantity of oxygen; thus, if freshly drawn venous blood be shaken in a bottle with pure oxygen, its color changes at once from purple to red. Carbonic acid exists, ready formed, in the venous blood before it reaches the lungs, while oxygen is absorbed during respiration, in a free state, in the arterial blood. *Carbonic acid* is not a direct product of oxidation, but it originates, in all probability, by a decomposition of the organic ingredients of the tissues, resulting in the production of carbonic acid on the one hand, and of various other substances which we need not treat of here. The *tissues* are by far the most important source of the carbonic acid of the blood. The next source is in the *blood* itself, for there is little doubt that some of the carbonic acid of the system is formed in the substance of the blood globules during their circulation. The third source is in the lungs; for, when the blood comes in contact with the pulmonary tissue, which is permeated everywhere by pneumic acid in a soluble form, its alkaline carbonates and bi-carbonates are decomposed with the production, on one hand, of the pneumates of soda and potash, and on the other of free carbonic acid, which is then exhaled. If the carbonic acid, which is produced in the body by the processes of nutritition, be allowed to collect in too large a quantity, it becomes a poisonous agent; for nearly 27,360 cubic inches of carbonic acid should be exhaled from the lungs per day, and from one-thirtieth to one-sixtieth of this amount by the skin. Under ordinary circumstances the carbonic acid is removed by exhalation through the lungs and skin as fast as it is produced in the interior of the body; but, if its exhalation be suspended, or seriously impeded, while its production continues, it accumulates in the blood and tissues, and terminates life by a rapid deterioration of the circulating fluid, and more particularly by its poisonous effect on the nervous system. Narcotics produce similar effects: Prussic-acid probably produces an increased production of carbonic acid in the blood itself; Belladonna, Stramonium, and others, more particularly in the tissues, and Opium and other drugs prevent its rapid elimination through the lungs.

The action of carbonic-acid gas, when inhaled, is very similar to the effects of narcotic remedies; in fact, it produces specific narcotic actions when taken internally: it causes throbbing headache, with a feeling of fullness and tightness across the temples and in the occipital regions, giddiness, loss of muscular power, tightness of the chest, augmented action of the heart, or palpitation; the ideas become confused, and the memory partially fails; buzzing in the ears occurs, vision is impaired but the eyes retain their lustre, and a strong tendency to sleep succeeds, or actual syncope ensues; the pulse may fall below its natural standard, the respiration become slow and laborious, the surface cold, and often livid; delirium, convulsions with foaming at the mouth, and vomiting may come on, terminating only in death, while *fluidity and darkness of the blood*, engorgement of the cerebral and spinal vessels, with exudations of serum or of blood may be found in various parts. In order to form some idea of the injurious effects of an excess of carbonic acid in the system, M. Bernard rapidly injected a solution of Bi-carbonate of Soda into the jugular vein of a rabbit, and found that it became decomposed in the lungs, with so rapid a development of carbonic acid that the gas accumulated in the pulmonary vessels and cavities of the heart to such an extent as to cause death by stoppage of the circulation. In the normal condition, however, the carbonates and bi-carbonates of the blood arrive so slowly at the lungs that, as fast as they are decomposed there, the carbonic acid is readily exhaled by expiration and produces no deleterious effect on the circulation. But in some diseases, especially in typhoid, scarlet, and other septic fevers, this is not the case; carbonic acid and other deleterious substances accumulate more rapidly than they are excreted; they poison and liquify the blood. If the quantity in the system be large, but not overwhelming, reactive fever ensues, with many signs of narcotic poisoning; if the quantity be excessive, all the signs of malignant fever arise, with stupor, petechiæ, hæmorrhages, &c. Poisoning with *Prussic-acid* resembles intense poisoning with Carbonic-acid: thus, where insensibility is not immediately produced by it, there is faintness, giddiness, debility, and perhaps convulsions, followed by insensibility; the eyes are fixed and glistening, pupils dilated, skin cold, with clammy perspiration, and convulsive respiration. After death the face is either livid or pale, the lips and nails blue, the skin of the neck, back, and shoulders much discolored; the eyes have the peculiar brilliant and glistening appearance, also common in cases of suffocation from fumes of charcoal; involuntary evacuations may take place from the bowels and bladder; the vessels of the brain are turgescent, the lungs congested with a very dark colored blood, the bronchial tubes filled to their extremities with bloody froth; the blood is generally dark, fluid, and sometimes of a purplish color. The whole presents a marked similarity to the appearances found after death in typhus, scarlet, or miasmatic fevers and malignant small-pox. In addition to the accumulation of carbonic acid gas in the blood in these diseases, it is probable that a peculiar virulent poison is also developed in the blood in each destructive form of fever; just as Atropine is found in Belladonna, Veratrine in various plants, and Morphine in Opium. Although we do not suppose that Prussic-acid has anything to do with the origin of these fevers, yet it has been found in the blood where none had been taken into the stomach, and the blood-poisons above alluded to, resemble it somewhat in their action. Thus, Taylor has noticed that the organs of persons who have died from natural causes occasionally exhale the odor of Prussic-acid; cheese, which is an albuminous substance, when exposed to the action of water and the sun, disengages ammonia, and if heated in this state with alcohol, yields traces of hydrocyanic acid; in the decomposition of animal matters, cyanogen is frequently generated. Pereira once detected prussic acid, or rather prussiate of iron, in the greenish thin discharge from an ulcer; cyanogen has been found in the urine, menstrual fluid, and perspiration. It is possible, in some weakly, nervous, and dyspeptic patients, that small quantities of prussic acid may be formed in the system, and cause a great feeling of sinking, debility, nervousness, cramps, &c. When large quantities are found in the blood, together with an excess of carbonic acid or carbonic oxide, we may have all the phenomena of low and malignant fever arising.

The effects of Belladonna *on the blood* are not as intense as those of Prussic-acid, and there is greater reaction of the system against it; it seems, at first, to cause an intense arterial and inflammatory condition, but, in fact, causes what may be termed a tumultuous conversion of arterial blood into venous, for, after ten or twelve hours, the apparently increased arterial action ceases, and excessive and predominant venosity ensues; the previous redness of the face gives place to lividity, the veins are over-crowded with dark blood, and profuse urination, aided or not by perspiration, eliminates the poison from the body and restores the balance of the system. In excessive doses, the effects of Belladonna are very much like those of the Prussic- or Carbonic acids, viz.: paralysis of the nervous system and decomposition of the blood, for blue spots and petechiæ form on the skin, decomposed, brown, and offensive blood may exude from various parts, and the patient becomes soporose and prostrate. From the above it is as difficult to understand the antidotal effects of Belladonna against scarlet fever as it is, those of Mercury against lues, and Quinine against fever and ague; but, according to Pereira, *Chlorine and Ammonia* are antidotes to Prussic-acid, and of these Chlorine is by far the best, while both of these remedies have been used largely and apparently successfully against scarlet fever. Pereira says Chlorine should be applied both internally and externally; Chlorine water should be given in doses of one or two teaspoonsful, properly diluted with water, and the patient should be allowed to inhale, very cautiously, air impregnated with Chlorine gas, developed by the action of dilute hydrochloric acid on chloride of lime. If Ammonia is used, and Pereira says it is certainly inferior to Chlorine, the liquor Ammoniæ diluted with eight or ten parts of water should be exhibited, and the vapor of Ammonia or its carbonate inhaled; the latter practice, he adds, is most important, and should not be omitted, although great caution is requisite in the employment of it. One or both of these plans may be used in very malignant cases of scarlet fever, in place of ordinary disinfectants.

To return to the consideration of Belladonna in scarlet fever, we give the experience of the German homœopathists, as detailed in "Rückert's Clinique." Gross reports a case in which tincture of Bellad., in drop-doses, was given every two hours, and claims that recovery took place the next day. Notwithstanding Gross' great reputation among the strict homœopathists, we regard the case as a doubtful one; but it shows that one who formerly gave the highest dilutions is not afraid to use rational doses. He reports another case, treated in the same way, and claims so completely to have broken up the case that the eruption did not appear at all. Seidel gave one dose, of one drop of the tincture of Bellad., as a preventive, but the eruption appeared abundantly, attended with delirium; still the case recovered on the fourth day. Perhaps if he had repeated his doses every two hours, like Gross, he would have been more successful. He publishes three other cases, treated with the twenty-fourth and thirtieth dilutions, in which the disease increased considerably for three or four days, and then subsided; the attack, doubtless, pursuing the natural course of mild scarlet fever uninfluenced by the treatment. Tietze reports a mild case, treated with Bellad., 30, with recovery on the fifth day, as doubtless would have occurred if nothing had been given. Trinks gives a similar case, convalescent on the sixth day, and treated with Bellad., 30; Kasemann reports a mild case, convalescent on the fifth day, treated with Bellad., 30; Müller, four cases, with Bellad., 30; Sonnenberg a similar case, and Gross another; Fleischmann, a slight case, treated with Bellad., 6; Schwarze, a mild case, with Bellad., 30, and Coffea, 3. If these examples prove anything, they show how little medicine need be given in mild cases; we are not told how much more comfortable the patients might have been in the meantime if more decided palliative means had been used. Müller treated two severe cases with tincture of Bellad., every two hours, with recovery in ten days; Schelling, a case, quickly followed by dropsy, cured with Aconite and Bellad.; also a doubtful case, complicated with erysipelatous inflammation of the leg, which progressed unchecked by high dilutions of Rhus, Merc. and Rhus, and then seemed to yield to more rational doses of Belladonna. We must here confess our surprise at the small number of cases of severe or malignant scarlet fever treated with Belladonna reported by the German homœopathists from the year 1822 to 1857.

If some of the homœopathists have used Belladonna in ridiculously small doses, some of the dominant school have given it in almost or quite dangerously large quantities; thus, Dr. Gardner, of Edinburgh, says: without regarding the opinions of the extreme homœopathists, he proceeded to try it in malignant scarlet fever, giving it in efficient doses; he was certain that the extract he used was good, for he always tested a grain or two on the eye-lids, and found it to produce full dilatation of the pupil in a minute or two. Without reckoning slight cases of scarlet fever and sore throat, he has treated upwards of thirty cases, with symptoms more or less grave, by means of Belladonna; in very many of these he should formerly have entertained no hope of seeing the patient pass through the attack, so malignant was the aspect of its approach. He says he need not enumerate the peculiar symptoms which characterize fatal scarlet fever, for these are well known to every experienced practitioner. Without Belladonna, he has often watched with despair these fatal tokens—they allow so little room for our anxious anticipations being negatived; but with Belladonna he has not yet met with a fatal case. Moreover, he continues, it is well known that in no inconsiderable proportion of cases, whether severe or slight, very inconvenient sequelæ occur on the subsidence of the fever, such as arthritic pains, œdema of the limbs, anasarca, and even hydrocephalus; in no case treated with Belladonna has he met with such sequelæ. He administers it, according to the ability of the patient to bear it, in doses of half a grain to a whole grain of good, but four or five years old extract, every three, four, or six hours: the dilatation of the pupil and amount of stupor produced being the basis of discrimination as to the size and repetition of the doses; he does not allow low delirium, even from the first, nor indeed any other symptom, to deter him from giving Belladonna, and he uses no other medicine whatever, except an occasional dose of Castor-oil to secure a daily action of the bowels. Making every allowance for the many sources of fallacy necessarily incident to an opinion, he knows nothing in the whole compass of medicine in which he has more confidence. He has recommended this plan of treating scarlet fever to several medical friends, and their reports of its effects have been uniformly favorable. Dr. Green, of Peckham, England, corroborates the experience of Dr. Gardner as to the value of Belladonna in large doses in scarlet fever; the quantity he gives to persons above puberty is one-sixth of a grain, every four hours; for children, he rubs one grain with five grains of sugar, and of this gives one-sixth or one-twelfth of a grain, also every four hours; for infants, it should be used in extremely minute doses.—*Braithwaite's Retrospect*, No. 24.

Opium is a narcotic, without the excessively stimulating and irritating properties of Belladonna and Stramonium, nor the greatly depressing powers of Aconite, Digitalis, or Tobacco; but it acts specifically on the skin, for nothing is better established than its power of exciting perspiration; another very common effect of it is an intolerable itching of the skin, and so intense is the irritation arising from this cause, in some instances, that the anodyne and composing influence of the drug is entirely annulled, and the patient tosses about the bed unable to find comfort in any position, and rubs and scratches every part of the body with violence. This itching, Stille says, is quite independent of the cutaneous eruptions which opiates frequently occasion, and which usually consist of *slightly elevated and reddish patches*, resembling those of measles, or still more prominent and distinct, like the wheals of urticaria; the latter, as well as prurigo and eczema, are not unfrequently developed around the margin of the blistered surface upon which a salt of Morphia has been sprinkled, and give rise to a very annoying degree of itching. This specific action upon the skin has led some physicians to use Opium in measles and scarlet fever; others use it with the idea of producing perspiration and relaxation of the skin, and thus restoring its functions in these diseases.

The *ultimate* action of Opium on the blood is similar to that of Carbonic-acid and other narcotics; that it is absorbed into the blood is evident, for Manuel detected morphia in the blood and urine of a person poisoned with Opium, while the milk of nurses under its influence has produced its peculiar effects on the nursing child. From the primary action of Opium the blood may retain its florid color for a time, and give a bright tint to the complexion during the stage of excitement; but in its secondary effects, the change from venous to arterial blood is less thoroughly effected, and it becomes darker hued; from large doses the venous hue upon the surface, and particularly in the face, is often conspicuous; if death ensues, the vessels of the cerebro-spinal axis are gorged with *black* blood, and the lungs, heart, liver, and spleen are, in most cases, distended with *dark* and *fluid blood.* In a person stupid from the effects of Opium it is surprising to notice the change in the color of the surface if the patient be roused: that which was *almost purplish, from the venous* hue of the blood, then reassumes in a considerable degree its natural appearance, because more oxygen has been supplied to the lungs, and some of the carbonic acid got rid of; but, the instant the patient is permitted to lie down and sleep, the *dark* suffusion of the face returns. It is evident from the above that Opium is antagonistic to the true arterial inflammatory process, and, if properly aided and controlled by Aconite, Veratrum-viride, or Digitalis, it ought to become one of the most prominent dominant school remedies against many inflammations. Again, Opium acts somewhat like Belladonna on the kidneys—viz., it first lessens the quantity of urine, and subsequently increases it. Thus, Wood says that, in the greater number of instances, the urine is diminished, but he has sometimes known it to be greatly increased, particularly by the salts of Morphia; indeed, he has seen few diuretics act more copiously than this for a short time, and the celebrated Graves has rendered himself renowned by his treatment of dropsy with Opium. The action of Opium on the *brain* is too well known to require much explanation: It often causes a universal feeling of delicious ease and comfort, with an elevation and expansion of the whole moral and intellectual nature; if he does not sleep, the patient may lie calmly and placidly, without mental effort or uneasiness, submitting himself to a current of vague, but generally pleasing fancies; if light sleep occurs there will be a constant succession of dreams, having the vividness almost of reality, and usually pleasant in their character. But repeatedly it acts disagreeably, and horrible dreams and fancies occur, bordering on delirium or insanity; when it exercises its full soporific influence the sleep is usually profound and dreamless, and continues for about eight or ten hours. It lessens all the mucous secretions quite as much as it increases those of the skin, while its constipating effects and its suppression of the secretion of bile to the extent of causing white stools are well known. With these prefatory remarks we proceed to the homœopathic experience with Opium in scarlet fever. Hahnemann used it when there was burning fever, sleepy stupefaction, agonizing restlessness, with vomiting, *diarrhœa*, and even convulsions. Some of these indications seem more or less antipathic, but he also used it when there was constipation. Trinks gave it when there was a *status nerv. stupid.*, in which the patient was in a deep sleep, or kind of stupor, from which it was difficult to arouse him, attended with slight spasms of the face and limbs, with congestion to the head, the face being bloated and red, the whole surface covered with perspiration, the respiration quick and superficial, the pulse full and quick; he often alternated it with Aconite. Some modern physicians assume that small doses of Opium act oppositely to large doses; that a small quantity will arouse, stimulate, and prevent the patient from sleeping;—Aconite modifies and controls its action in many important points, especially in modifying congestion to the brain. Hartmann advises it when a soporose condition alternates with raging delirium; when the eyes are red, wild, sparkling, and the face reddened, but becomes pale and pinched when sopor sets in. The delirium against which he found it useful was attended with spasmodic movements of the limbs or whole body; at times *diarrhœa* was present, at other constipation. He claims to have been very successful with it, and some have insisted that many of his indications are antipathic. Lorbach found it indicated not only where there was coma with dark redness of the face, slow respiration, slow and intermitting pulse, and slight twitchings of the muscles of the face; but also when there were violent *convulsions*, great redness of the face, squinting, profuse sweats, slow pulse, and deep, often snoring respiration; he adds that the presence of a profuse and very offensive *diarrhœa* is no contra-indication. He alternated Hyosc. with Opium when the convulsions were severe, but, as he gave his small doses only every one or two hours, it is not probable that the spasms were controlled very quickly. Belladonna, although quite as much, or even seemingly more indicated, never relieved the convulsions in his hands. In allopathic practice it has not been much used in scarlet fever, but it has, and successfully, in typhus and small-pox. Graves used it, combined or alternated with Tartar

Emetic, when there was violent delirium, furious aspect, suffusion of the eyes, constant raving and muttering, with perfect sleeplessness; Louis found it effectual, in small doses, in moderating subsultus and delirium in mild cases of typhus, and suggests that it should be used in severe cases, and in other fevers. Sydenham, Cullen, and Hildebrandt used it against fevers with maniacal delirium; in simple delirium with watchfulness and subsultus; in nervous states and low delirium, and profuse discharges from the bowels. These eminent men generally used preparatory evacuant treatment, or combined it with Nitre or some other sedative to the circulation. (The use of Opium in small-pox has been given on page 324.)

Stimulants and Tonics.—The homœopathists use Phosphorus, Arsenicum, Rhus, Arnica, Coffea, Muriatic-acid, Zinc, and have adopted Carbonate of Ammonia and Camphor. In the dominant school, Quinine, Wine, Iron, Carbonate of Ammonia, Capsicum, &c., are the favorites in the malignant forms of the disease.

Phosphorus.—The action of this remedy has already been touched upon on page 213. Pereira says, in small doses, it excites the nervous, vascular, and secreting organs; often creates an agreeable feeling of warmth at the epigastrium, increases the frequency and fullness of the pulse, augments the heat of the skin, heightens the mental activity and the muscular powers, and operates as a powerful sudorific and diuretic. From its offensive taste in any except very minute doses it is rarely employed in the dominant practice in England and America; but it has been strongly recommended by German physicians in many cases attended with great prostration of the vital powers, as in the latter stages of typhus and scarlet fevers, and in dropsies; in some of the exanthemata, as measles and scarlet fever, it has been exhibited to promote the appearance of the eruption when this has receded from the skin. Phosphorus is a natural constituent of the human body, especially of the brain and nerves, in which as much as from 1.65 to 3.40 exists normally. Phosphoric acid is present largely and normally in the muscular juice, for Weber found from 40 to 47 per cent. in the ash of flesh, and 2 per cent. in that of the serum of the blood; in healthy urine Winter found that from 3.765 to 5.180 grammes, or from 55 to 78 grains of phosphoric acid were eliminated from the body in twenty-four hours. In fact, so abundant and important are the phosphates to the animal economy that Lehmann says that, wherever free acids occur in the parenchyma of the organs, the acid *phosphates* are invariably present; and the proposition may be established, that in animal juices which exhibit an acid reaction, the *soluble phosphates* are especially accumulated. These facts are dwelt upon here to show how congenial, natural, and essential Phosphorus and the phosphates are to the human body, and to raise the conjecture that they may be as frequently required in disease as Iron is now given by many physicians. Phosphoric-acid is at once more powerful than strong Sulphuric-acid, and less irritant than weak Vinegar, so that it can and does innocently traverse every part of the body. Professor Wilson, of Edinburgh, says that Phosphorus can imperceptibly and quickly pass from a condition of great chemical activity to one of great chemical inertness, and he suggests this susceptibility of change as one reason why phosphorus is a predominant organismal element. Phosphorus, in virtue of its mutability and mobility, can follow the blood in its changes; may oxydize in one great set of capillaries, and be indifferent to oxygen in another; may occur in the brain in the vitreous form, changing as quickly as the intellect or imagination demands, and literally flaming, that thoughts may breathe and words may burn; and may be present in the bones in its amorphous form, content, like an impassive caryatid, to sustain upon its unwearied shoulders the mere dead weight of stones of flesh. And what is said here of the brain, as contrasted with the bones, will apply with equal or similar force to many other organs of the body: all throughout the living system we may believe that phosphorus is found, at the centres of vital action in an active condition, and at its outlying points in a passive condition. Phosphorus, Phosphoric-acid, and Iron may become as necessary in some states of the system as beef, bread, wine, or Iron. Trinks used it in scarlet fever, when the disease took a turn which threatened to affect the lungs; when an incessant spasmodic cough occurred, with inflammatory spasm of the throat and larynx, excessive anxiety, sensation of fainting, nausea, great acceleration of breathing, rapid, small, and failing pulse, and threatening of paralysis of the lungs sat in. The celebrated Dr. Wolf, of Dresden, gave it successfully under like circumstances. Hartmann relied upon it when there was considerable anxiety, groaning, and tossing about, although the eruption was out fully. Lobethal used it when there was difficulty of breathing, oppression of the chest, and rattling of mucus, leading to the fear of catarrhal suffocation.

Iron.—The Citrate of Iron and the tincture of the Sesquichloride have been highly recommended, in view of their tonic properties. Dr. Bishop, of Devonport, states that he has treated fifty-one cases in this way, with but one death. He uses these tonics from the commencement, and makes no change, even if there be serious complications present. The Muriate tincture of Iron is thought most effectual in what has been called acute desquamative nephritis following scarlatina. This condition is often marked by high fever, great prostration, with an occasional tendency to a typhoid condition, brown and dry tongue, gum-sordes, stupor, great scantiness of urine, constipation, and torpor of all the natural emunctories. The urine is very scant, high colored, sometimes offensive, and, upon microscopic examination, will be found to be loaded with perfect and imperfect blood-corpuscles, and occasionally epithelial casts. After the first violence of the fever has departed the Muriate tincture of Iron will act very happily; but Aconite and Digitalis, in one to three-drop doses, will be found very valuable adjuncts. Dr. Mead, of Bradford, England, being much struck with the analogy between the symptoms of scarlet fever and erysipelas, very successfully applied the tincture of Iron treatment, said to be so useful in the latter, giving from five to fifteen minims, according to the age of the patient, every three or four hours; he lost only one case during the whole of one spring and winter, and claims that almost all the cases in which he employed this treatment recovered with unusual rapidity. Somewhat of the benefit from the use of Muriate tincture of Iron may arise from the presence of Muriatic-acid, which, like the Phosphoric, is so useful in typhoid fevers, and the rest to the presence of Iron, which is as much a tonic to the blood as Phosphorus is to both the blood and nerves; both are natural constituents of the human body, and, not only congenial to it, but absolutely necessary to its existence. Iron, too, produces almost an opposite state of the blood to that caused by Carbonic- and Prussic-acid, and the narcotics generally, and that which obtains in low, typhoid, and septic fevers, and hence may prove a true antipathic remedy to some forms of malignant, putrid, septic fevers, such as malignant small-pox, measles, scarlet, typhus, typhoid, petechial, and hæmorrhagic fevers. It should be fully recognized that, in many cases, Iron, like Cod-liver Oil and Phosphorus, is a *nutrient* rather than a drug, since it furnishes one of the most important elements of the organism, and the one which is frequently deficient in the diseases for which it forms a most effectual and, as it were, specific remedy. An increase in the proportion of iron is found in the blood of those who use it, and, on chemical examination, it is found organically incorporated with the red globules of the blood, and not merely dissolved or suspended in the serum, as is the case with many other medicines. According to Stille, the most evident effect of Iron is that, during its administration, the blood becomes redder and its red globules more abundant. The red globules appear to be the organs to which Iron is especially directed, and by which the activity of animal as well as of organic life is sustained at the highest point. These bodies it is which, by contact with the inspired air in the lungs, attract and become impregnated by oxygen, the essential agent in all the compositions and decompositions which sustain life in the tissues, acquiring thereby the scarlet hue of arterial blood, which they lose with their oxygen in their passage through the tissues to the venous system. Thus it would appear that the activity of nutrition, and probably, also, of calorification, is dependent upon the iron in the blood, and that, when the red globules which contain it are most abundant, all the functions of the animal economy attain their highest degree of activity and vigor, such as is displayed in persons of a sanguine temperament. Liebig first propounded the theory that the red globules of the blood carry oxygen from the lungs to the tissues, and carbonic acid from the tissues to the lungs, and in performing which service they wear by turns the scarlet hue of arterial, and the crimson color of venous blood. It is evident, from the above, that Iron is a direct chemical antidote against that state of blood which is produced by the Carbonic and Prussic-acids and the narcotics; and hence, if rightly applied, its stimulating action being modified by proper antecedent treatment, or controlled by evacuant, sedative, or cooling medicines, it may be safely and usefully given when there is asthenic activity of the circulation, with heat of the skin and venous congestion of various organs. Stille goes on to say that Iron, on entering the blood-vessels, combines immediately with the corpuscules which have not yet acquired, or which have lost more or less of the ferruginous element. It enters the blood as a chloride, from its combination with the muriatic acid of the gastric juice, and hence its action is often more similar to that of the Muriate tincture of Iron than any other preparation; but it is decomposed in the blood, combines with the corpuscules as a carbonate of the protoxide of iron, and in the lungs gives up carbonic acid and absorbs oxygen, and is thereby converted into a peroxide. The white corpuscules are naturally destitute of iron; but, when once saturated with it, neither they nor the red corpuscules can receive any more. The mildest and most appropriate preparation of Iron is the *Tartrate of Iron* and *Potassa*, or combination of Cream of Tartar and hydrated Sesquioxide of Iron. According to Stille, among the compounds of Iron with organic acids this is by far the most important, for it is one of the most valuable of the chalybeate preparations. As Mialhe and Quevenne have remarked, it is at once the richest in iron, the most agreeable to the taste, the least irritating to the bowels and oppressive to the chest, the least apt to cause constipation and overheating of the system, and the most readily absorbed of all the soluble preparations of Iron. According to Mialhe, other soluble compounds of Iron are precipitated in the stomach, and so much of them only can be absorbed as is redissolved by an excess of acid. He claims to have shown that, although this salt, like others of its class, is precipitated in the stomach, yet, on reaching the intestines, and there coming in contact with the normal alkaline secretions of the bowels, it is not decomposed; and as the natural acids of the stomach, which caused its precipitation in that organ, unite with the alkaline bases, the iron resumes the solubility which it had temporarily lost, and becomes apt for absorption throughout the whole intestinal tube, so that it can be administered as effectually by the rectum as the mouth. Stille says, if this view of its operation be correct, the medicine must possess the singular advantage of not being dependent, like the other most useful preparations, upon the gastric acids for absorption. Hence, if Iron be useful at all in scarlet fever, it will be safest to commence with the Tartrate; then, if necessary, change to the Citrate or Lactate, and finally resort to the Muriate tincture. Lactic acid is normally present in the stomach, and the *Lactate* is regarded by some authorities as preferable to other salts of Iron, because its acid is presumed to be the same that naturally combines with the metal in the stomach. The *Citrate* is even more tasteless than the Tartrate of Iron and Potassa, and thus is regarded as an excellent remedy when the stomach is delicate; but it is less adapted in febrile and congestive affections. Some of the benefit of the preparations of Iron arises from the presence of Tartaric, Citric, and Muriatic-acids, all of which may prove more or less useful in scarlet fever unaided by other remedies.

Quinine.—Recourse has been had to Quinine in the treatment of scarlatina, and it has been recommended to commence with it on the occurrence of the first symptoms of the disease. Though this recommendation is supported by the assurance of the author (Dr. Morrison, of Lawrenceville, Virginia) that of all the modes of treatment he has ever seen tried this is the most efficacious, it would be safest to restrict its use to those severe cases where reaction fails to take place, or the patient is in danger of sinking. If the eruption has been very severe and the fever violent, and the patient shows signs of exhaustion, or if the eruption be disposed to assume a livid hue, recourse might safely be had to Quinine at once. Dr. Caspar Morris, of Philadelphia, who has had a very large experience in the treatment of scarlet fever, says that, while he desires to caution against the resort to those remedies which directly exhaust the vital power, he would enter an equally strong protest against the premature employment of stimulating remedies. If malignant symptoms are present from the first, we must immediately adopt the stimulation necessary to counteract their tendency; but do not let the fear of their future occurrence induce a premature resort to them as a preventive. These remarks are especially applicable to the use of Quinine. *Wine whey* is safer, for it is transient in its influence, and *Capsicum* gives rise to no febrile reaction; but *Quinine* produces a more permanent impression upon the nervous system, and has a stronger tendency to excite local inflammation; properly applied, it may be the sheet-anchor of our hope, but the very power which renders it so, causes it, when misused, to be most pernicious. He says it should be given, when required, in full doses, at long intervals, leaving the stomach free to receive animal broth, wine whey, or brandy, if required; these latter are at times most conveniently given in arrowroot, or some of the usual farinaceous articles of diet. Where there is much tendency to collapse, he says, warm wine-whey or brandy and water may be given internally. But Dr. P. Hood, of London, is the most earnest advocate for the use of Quinine in scarlet fever; he precedes it, however, with emetics and purgatives. He says, in his little treatise "On the Successful Treatment of Scarlet Fever," that, as he regards Quinine to be the sheet-anchor in scarlet fever, he is relieved of all anxiety as to the result of the disease when he has once fairly established the regularity of its administration. Formerly he was in the habit of prescribing it without paying the attention which he has since found necessary to the previous exhibition of an emetic and purgative. Medicines of the latter kind he has, however, found to be of the greatest efficacy in preventing subsequent complications and ensuring a favorable termination of the disease. Though he claims never to have lost a patient under the former course of treatment, yet he often had to contend against complications that followed the subduction of the primary disease; hence he must have treated mild cases, which only are followed by dropsy, with Quinine and other severe remedies. Some of his cases, he says, were of the most severe kind, and he is now disposed to attribute *much of this severity* to the use of the very remedy (viz., Quinine) which he now finds so eminently advantageous in preventing any such description of sequelæ or complications. The natural conclusion of this is, that some of his cases recovered in spite of being greatly aggravated by his treatment. But he goes on to say that, when proper attention has been paid to the evacuation of the bowels, and the system by such means is relieved from all poisonous excrementitious matters, Quinine, in combination with the *dilute Sulphuric-acid*, will then be found to produce its antiseptic and febrifuge effects in the most satisfactory manner: the accelerated action of the heart will abate, the skin become cooler, and the nervous irritability, so strikingly displayed as the result of some poisonous influence pervading the system, will be tranquillized; the rash will soon fade (it seldom lasts longer than three days), and the swelling of the tonsils will diminish and subside. One cannot resist the supposition that Dr. Hood treats even mild cases with Quinine, and they recover in spite of the disease and unnecessarily severe treatment. He also asserts that no superficial ulceration will occur on the tonsils, the mucous membrane of the mouth and throat will assume a healthier hue, and the swelling of the face and eye-lids soon subside. Conviction is thus forced on his mind—but not upon that of all others—that Quinine is the antidote to the specific poison of scarlet fever, provided it be so administered as to enable it to exercise its most valuable properties in the way sought for. This, however, it will not do, unless the system, by the use of purgatives, is kept free from effete matters, which otherwise will most prejudicially interfere with its action. When this most important preliminary object has not been attained, Quinine, instead of allaying the rapid action of the heart, accelerates it; at the same time rendering the skin hotter, and the rash more vivid in color, increasing the swelling of the face and eye-lids, and injuriously affecting the internal mucous membranes; the eyes acquire additional brilliancy; the patient complains of frontal headache, and his restlessness becomes painful to witness. If these symptoms are allowed to continue, delirium of an active kind will supervene, and one or the other of the vital organs of the body will soon suffer severely from the Quinine. He has no doubt that Quinine, having been found unsuitable as an *early* remedy in scarlet fever, except in its more malignant forms, has been the cause of its curative power being undervalued in other stages of the disease by those who were unacquainted with the manner of bringing the system to *tolerate* its administration; and that, from the occurrence of the stimulating effects in producing a train of unfavorable symptoms, as above noticed, it has not been universally employed. It cannot, however, have failed to have struck many that scarlet fever, which shows so great a facility in assuming a low or typhoid character, would be best combatted by such a remedy as Quinine, in consequence of its great antiseptic powers.

ACIDS.—The practical application of some of this class of remedies has already been touched upon, but the spirit of their action has not yet been given; and, as they are frequently regarded as tonics, here will be a proper place to turn our consideration to them. They play a most important part in the organism. The gastric juice is distinguished for its acidity, *muriatic* and *lactic acids* being predominant; the acidity of the muscular juice is equally marked, lactic acid alone being present; the parenchymatous fluids of the spleen, thymus gland, smooth muscles, liver, and supra-renal capsules all contain free acid, the *acid phosphates* being internally present; the serum of the blood is always alkaline, but the contents of the red blood-corpuscules have either an acid reaction, or else contain substances which are able to saturate alkalies; the urine, it is well known, is always acid in health, mainly arising from the presence of *acid phosphate of soda*, although no less than thirty-one grains of *sulphuric acid* are secreted by the kidneys in twenty-four hours, also from fifty-two to seventy-five grains of *phosphoric-acid*, and from seven and a half to fifteen grains of *uric acid*—the acidity of urine also often increases rapidly after its discharge, owing to the formation of *lactic* or *acetic acid* in it.

From the above it is evident that there must be a proper supply of acids to the system for the maintenance of health; sometimes the supply must be diminished, at others increased. Muriatic- and Phosphoric-acids are regarded as powerful tonics; Sulphuric as the most efficient astringent; Nitric as an alterative and hepatic remedy.

In the healthy state, when the stomach is empty, the fluid which moistens its surface is slightly alkaline or neutral; the contact of food excites the secretion of gastric juice, in which *muriatic* acid exists in conjunction with a certain quantity of *lactic* acid. This acid fluid is nature's solvent for the nitrogenous or *albuminous* constituents only of the food; while the saliva, pancreatic and intestinal juices, which are all alkaline, digest the *starchy* elements. The acid gastric juice gradually dissolves the albuminous portions, and, as the food becomes more and more digested, the acidity of the gastric fluid increases; the acid passes out of the stomach with the chyme, and the larger portion of it is then neutralized by the alkaline secretions of the liver, pancreas, and small intestines, so that the contents of the small bowels, when examined a little way down, are generally, or ought to be, slightly alkaline or neutral.

Excessive acidity of the stomach may be excited in a four-fold manner: *First,* Acid may be poured out in excess by the glands of the stomach; *Second,* It may be taken in with the food; *Third,* It may be generated from the food in the stomach by some fermentative process; *Fourth,* The natural function of the saliva is to convert starchy substances instantaneously into sugar, which sugar is subsequently converted into *lactic acid.* Hence the withholding and giving of acids becomes necessary in some diseases. Acetic and Phosphoric acids form very soluble compounds with albumen and fibrin. Acids are absorbed into the blood, and are thrown out of the system by the excreting organs, especially by the kidneys, the secretions of which they render preternaturally acid. But they do not enter the blood in the form of acids, for the blood is always alkaline, and does not lose its alkaline properties by transmitting them; they enter into combination with various bases, and have their acid properties neutralized. The acids unite in the alimentary canal, not only with the albuminous substances of the food, secretions, and tissues, and with mucus, but also with the alkaline (soda) and earthy bases (lime and magnesia) which normally exist in the saliva, bile, and pancreatic juice; and in this way they become neutralized, and form compounds and salts, some of which are soluble and others insoluble—the former are absorbed into the blood, the latter are rejected. It is important to remember that acids enter the blood in combination with bases, so that they act on the stomach and bowels as acids, but in the blood as *salts.* It must not be inferred, however, that the influence of the acids on the blood and general system is identical with that of the salts of the same acids; for it must be remembered that the acids deprive the system of part of its alkaline and earthy bases, which are employed in neutralizing and conducting the acids safely out of the system, and which, but for the administration of the latter, would have been otherwise applied to the purposes of the economy. Now these bases, though obtained directly from the saliva, the bile (chiefly), and the pancreatic juice, are indirectly derived from the blood, so that, in a secondary way, at least, the acids must modify the composition of the blood—*i. e.*, render it less alkaline than it is normally, and correct an excess of alkali, which obtains in some diseases. Several of the free vegetable acids, when administered by the mouth, are subsequently detected in the urine in combination with an alkali; but, when given combined with alkali, in the shape of a salt, carbonates of the alkali are found in the urine. The free vegetable acids therefore rob the system of alkaline matter, while the salts of the same acids deprive the system of oxygen. From the preceding remarks it may be inferred that the precise changes effected in the blood by the internal administration of acids are complicated and somewhat obscure; but they lessen preternatural heat, and reduce the frequency and force of the pulse, check profuse perspiration and some hæmorrhages, allay distressing itching and irritation of the skin, and remove some dyscrasias. In some so-called putrid fevers they have frequently proved serviceable by removing basic matter from the system, and checking some decompositions of the fluids.

Sulphuric-acid exhibits some of the antipsoric and antidyscratic effects of Sulphur; in small doses it increases the appetite, promotes digestion and nutrition, at the same time that it reduces the frequency and force of the pulse, and diminishes the temperature of the body. Christison states that it is also diuretic, and that it sometimes succeeds in promoting an increased secretion of urine in dropsical affections when other powerful diuretics have failed. Hence, Wood concludes that it may be regarded as tonic, astringent, refrigerant, and diuretic. It has long been noticed that this acid is peculiarly apt to give astringency to its salts, more so, indeed, than any other mineral acid, as is evinced in the effects of alum, or sulphate of alumina, and sulphates of iron, copper, zinc, &c. As soda and potash are abundantly present in the system, it is probable the sulphates of soda and potash are formed in the blood.

The homœopathists claim that the severe effects of the mineral acids are somewhat similar to the acrid and corrosive effects of intense or malignant scarlet fever; for they may produce burning pain and inflammation in the mouth, fauces, and stomach, with nausea, and vomiting of bloody or dark colored liquids, severe pains in the bowels, and bloody stools; the voice often becomes hoarse from inflammation of the glottis; the breath sometimes fetid from the decomposition of the destroyed tissues, with great prostration, cold surface, feeble and

www.ingramcontent.com/pod-product-compliance
Lightning Source LLC
LaVergne TN
LVHW020925110826
845150LV00004B/767

* 9 7 8 1 4 2 5 5 5 3 9 5 1 *